Lifestyle Behavior and Neural Implications

Lifestyle Behavior and Neural Implications

Edited by Rachel Hughes

hayle medical

New York

Hayle Medical,
750 Third Avenue, 9th Floor,
New York, NY 10017, USA

Visit us on the World Wide Web at:
www.haylemedical.com

ISBN: 978-1-64647-515-5

Cataloging-in-Publication Data

Lifestyle behavior and neural implications / edited by Rachel Hughes.
p. cm.
Includes bibliographical references and index.
ISBN 978-1-64647-515-5
1. Health behavior. 2. Lifestyles. 3. Nervous system--Diseases. I. Hughes, Rachel.
RA776.9 .L54 2023
613--dc23

Table of Contents

Preface

Lifestyle refers to the behaviors, interests, beliefs and behavioral orientations of a person, group or culture. Lifestyle behaviors are daily activities that are influenced by a person's knowledge, values and norms along with the cultural and socio-economic factors. These behaviors affect general health as well as body weight of an individual. A wide variety of social characteristics influence these lifestyle behaviors. Adequate physical activity and balanced diet can aid in preventing cardiovascular diseases like type 2 diabetes, coronary heart disease and hypertension. Unhealthy lifestyle behaviors have significant effect on brain health and may possibly damage the neural pathways. An active lifestyle is also beneficial for preserving neurological and cognitive health across the age groups particularly in higher order processes like cognitive inhibition, task switching and working memory. This book aims to shed light on some of the unexplored aspects of lifestyle behaviors and their neural implications. It will serve as a reference to a broad spectrum of readers.

Significant researches are present in this book. Intensive efforts have been employed by authors to make this book an outstanding discourse. This book contains the enlightening chapters which have been written on the basis of significant researches done by the experts.

Finally, I would also like to thank all the members involved in this book for being a team and meeting all the deadlines for the submission of their respective works. I would also like to thank my friends and family for being supportive in my efforts.

Editor

Cognition and Brain Activation in Response to Various Doses of Caffeine: A Near-Infrared Spectroscopy Study

Bin Zhang[1], Ying Liu[1], Xiaochun Wang[1], Yuqin Deng[2]* and Xinyan Zheng[1]*

[1] Shanghai University of Sport, Shanghai, China, [2] School of Sports Science, Nantong University, Nantong, China

***Correspondence:**
Yuqin Deng
yuqindeng@126.com
Xinyan Zheng
zhengxinyan0513@163.com

Caffeine, which is widely used for enhancing athletic performance, has been suggested to have a positive impact on cognition via stimulating the brain. However, no study published to date has explored the effects of different doses of caffeine ingestion on brain activation via cortical hemodynamics. The purpose of the present crossover, double-blind study was to investigate the effects of low, moderate, and high doses of caffeine ingestion on cognitive performance and brain activation. Ten healthy male subjects ingested placebo or caffeine (3, 6, or 9 mg/kg body mass). The effects of each treatment condition were evaluated by Stroop tasks before and 60 min after the ingestion of caffeine. Reaction time (RT) and accuracy of responses to congruent and incongruent stimuli were assessed. As an index of brain activation with cognition, levels of oxygenated hemoglobin (HbO) were measured via near-infrared spectroscopy. A 4 × 2 mixed ANOVA revealed that there were significant interaction effects for RT in both incongruent and congruent conditions ($P < 0.01$, $P\eta^2 = 0.384$; $P < 0.05$, $P\eta^2 = 0.259$; and $P < 0.05$, $Pr^2 = 0.309$). Both 3 and 6 mg/kg of caffeine ingestion significantly decreased RT to incongruent stimuli. The only dose of caffeine to decrease RT in response to congruent stimuli was 3 mg/kg. None of the doses of caffeine administered affected accuracy of responses to incongruent or congruent stimuli. Under the congruent stimulus condition, ingestion of 3 mg/kg of caffeine significantly increased mean HbO in the dorsolateral prefrontal cortex, frontal pole area, ventrolateral prefrontal cortex ($P < 0.01$, $P\eta^2 = 0.319$; $P < 0.05$, $P\eta^2 = 0.263$; and $P < 0.05$, $P\eta^2 = 0.259$, respectively). None of the doses of caffeine investigated affected HbO under the incongruent stimulus condition. Ingestion of low-dose caffeine has greater effects on cognition and brain activation than moderate and high doses of caffeine, suggesting that low-dose caffeine may be a selective supplement in enhancing executive function and prefrontal activities.

Keywords: caffeine, different doses, cognition, brain activation, near-infrared spectroscopy

INTRODUCTION

Caffeine is widely used by athletes for improving exercise performance. Administration of 3–13 mg/kg body mass caffeine increases exercise performance during intensive running or cycling by 20–50% (Sökmen et al., 2008). Graham and Spriet (1995) investigated the effects of low, moderate, and high doses of caffeine on prolonged exercise capacity. They found that ingestion of 3 or 6 mg/kg of caffeine improved time to exhaustion, whereas 9 mg/kg of caffeine did not. There results indicated that the effect of low-dose caffeine ingestion had the similar ergogenic effect as moderate dose, which could improve physical ability. Excellence in sport performance requires not only physical and motor capabilities but also sensory–cognitive skills (Moscatelli et al., 2016). However, to our knowledge, no study examined the effects of low, moderate, and high doses of caffeine on cognition until now.

Stimulation of the central nervous system (CNS) has been proposed to explain caffeine's ergogenic effects (Kalmar and Cafarelli, 2004). Caffeine acts as a central stimulant and enhances cognitive and psychomotor functioning, particularly during mental and physical fatigue, through effects that enhance alertness and vigilance. These findings suggest that the exercise performance-enhancing effects of caffeine stem from the compound's ability to alter CNS function (Hogervorst et al., 2008).

The action of caffeine on the brain suggests an effect on cognitive performance. Cognition includes executive functioning (EF), decision making, and creativity. Executive functioning is important during exercise and can be affected by prolonged exercise (Yanagisawa et al., 2010). Reports in the scientific literature present inconsistent findings in relation to the effects of caffeine ingestion on the Stroop task performance, a measure of executive function. Some studies involving cognitive inhibition or interference conditions report faster or potential fast reaction times (RTs) with the use of caffeine (Hasenfratz and Bättig, 1992; Kenemans et al., 1999; Hogervorst et al., 2008; Dixit et al., 2012; Dodd et al., 2015; Souissi et al., 2019), whereas others report no change at all (Edwards et al., 1996; Bottoms et al., 2013). Differences in outcomes between studies may be related to the sensitivity of the cognitive tests used or the dose of caffeine administered, and more studies need to examine effects of caffeine on cognition.

The effects of caffeine on cognition may be related to the enhancement of brain activation. Early studies postulated that the effects of caffeine on brain activation depend on the complex interaction of neuronal and vascular responses. These responses may vary among brain regions, introducing an additional layer of complexity (Laurienti et al., 2003; Koppestaetter et al., 2010). Caffeine acts as a non-adenosine receptor antagonist. It blocks adenosine receptors and excites neuro-stimulants (Dunwiddie and Masino, 2001). Moreover, caffeine acts as a vasoconstrictor via blocking adenosine 2A and 2B receptors, resulting in decreased cerebral blood flow (CBF) (Laurienti et al., 2002; Pelligrion et al., 2010). The interaction of caffeine with neural and vascular systems has direct effects on neural connectivity during resting states as well as cognitive activation (Haller et al., 2014).

Brain activation is measured using neuroimaging techniques such as functional magnetic resonance imaging (fMRI) and near-infrared spectroscopy (NIRS). Using blood oxygen level-dependent (BOLD) fMRI, Diukova et al. (2012) found that caffeine ingestion increased activity in the frontal cortex. The BOLD signal is a complex functional measurement of changes in neural activity, oxygen metabolism, cerebral blood volume, and CBF (Buxton et al., 2004). The balance between blood levels of oxygenated hemoglobin (HbO) and deoxygenated hemoglobin (HbR) is a critical determinant of the BOLD response. Levels of HbO and HbR may be measured with NIRS to investigate components underlying the BOLD response. NIRS studies that evaluated the responses of participants on various tests of cognition have reported conflicting results for the effects of caffeine on HbO and HbR (Niioka and Sasaki, 2003; Higashi et al., 2004; Heilbronner et al., 2015).

To our knowledge, no NIRS-based study published to date has explored the effects of low, moderate, and high doses of caffeine on brain activation during cognitive tasks. The purpose of the present study was to investigate the effects of various doses of caffeine ingestion on brain activation and cognitive performance. We hypothesized that low-dose caffeine ingestion had similar effects as moderate dose, which could improve executive functioning and brain activation.

MATERIALS AND METHODS

Subjects

Ten healthy, non-smoking male subjects (age 20 $\pm$ 1 year, height 1.73 $\pm$ 0.20 m, and weight 70.5 $\pm$ 4.8 kg) participated in this study. They were non-users (ingesting $<$ 50 mg of caffeine/day). The sample size used was calculated by G-Power software [effect size (ES) = 0.15, power = 0.80; Faul et al., 2007]. Subjects were required to visit the laboratory with an empty belly and to abstain from drinking beverages containing caffeine and from use of other psychoactive substances or medication for at least 24 h before every experimental trial. All subjects were fully informed of the nature and possible risks of the study. After that, written informed consent was obtained from all subjects before study enrollment. The study followed the ethical guidelines of the Declaration of Helsinki and was approved by the local ethics committee at Shanghai University in Sport, Shanghai, China (No. 2016008).

Protocol

Subjects visited the laboratory four times, at the same time of day. When participants arrived in the dimly lit room where experiments were to be conducted, they were seated in a comfortable chair in front of a computer monitor. After the NIRS optode grid had been positioned on the subjects' head, they performed the Stroop familiarization trial. In order to obtain baseline measurements of performance on the Stroop task, each subject sat quietly for 5 min and watched a black screen. At that point, the NIRS recording was paused, and participants ingested capsules containing placebo (calcium carbonate; CON) or 3 mg/kg (CAF3), 6 mg/kg (CAF6), or 9 mg/kg (CAF9) of caffeine with 200 ml of water (PRE). After a 60-min delay, during which the optode grid remained in place, participants once again performed the same Stroop task (POST). The crossover, double-blind design was used in the present study. All subjects completed all experiment conditions, which were separated by 1 week to ensure drug washout period.

Drugs

Caffeine hydrate (Wako Pure Chemical Industries, Ltd., Osaka, Japan) and calcium carbonate, which are white powder, were used in this study. The dosage of each condition was calculated according to the weight. In the CON condition, 9 mg/kg of calcium carbonate was put into three red capsules. In the CAF3 condition, both 3 mg/kg of caffeine and 6 mg/kg of calcium carbonate were put into three red capsules. In the CAF6 condition, both 6 mg/kg of caffeine and 3 mg/kg of calcium carbonate were put into three red capsules. In the CAF9 condition, 9 mg/kg of caffeine was put into three red capsules. In this way, researchers and subjects could not identify caffeine according to the appearance and taste of the capsule.

Stroop Task

The Stroop task is widely used to evaluate selective attention, cognitive flexibility, and processing speed (Pauw et al., 2015). It was programmed and performed on E-prime 1.0 software (Psychology Software Tools, Pittsburgh, PA, United States). Each trial was displayed as follows: a fixed cross in the center of the screen for 500 ms and a stimulus duration for 500 ms. There were two kinds of stimuli in current study: congruent and incongruent conditions. The congruent condition is composed of three Chinese color words (i.e., 绿 for green, 蓝 for blue, and 红 for red), whose color was the same to the meaning of the color words (e.g., "green" word was presented in green). And the incongruent condition consisted of the same three-color words, whose color was completely different from the meaning of the color words (e.g., "green" words were presented in blue or red). Subjects were required to figure out the presenting color of each word by using the numeric keypad as the response apparatus. And the numeric keypad featured digits "1," "2," and "3" from left to right, which correspond to the responses of "blue," "green," and "red," respectively. The subjects used the index, middle, and ring fingers of their right hand for the response of digits "1," "2," and "3." According to the previous Stroop task, the RTs on figuring out the color in the incongruent condition were longer than those in the congruent condition, as the processing of word meaning in the incongruent condition interferes with the color recognition (e.g., when "green" words were presented in red, the meaning of the green word impedes the recognition of red; Stroop, 1935; Pauw et al., 2015).

Participants performed two blocks of 120 trials. Each block included 60 congruent and 60 incongruent trials, which were randomly presented. To prevent participants from anticipating a stimulus, the interval between appearance of the fixed cross and presentation of the stimulus was randomly differed between 300 and 800 ms, with the fixed inter-stimulus interval (ISI) duration of 1,500 ms. Both RT and accuracy (ACC) were recorded for further analysis.

Hemodynamic Data Acquisition

We used a multichannel, continuous wave, NIRS instrument (NIRScout, NIRx Medical Technologies LLC, Minneapolis, MN, United States) for monitoring hemodynamic activity during performance of the task and during the resting state. The sampling rate was 3.91 Hz. The NIRS probe included 16 dual-wavelength sources (780 and 830 nm) and 15 optical detectors, which covered the frontal and parietal areas bilaterally (**Figure 1**). One emitter and one detector (3 cm apart) formed a channel. Forty channels were assessed: 20 distributed throughout the frontal area and 20 distributed throughout parietal areas. The correspondence between NIRS channel locations and specific brain regions was established by Okamoto et al. (2004, 2009) and Tsuzuki et al. (2007). Probes were set according to a 10/20 electroencephalogram system, with some adjustments to ensure that each emitter was 3 cm away from its corresponding detector (Chen et al., 2018).

Hemodynamic Data Analysis

Optical data were transformed into hemoglobin signals with arbitrary units in accordance with the modified Beer–Lambert law (Cope et al., 1988). It has been reported that HbO signals have a better signal-to-noise ratio than HbR signals (Niu et al., 2013; Schaeffer et al., 2014), so we used only HbO measurements to analysis. The HbO data were analyzed with nirsLAB software. After discontinuous shifts were removed from the time series dataset, HbO signals were bandpass-filtered between 0.01 and 0.2 Hz to remove baseline drift and physiological noise (e.g., heartbeats). Bandpass filtering was performed by a high-pass filter with a cutoff frequency of 0.01 Hz to remove low-frequency noise, such as head movement, and by a low-pass filter with a cutoff frequency of 0.2 Hz to attenuate high-frequency noise and cardiovascular artifacts (Huppert et al., 2009; Yunjie et al., 2012). Then, each subject's HbO during a given session was calculated. Hemodynamic data were then baseline-corrected based on the mean value of all signals from each block (5 s before to 15 s after the block). The HbO data were then averaged across subjects (Chen et al., 2018).

The region of interest (ROI) channels were defined as those channels with maximal HbO. After HbO was averaged across subjects, mean HbO during the congruent and incongruent conditions was subtracted from mean HbO during the resting state. The mean difference between the single-cognitive task and resting state sessions was arranged according to descending magnitude, for each channel (Chen et al., 2018). We defined channels of interest as the top 30% of channels (greatest values). The multichannel NIRS space was transformed into traditional Montreal Neurological Institute space (Cutini et al., 2011). Channels of interest were related to three ROIs on the basis of their spatial distribution relative to the automated anatomical labeling template (**Table 1**). HbO values were then averaged through channels within a given ROI.

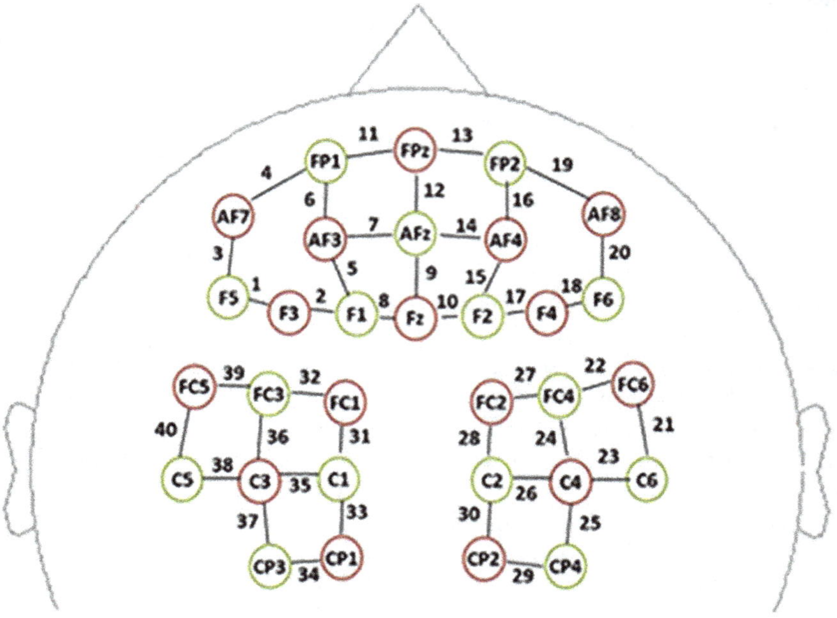

FIGURE 1 | The spatial profile of functional near-infrared spectral imaging (fNIRS) probes. The red circles indicate the 16 optical sources, the green circles indicate the 15 detectors, and the black numbers (1–40) indicate fNIRS channels. The optical sources and detectors were positioned on the international 10–20 standard positions.

Data Analysis

Statistical analyses were conducted with SPSS 20.0 software (SPSS Inc., Chicago, IL, United States). One-sample Kolmogorov–Smirnov test was used to test whether data were normally distributed. When data are not normally distributed, statistical analysis was performed on the logarithmic transformation of the data. RT, ACC and mean HbO data for all frequencies in a given ROI were subjected to repeated-measures three-way ANOVA with dose (CON/CAF3/CAF6/CAF9), time (PRE/POST), and condition (incongruent/congruent) as within subject factors to examine whether the general tendencies for the Stroop task could be reproduced in all conditions. Then alterations in RT, ACC, and averaged HbO data for all frequencies in a given ROI were subjected to 4 × 2 repeated-measures ANOVAs. For cases in which the assumption of sphericity was violated, the Greenhouse–Geisser correction was used to reduce the likelihood of a Type I error. If significant main or interaction effects were found, *post-hoc* analyses were carried out with a Bonferroni correction. Partial eta^2 ($P\eta^2$) was used as a measure of ES in the case of ANOVA. The criteria to interpret the magnitude of ES were as follows: small ($P\eta^2 = 0.01$), medium ($P\eta^2 = 0.06$), or large ($P\eta2 = 0.14$; Cohen, 1992). Data are presented as mean ± SD. Statistical significance was accepted at $P < 0.05$.

TABLE 1 | Stroop task-related regions of interest (ROIs).

ROI	Channels	Hemisphere	Location
1	5,7,14,15	Bilateral	DLPFC
2	6,11,13,14	Bilateral	FPA
3	3,4,19,20	Bilateral	VLPFC

DLPFC, dorsolateral prefrontal cortex; FPA, frontal pole area; VLPFC, ventrolateral prefrontal cortex.

RESULTS

Stroop Task Performance

The three-way ANOVA for RT and ACC demonstrated no significant interaction effects ($P = 0.201$, $P\eta^2 = 0.155$; and $P = 0.201$, $P\eta^2 = 0.155$, respectively). The ANOVA revealed that there were significant main effects of condition for RT ($P < 0.001$, $P\eta^2 = 0.882$) and ACC ($P < 0.01$, $P\eta^2 = 0.567$). These results confirmed that Stroop interference could be generally observed between the congruent and incongruent conditions.

Incongruent Condition

A 4 × 2 mixed ANOVA revealed that there was a significant interaction for RT [$F(3, 27) = 5.61$, $P < 0.01$, $P\eta^2 = 0.384$, **Table 2**]. RT of 60 min after the administration was significantly decreased after treatment with 3 mg/kg (PRE, 685.43 ± 85.95 ms; POST, 649.70 ± 96.53 ms, $P < 0.05$) or 6 mg/kg (PRE, 658.83 ± 71.93 ms; POST, 624.10 ± 84.57 ms, $P < 0.05$). There was no significant difference in RT between CAF3 and CAF6. Treatment with 9 mg/kg of caffeine did not affect RT. There was no significant interaction for ACC (**Table 2**).

Congruent Condition

We found a significant interaction for RT [$F(3, 27) = 3.14$, $P < 0.05$, $P\eta^2 = 0.259$, **Table 2**]. RT had decreased significantly at 60 min after the administration of 3 mg/kg of caffeine (PRE,

TABLE 2 | The reaction time and accuracy rate of the Stroop test.

Measurements	Condition	Dose (mg/kg)	PRE	95%CI	POST	95%CI
	Incongruent (ms)	0	643.18 ± 82.80	583.95–702.42	669.18 ± 72.47	617.34–721.02
		3	685.43 ± 85.95	623.94–746.91	649.70 ± 96.53#	580.65–718.75
		6	658.83 ± 71.93	607.37–710.28	624.10 ± 84.56#	563.61–684.59
Reaction time		9	654.54 ± 93.05	587.98–721.11	649.65 ± 104.41	574.95–724.33
	Congruent (ms)	0	582.54 ± 82.05	523.84–641.23	608.85 ± 79.50	551.98–665.72
		3	580.66 ± 79.39	523.86–637.44	553.60 ± 78.32#	497.57–609.63
		6	576.28 ± 67.48	528.01–624.55	580.37 ± 66.12	533.07–627.66
		9	585.74 ± 67.94	537.14–634.34	574.05 ± 78.29	518.03–630.05
	Incongruent	0	0.92 ± 0.07	0.87–0.96	0.95 ± 0.07	0.91–1.00
		3	0.94 ± 0.06	0.90–0.98	0.94 ± 0.04	0.91–0.97
		6	0.95 ± 0.04	0.92–0.97	0.93 ± 0.06	0.89–0.98
Accuracy rate		9	0.92 ± 0.05	0.89–0.96	0.95 ± 0.06	0.91–0.99
	Congruent	0	0.96 ± 0.03	0.93–0.98	0.96 ± 0.05	0.92–1.00
		3	0.97 ± 0.04	0.94–0.99	0.99 ± 0.01	0.98–1.00
		6	0.98 ± 0.04	0.95–1.00	0.98 ± 0.02	0.97–1.00
		9	0.96 ± 0.03	0.94–0.98	0.97 ± 0.03	0.95–0.99

PRE, before administration; POST, after administration. #Significant PRE vs. POST ($p < 0.05$). Values are mean ± SD.

580.66 ± 79.39 ms; POST, 553.60 ± 78.32 ms, $P < 0.01$). However, the administration of caffeine at doses of 6 or 9 mg/kg did not affect RT. We found no significant interaction for ACC (**Table 2**).

Near-Infrared Spectroscopy

The three-way ANOVA for ROI-1 [dorsolateral prefrontal cortex (DLPFC)], ROI-2 [frontal pole area (FPA)], and ROI-3 [ventrolateral prefrontal cortex (VLPFC)] demonstrated no significant interaction effects ($P = 0.09$, $P\eta^2 = 0.230$; $P = 0.224$, $P\eta^2 = 0.154$; and $P = 0.633$, $P\eta^2 = 0.061$, respectively). The ANOVA revealed that there was a significant main effect of condition for ROI-1 ($P < 0.05$, $P\eta^2 = 0.394$).

Incongruent Condition

A 4 × 2 mixed ANOVA revealed that there was no significant interaction for mean HbO in ROI-1 (**Figure 2A**), ROI-2 (**Figure 2B**), or ROI-3 (**Figure 2C**).

Congruent Condition

We found a significant interaction for mean HbO in ROI-1 [$F(3, 27) = 4.21$, $P < 0.01$, $P\eta^2 = 0.319$, **Figure 3A**]. In the CON group, mean HbO had significantly decreased at 60 min after administration of the placebo, as compared with baseline values. At 60 min after the administration of 3 mg/kg of caffeine, mean HbO had significantly increased. The administration of caffeine at doses of 6 or 9 mg/kg did not affect mean HbO.

A 4 × 2 mixed ANOVA revealed that there was a significant interaction for the mean HbO in ROI-2 [$F(3, 27) = 3.21$, $P < 0.05$, $P\eta^2 = 0.263$, **Figure 3B**]. Compared with baseline values, mean HbO after 60 min showed a significant decrease in the CON group. At 60 min after the administration of 3 mg/kg of caffeine, mean HbO had significantly increased. Treatment with caffeine at doses of 6 or 9 mg/kg did not affect mean HbO.

Two-factor ANOVA of mean HbO showed significant effects of dose × time [$F(3, 27) = 4.02$, $P < 0.05$, $P\eta^2 = 0.309$, **Figure 3C**]. Compared with baseline values, mean HbO had significantly decreased at 60 min in the CON group. At 60 min after treatment with 3 mg/kg of caffeine, mean HbO had significantly increased. Treatment with caffeine at doses of 6 or 9 mg/kg did not affect mean HbO.

DISCUSSION

This novel study investigated the effects of ingestion of low, moderate, or high doses of caffeine typically used by athletes on cognition and brain activation using NIRS. We found that ingestion of low doses of caffeine, but not moderate or high doses caffeine, decreased RT on the Stroop task, under the congruent and incongruent conditions, and increased mean HbO in three ROIs under the congruent condition. Ingestion of moderate doses caffeine only decreased RT on the Stroop task, under the incongruent conditions.

Low doses (≤3 mg/kg) of caffeine have been reported to improve cognition during and after strenuous exercise (Hogervorst et al., 1999, 2008). Ingestion of 3 mg/kg of caffeine, but not 6 or 9 mg/kg, decreased RT under the congruent condition on the Stroop task. This result suggests that low-dose caffeine may represent "a direct and specific 'perceptual-motor' speed or efficiency factor" (Nehlig, 2010). After consumption of low doses of caffeine, participants in our study showed decreased RT, accompanied by a significant decrease in interference effects. These findings are similar to those reported by Kenemans et al. (1999).

In this study, the ingestion of 6 mg/kg of caffeine decreased RT on the Stroop task under the incongruent condition. Nonetheless, the beneficial effects of 6 mg/kg of caffeine on cognitive performance are in dispute. Similar to the present study, Souissi et al. (2019) found that 6 mg/kg of caffeine ingestion improved RT and attention. Moreover, Ali et al. (2015) showed that 6 mg/kg of caffeine induced a tendency toward improvement in performance on the Stroop task among female athletes engaged in team

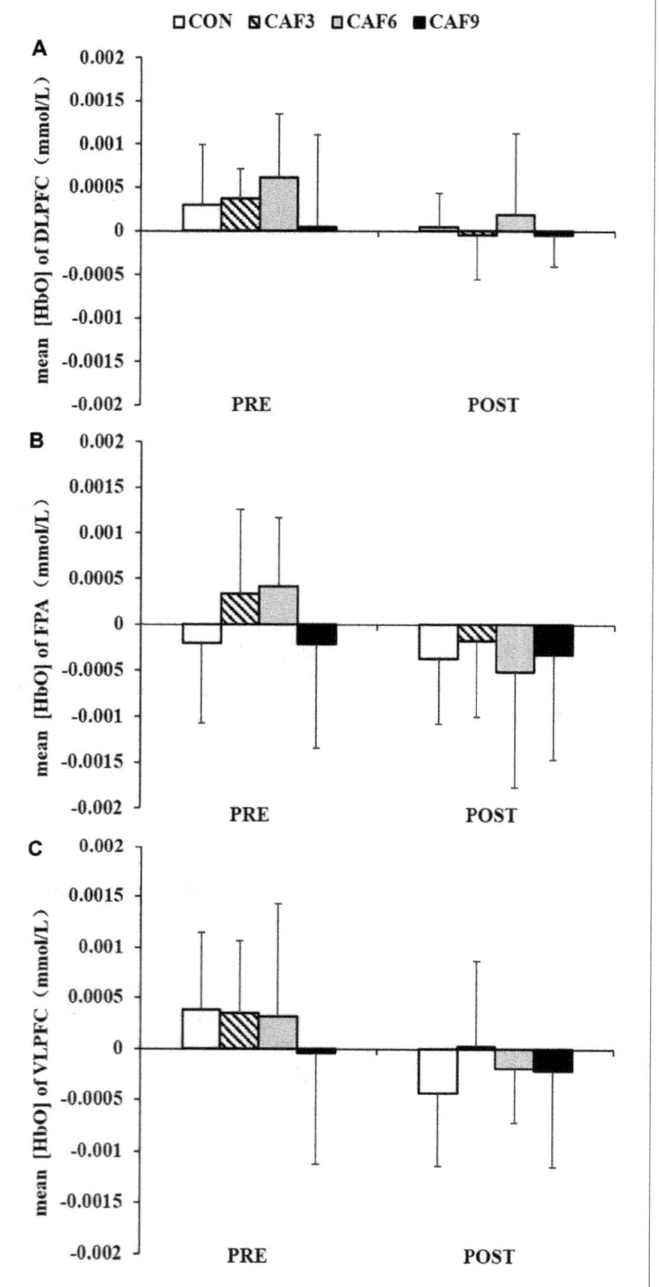

FIGURE 2 | Changes in the mean [HbO] of incongruent condition in the DLPFC **(A)**, FPA **(B)**, and VLPFC **(C)**. HbO, oxygenated hemoglobin; DLPFC, dorsolateral prefrontal cortex; FPA, frontal pole area; VLPFC, ventrolateral prefrontal cortex; PRE, before administration; POST, after administration. Values are mean ± SD.

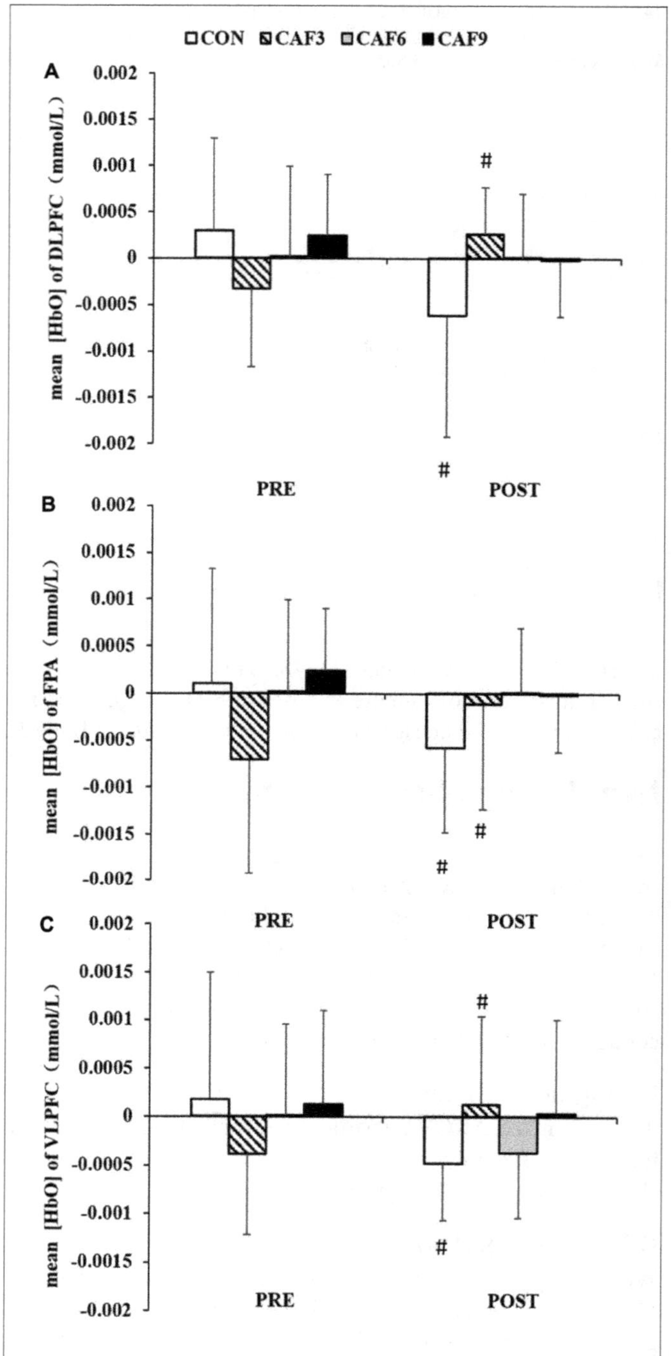

FIGURE 3 | Changes in the mean [HbO] of congruent condition in DLPFC **(A)**, FPA **(B)**, and VLPFC **(C)**. HbO, oxygenated hemoglobin; DLPFC, dorsolateral prefrontal cortex; FPA, frontal pole area; VLPFC, ventrolateral prefrontal cortex; PRE, before administration; POST, after administration. [#]Significant PRE vs. POST ($P < 0.05$). Values are mean ± SD.

sports. This discrepancy in results may reflect methodological differences related to the specific protocol used or the gender of the study participants. Moreover, we observed that high doses of caffeine had no effect on cognitive performance. One possible explanation for this finding is that the ingestion of high doses of caffeine induces side effects such as gastrointestinal upset, nervousness, mental confusion, and inability to focus (Graham and Spriet, 1995). Our data suggest that ingestion of low or moderate doses of caffeine ingestion decreases interference with successful performance on the Stroop task. As 3 mg/kg of caffeine improved performance on simple as well as complex cognitive tasks, we suggest that low-dose caffeine has a greater impact on cognition than moderate or high doses of caffeine.

Previous studies have reported the activation of the lateral prefrontal cortex (LPFC) upon execution of the Stroop task. Banich et al. (2000, 2001) suggested that LPFC activation may reflect interference processing and/or response inhibition. This may result in greater activation of relevant LPFC in the incongruent condition compared with the congruent condition. Milham et al. (2003) reported that during the Stroop task, the DLPFC in the LPFC is the primary region involved in the implementation of top-down attention control. Additionally, according to Krompinger and Simons (2011), the DLPFC resolves conflicts that occur during information processing of incongruent stimuli during the Stroop task. Therefore, the Stroop performance is more related to activation of the DLPFC. In the present study, we found a significant main effect of condition for the mean HbO of the DLPFC: the mean HbO in the incongruent condition was higher than in the congruent condition. These Stroop effect findings are similar to those in previous functional NIRS (fNIRS) studies, which suggested that executive functioning is associated with activation of DLPFC (Xu et al., 2017; Kujach et al., 2018). Interestingly, we found different results with previous two fNIRS studies (Xu et al., 2017; Kujach et al., 2018): the present Stroop task failed to activated the FPA and the VLPFC. But DLPFC activation in the present study is consistent with that of a previous meta-analysis review on Stroop task-related fMRI, in which FPA and VLPFC also could not be significantly activated (Nee et al., 2007; Huang et al., 2020). Thus, more fNIRS or fMRI neuroimaging studies are needed to clarify the roles of FPA and VLPFC in the Stroop task.

That caffeine improved the Stroop task performance may be related to activation of LPFC. Different from our hypothesis, caffeine ingestion failed to affect the mean HbO in the DLPFC, FPA, and VLPFC under the incongruent condition, whereas under the congruent condition, ingestion of 3 mg/kg of caffeine increased mean HbO in the DLPFC, FPA, and VLPFC. Combining the above-mentioned opposite pattern in which the mean HbO of DLPFC in the incongruent condition was higher than that in the congruent condition, indicated that mean HbO of LPFC, especially DLPFC, has been increased during Stroop-interference processing in the incongruent condition, whereas following caffeine ingestion, the significant reduction was found in the activation of LPFC. On the other hand, in the congruent condition, in which the cognitive processing is less demanding than in the incongruent condition, HbO of DLPFC has been less activated, whereas mean HbO in the DLPFC, FPA, and VLPFC was increased after the ingestion of 3 mg/kg of caffeine. These results demonstrate that under high cognitive processing, the effects of caffeine on LPFC activation have been attenuated by higher demanding processing, whereas under low cognitive tasks, the effects of caffeine on LPFC activation are more pronounced, because the congruent condition in Stroop task involved less demanding processing. The present results provide new evidences for previous studies that caffeine improvement of brain activation is induced more easily at the moment of the lowest values (Niioka and Sasaki, 2003; Souissi et al., 2019).

In the present study, under the congruent condition, no doses of caffeine ingestion affect the mean HbO. These results contrast with those of previous studies, which found that ingestion of 75 or 200 mg of caffeine was associated with decreased mean HbO on the Stroop task (Niioka and Sasaki, 2003; Dodd et al., 2015). This discrepancy in results may reflect methodological differences related to the specific protocol used. Therefore, use of the Stroop task should be standardized in future studies for investigating the effects of drugs on cerebral hemodynamic responses. Furthermore, under the congruent condition used, ingestion of 3 mg/kg of caffeine increased mean HbO in the DLPFC, FPA, and VLPFC. These results are consistent with those of a previous fMRI study, which showed that ingestion of low-dose caffeine enhanced neuro-activation in the frontal cortex (Diukova et al., 2012).

The increase in mean HbO during the Stroop task observed in this study after ingestion of low-dose caffeine may be related to an increase in regional cerebral blood volume (rCBV). Caffeine acts as an adenosine receptor antagonist and consequently as an excitatory neuro-stimulant, thus enhancing neural activity (Dunwiddie and Masino, 2001) and increasing rCBV. These findings are in line with a report by Higashi et al. (2004) that ingestion of 180 mg of caffeine maintained an increase in frontal rCBV during performance of an arithmetic task. Caffeine also regulates cerebral perfusion and acts as a vasoconstrictor, decreasing CBF via the blockade of A2A and A2B receptors (Laurienti et al., 2002; Pelligrion et al., 2010). Our observation that ingestion of low-dose caffeine increases mean HbO suggests that caffeine increases in rCBF via exciting neuro-stimulants outweigh caffeine decreases in rCBF via decreasing CBF. Along these lines, the lack of any observed effect of 6 or 9 mg/kg of caffeine on mean HbO suggests that, at these doses, the increase in rCBV may be equivalent to the decrease in CBF.

Moderate-to-high doses of caffeine administrated 1 h before and during exercise have been known to increase endurance athletic performance. In contrast, recent evidence has shown an ergogenic effect of low and extremely low doses of caffeine taken late during a period of prolonged exercise (Hogervorst et al., 1999; Jenkins et al., 2008). Furthermore, low doses of caffeine do not affect peripheral whole-body responses to exercise and are associated with few, if any, side effects; Spriet (2014) suggested that low doses of caffeine ingestion improve exercise performance In this study, we observed that ingestion of low-dose caffeine had greater effect on cognition and brain activation than had moderate and high doses, which means that low doses of caffeine have greater effect on stimulating the CNS. We suggest that ingestion of low-dose caffeine before and/or during exercise may induce more ergogenic effects than use of moderate or high doses.

Limitation

The present study maintained a few limitations. We used G-power to estimate the sample size, and the numbers of subjects in this study met the minimum sample size requirements. However, more samples are needed in the future research so that the research results can be further verified and repeated. In the double-blind designed study, it is best to ask subjects which dose they think they ingested in each trail after completion of all groups and to outline why they identified which trial as which. However, in the present study, we did not note the responses of the subjects, so we could not assess the efficacy of blinding.

Although four conditions in the present study are difficultly for participants to identify, we should value the assessment of blinding in future studies. Moreover, only Stroop task was used to measure executive function. There are other cognitive tasks on executive function, such as n-back and switching task. Therefore, more tasks are need to measure to ensure effects of various doses of caffeine ingestion on executive function in the future.

CONCLUSION

The present study found that ingestion of 3 mg/kg of caffeine improved performance on the Stroop task under both the incongruent and congruent conditions and increased mean HbO under the congruent condition. Ingestion of 6 mg/kg of caffeine improved performance on the Stroop task under the incongruent condition. These results demonstrate that ingestion of low-dose caffeine has greater effects on cognition and brain activation than moderate and high doses of caffeine, suggesting that low-dose caffeine may be a selective supplement in enhancing executive function and prefrontal activities.

ETHICS STATEMENT

The study followed the ethical guidelines of the Declaration of Helsinki and was approved by the local Ethics Committee at the Shanghai University in Sport, Shanghai, China (No. 2016008). The patients/participants provided their written informed consent to participate in this study.

AUTHOR CONTRIBUTIONS

XZ and YD conceived and supervised the study and designed the experiments. BZ and YL carried out the experiments. YL and XW analyzed the data. BZ wrote the manuscript. All authors contributed to the article and approved the submitted version.

REFERENCES

Ali, A., O'Donnell, J., Von Hurst, P., Foskett, A., Holland, S., Rutherfurd-Markwick, K., et al. (2015). Caffeine ingestion enhances perceptual responses during intermittent exercise in female team-game players. *J. Sports. Sci.* 34, 330–341. doi: 10.1080/02640414.2015.1052746

Banich, M. T., Milham, M. P., Atchley, R., Cohen, N. J., Webb, A., Wszalek, T. A., et al. (2000). fMRI studies of Stroop tasks reveal unique roles of anterior and posterior brain systems in attentional selection. *J. Cogn. Neurosci.* 12, 988–1000. doi: 10.1162/08989290051137521

Banich, M. T., Milham, M. P., Jacobson, B. L., Webb, A., Wszalek, T., Cohen, N. J., et al. (2001). Attentional selection and the processing of task-irrelevant information: insights from fMRI examinations of the Stroop task. *Prog. Brain. Res.* 134, 459–470. doi: 10.1016/S0079-6123(01)34030-X

Bottoms, L., Greenhalgh, A., and Gregory, K. (2013). The effect of caffeine ingestion on skill maintenance and fatigue in epee fencers. *J. Sports. Sci.* 31, 1091–1099. doi: 10.1080/02640414.2013.764466

Buxton, R. B., Uludaǒ, K., Dubowitz, D. J., and Liu, T. T. (2004). Modeling the hemodynamic response to brain activation. *Neuroimage* 23, S220–S233. doi: 10.1016/j.neuroimage.2004.07.013

Chen, Y., Yu, Y., Niu, R., and Liu, Y. (2018). Selective effects of postural control on spatial vs. nonspatial working memory: a functional near- infrared spectral imaging study. *Front. Hum. Neurosci.* 12:243. doi: 10.3389/fnhum.2018.00243

Cohen, J. (1992). A power primer. *Psychol. Bull.* 112, 155–159. doi: 10.1037/0033-2909.112.1.155

Cope, M., Delpy, D. T., Reynolds, E. O., Wray, S., and van der Zee, P. (1988). Methods of quantitating cerebral near infrared spectroscopy data. *Adv. Exp. Med. Biol.* 222, 183–189. doi: 10.1007/978-1-4615-9510-6_21

Cutini, S., Scatturin, P., and Zorzi, M. (2011). A new method based on ICBM152 head surface for probe placement in multichannel fNIRS. *Neuroimage* 54, 919–927. doi: 10.1016/j.neuroimage.2010.09.030

Diukova, A., Ware, J., Smith, J. E., Evans, C. J., Murphy, K., Rogers, P. J., et al. (2012). Separating neural and vascular effects of caffeine using simultaneous EEG-fMRI: differential effects of caffeine on cognitive and sensorimotor brain responses. *Neuroimage* 62, 239–249. doi: 10.1016/j.neuroimage.2012.04.041

Dixit, A., Goyal, A., Thawani, R., and Vaney, N. (2012). Effect of caffeine on information processing: evidence from Stroop task. *Indian. J. Psychol. Med.* 34, 218–222. doi: 10.4103/0253-7176.106013

Dodd, F. L., Kennedy, D. O., Riby, L. M., and Haskell-Ramsay, C. F. (2015). A double-blind, placebo-controlled study evaluating the effects of caffeine and L-theanine both alone and in combination on cerebral blood flow, cognition and mood. *Psychopharmacology* 232, 2563–2576. doi: 10.1007/s00213-015-3895-0

Dunwiddie, T. V., and Masino, S. A. (2001). The role and regulation of adenosine in the central nervous system. *Annu. Rev. Neurosci.* 24, 31–55. doi: 10.1146/annurev.neuro.24.1.31

Edwards, S., Brice, C., Craig, C., and Penri-Jones, R. (1996). Effects of caffeine, practice, and mode of presentation on Stroop task performance. *Pharmacol. Biochem. Behav.* 54, 309–315. doi: 10.1016/0091-3057(95)02116-7

Faul, F., Erdfelder, E., Lang, A. G., and Buchner, A. (2007). G*Power 3: a flexible statistical power analysis program for the social, behavioral, and biomedical sciences. *Behav Res Method.* 39, 175–191. doi: 10.3758/bf03193146

Graham, T. E., and Spriet, L. L. (1995). Metabolic, catecholamine, and exercise performance responses to various doses of caffeine. *J. Appl. Physiol.* 78, 867–874. doi: 10.1152/jappl.1995.78.3.867

Haller, S., Montandon, M. L., Rodriguez, C., Moser, D., Hofmeister, J., Sinanaj, I., et al. (2014). Acute caffeine administration effect on brain activation patterns in mild cognitive impairment. *J. Alzheimers. Dis.* 41, 101–112. doi: 10.3233/JAD-132360

Hasenfratz, M., and Bättig, K. (1992). Action profiles of smoking and caffeine: stroop effect. EEG, and peripheral physiology. *Pharmacol. Biochem. Behav.* 42, 155–161. doi: 10.1016/0091-3057(92)90459-S

Heilbronner, U., Hinrichs, H., Heinze, H. J., and Zaehle, T. (2015). Caffeine differentially alters cortical hemodynamic activity during working memory: a near infrared spectroscopy study. *BMC Res. Notes.* 8:520. doi: 10.1186/s13104-015-1491-3

Higashi, T., Sone, Y., Ogawa, K., Kitamura, Y. T., Saiki, K., Sagawa, S., et al. (2004). Changes in regional cerebral blood volume in frontal cortex during mental work with and without caffeine intake: functional monitoring using near-infrared spectroscopy. *J. Biomed. Opt.* 9, 788–793. doi: 10.1117/1.1755233

Hogervorst, E., Bandelow, S., Schmitt, J., Jentjens, R., Oliveira, M., Allgrove, J., et al. (2008). Caffeine improves physical and cognitive performance during exhaustive exercise. *Med. Sci. Sports. Exerc.* 40, 1841–1851. doi: 10.1249/MSS.0b013e31817bb8b7

Hogervorst, E., Riedel, W. J., Kovacs, E., Brouns, F., and Jolles, J. (1999). Caffeine improves cognitive performance after strenuous physical exercise. *Int. J. Sports. Med.* 20, 354–361. doi: 10.1055/s-2007-971144

Huang, Y., Su, L., and Ma, Q. (2020). The Stroop effect: an activation likelihood estimation meta-analysis in healthy young adults. *Neurosci. Lett.* 716:134683. doi: 10.1016/j.neulet.2019.134683

Huppert, T. J., Diamond, S. G., Franceschini, M. A., and Boas, D. A. (2009). HomER: a review of time-series analysis methods for near-infrared spectroscopy of the brain. *Appl. Opt.* 48:D280. doi: 10.1364/AO.48.00D280

Jenkins, N. T., Trilk, J. L., Singhal, A., O'Connor, P. J., and Cureton, K. J. (2008). Ergogenic effects of low doses of caffeine on cycling performance. *Int. J. Sport. Nutr. Exerc. Metab.* 18, 328–342. doi: 10.1123/ijsnem.18.3.328

Kalmar, J. M., and Cafarelli, E. (2004). Caffeine: a valuable tool to study central fatigue in humans? *Exerc. Sport. Sci. Rev.* 32, 143–147. doi: 10.1097/00003677-200410000-00004

Kenemans, J. L., Wieleman, J. S., Zeegers, M. N., and Verbater, M. N. (1999). Caffeine and stroop interference. *Pharmacol. Biochem. Behav.* 63, 589–598. doi: 10.1016/S0091-3057(99)00022-2

Koppestaetter, F., Poeppel, T. D., Siedentopf, C. M., Ischebeck, A., Kolbitsch, C., Mottaghy, F. M., et al. (2010). Caffeine and cognition in functional magnetic resonance imaging. *J. Alzheimers. Dis.* 20, S71–S84. doi: 10.3233/JAD-2010-1417

Krompinger, J. W., and Simons, R. F. (2011). Cognitive inefficiency in depressive undergraduates: stroop processing and ERPs. *Biol. Psychol.* 86, 239–246. doi: 10.1016/j.biopsycho.2010.12.004

Kujach, S., Byun, K., Hyodo, K., Suwabe, K., Fukuie, T., Laskowski, R., et al. (2018). A transferable high-intensity intermittent exercise improves executive performance in association with dorsolateral prefrontal activation in young adults. *Neuroimage.* 169, 117–125. doi: 10.1016/j.neuroimage.2017.12.003

Laurienti, P. J., Field, A. S., Burdette, J. H., Maldjian, J. A., Yen, Y. F., Moody, D. M., et al. (2002). Dietary caffeine consumption modulates fMRI measures. *Neuroimage.* 17, 751–757. doi: 10.1006/nimg.2002.1237

Laurienti, P. J., Field, A. S., Burdette, J. H., Maldjian, J. A., Yen, Y. F., Moody, D. M., et al. (2003). Relationship between caffeine-induced changes in resting cerebral perfusion and blood oxygenation level-dependent signal. *AJNR Am. J. Neuroradiol.* 24, 1607–1611.

Milham, M. P., Banich, M. T., Claus, E. D., and Cohen, N. J. (2003). Practice-related effects demonstrate complementary roles of anterior cingulated and prefrontal cortices in attentional control. *Neuroimage* 18, 483–493. doi: 10.1016/S1053-8119(02)00050-2

Moscatelli, F., Messina, G., Valenzano, A., Petito, A., Triggian, A. I., Messina, A. et al. (2016). Differences in corticospinal system activity and reaction response between karate athletes and non-athletes. *Neurol. Sci.* 37, 1947–1953. doi: 10.1007/s10072-016-2693-8

Nee, D. E., Wager, T. D., and Jonides, J. (2007). Interference resolution: insights from a meta-analysis of neuroimaging tasks. *Cogn. Affect. Behav. Neurosci.* 7, 1–17. doi: 10.3758/cabn.7.1.1

Nehlig, A. (2010). Is caffeine a cognitive enhancer? *J. Alzheimers. Dis.* 20, S85–S94. doi: 10.3233/JAD-2010-091315

Niioka, T., and Sasaki, M. (2003). Individual cerebral hemodynamic response to caffeine was related to performance on a newly developed stroop color-word task. *Opt. Rev.* 10, 607–608. doi: 10.1007/s10043-003-0607-5

Niu, H. J., Li, X., Chen, Y. J., Ma, C., Zhang, J. Y., Zhang, Z. J., et al. (2013). Reduced frontal activation during a working memory task in mild cognitive impairment: a non-invasive near-infrared spectroscopy study. *CNS Neurosci. Ther.* 19, 125–131. doi: 10.1111/cns.12046

Okamoto, M., Dan, H., Sakamoto, K., Takeo, K., Shimizu, K., Kohno, S., et al. (2004). Three-dimensional probabilistic anatomical cranio-cerebral correlation via the international 10-20 system oriented for transcranial functional brain mapping. *Neuroimage* 21, 99–111. doi: 10.1016/j.neuroimage.2003.08.026

Okamoto, M., Tsuzuki, D., Clowney, L., Dan, H., Singh, A. K., Dan, I., et al. (2009). Structural atlas-based spatial registration for functional near-infrared spectroscopy enabling inter-study data integration. *Clin. Neurophysiol.* 120, 1320–1328. doi: 10.1016/j.clinph.2009.01.023

Pauw, K. D., Roelands, B., Knaepen, K., Polfliet, M., Stiens, J., Meeusen, R., et al. (2015). Effects of caffeine and maltodextrin mouth rinsing on P300, brain imaging and cognitive performance. *J. Appl. Physiol.* 118, 776–782. doi: 10.1152/japplphysiol.01050.2014

Pelligrion, D. A., Xu, H. L., and Vetri, F. (2010). Caffeine and the control of cerebral hemodynamics. *J. Alzheimers. Dis.* 20, S51–S62. doi: 10.3233/JAD-2010-091261

Schaeffer, J. D., Yennu, A. S., Gandy, K. C., Tian, F., Liu, H., Park, H., et al. (2014). An fNIRS investigation of associative recognition in the prefrontal cortex with a rapid event-related design. *J. Neurosci. Methods* 235, 308–315. doi: 10.1016/j.jneumeth.2014.07.011

Sökmen, B., Armstrong, L. E., Kraemer, W. J., Casa, D. J., Dias, J. C., Judelson, D. A., et al. (2008). Caffeine use in sports: considerations for the athlete. *J. Strength. Cond. Res.* 22, 978–986. doi: 10.1519/JSC.0b013e3181660cec

Souissi, Y., Souissi, M., and Chtourou, H. (2019). Effects of caffeine ingestion on the diurnal variation of cognitive and repeated high-intensity performances. *Pharmacol. Biochem. Behav.* 177, 69–74. doi: 10.1016/j.pbb.2019.01.001

Spriet, L. L. (2014). Exercise and sport performance with low doses of caffeine. *Sports Med.* 44, S175–S184. doi: 10.1007/s40279-014-0257-8

Stroop, J. R. (1935). Studies of interference in serial verbal reactions. *J. Exp. Psychol.* 18, 643–662. doi: 10.1037/h0054651

Tsuzuki, D., Jurcak, V., Singh, A. K., Okamoto, M., Watanabe, E., Dan, I., et al. (2007). Virtual spatial registration of stand-alone fNIRS data to MNI space. *Neuroimage* 34, 1506–1518. doi: 10.1016/j.neuroimage.2006.10.043

Xu, X., Deng, Z. Y., Huang, Q., Zhang, W. X., Qi, C. Z., Huang, J. A., et al. (2017). Prefrontal cortex-mediated executive function as assessed by Stroop task performance associateds with weight loss among overweight and obese adolescents and young adults. *Beha. Brain. Res.* 312, 240–248. doi: 10.1016/j.bbr.2016.12.040

Yanagisawa, H., Dan, I., Tsuzuki, D., Kato, M., Okamoto, M., Kyutoku, Y., et al. (2010). Acute moderate exercise elicits increased dorsolateral prefrontal activation and improves cognitive performance with Stroop test. *Neuroimage* 50, 1702–1710. doi: 10.1016/j.neuroimage.2009.12.023

Yunjie, T., Lia Maria, H., Licata, S. C., and Blaise Deb, F. (2012). Low-frequency oscillations measured in the periphery with near-infrared spectroscopy are strongly correlated with blood oxygen level-dependent functional magnetic resonance imaging signals. *J. Biomed. Opt.* 17:106004. doi: 10.1117/1.JBO.17.10.106004

2

Exercise Intervention in PTSD: A Narrative Review and Rationale for Implementation

Nicole J. Hegberg[1], *Jasmeet P. Hayes*[2,3] *and Scott M. Hayes*[1,2,3*]

[1] *VA Boston Healthcare System, Memory Disorders Research Center, Boston University School of Medicine, Boston, MA, United States,* [2] *Department of Psychology, The Ohio State University, Columbus, OH, United States,* [3] *Chronic Brain Injury Initiative, The Ohio State University, Columbus, OH, United States*

Correspondence:
Scott M. Hayes
hayes.1074@osu.edu

Posttraumatic stress disorder (PTSD) is a prominent mental health problem in veteran and community populations. There is accumulating evidence to suggest that aerobic exercise may serve as an effective treatment option for individuals with PTSD. The purpose of this review is to summarize the existing literature exploring aerobic exercise and PTSD and briefly discuss potential mechanisms of PTSD symptom reduction. A search of electronic databases and reference sections of relevant articles published through October 1, 2018 revealed 19 relevant studies that examined aerobic exercise and PTSD symptomatology. A narrative review of extant studies provides encouraging evidence that aerobic exercise interventions alone or as an adjunct to standard treatment may positively impact PTSD symptoms. Potential mechanisms by which aerobic exercise could exert a positive impact in PTSD include exposure and desensitization to internal arousal cues, enhanced cognitive function, exercise-induced neuroplasticity, normalization of hypothalamic pituitary axis (HPA) function, and reductions in inflammatory markers. Randomized clinical trials and translational neuroscience approaches are required to clarify the efficacy of exercise intervention for PTSD and elucidate potential mechanisms of exercise-induced PTSD symptom reduction.

Keywords: aerobic exercise, physical activity, fitness, emotion regulation, cognition, MRI, fMRI, PTSD

INTRODUCTION

Posttraumatic stress disorder (PTSD) can develop after exposure to life-threatening and highly distressing events such as military combat, accidents, assault, or natural, or human-caused disasters. PTSD is a prominent mental health problem in veteran and community populations, affecting 7.6% of OEF/OIF veterans (1) and 3.5% of adult Americans (2). According to the DSM-5, the diagnosis of PTSD is characterized by four broad symptom clusters that include intense reliving of the traumatic event through disruptive memories and nightmares, avoidance of reminders of the event, negative cognitions and mood, and hyperarousal. The impact of PTSD is multi-faceted. In addition to the characteristic symptoms of PTSD, impaired cognitive performance (3, 4) and alterations in brain structure and function (5, 6) are well-documented. Further, individuals with PTSD have increased rates of health-care utilization, loss of productivity, and major chronic diseases (7, 8). For instance, individuals with PTSD have higher rates of diabetes, obesity, and metabolic syndrome (9–12). Moreover, individuals with PTSD exhibit reduced participation in regular physical activity relative to pre-PTSD time periods (13), which likely contributes to the medical, cognitive, and neural comorbidities associated with sedentary behavior (14–16).

Although there are evidence-based psychological and pharmacological (17) treatments that have proven to be effective in treating the characteristic symptoms of PTSD, there are often barriers to treatment initiation among those suffering from PTSD, including stigma, motivation, cost, and access to care (18). While exercise is not without its barriers, such as limited motivation, self-efficacy, or time, it is one intervention that is broadly accessible, low-cost, and could avoid the negative connotations associated with traditional mental health treatment approaches (19). Given the constellation of psychiatric, cognitive, and general health issues associated with PTSD, it is important to consider the case for aerobic exercise for the treatment of PTSD, which may have the potential to enhance functioning in each of these areas. Indeed, aerobic exercise has the potential to exert a positive impact on PTSD via both psychological and neurophysiological mechanisms, such as exposure and desensitization to internal arousal cues, enhanced cognitive function, exercise-induced neuroplasticity, normalization of hypothalamic pituitary axis (HPA) function, and reductions in inflammatory markers.

The notion that physical activity and exercise are viable treatments for PTSD has been gaining momentum in the research community (20–25). The terms are often used interchangeably but are distinct from one another. Physical activity is "any bodily movement produced by skeletal muscles that results in energy expenditure" [(26), p 126]. Physical activity can be in the form of walking, cycling, sport, household or occupational activities, and can vary widely in the amount of energy expenditure (see **Table 1** for description of exercise intensities). Regular physical activity often results in improved balance, coordination, musculoskeletal strength, and/or aerobic fitness, depending on the type. The term exercise is commonly used in the literature and refers to a subcategory of physical activity that is planned, structured, repetitive, and intended to improve or maintain physical fitness (26). Cardiorespiratory fitness is one type of physical fitness that refers to the ability to perform large-muscle, dynamic, moderate to high-intensity physical activity for a prolonged period, and depends on the cardiovascular, respiratory, and skeletal muscle systems. Regular physical activity and/or exercise that is tailored to improve cardiorespiratory fitness, such as walking, dancing, or cycling, has significant health benefits such as reducing the risk of cardiovascular disease, diabetes, and obesity (28). Benefits of regular physical activity and/or exercise also extend to mental health (29–31). In fact, research suggests aerobic exercise, which improves cardiorespiratory fitness, is an effective treatment for depression, anxiety, and schizophrenia (32–36) through both physiological and psychological mechanisms, and may be comparable or superior to other common treatments, such as psychotherapy and pharmacology (37–39). Although PTSD shares some symptomatic overlap with depression and anxiety disorders, there is consensus that PTSD is a distinct disorder, in terms of etiology, symptomatology, and neurobiological correlates. Treatments that are highly efficacious for the treatment of depression may be less effective in PTSD treatment. Therefore, the purpose of this review is to provide a summary of the extant literature examining the impact of exercise on PTSD specifically. We discuss possible mechanisms underlying the potential link between aerobic exercise and PTSD symptoms, and conclude with future directions for aerobic exercise studies in PTSD.

TABLE 1 | Exercise intensities.

Intensity	Percentage of Maximal HR*	Oxygen Consumption*	Examples
Light	57–63%	<3 METs	Slow walk, household chores
Moderate	64–76%	3–6 METs	Brisk walk, slow jog, easy bike riding, tennis
Vigorous	77–95%	>6 METs	Running, hard bike riding, fast swimming, basketball, soccer

Values from Garber et al. (27). HR, heart rate; MET, metabolic equivalent.

METHODS

For this narrative review, we focused on aerobic exercise studies targeting enhancement of cardiorespiratory fitness. To identify studies examining the impact of aerobic exercise on PTSD symptoms, we completed a search of electronic databases (PubMed, Google Scholar, PsycINFO) for relevant studies published through October 1, 2018 using the search terms "PTSD" and "exercise' or "physical activity" or "walking" or "cycling" or "high intensity interval training" or "aerobic fitness" or "cardiorespiratory fitness." We also searched the reference section of relevant articles. To be included in the review, studies had to include an assessment of PTSD symptomatology (in trauma-exposed community or clinical samples) and metrics of aerobic physical activity or exercise or implement an aerobically based exercise intervention in patients with PTSD (or assess PTSD symptoms). If the intervention was combined with an aerobic component (e.g., aerobic + resistance training), we included it in our review. We excluded other exercise interventions that have been explored in the context of PTSD, such as yoga (40), which typically elicits smaller changes in cardiorespiratory fitness than aerobic-focused exercise programs or have a dearth of studies to draw upon for review (e.g., resistance training alone). Our search revealed 19 relevant studies (nine observational and 10 intervention) that examine aerobic exercise and PTSD symptomatology in community and clinical samples of trauma-exposed individuals with methodology exploring correlational, preventative, and treatment effects.

RESULTS AND DISCUSSION

Observational Research

An aggregate of correlational studies suggests that exercise reduces PTSD symptoms (see **Table 2**). Of note, the majority of studies assessed PTSD using DSM-IV criteria or using PTSD questionnaires that assess the three broad symptom clusters defined in the DSM-IV (re-experiencing, avoidance/numbing, and hyperarousal). In one prospective study of 38,883 randomly selected U.S. veterans (77% male), 96% of which did not have PTSD at baseline, participants who reported engaging in

TABLE 2 | Observational studies of exercise and PTSD.

Study	*N*	Age	Gender	Ethnicity	Population/ Dx criteria	Study Design	EX Type/ Measure	Outcome Measure	Results	Significance
Arnson et al. (41)	55	Mean: 49.7 ± 7.5 Range: 19–60	0% female	NR	Israeli veterans/ DSM-IV PTSD	CS	Self-reported EX/ (single item: regular, infrequent, or none)	CAPS	Severity of PTSD did not differ across EX groups	$p = 0.52$
Bosch et al. (42)	76	Mean: 36.4 ± 9.9 Range: NR	18% female	58% white	OEF/OIF/OND veterans/ DSM-IV-TR full or subthreshold PTSD	Longitudinal	Self-reported EX/ (dichotomous variable: engaging in exercise or not)	PCL-M 1 year FU	Baseline EX not significantly related to PTSD sxs at FU	$p = 0.57$
Bourn et al. (43)	239	Mean: 50 ± 15.3 Range: 21–83	9% female	88% white	U.S. Veterans/ CAPS full or subthreshold PTSD	CS	Self-reported EX/GLTEQ	CAPS	Among those reporting high levels of pain severity and interference, individuals who reported being active reported fewer PTSD sxs than those who reported being inactive	*
Davidson et al. (44)	346	Mean: 45.5 ± 14.27 Range: NR	19% female	60% white	U.S. veterans/ residential treatment for PTSD	CS	Self-reported EX/ (single item: days of EX per week)	PCL-M	EX not correlated with PTSD sxs	n.s.
Harte et al. (45)	108	Mean: 23.9 ± 10.22 Range: 18–62	42% female	92% white	Trauma-exposed community/ DSM-IV Criterion A	CS	Self-reported EX/ EHQ-R	PDS	Vigorous, but not light- or moderate-intensity EX, was significantly and inversely related to hyperarousal PTSD sxs	*
LeardMann et al. (46)	38,883	Mean: NR Range: NR	23% female	83% white	U.S. Veterans/ PCL-C	Longitudinal	Self-reported EX/ 2001 National Health Interview Survey	PCL-C	Engaging in vigorous EX (≥20 min, 2 + times/wk) resulted in: Decreased odds of developing sxs; Decreased odds of having persistent PTSD sxs at follow up	 OR = 0.58 [0.049–0.70] OR = 0.59 [0.42–0.83]
Rosenbaum et al. (47)	76	Mean: 47.6 ± 11.9 Range: NR	17% female	NR	Inpatient/ DSM-IV PTSD	CS	Self-reported EX/ IPAQ-SF	PCL-C	Total walking time negatively associated with PTSD sxs; moderate and vigorous EX not significantly correlated with PTSD sxs	*** n.s.
Vujanovic et al. (48)	86	Mean: 24.3 ± 10.54 Range: NR	58% female	89.5% white	Trauma-exposed community/ DSM-IV Criterion A	CS	Self-reported EX/ EHQ-R	PDS	Regular smokers who also endorsed a high level of weekly EX had fewer PTSD sxs than low-level exercisers	*
Whitworth et al. (49)	182	Mean: 34.6 ± 13.3 Range: 18–69	72% female; 1% other	63.2% white	Adults/ PTSD per PCL-C	Longitudinal	Self-reported EX/ GLTEQ	PCL-C 3 month FU	Total EX: - Directly related to avoid/numbing at FU Indirectly associated with total PTSD sxs through alcohol use at FU Strenuous EX: - Directly related to avoid/numbing and hyperarousal sxs at FU - Indirectly related to total PTSD, avoid/numbing, and hyperarousal sxs through sleep at FU	* 95% CI [0.18–1.42] * 95% CI [−2.43 to −0.05] 95% CI [−1.88 to −0.07]

CAPS, Clinician-Administered PTSD Scale; CS, cross-sectional; Dx, diagnostic; EHQ-R, Exercise Habits Questionnaire- Revised; EX, exercise; FU, follow-up; GLTEQ, Godin Leisure-Time Exercise Questionnaire; IPAQ-SF, International Physical Activity Questionnaire- Short Form; NA, not applicable; NR, not reported; n.s., not significant; PCL-C, Posttraumatic Stress Disorder Checklist–Civilian Version; PCL-M, Posttraumatic Stress Disorder Checklist–Military Version; PDS, Posttraumatic Diagnostic Scale; sxs, symptoms; +, sample deemed too small to conduct traditional significance tests. No observational studies assessed cardiorespiratory fitness. **p* < 0.05; ****p* < 0.001.

vigorous exercise ($\geq$ 20 min, two or more times per week), but not combined light or moderate intensity, had significantly decreased odds of developing new PTSD symptoms (odds ratio [OR] 50.58, 95% confidence interval [CI] 0.49, 0.70) or having persistent symptoms (OR 50.59, 95% CI 0.42, 0.83) at 3–5 year follow-up (46). Similarly, Harte et al. (45) found in a cross-sectional analysis of community recruited trauma-exposed adults ($N = 108$; mean age $= 23.9$; 58% male; 81.7% white) that self-reported vigorous-intensity exercise, but not light- or moderate-intensity exercise, was significantly and inversely associated with PTSD hyperarousal symptom severity on a self-report questionnaire (Posttraumatic Diagnostic Scale [PDS]; $\beta = -0.22$, $p = 0.04$). One caveat was that the participants in the study endorsed relatively low levels of PTSD symptomatology (PDS total score: $M = 7.6$, $SD = 8.75$) and did not suffer from other psychopathology, suggesting the findings may not be reflective of associations in clinical samples with greater severity of PTSD or other co-morbid conditions.

The link between vigorous-intensity exercise and PTSD was further supported by Whitworth et al. (49) who longitudinally assessed 182 community-recruited adults with PTSD (mean age: 34.6 ± 13.3, 72% female, 63% white) at baseline and 3 month follow-up. Findings suggested that those who reported engaging in vigorous-intensity exercise (vigorous running or cycling) but not moderate intensity exercise (non-exhaustive sports) on the Godin Leisure-Time Questionnaire (GLTEQ) had fewer avoidance/numbing ($\beta = -2.18$, $p = 0.05$) and hyperarousal ($\beta = -1.87$, $p = 0.03$) symptoms at follow-up, assessed with the PTSD Checklist-Civilian screening (PCL-C). For those participants reporting both moderate- and vigorous-intensity exercise, the longitudinal association between total exercise and PTSD was observed only for avoidance/numbing symptoms ($\beta = -1.76$, $p = 0.05$). Moderate-intensity activity alone was not associated with total PTSD symptoms or any of the symptom clusters at follow-up. Taken together, the findings suggest that those with low levels of PTSD who engage in vigorous-intensity activity may see the most profound effects on hyperarousal symptoms, whereas there may be more widespread symptom effects as PTSD severity increases.

In contrast to the evidence supporting the link between vigorous-intensity exercise and PTSD, a cross-sectional study found that light-intensity exercise (time spent walking) endorsed on a self-report questionnaire (International Physical Activity Questionnaire- Short Form; IPAQ-SF) was significantly and negatively correlated with PTSD symptoms ($\beta = -0.4$; $t = -3.4$; $p < 0.001$) in an inpatient clinical sample ($N = 76$; mean age $= 47.6$; 83% male), but moderate- and vigorous-intensity exercise were not (47). There are also studies that have failed to establish a significant association between exercise and PTSD symptomatology (41, 42, 44). However, methodological limitations may explain these inconsistencies. For example, studies that failed to detect a significant association measured exercise with a single-item questionnaire or variable (e.g., assessing engagement in exercise or not, or number of days per week of exercise), whereas studies that have found significant effects used validated, multiple-item exercise assessment measures. A single-item measure does not capture frequency, intensity, and time (duration) and type of exercise, and therefore may not be adequate to assess behaviors that promote alterations in cardiorespiratory fitness or the effectiveness of aerobic exercise.

Additional cross-sectional studies highlight co-morbid health concerns as moderators of the association between exercise and PTSD symptoms. For instance, it has been shown that exercise moderates the association between regular smoking and PTSD symptoms in a non-clinical sample of trauma-exposed individuals ($N = 86$; mean age $= 24.3$; 42.9% male, 89.5% white), such that regular smokers who also endorsed high levels of weekly exercise had fewer hyperarousal ($\beta = -0.33$, $p = 0.05$), and avoidance ($\beta = -0.38$, $p = 0.04$) symptoms of PTSD than their low-level exercise counterparts (48). Moderating effects have also been observed in clinical samples with PTSD. Despite no main effect of exercise on PTSD severity in PTSD treatment-seeking veterans ($N = 239$; mean age $= 50$; 91.1% male; 87.5% white), among veterans who endorsed high levels of pain severity ($\beta = -0.031$, $p = 0.031$) and pain interference ($\beta = -0.142$, $p = 0.025$), those who reported being physically active reported fewer PTSD symptoms than those who reported being inactive (43).

The observational research provides promising support for the association between exercise and PTSD along with indications of some variables that could influence this association. These studies suggest that the effect of exercise may vary by disorder severity and/or co-morbid health concerns, which might also serve as a marker for disorder severity. Further, findings suggest that exercise might target different symptoms based on intensity (i.e., vigorous-intensity and hyperarousal symptoms), which may provide insight into potential mechanisms of action. For instance, it may be that vigorous-intensity exercise allows for exposure and desensitization to arousal cues, thereby reducing the heightened response to these cues often seen in hyperarousal. These observational studies, however, are not without their limitations. Many of the studies rely on retrospective self-report measures of exercise, which may be prone to bias, inaccuracies, and misunderstanding of questions [e.g., (50–52)]. Several studies did not report time since the traumatic event, and thus the extent to which chronicity of PTSD symptoms relates to the benefits of exercise is unknown. Moreover, given the cross-sectional nature of many of these studies, the directionality of the relationship between exercise and PTSD symptoms is unknown. That is, an association between exercise and PTSD symptoms might suggest that exercise leads to a reduction in PTSD symptoms, but it does not rule out the possibility that those individuals with lower levels of PTSD tend to exercise more.

Intervention Research

We identified 10 published studies that explored the impact of exercise interventions on PTSD symptoms, using a randomized clinical trial (RCT), quasi-RCT, or single-group intervention design. These studies suggest that exercise may be effective as a stand-alone treatment or as an augmentation to traditional PTSD treatment (see **Table 3**).

TABLE 3 | Exercise intervention studies and PTSD.

Study	*N*	Age	Gender	Ethnicity	Population/ Dx criteria	EX Type/ Measure	Fitness indices	Control	Outcome Measure	Results	*p*
Babson et al. (53)	217	Mean: 52.2 ± 7.06 Range: 24–70	0% female	NR	U.S. veterans/ residential treatment for PTSD	Cycling while in group cycling program/ cyclometer on road bike; no specifications about frequency, intensity or duration	NA	None	PCL-M	For those reporting poor baseline sleep quality, time spend cycling improved hyperarousal PTSD sxs	*
Diaz and Motta (54)	12	Mean: 15.42 ± 0.79 Range: 14–17	100% female	17% white	Residential treatment center/ DSM-IV PTSD	5 week aerobic EX program (25 min moderate walking 60–90% HR at completion, 3x/wk)	NA	None	CPSS; TSCC	Reduced PTSD sxs and trauma severity; 1 month follow up mixed for 3 participants remaining at facility	* *
Fetzner and Asmundson (55)	33	Mean: 36.9 ± 11.2 Range: NR	76% female	79% white	Community sample/ DSM-IV-TR full or subthreshold PTSD	2 week aerobic EX program (20 min EX at 60-80% HR, 6x/intervention) with attentional focus (distraction or somatic sensations)	YMCA ergometer bike test at baseline	EX program without attentional focus	PCL-C	Reduced PTSD symptoms regardless of attentional focus	**
Goldstein et al. (56)	47	Mean: 46.8 ± 14.93 Range: 24–69	19% female	40% white	U.S. veterans/ DSM-IV full or subthreshold PTSD	12 week EX program (3, 1hr exercise sessions combining aerobic and resistance exercise and yoga movements)	NA	Waitlist	CAPS	Those participating in EX program reported greater reduction in PTSD sx severity compared to waitlist controls	*
LeBouthillier et al. (57)	32	Mean: 36.75 ± 11.3 Range: NR	75% female	78% white	Community sample/ DSM-IV-TR full or subthreshold PTSD	2 week aerobic EX program (20 min EX at 60–80% HR, 6x/intervention)	Baseline YMCA ergometer bike test (VO_2 max)	None	PCL-C	Those with lower baseline fitness reported a greater reduction in avoidance and hyperarousal PTSD sxs, compared to those with higher baseline fitness	**
Manger and Motta (58)	9	Mean: 48.1 Range: NR	NR	NR	Community sample/ CAPS ≥ 20	10 week aerobic EX program (2–3x/wk, 30 min walk or jog at moderate intensity (60–80% max HR), 10 min cool down ≥12x/intervention)	NA	None	PDS	Reduced PTSD sxs after intervention and at 1-month follow-up	*
Newman and Motta (59)	11	Mean: 15.7 Range: 14–17	100% female	36% white	Residential treatment center/ DSM-IV PTSD	8-week aerobic EX program (40 min with 20 min at 60–80% max HR, 3x/wk)	NA	None	CPTSDI; PTSD-RI	Reduced PTSD sxs compared to baseline; fewer individuals met criteria for PTSD	*** ***
Powers et al. (60)	9	Mean: 34 ± 11.82	89% female	89% white	Community sample/ DSM-IV PTSD	12 session moderate aerobic EX (stationary cycling at 70% age predicted HR) plus PE	NA	PE	PSSI	Greater reduction in PTSD sxs	+ $d = 2.65$
Rosenbaum et al. (61)	81	Mean: 48 ± 12.1 Range: 23–73	16% female	NR	Inpatient population/ DSM-IV-TR PTSD	12 week EX program (progressive resistance training 30 min, 3x/wk and walking 10,000 steps/day) + inpatient care as usual	6-min walk test, resting HR, blood pressure	Inpatient care as usual	PCL-C	Greater reduction in PTSD sxs; groups did not differ in fitness level post intervention (no pre- to post-intervention fitness analyses)	*
Shivakumar et al. (62)	16	Median: 34	100% female	14% white	U.S. veterans/ CAPS ≥ 45	12 week aerobic EX program (brisk walking at 3 mi/hr for 30–40 min, 4x/wk)	NA	None	CAPS; PCL	Improved overall PTSD symptoms	*

CAPS, Clinician-Administered PTSD Scale; CPSS, Child PTSD Symptom Scale; CPTSDI, Child PTSD Inventory; Dx, diagnostic; EHQ-R, Exercise Habits Questionnaire- Revised; EX, exercise; GLTEQ, Godin Leisure-Time Exercise Questionnaire; IPAQ-SF, International Physical Activity Questionnaire- Short Form; NA, not applicable; NR, not reported; n.s., not significant; PCL-C, Posttraumatic Stress Disorder Checklist–Civilian Version; PCL-M, Posttraumatic Stress Disorder Checklist–Military Version; PDS, Posttraumatic Diagnostic Scale; PE, prolonged exposure therapy; PSSI, PTSD Symptom Scale-Interview; PTSD-RI, UCLA PTSD Reaction Index for DSM-IV; sxs, symptoms; TSCC, Trauma Symptom Checklist for Children; +, sample deemed too small to conduct traditional significance tests. *$p < 0.05$; **$p < 0.01$; ***$p < 0.001$.

Exercise Only

One of the first studies in this area (58) assessed the impact of a 10 week aerobic exercise program with multiple baselines on PTSD, anxiety, and depression in 9 non-exercising community members who reported severe PTSD symptomatology in response to a trauma occurring at least 3 months prior during a structured interview [Clinician-Administered PTSD Scale [CAPS]: $M = 63.67 \pm 25.95$ (63)]. After the intervention, which included at least 12, 30-min moderate intensity (60–80% max HR) exercise sessions over 10 weeks, and at one-month follow up (participants refrained from exercising between intervention and follow up), participants who completed the exercise intervention reported significant reductions in PTSD [$t_{(8)} = 3.49, p = 0.008$ and $t_{(8)} = 3.30, p = 0.011$, respectively], as well as depression symptomatology [$t_{(8)} = 4.26, p = 0.003$ and $t_{(8)} = 3.05, p = 0.016$, respectively] and trait anxiety [$t_{(8)} = 3.07$, $p = 0.002$ and $t_{(8)} = 2.31$, $p = 0.050$, respectively]. The researchers followed up this initial study with another multiple baseline intervention in a sample of institutionalized female adolescents ($N = 11$; age: range 14–17 years; 36% white) who met DSM-IV criteria for PTSD based on a clinical administered scale [Children's PTSD Inventory [CPTSDI]; (64)]. Results from the study showed that, compared to baseline, participants who engaged in an 8 week aerobic exercise program (three times per week, 40 min with 20 min at 60–80% maximum heart rate) at an average of 3 years following the experienced trauma reported reduced PTSD symptomatology after the intervention [$t_{(10)} = 23.56$, $p < 0.001$] such that fewer individuals met full criteria for PTSD (59). Further, at 1 month follow-up, PTSD symptomatology increased but did not revert to baseline level, suggesting that reductions may have been at least partly dependent on the exercise intervention. Similarly, another study (54) of 12 institutionalized female adolescents (age range: 14–17 years; 100% female; 17% white) who met criteria for PTSD based on self-report [≥11; Child PTSD Symptom Scale [CPSS]; (65)], with no clear duration since experiencing trauma, showed that a shorter, 5 week aerobic exercise intervention (three times per week, 25 min of moderate-intensity walking: 60–90% maximum heart rate at completion) also resulted in significant reductions in self-reported PTSD symptoms (CPSS) and trauma symptom severity [Trauma Symptom Checklist for Children [TSCC]; (66)]. Only three participants remained at the facility at 1 month follow up and all continued to report significantly less PTSD symptoms and trauma symptom severity compared to baseline.

A more recent study conducted by Shivakumar et al. (62) resulted in similar findings. A small convenience sample of female veterans who reported PTSD symptomatology on the CAPS (≥45; $N = 16$; median age = 34; 14% white, 50% military sexual trauma) and completed a 12 week moderate-intensity exercise program (30–40 min of brisk walking at 3 mph, four times per week) reported significant reductions in overall PTSD symptomatology based on two separate assessments of symptoms (CAPS & PCL; $z = -2.395$, $p = 0.017$ and $F_{(2, 12)} = 9.42$, $p = 0.03$, respectively). In a larger study of male veterans in a 60- to 90-day residential treatment program ($N = 217$; mean age = 52 years), time spent cycling in a non-standardized group bicycling program reduced hyperarousal symptoms at discharge ($\beta = 0.24$, $p = 0.002$), but only for those who reported poor baseline sleep quality (53). Findings suggest that only select individuals might benefit from unstandardized exercise with no clear frequency, intensity, or duration. Authors did not report when the interventions occurred in relation to the participants' experienced trauma(s) in either of these two studies.

Studies with larger sample sizes and randomized conditions show further promise for the beneficial effects of aerobic exercise on PTSD. Fetzner and Asmundson (55) examined the influence of aerobic training and attentional focus to somatic sensations on PTSD symptoms in a community sample ($N = 33$; mean age = 37, 75% female). The exercise program consisted of six, 20-min moderate-intensity aerobic exercise sessions (60–80% heart rate) over 2 weeks. It was implemented, on average, 8 years following the participants' experienced trauma with most occurring 1–4 years prior to intervention. The results indicated that the aerobic exercise training, regardless of attentional focus, reduced total self-reported PTSD symptoms on a questionnaire (PCL-C; $p < 0.01$), which was driven by reductions in avoidance symptoms ($p < 0.01$). Another article published from these data (57) suggested that participants with lower fitness at baseline, measured using the YMCA ergometer bike test which assesses submaximal VO_2 maximum, reported a greater reduction in PTSD symptoms compared to their higher-fit peers ($\beta = 0.10$, $p < 0.10$). These results suggest that individuals with low fitness may preferentially benefit from the effects of aerobic exercise on PTSD. Finally, a randomized study conducted in a veteran population ($N = 47$; mean age = 46.8; 19% female) explored the impact of a 12 week aerobic exercise program (at least three, 1 hour sessions per week of moderate-intensity aerobic and anaerobic exercise), compared to waitlist control, on self-reported symptoms of PTSD [CAPS; (56)]. There was no indication when intervention took place in relation to experienced trauma. Results revealed that participants who completed the exercise program reported greater reduction in PTSD symptom severity compared to waitlist controls [$F_{(1, 35.3)} = 4.64$, $p = 0.038$]. Further, hyperarousal symptoms were the only cluster that benefitted significantly from the exercise intervention [$F_{(1, 35.2)} = 4.40$, $p = 0.044$]. Additional findings from the same sample suggest that the exercise program was also associated with increased self-reported mindfulness and interoceptive awareness (67).

Exercise Plus Standard PTSD Treatment

Two additional studies examined the effect of aerobic exercise training on PTSD symptoms in conjunction with other forms of treatment. A study conducted by Powers et al. (60) compared PTSD symptom changes in community adults with PTSD ($N = 9$; mean age = 34; 89% female) who were assigned to moderate-intensity aerobic exercise (stationary cycling; 70% age predicted heart rate max) prior to 12 prolonged exposure therapy sessions (an evidence-based treatment for PTSD) or to prolonged exposure therapy only ($d = 2.65$, $SE = 0.92$). The results indicated that the group who exercised prior to therapy showed greater improvement in PTSD symptoms relative to the group only participating in therapy.

In another study, inpatients with PTSD ($N = 81$; mean age: 48; 84% male; BMI = 30.1 obese) were assigned to either a 12 week exercise program that included three, 30-min sessions per week of progressive resistance training, walking (daily step count goal = 10,000 steps), and "care as usual" to "care as usual" alone (68). Individuals in the exercise group had significantly greater symptom reduction on a self-report measure of PTSD (PCL-C; *mean difference* = −5.4, 95% CI −10.5 to −0.3, $p = 0.04$), as well as greater reductions on measures of depression, anxiety, stress, weight, percent body fat, and weight circumference compared to the "care as usual" group. The reductions in PTSD symptomatology occurred despite the finding that there were no between-group differences in indicators of cardiorespiratory fitness as measured by the 6-min walk test, resting heart rate, and blood pressure. Pre-to post-intervention within-group differences in cardiorespiratory fitness were not measured. Results from these two studies converge to suggest that exercise combined with other forms of treatment may reduce symptoms above and beyond symptom reduction with standard treatments alone.

The intervention studies to date suggest that exercise may in fact lead to reduction in symptoms among individuals with PTSD. While the existing studies are promising in this regard, many of the studies have small sample sizes. In addition, six of the ten intervention studies lack control groups, and thus do not account for other variables that may contribute to symptom improvement. This is important to note given that in some cases symptoms of PTSD resolve without intervention and only a percentage of the population requires treatment for PTSD symptom resolution. However, half of these studies were conducted in the context of residential treatment programs suggesting the participants were likely constituents that would, in fact, benefit from treatment to promote symptom reduction.

General Discussion

To summarize, both observational and intervention studies provide support for the notion that aerobic exercise, either alone or in combination with standard treatments, exerts positive mental health benefits among individuals with PTSD. The results are encouraging as positive effects were observed in both civilian and military populations, as well as in both predominately female and male study samples. Based on the pattern of findings across studies and other existing areas of research we briefly review potential mechanisms by which aerobic exercise may exert a positive impact in PTSD symptoms, followed by the limitations of the current studies and potential future directions.

Exposure and Desensitization to Internal Arousal Cues

One of the core features of PTSD symptomatology is hyperarousal, which results in sensitivity to physiological arousal cues. Research suggests that repeated exposure to these physiological cues, such as rapid heartbeat, in the context of exercise may increase tolerance of and facilitate desensitization to the physiological sensations (32, 69, 70). However, existing research has focused on this mechanism in anxiety disorders and this effect has been largely unexplored in individuals with PTSD. Nevertheless, the possibility that exercise could result in desensitization to physiological arousal cues in a clinical PTSD sample is consistent with the findings reviewed that suggest that those who engage in vigorous-intensity exercise have fewer hyperarousal symptoms of PTSD (45, 49, 53). In other words, it may be that the vigorous activity, which by definition elicits the greatest increase in physiological arousal cues, is a means of exposure, and reduces the individuals' subjective heightened response to these cues in other (non-exercising) contexts. While we are not aware of quantitative evidence of this exercise-related exposure effect in PTSD populations, a recent case study suggested that this type of exposure might contribute to the therapeutic effects of exercise on PTSD. More specifically, the case study revealed that an individual with PTSD who participated in a 3 month exercise program (2x/week for a total of 90 min) became more aware that his bodily sensations, like pain or fast heartbeat, were not necessarily catastrophic or related to a traumatic event (71). Taken together, it is reasonable to hypothesize that exposure to arousal cues may partly explain the beneficial effect of exercise on PTSD symptomatology.

Improved Cognitive Function

A well-replicated finding in the PTSD literature is that of disrupted cognitive control in individuals with PTSD, evidenced by greater distractibility from task irrelevant stimuli and difficulty inhibiting responses to task irrelevant stimuli (72–74). At the center of the cognitive control disturbance is difficulty disengaging attention from salient stimuli that may be interpreted as potentially threatening, even if neutral or positively valenced (75, 76). This impairment in cognitive control may contribute to the maintenance of PTSD symptoms, such as hypervigilance and avoidance (77). In addition to impairments in cognitive control, PTSD is also associated with reduced learning and memory. In particular, individuals with PTSD show reduced encoding of specific episodic details, including autobiographical memories, as well as increased false memory and reduced extinction learning, which also has implications for the maintenance of PTSD symptoms.

To date, we are not aware of any aerobic exercise studies in PTSD that used cognitive outcome measures. Nevertheless, PTSD-related cognitive impairment and the maintenance of PTSD symptoms may be alleviated by improvements in cognition that are often associated with aerobic exercise. To date, the majority of studies on aerobic exercise and cognition have focused on older adults. For instance, extant research among healthy older adults suggests that cardiorespiratory fitness and aerobic exercise positively affect executive function (78, 79) and episodic memory (80–83)—the same cognitive functions negatively impacted by PTSD. Although speculative, it may be the case that aerobic exercise improves executive function and episodic memory function in PTSD, which are deficits that contribute to the core psychiatric symptoms of PTSD, such as re-experiencing, avoidance, and hyperarousal.

Alterations in Brain Structure and Function

The presence and severity of PTSD symptoms have been linked to structural gray and white matter abnormalities in the medial temporal lobes and fronto-parietal regions, which underpin executive function and episodic memory. For instance, gray matter changes associated with PTSD include reduced volume in the hippocampus and the anterior cingulate (84–86), reduced volume or cortical thickness in the precuneus, insula, and ventromedial and lateral prefrontal cortex (87, 88). A preliminary quantitative meta-analysis of seven adult onset PTSD studies (89) revealed white matter abnormalities in the cingulum bundle, a white matter tract that links the anterior medial prefrontal cortex to the medial temporal lobes, and the superior longitudinal fasciculus, which connects the frontal and parietal lobes (90). These structural alterations co-occur with functional brain alterations in PTSD, which include alterations in activation and connectivity in amygdala, hippocampal, orbitofrontal cortex and dorsal anterior cingulate cortex (3, 6, 91, 92).

We are not aware of any exercise intervention studies in PTSD that assess brain structure or function. However, there is overlap among the neural correlates of PTSD and the brain regions impacted by aerobic exercise (93), suggesting that exercise-induced brain changes may be a mechanism by which aerobic exercise positively impacts PTSD symptomatology. For instance, aerobic training studies in older adults have revealed increased volume of prefrontal regions, including anterior cingulate cortex, during aerobic training (exercising at up to 70% of their heart rate reserve; HRR) relative to a non-aerobic stretching control group (94). Another study found that increases in physical activity resulting from exercise training were associated with gray matter volume increases in the cingulate gyrus (including both anterior and posterior cingulate cortex), left superior frontal gyrus, left medial parietal cortex, among others (95). After participation in an aerobic exercise program in another study, older adults demonstrated an approximately 2% increase in hippocampal volume, whereas a *decrease* of roughly 1.4% was observed in the stretching control group (96). Increased hippocampal volume may in part be explained by exercise associated increases in neurogenesis in the dentate gyrus subfield of the hippocampus (97, 98), which is negatively impacted in PTSD (84). Cardiorespiratory fitness and aerobic exercise have been positively associated with fronto-parietal and medial temporal lobe white matter tracts including the fornix, cingulum bundle and superior longitudinal fasciculus (99–102). Functional brain alterations have also been associated with aerobic fitness (103–105), and aerobic exercise has been shown to impact activation in many of the same regions implicated in PTSD (93, 106, 107).

Normalization of Hypothalamic Pituitary Axis (HPA) Axis Function

The HPA axis is a neuroendocrine system that regulates reactions to stress and physiological processes. In the context of stress, the hypothalamus releases corticotrophin releasing hormone (CRH), which stimulates the pituitary gland to release adrenocorticotropic hormone (ACTH). Ultimately, cortisol is released by the adrenal cortex, which regulates the system by providing negative feedback to the hypothalamus and pituitary gland. Alterations in the HPA axis are a relatively reliable finding in the PTSD literature. More specifically, a recent review of the neuroendocrine characteristics of PTSD indicated that individuals with PTSD tend to express low basal cortisol levels, which is associated with increased levels of CRH, and an exaggerated HPA axis negative feedback loop, while peripheral and central catecholamine levels are increased (108). Further, a review of studies that assess the acute response to laboratory stressors suggests that the HPA axis response among those with PTSD is characterized by an exaggerated cortisol response (109).

Normalization of the HPA axis may be a therapeutic target for PTSD based on its association with PTSD symptom improvement (110, 111). In fact, acute and regular aerobic exercise exert positive effects on the HPA axis, which may promote normalization and reduction in PTSD symptoms. For instance, an early review suggests that acute exercise induces the secretion of ACTH which stimulates the release of cortisol (112). Findings from more recent intervention studies suggest that acute moderate- and vigorous-intensity, but not low-intensity, exercise result in increased levels of cortisol (113, 114), which might target the low basal cortisol levels seen in PTSD populations. Additional research conducted in healthy or other clinical populations provides evidence that acute and regular exercise regulate or improve one's stress-related activation of the HPA axis, including a blunted cortisol response (115–118). The extent to which these findings translate to the PTSD-related HPA axis alterations is unclear because to our knowledge, this effect has only been explored in healthy populations or clinical populations with HPA axis alterations that differ from those observed in PTSD.

Activation of the Immune System and Reduced Inflammation

The activation of the HPA axis has pro-inflammatory implications for the immune system (119). While the understanding of the role of inflammation in the etiology and maintenance of PTSD is limited, there is evidence to suggest that PTSD is characterized by increased inflammatory activity. More specifically, a meta-analysis comparing individuals with PTSD and healthy controls, found that PTSD was associated with elevations in pro-inflammatory cytokines such as interleukin-1 beta (IL-1β), interleukin-6 (IL-6), tumor necrosis factor-alpha (TNF-α), interferon-gamma [INF-γ; (120)]. There is also evidence to suggest that there is increased c-reactive protein (CRP), decreased anti-inflammatory markers (e.g., interleukin-8 [IL-8], interleukin-2 [IL-2]) as well as alterations in cell function and genes related to inflammation in populations with PTSD (119, 121–123).

Interestingly, exercise has been shown to influence these same inflammatory pathways in a manner that could possibly counteract some of the augmentations documented in PTSD. For example, regular aerobic exercise can increase factors involved in immunomodulatory function and diminish pro-inflammatory signaling, through downstream anti-inflammatory effects of acute production of IL-6 (124–127). There is also evidence to suggest that inflammatory alterations might partly explain the effect of exercise on sleep quality (128), which has shown to both moderate and mediate the association between aerobic exercise and PTSD (49, 53). Pro-inflammatory cytokines that are modulated by exercise play a crucial role in sleep regulation, with low concentrations of IL-1 and TNF-α associated with enhanced non-REM sleep (128–130), and high levels linked to sleep disorders. Taken together, the favorable effects of exercise on inflammation and the role of inflammation in sleep regulation support the notion that exercise may be an effective tool for improving PTSD symptoms but requires additional study to directly test this assertion.

Limitations

Although the current review of the literature is encouraging, the extant studies have limitations. For instance, many of the studies had small sample sizes, restricted age ranges and/or ethnicities (many predominantly white samples), focused on either females or males, and/or relied on convenience sampling for recruitment. In addition, the populations from these studies are quite variable in terms of severity of PTSD symptoms (ranging from inpatient to trauma-exposed without PTSD), veteran status, and whether they are seeking treatment. While these factors limit the generalizability of each study to dissimilar populations, the positive association between exercise and PTSD across these variable samples provides some evidence for the generalizability of the findings. There are also considerable limitations related to the heterogeneity in research methodology. In terms of measurement, PTSD was assessed using many different self-report measures of PTSD symptoms and only select studies reported on time since traumatic event, which could impact the benefits of exercise on PTSD. There is substantial variability in the exercise measures and protocols administered across studies. First, single-item measures of exercise may hinder the detection of significant findings due to the oversimplification of exercise. Second, many of the studies rely on retrospective self-report measures of exercise, which may be prone to bias, inaccuracies, and misunderstanding of questions [e.g., (50–52)], rather than objective measures of exercise or fitness levels. In addition, the majority of the existing intervention studies failed to implement rigorous pre- and post- intervention fitness assessments and few included a control group. Therefore, some of these early studies are not able to demonstrate that alterations in PTSD were specific to alterations in fitness (as opposed to common factors). As more randomized clinical trials of exercise and PTSD appear in the literature, it will be possible to complete a quantitative meta-analysis of the effects of aerobic exercise on PTSD symptoms. However, given the heterogeneity in the study methods outlined above, and in particular the lack of an adequate number of studies that included a control group, we felt a quantitative analysis of the literature was not appropriate at this time. Nevertheless, these early and promising findings as well as the consideration of some of the potential mechanisms by which exercise could exert a positive impact in PTSD provide motivation for further investigation.

Future Directions

While there is evidence that aerobic exercise may positively impact PTSD symptoms, appropriately powered randomized clinical trials are required to more firmly establish the relationship between exercise and PTSD. At a minimum, aerobic exercise interventions should adhere to CDC's recommended guidelines for cardiovascular fitness-improving activity (i.e., 150 min of moderate-intensity or 75 min of vigorous-intensity exercise per week). Future studies should implement gold standard pre- and post-intervention diagnostic interviews to determine the presence and severity of PTSD symptomatology, such as the Clinician-Administered PTSD Scale for DSM-5 (CAPS-5) and a progressive, graded exercise test to assess cardiorespiratory fitness. Objective assessment of exercise adherence could be assessed through the use of accelerometers paired with chest-strap heart rate monitors (shown to be superior to wrist-based heart rate monitors), which would allow researchers to objectively assess the frequency, intensity, and time (duration) of exercise during the intervention. Moreover, use of accelerometers would also provide insight about non-exercise related physical activity, such as occupational, domestic, or travel-related physical activity, which could potentially moderate treatment effects. Given the constellation of psychiatric, cognitive, neural, and general health markers of PTSD, it is also important to consider the use of cognitive, neuroimaging, and neurobiological outcome measures. These data may elucidate the mechanisms of exercise-induced symptom reduction in PTSD, and once clarified, may provide insight as to the dosage of exercise required to attenuate PTSD symptoms. Moreover, given the current state of the literature, we have focused exclusively on aerobic fitness. Other exercise interventions, which have yet to be thoroughly explored, including resistance training or combined aerobic and resistance training, could also elicit significant reductions in PTSD symptoms. Further research on exercise and PTSD using some of these suggestions would help to better understand the effects of exercise on PTSD and might shed light on the possible mechanisms by which exercise improves PTSD and its sequelae.

Conclusion

Aerobic exercise is a low-cost, widely accessible activity known to provide multiple health benefits, including cardiovascular health and musculoskeletal health, as well as reduced rates of co-morbidity and mortality (28). Moreover, aerobic exercise is not associated with the stigma of standard mental health treatment (19). There is growing evidence of the beneficial effects of exercise on mental health disorders, including depression and anxiety (32, 33, 35, 36). Our review of the literature suggests aerobic exercise may also reduce PTSD symptomatology across a variety of populations providing evidence for the clinical utility of exercise as a form of treatment. Additional RCTs are required to provide more definitive evidence of a causal relationship between exercise and PTSD. Nevertheless, we are not aware of any negative effects of exercise on PTSD symptoms. Thus, in the absence of medical contraindications for exercise, providers for patients with PTSD may consider prescribing aerobic exercise. To date, the precise mechanisms by which the beneficial effects of exercise may influence PTSD are unknown. However, there are multiple psychological, cognitive, and neurobiological routes that may underpin exercise-induced improvements in PTSD. Methodologically-rigorous research is required to provide more definitive evidence of a positive effect of aerobic exercise on PTSD and identify the mechanisms of exercise-induced alterations in PTSD.

AUTHOR CONTRIBUTIONS

SH generated the idea and outline for the project. NH completed the literature search and wrote the review, with JH and SH contributing conceptual guidance and writing.

ACKNOWLEDGMENTS

This work was supported by the National Institute on Aging of the National Institutes of Health (R21AG056921 awarded to SH), The Ohio State University Discovery Themes Chronic Brain Injury Initiative (SH and JH) and the Boston University Spivack Emerging Leaders in Neurosciences Award (SH). The content is solely the responsibility of the authors and does not necessarily represent the official views of the National Institutes of Health.

REFERENCES

Smith TC, Ryan MA, Wingard DL, Slymen DJ, Sallis JF, Kritz- Silverstein D. New onset and persistent symptoms of post-traumatic stress disorder self reported after deployment and combat exposures: prospective population based US military cohort study. *Br Med J.* (2008) 336:366–71. doi: 10.1136/bmj.39430.638241.AE

Kessler RC, Chiu WT, Demler O, Merikangas KR, Walters EE. Prevalence, severity, and comorbidity of 12-month DSM-IV disorders in the National Comorbidity Survey Replication. *Arch Gen Psychiatry.* (2005) 62:617–27. doi: 10.1001/archpsyc.62.6.617

Hayes JP, Vanelzakker MB, Shin LM. Emotion and cognition interactions in PTSD: a review of neurocognitive and neuroimaging studies. *Front Integr Neurosci.* (2012) 6:89. doi: 10.3389/fnint.2012.00089

Woon FL, Farrer TJ, Braman CR, Mabey JK, Hedges DW. A meta- analysis of the relationship between symptom severity of posttraumatic stress disorder and executive function. *Cogn Neuropsychiatry.* (2017) 22:1–16. doi: 10.1080/13546805.2016.1255603

Hayes JP, Hayes SM, Mikedis AM. Quantitative meta-analysis of neural activity in posttraumatic stress disorder. *Biol Mood Anxiety Disord.* (2012) 2:9. doi: 10.1186/2045-5380-2-9

Miller DR, Hayes SM, Hayes JP, Spielberg JM, Lafleche G, Verfaellie M. Default mode network subsystems are differentially disrupted in posttraumatic stress disorder. *Biol Psychiatry Cogn Neurosci Neuroimaging.* (2017) 2:363–71. doi: 10.1016/j.bpsc.2016.12.006

Boscarino JA. Diseases among men 20 years after exposure to severe stress: implications for clinical research and medical care. *Psychosom Med.* (1997) 59:605–14. doi: 10.1097/00006842-199711000-00008

Pacella ML, Hruska B, Delahanty DL. The physical health consequences of PTSD and PTSD symptoms: a meta-analytic review. *J Anxiety Disord.* (2013) 27:33–46. doi: 10.1016/j.janxdis.2012.08.004

Bartoli F, Crocamo C, Alamia A, Amidani F, Paggi E, Pini E, et al. Posttraumatic stress disorder and risk of obesity: systematic review and meta-analysis. *J Clin Psychiatry.* (2015) 76:e1253–61. doi: 10.4088/JCP.14r09199

Boscarino JA. Posttraumatic stress disorder and physical illness: results from clinical and epidemiologic studies. *Ann N Y Acad Sci.* (2004) 1032:141–53. doi: 10.1196/annals.1314.011

Rosenbaum S, Stubbs B, Ward PB, Steel Z, Lederman O, Vancampfort D. The prevalence and risk of metabolic syndrome and its components among people with posttraumatic stress disorder: a systematic review and meta- analysis. *Metabolism.* (2015) 64:926–33. doi: 10.1016/j.metabol.2015.04.009

Wolf EJ, Bovin MJ, Green JD, Mitchell KS, Stoop TB, Barretto KM, et al. Longitudinal associations between post-traumatic stress disorder and metabolic syndrome severity. *Psychol Med.* (2016) 46:2215–26. doi: 10.1017/S0033291716000817

de Assis MA, de Mello MF, Scorza FA, Cadrobbi MP, Schooedl AF, Gomes da Silva S, et al. Evaluation of physical activity habits in patients with posttraumatic stress disorder. *Clinics (Sao Paulo).* (2008). 63:473–8. doi: 10.1590/S1807-59322008000400010

Ford ES, Caspersen CJ. Sedentary behaviour and cardiovascular disease: a review of prospective studies. *Int J Epidemiol.* (2012) 41:1338–53. doi: 10.1093/ije/dys078

Vaynman S, Gomez-Pinilla F. Revenge of the "sit": how lifestyle impacts neuronal and cognitive health through molecular systems that interface energy metabolism with neuronal plasticity. *J Neurosci Res.* (2006) 84:699– 715. doi: 10.1002/jnr.20979

Voss MW, Carr LJ, Clark R, Weng T. (2014). Revenge of the "sit" II: does lifestyle impact neuronal and cognitive health through distinct mechanisms associated with sedentary behavior and physical activity? *Ment Health Phys Act.* 7:9–24. doi: 10.1016/j.mhpa.2014.01.001

Lancaster CL, Teeters JB, Gros DF, Back SE. Posttraumatic stress disorder: overview of evidence-based assessment and treatment. *J Clin Med.* (2016) 5:105. doi: 10.3390/jcm5110105

Sayer NA, Friedemann-Sanchez G, Spoont M, Murdoch M, Parker LE, Chiros C, et al. A qualitative study of determinants of PTSD treatment initiation in veterans. *Psychiatry.* (2009) 72:238–55. doi: 10.1521/psyc.2009.72.3.238

Dickstein BD, Vogt DS, Handa S, Litz BT. Targeting self-stigma in returning military personnel and veterans: a review of intervention strategies. *Mil Psychol.* (2010) 22:224. doi: 10.1080/08995600903417399

Vancampfort D, Stubbs B, Richards J, Ward PB, Firth J, Schuch FB, et al. Physical fitness in people with posttraumatic stress disorder: a systematic review. *Disabil Rehabil.* (2017) 39:2461–7. doi: 10.1080/09638288.2016.1226412

Caddick N, Smith B. Exercise is medicine for mental health in military veterans: a qualitative commentary. *Qual Res Sport Exerc Health.* (2017) 1–12. doi: 10.1080/2159676X.2017.1333033

Sornborger J, Fann A, Serpa JG, Ventrelle J, RDN M, Ming Foynes M, et al. Integrative therapy approaches for posttraumatic stress disorder: a special focus on treating veterans. *Focus.* (2017) 15:390–8. doi: 10.1176/appi.focus.20170026

Whitworth JW, Ciccolo JT. Exercise and post-traumatic stress disorder in military veterans: a systematic review. *Mil Med.* (2016) 181:953–60. doi: 10.7205/MILMED-D-15-00488

Hall KS, Hoerster KD, Yancy Jr WS. Post-traumatic stress disorder, physical activity, and eating behaviors. *Epidemiol Rev.* (2015) 37:103–15. doi: 10.1093/epirev/mxu011

McCash JA, Abraham S. Effects of aerobic exercise on patients with mental illness in a veterans inpatient psychiatric unit: a review of the literature. *Int J Stud Nurs.* (2017) 3:34. doi: 10.20849/ijsn.v3i1.235

Caspersen CJ, Powell KE, Christenson GM. Physical activity, exercise, and physical fitness: definitions and distinctions for health-related research. *Public Health Rep.* (1985) 100:126–31. doi: 10.2307/200 56429

Garber CE, Blissmer B, Deschenes MR, Franklin BA, Lamonte MJ, Lee I-M, et al. American College of Sports Medicine position stand. Quantity and quality of exercise for developing and maintaining cardiorespiratory, musculoskeletal, and neuromotor fitness in apparently healthy adults: guidance for prescribing exercise. *Med Sci Sports Exerc.* (2011) 43:1334–59. doi: 10.1249/MSS.0b013e318213fefb

Warburton DE, Nicol CW, Bredin SS. Health benefits of physical activity: the evidence. *CMAJ.* (2006) 174:801–9. doi: 10.1503/cmaj.051351

Kim YS, Park YS, Allegrante JP, Marks R, Ok H, Ok Cho K, et al. Relationship between physical activity and general mental health. *Prev Med.* (2012) 55:458–63. doi: 10.1016/j.ypmed.2012.08.021

Stathopoulou G, Powers MB, Berry AC, Smits JA, Otto MW. Exercise interventions for mental health: a quantitative and qualitative review. *Clin. Psychol.* (2006) 13:179–93. doi: 10.1111/j.1468-2850.2006.00021.x

Strohle A. Physical activity, exercise, depression and anxiety disorders. *J Neural Transm (Vienna).* (2009) 116:777–84. doi: 10.1007/s00702-008-0092-x

Asmundson GJ, Fetzner MG, Deboer LB, Powers MB, Otto MW, Smits JA. Let's get physical: a contemporary review of the anxiolytic effects of exercise for anxiety and its disorders. *Depress Anxiety.* (2013) 30:362–73. doi: 10.1002/da.22043

Dunn AL, Trivedi MH, O'Neal HA. Physical activity dose-response effects on outcomes of depression and anxiety. *Med Sci Sports Exerc.* (2001). 33 (Suppl. 6), S587–97; discussion 609-510. doi: 10.1097/00005768-200106001-00027

Firth J, Stubbs B, Rosenbaum S, Vancampfort D, Malchow B, Schuch F, et al. Aerobic exercise improves cognitive functioning in people with schizophrenia: a systematic review and meta-analysis. *Schizophr Bull.* (2017) 43:546–56. doi: 10.1093/schbul/sbw115

Herring MP, Jacob ML, Suveg C, Dishman RK, O'Connor PJ. Feasibility of exercise training for the short-term treatment of generalized anxiety disorder: a randomized controlled trial. *Psychother Psychosom.* (2012) 81:21– 8. doi: 10.1159/000327898

Schuch FB, Vancampfort D, Richards J, Rosenbaum S, Ward PB, Stubbs B. Exercise as a treatment for depression: a meta-analysis adjusting for publication bias. *J Psychiatr Res.* (2016) 77:42–51. doi: 10.1016/j.jpsychires.2016.02.023

Carek PJ, Laibstain SE, Carek SM. Exercise for the treatment of depression and anxiety. *Int J Psychiatry Med.* (2011) 41:15–28. doi: 10.2190/PM. 41.1.c

Petruzzello SJ, Landers DM, Hatfield BD, Kubitz KA, Salazar W. A meta-analysis on the anxiety-reducing effects of acute and chronic exercise. Outcomes and mechanisms. *Sports Med.* (1991) 11:143–82. doi: 10.2165/00007256-199111030-00002

Wipfli BM, Rethorst CD, Landers DM. The anxiolytic effects of exercise: a meta-analysis of randomized trials and dose-response analysis. *J Sport Exerc Psychol.* (2008) 30:392–410. doi: 10.1123/jsep.30.4.392

Mitchell KS, Dick AM, DiMartino DM, Smith BN, Niles B, Koenen KC, et al. A pilot study of a randomized controlled trial of yoga as an intervention for PTSD symptoms in women. *J Trauma Stress.* (2014) 27:121– 8. doi: 10.1002/ jts.21903

Arnson Y, Amital D, Fostick L, Silberman A, Polliack ML, Zohar J, et al. Physical activity protects male patients with post-traumatic stress disorder from developing severe fibromyalgia. *Clin Exp Rheumatol.* (2007) 25:529–33.

Bosch J, Weaver TL, Neylan TC, Herbst E, McCaslin SE. Impact of engagement in exercise on sleep quality among veterans with posttraumatic stress disorder symptoms. *Mil Med.* (2017) 182:e1745–50. doi: 10.7205/ MILMED-D-16-00385

Bourn LE, Sexton MB, Porter KE, Rauch SAM. Physical activity moderates the association between pain and PTSD in treatment-seeking veterans. *Pain Med.* (2016) 17:2134–41. doi: 10.1093/pm/pnw089

Davidson CL, Babson KA, Bonn-Miller MO, Souter T, Vannoy S. The impact of exercise on suicide risk: examining pathways through depression, PTSD, and sleep in an inpatient sample of veterans. *Suicide Life Threat Behav.* (2013) 43:279–89. doi: 10.1111/sltb.12014

Harte CB, Vujanovic AA, Potter CM. Association between exercise and posttraumatic stress symptoms among trauma-exposed adults. *Eval Health Prof.* (2015) 38:42–52. doi: 10.1177/0163278713494774

LeardMann CA, Kelton ML, Smith B, Littman AJ, Boyko EJ, Wells TS, et al. Prospectively assessed posttraumatic stress disorder and associated physical activity. *Public Health Rep.* (2011) 126:371–83. doi: 10.1177/003335491112600311

Rosenbaum S, Vancampfort D, Tiedemann A, Stubbs B, Steel Z, Ward PB, et al. Among inpatients, posttraumatic stress disorder symptom severity is negatively associated with time spent walking. *J Nerv Ment Dis.* (2016) 204:15–9. doi: 10.1097/NMD.0000000000000415

Vujanovic AA, Farris SG, Harte CB, Smits JA, Zvolensky MJ. Smoking status and exercise in relation to PTSD symptoms: a test among trauma-exposed adults. *Ment Health Phys Act.* (2013) 6:132–8. doi: 10.1016/j.mhpa.2012.12.001

Whitworth JW, Craft LL, Dunsiger SI, Ciccolo JT. Direct and indirect effects of exercise on posttraumatic stress disorder symptoms: a longitudinal study. *Gen Hosp Psychiatry.* (2017) 49:56–62. doi: 10.1016/j.genhosppsych.2017.06.012

Prince SA, Adamo KB, Hamel ME, Hardt J, Connor Gorber S, Tremblay M. A comparison of direct versus self-report measures for assessing physical activity in adults: a systematic review. *Int J Behav Nutr Phys Act.* (2008). 5:56. doi: 10.1186/1479-5868-5-56

Rzewnicki R, Auweele YV, De Bourdeaudhuij I. Addressing overreporting on the International Physical Activity Questionnaire (IPAQ) telephone survey with a population sample. *Public Health Nutr.* (2003) 6:299–305. doi: 10.1079/ PHN2002427

Shephard RJ. Limits to the measurement of habitual physical activity by questionnaires. *Br J Sports Med.* (2003) 37:197–206. doi: 10.1136/ bjsm.37.3.197

Babson KA, Heinz AJ, Ramirez G, Puckett M, Irons JG, Bonn-Miller MO, et al. The interactive role of exercise and sleep on veteran recovery from symptoms of PTSD. *Ment Health Phys Act.* (2015) 8:15–20. doi: 10.1016/j. mhpa.2014.12.002

Diaz AB, Motta R. The effects of an aerobic exercise program on posttraumatic stress disorder symptom severity in adolescents. *Int J Emerg Ment Health.* (2008) 10:49–59.

Fetzner MG, Asmundson GJ. Aerobic exercise reduces symptoms of posttraumatic stress disorder: a randomized controlled trial. *Cogn Behav Ther.* (2015) 44:301–13. doi: 10.1080/16506073.2014.916745

Goldstein LA, Mehling WE, Metzler TJ, Cohen BE, Barnes DE, Choucroun GJ, et al. Veterans group exercise: a randomized pilot trial of an integrative exercise program for veterans with post-traumatic stress. *J Affect Disord.* (2018) 227:345–52. doi: 10.1016/j.jad.2017.11.002

LeBouthillier DM, Fetzner MG, Asmundson GJ. Lower cardiorespiratory fitness is associated with greater reduction in PTSD symptoms and anxiety sensitivity following aerobic exercise. *Ment Health Phys Act.* (2016) 10:33–9. doi: 10.1016/j. mhpa.2015.11.001

Manger TA, Motta RW. The impact of an exercise program on posttraumatic stress disorder, anxiety, and depression. *Int J Emerg Ment Health.* (2005) 7:49–57.

Newman CL, Motta RW. The effects of arobic exercise on childhood PTSD, anxiety, and depression. *Int J Emerg Ment Health.* (2007) 9:133–58.

Powers MB, Medina JL, Burns S, Kauffman BY, Monfils M, Asmundson GJ, et al. Exercise augmentation of exposure therapy for PTSD: rationale and pilot efficacy data. *Cogn Behav Ther.* (2015) 44:314–27. doi: 10.1080/16506073.2015.1012740

Rosenbaum S, Vancampfort D, Steel Z, Newby J, Ward PB, Stubbs B. Physical activity in the treatment of post-traumatic stress disorder: a systematic review and meta-analysis. *Psychiatry Res.* (2015) 230:130–6. doi: 10.1016/j. psychres.2015.10.017

Shivakumar G, Anderson EH, Surís AM, North CS. Exercise for PTSD in women veterans: a proof-of-concept study. *Mil Med.* (2017) 182:e1809. doi: 10.7205/ MILMED-D-16-00440

Blake D, Weathers F, Nagy L, Kaloupek D, Charney D, Keane T. *Clinician Administered PTSD Scale (revised).* (1997). Boston, MA: Behavioral Science Division, Boston National Center for Post-Traumatic Stress Disorder.

Saigh P. *Children's PTSD Inventory (DSM-IV Version).* (1998). New York, NY.

Foa EB, Johnson K, Feeny N, Treadwell K. The Child PTSD Symptom Scale (CPSS): preliminary psychometrics of a measure for children with PTSD. *J Clin. Child Psychol.* (2001) 30:376–84. doi: 10.1207/S15374424JCCP 3003_9

Briere, J. (1996). *Trauma Symptom Checklist for Children (TSCC): Professional manual.* Odessa: Psychological Assessment Resources.

Mehling WE, Chesney MA, Metzler TJ, Goldstein LA, Maguen S, Geronimo C, et al. A 12-week integrative exercise program improves self-reported mindfulness and interoceptive awareness in war veterans with posttraumatic stress symptoms J Clinical Psychol. (2017) 74:554–65. doi: 10.1002/jclp.22549

Rosenbaum S, Sherrington C, Tiedemann A. Exercise augmentation compared with usual care for post-traumatic stress disorder: a randomized controlled trial. *Acta Psychiatr Scand.* (2015) 131:350–9. doi: 10.1111/acps.12371

Anderson E, Shivakumar G. Effects of exercise and physical activity on anxiety. *Front Psychiatry.* (2013) 4:27. doi: 10.3389/fpsyt.2013.00027

Broman-Fulks JJ, Storey KM. Evaluation of a brief aerobic exercise intervention for high anxiety sensitivity. *Anxiety Stress Coping.* (2008) 21:117–28. doi: 10.1080/10615800701762675

Ley C, Rato Barrio M, Koch A. "In the Sport I Am Here": therapeutic processes and health effects of sport and exercise on PTSD. *Qual Health Res.* 28:491– 507. doi: 10.1177/1049732317744533

Hayes JP, Labar KS, Petty CM, McCarthy G, Morey RA. Alterations in the neural circuitry for emotion and attention associated with posttraumatic stress symptomatology. *Psychiatry Res.* (2009) 172:7–15. doi: 10.1016/j. pscychresns.2008.05.005

Pineles SL, Shipherd JC, Mostoufi SM, Abramovitz SM, Yovel Attentional biases in PTSD: more evidence for interference. *Behav Res Ther.* (2009) 47:1050–7. doi: 10.1016/j.brat.2009. 08.001

Pineles SL, Shipherd JC, Welch LP, Yovel I. The role of attentional biases in PTSD: is it interference or facilitation? *Behav Res Ther.* (2007) 45:1903–13. doi: 10.1016/j.brat.2006.08.021

Aupperle RL, Melrose AJ, Stein MB, Paulus MP. Executive function and PTSD: disengaging from trauma. *Neuropharmacology.* (2012) 62:686–94. doi: 10.1016/j.neuropharm.2011.02.008

Block SR, Liberzon I. Attentional processes in posttraumatic stress disorder and the associated changes in neural functioning. *Exp Neurol.* (2016) 284:153–67. doi: 10.1016/j.expneurol.2016.05.009

Weierich MR, Treat TA, Hollingworth A. Theories and measurement of visual attentional processing in anxiety. *Cogn Emot.* (2008) 22:985–1018. doi: 10.1080/02699930701597601

Colcombe S, Kramer AF. Fitness effects on the cognitive function of older adults: a meta-analytic study. *Psychol Sci.* (2003) 14:125–30. doi: 10.1111/1467-9280. t01-1-01430

Guiney H, Machado L. Benefits of regular aerobic exercise for executive functioning in healthy populations. *Psychon Bull Rev.* (2013) 20:73–86. doi: 10.3758/s13423-012-0345-4

Cox EP, O'Dwyer N, Cook R, Vetter M, Cheng HL, Rooney K, et al. Relationship between physical activity and cognitive function in apparently healthy young to middle-aged adults: a systematic review. *J Sci Med Sport.* (2016) 19:616–28. doi: 10.1016/j.jsams.2015.09.003

Hayes SM, Alosco ML, Hayes JP, Cadden M, Peterson KM, Allsup K, et al. Physical activity is positively associated with episodic memory in aging. *J Int Neuropsychol Soc.* (2015) 21:780–90. doi: 10.1017/S1355617715000910

Hayes SM, Forman DE, Verfaellie M. Cardiorespiratory fitness is associated with cognitive performance in older but not younger adults. *J Gerontol B Psychol Sci Soc Sci.* (2016) 71:474–82. doi: 10.1093/geronb/gbu167

Smith PJ, Blumenthal JA, Hoffman BM, Cooper H, Strauman TA, Welsh- Bohmer K, et al. Aerobic exercise and neurocognitive performance: a meta- analytic review of randomized controlled trials. *Psychosom Med.* (2010) 72:239–52. doi: 10.1097/PSY.0b013e3181d14633

Hayes JP, Hayes S, Miller DR, Lafleche G, Logue MW, Verfaellie M. Automated measurement of hippocampal subfields in PTSD: evidence for smaller dentate gyrus volume. *J Psychiatr Res.* (2017) 95:247–52. doi: 10.1016/j.jpsychires.2017.09.007

Logue MW, van Rooij SJ, Dennis EL, Davis SL, Hayes JP, Stevens JS, et al. Smaller hippocampal volume in posttraumatic stress disorder: a multisite ENIGMA-PGC study: subcortical volumetry results from posttraumatic stress disorder consortia. *Biol Psychiatry.* (2018) 83:244–53. doi: 10.1016/j.biopsych.2017.09.006

O'Doherty DC, Chitty KM, Saddiqui S, Bennett MR, Lagopoulos J. A systematic review and meta-analysis of magnetic resonance imaging measurement of structural volumes in posttraumatic stress disorder. *Psychiatry Res.* (2015) 232:1–33. doi: 10.1016/j.pscychresns.2015.01.002

Karl A, Schaefer M, Malta LS, Dorfel D, Rohleder N, Werner A. A meta- analysis of structural brain abnormalities in PTSD. *Neurosci Biobehav Rev.* (2006) 30:1004–31. doi: 10.1016/j.neubiorev.2006.03.004

Shin LM, Rauch SL, Pitman RK. Amygdala, medial prefrontal cortex, and hippocampal function in PTSD. *Ann N Y Acad Sci.* (2006) 1071:67–79. doi: 10.1196/annals.1364.007

Daniels JK, Lamke JP, Gaebler M, Walter H, Scheel M. White matter integrity and its relationship to PTSD and childhood trauma—a systematic review and meta-analysis. *Depress Anxiety.* (2013) 30:207–16. doi: 10.1002/da.22044

Schmahmann JD, Pandya DN. Cerebral white matter–historical evolution of facts and notions concerning the organization of the fiber pathways of the brain. *J Hist Neurosci.* (2007) 16:237–67. doi: 10.1080/09647040500495896

Sripada RK, King AP, Garfinkel SN, Wang X, Sripada CS, Welsh RC, et al. Altered resting-state amygdala functional connectivity in men with posttraumatic stress disorder. *J Psychiatry Neurosci.* (2012) 37:241–9. doi: 10.1503/jpn.110069

Sripada RK, King AP, Welsh RC, Garfinkel SN, Wang X, Sripada CS, et al. Neural dysregulation in posttraumatic stress disorder: evidence for disrupted equilibrium between salience and default mode brain networks. *Psychosom Med.* (2012) 74:904–11. doi: 10.1097/PSY.0b013e318273bf33

Hayes SM, Hayes JP, Cadden M, Verfaellie M. A review of cardiorespiratory fitness-related neuroplasticity in the aging brain. *Front Aging Neurosci.* (2013) 5:31. doi: 10.3389/fnagi.2013.00031

Colcombe SJ, Erickson KI, Scalf PE, Kim JS, Prakash R, McAuley E, et al. Aerobic exercise training increases brain volume in aging humans. *J Gerontol A Biol Sci Med Sci.* (2006) 61:1166–70. doi: 10.1093/gerona/61.11.1166

Ruscheweyh R, Willemer C, Kruger K, Duning T, Warnecke T, Sommer J, et al. Physical activity and memory functions: an interventional study. *Neurobiol Aging.* (2011) 32:1304–19. doi: 10.1016/j.neurobiolaging.2009.08.001

Erickson KI, Voss MW, Prakash RS, Basak C, Szabo A, Chaddock L, et al. Exercise training increases size of hippocampus and improves memory. *Proc Natl Acad Sci USA.* (2011) 108:3017–22. doi: 10.1073/pnas.1015950108

Firth J, Stubbs B, Vancampfort D, Schuch F, Lagopoulos J, Rosenbaum S, et al. Effect of aerobic exercise on hippocampal volume in humans: a systematic review and meta-analysis. *Neuroimage.* (2018) 166:230–8. doi: 10.1016/j.neuroimage.2017.11.007

Pereira AC, Huddleston DE, Brickman AM, Sosunov AA, Hen R, McKhann GM, et al. An *in vivo* correlate of exercise-induced neurogenesis in the adult dentate gyrus. *Proc Natl Acad Sci USA.* (2007) 104:5638–43. doi: 10.1073/pnas.0611721104

Burzynska AZ, Chaddock-Heyman L, Voss MW, Wong CN, Gothe NP, Olson EA, et al. Physical activity and cardiorespiratory fitness are beneficial for white matter in low-fit older adults. *PLoS ONE.* (2014) 9:e107413. doi: 10.1371/journal.pone.0107413

Burzynska AZ, Jiao Y, Knecht AM, Fanning J, Awick EA, Chen T, et al. White matter integrity declined over 6-months, but dance intervention improved integrity of the fornix of older adults. *Front Aging Neurosci.* (2017) 9:59. doi: 10.3389/fnagi.2017.00059

Hayes SM, Salat DH, Forman DE, Sperling RA, Verfaellie M. Cardiorespiratory fitness is associated with white matter integrity in aging. *Ann Clin Transl Neurol.* (2015) 2:688–98. doi: 10.1002/acn3.204

Voss MW, Heo S, Prakash RS, Erickson KI, Alves H, Chaddock L, et al. The influence of aerobic fitness on cerebral white matter integrity and cognitive function in older adults: results of a one-year exercise intervention. *Hum Brain Mapp.* (2012) 34:2972–85. doi: 10.1002/hbm.22119

Hayes SM, Hayes JP, Williams VJ, Liu H, Verfaellie M. FMRI activity during associative encoding is correlated with cardiorespiratory fitness and source memory performance in older adults. *Cortex.* (2017) 91:208–20. doi: 10.1016/j.cortex.2017.01.002

Prakash RS, Voss MW, Erickson KI, Lewis J, Chaddock L, Malkowski E, et al. Cardiorespiratory fitness and attentional control in the aging brain. *Front Human Neurosci.* (2011) 5:12. doi: 10.3389/fnhum.2010.00229

Wong CN, Chaddock-Heyman L, Voss MW, Burzynska AZ, Basak C, Erickson KI, et al. Brain activation during dual-task processing is associated with cardiorespiratory fitness and performance in older adults. *Front Aging Neurosci.* (2015) 7:154. doi: 10.3389/fnagi.2015.00154

Smith JC, Nielson KA, Antuono P, Lyons JA, Hanson RJ, Butts AM, et al. Semantic memory functional MRI and cognitive function after exercise intervention in mild cognitive impairment. *J Alzheimers Dis.* (2013) 37:197– 215. doi: 10.3233/JAD-130467

Voss MW, Prakash RS, Erickson KI, Basak C, Chaddock L, Kim JS, et al. Plasticity of brain networks in a randomized intervention trial of exercise training in older adults. *Front Aging Neurosci.* (2010) 2:32. doi: 10.3389/fnagi.2010.00032

Daskalakis NP, McGill MA, Lehrner A, Yehuda R. Endocrine aspects of PTSD: Hypothalamic-Pituitary-Adrenal (HPA) axis and beyond. *Compr Guide Post-Traum Stress Disord.*(2016) 245–60. doi: 10.1007/978-3-319-08359-9_130

De Kloet C, Vermetten E, Geuze E, Kavelaars A, Heijnen C, Westenberg H. Assessment of HPA-axis function in posttraumatic stress disorder: pharmacological and non-pharmacological challenge tests, a review. *J Psychiatr Res.* (2006) 40:550–67. doi: 10.1016/j.jpsychires.2005.08.002

Childs E, de Wit H. Regular exercise is associated with emotional resilience to acute stress in healthy adults. *Front Physiol.* (2014) 5:161. doi: 10.3389/fphys.2014.00161

Olff M, de Vries G-J, Güzelcan Y, Assies J, Gersons BP. Changes in cortisol and DHEA plasma levels after psychotherapy for PTSD. *Psychoneuroendocrinology.* (2007) 32:619–26. doi: 10.1016/j.psyneuen.2007.04.001

Galbo H. The hormonal response to exercise. *Diabetes Metab Res.* (1986) 1:385–408. doi: 10.1002/dmr.5610010404

Chatzinikolaou A, Fatouros IG, Gourgoulis V, Avloniti A, Jamurtas AZ, Nikolaidis MG, et al. Time course of changes in performance and inflammatory responses after acute plyometric exercise. *J Strength Cond Res.* (2010) 24:1389–98. doi: 10.1519/JSC.0b013e3181d1d318

Hill E, Zack E, Battaglini C, Viru M, Viru A, Hackney A. Exercise and circulating cortisol levels: the intensity threshold effect. *J Endocrinol Invest.* (2008) 31:587–91. doi: 10.1007/BF03345606

Nabkasorn C, Miyai N, Sootmongkol A, Junprasert S, Yamamoto H, Arita M, et al. Effects of physical exercise on depression, neuroendocrine stress hormones and physiological fitness in adolescent females with depressive symptoms. *Eur J Public Health.* (2006) 16:179–84. doi: 10.1093/eurpub/cki159

Stranahan AM, Lee K, Mattson MP. Central mechanisms of HPA axis regulation by voluntary exercise. *Neuromolecular Med.* (2008) 10:118–27. doi: 10.1007/s12017-008-8027-0

Wunsch K, Wurst R, Kasten N, von Dawans B, Strahler J, Fuchs R. The influence of habitual and acute exercise on SNS and HPA axis responses to psychosocial stress–a randomized, controlled trial. *Psychoneuroendocrinology.* (2017) 83:77. doi: 10.1016/j.psyneuen.2017.07.445

Zschucke E, Renneberg B, Dimeo F, Wüstenberg T, Ströhle A. The stress-buffering effect of acute exercise: evidence for HPA axis negative feedback. *Psychoneuroendocrinology.* (2015) 51:414–25. doi: 10.1016/j.psyneuen.2014.10.019

Michopoulos V, Powers A, Gillespie CF, Ressler KJ, Jovanovic T. Inflammation in fear-and anxiety-based disorders: PTSD, GAD, and beyond. *Neuropsychopharmacology.* (2016) 42:254. doi: 10.1038/npp.2016.146

Passos IC, Vasconcelos-Moreno MP, Costa LG, Kunz M, Brietzke E, Quevedo J, et al. Inflammatory markers in post-traumatic stress disorder: a systematic review, meta-analysis, and meta-regression. *Lancet Psychiatry.* (2015) 2:1002–12. doi: 10.1016/S2215-0366(15)00309-0

Altemus M, Dhabhar FS, Yang R. Immune function in PTSD. *Ann N Y Acad Sci.* (2006) 1071:167–83. doi: 10.1196/annals.1364.013

Groer MW, Kane B, Williams SN, Duffy A. Relationship of PTSD symptoms with combat exposure, stress, and inflammation in american soldiers. *Biol Res Nurs.* (2015) 17:303–10. doi: 10.1177/1099800414544949

Plantinga L, Bremner JD, Miller AH, Jones DP, Veledar E, Goldberg J, et al. Association between posttraumatic stress disorder and inflammation: a twin study. *Brain Behav Immun.* (2013) 30:125–32. doi: 10.1016/j.bbi.2013. 01.081

Archer T, Fredriksson A, Schütz E, Kostrzewa RM. Influence of physical exercise on neuroimmunological functioning and health: aging and stress. *Neurotox Res.* (2011) 20:69–83. doi: 10.1007/s12640-010-9224-9

Gleeson M, Bishop NC, Stensel DJ, Lindley MR, Mastana SS, Nimmo MA. The anti-inflammatory effects of exercise: mechanisms and implications for the prevention and treatment of disease. *Nat Rev Immunol.* (2011) 11:607–15. doi: 10.1038/nri3041

Kasapis C, Thompson PD. The effects of physical activity on serum C- reactive protein and inflammatory markers: a systematic review. *J Am Coll Cardiol.* (2005) 45:1563–9. doi: 10.1016/j.jacc.2004.12.077

Walsh NP, Gleeson M, Shephard RJ, Gleeson M, Woods JA, Bishop N, et al. Position statement part one: immune function and exercise. *Exerc Immunol Rev.* (2011) 17:6–63.

Santos R, Tufik S, De Mello M. Exercise, sleep and cytokines: is there a relation? *Sleep Med Rev.* (2007) 11:231–9. doi: 10.1016/j.smrv.2007.03.003

Krueger JM, Obál F, Fang J, Kubota T, Taishi P. The role of cytokines in physiological sleep regulation. *Ann N Y Acad Sci.* (2001) 933:211–21. doi: 10.1111/j.1749-6632.2001.tb05826.x

Rockstrom MD, Chen L, Taishi P, Nguyen JT, Gibbons CM, Veasey SC, et al. Tumor necrosis factor alpha in sleep regulation. *Sleep Med Rev.* (2017) 30:1e10.

3

Effects of Acute and Chronic Exercises on Executive Function in Children and Adolescents: A Systemic Review and Meta-Analysis

Shijie Liu [1], Qian Yu [2], Zaimin Li [3], Paolo Marcello Cunha [4], Yanjie Zhang [5], Zhaowei Kong [6], Wang Lin [7], Sitong Chen [1] and Yujun Cai [1]*

[1] School of Physical Education and Sport Training, Shanghai University of Sport, Shanghai, China, [2] Exercise and Mental Health Laboratory, School of Psychology, Shenzhen University, Shenzhen, China, [3] School of Wushu, Chengdu Sport University, Chengdu, China, [4] Metabolism, Nutrition, and Exercise Laboratory, Londrina State University, Londrina, Brazil, [5] Health and Exercise Science Laboratory, Institute of Sports Science, Seoul National University, Seoul, South Korea, [6] Faculty of Education, University of Macao, Macao, China, [7] Department of Physical Education, Wuhan University of Technology, Wuhan, China

***Correspondence:**
Yujun Cai
caiyujun@sus.edu.cn

Background: Physical exercises can affect executive function both acutely and chronically, with different mechanisms for each moment. Currently, only a few reviews have elaborated on the premise that different types of exercises have different mechanisms for improving executive function. Therefore, the primary purpose of our systematic review was to analyze the effects of acute and chronic exercises on executive function in children and adolescents.

Objective: We identified acute and chronic exercise studies and randomized controlled trials (RCTs) of executive function in children and adolescents that reported overall effect, heterogeneity, and publication bias of acute and chronic exercises on executive function.

Methods: We searched for RCTs of exercise interventions in children and adolescents from databases including PubMed, Web of Science, Scopus, The Cochrane Library, CNKI (China National Knowledge Infrastructure), and Wanfang, from January 1 2009 to December 31 2019. We performed methodological quality evaluations on the included literature using the Physiotherapy Evidence Database Scale (PEDro) and graded evidence with a meta-analysis using Stata 12.0 software.

Results: In total, 36 RCTs were included (14 acute exercises, 22 chronic exercises); the overall results of the meta-analysis (4,577 students) indicated that acute exercises significantly improved working memory (standardized mean difference (SMD) = −0.72; 95% confidence interval (CI) −0.89 to −0.56; $p < 0.001$), inhibitory control (SMD = −0.25; 95% CI −0.40 to −0.09; $p = 0.002$), and cognitive flexibility (SMD = −0.34; 95% CI −0.55 to −0.14; $p < 0.005$), whereas chronic exercises significantly improved working memory (SMD = −0.54; 95% CI −0.74 to −0.33; $p < 0.001$), inhibitory control (SMD = −0.30; 95% CI −0.38 to −0.22; $p < 0.001$), and cognitive flexibility (SMD = −0.34, 95 % CI −0.48 to −0.20, $p < 0.001$).

Conclusion: Acute and chronic exercises can effectively improve the executive function of children and adolescents. The effects on inhibitory control and cognitive flexibility are considered as small effect sizes, while the effects on working memory are considered as moderate effect size. Limited by the quantity and quality of the included studies, the above conclusions need to be verified with more high-quality studies.

Keywords: executive function, acute exercise, chronic exercise, cognitive, adolescents

INTRODUCTION

A sedentary lifestyle and physical inactivity (insufficient exercises time) are prevalent among children and adolescents (Sisson et al., 2009; Qi et al., 2019) and are negatively linked with their physical and psycho-cognitive health (Tremblay et al., 2011; Flashner et al., 2019). Specifically, these unhealthy lifestyle behaviors result in obesity (Rey-Lopez, 2008), uncoordinated movements (Ferguson et al., 2014; Flashner et al., 2019; Kong et al., 2019; Riquelme et al., 2019), negative emotions (depression, anxiety, suicide attempts) (Berardelli et al., 2018; Thivel et al., 2018; Padulo et al., 2019) and a severe deficit of cognitive functions (Torrens-Burton et al., 2017; Koolhaas et al., 2019; Loprinzi et al., 2019). Among the components of cognitive functioning, inhibitory control, working memory, and cognitive flexibility play a critical role in the development of school-age children and their educational achievement or academic performance (Best, 2010; Willoughby et al., 2012).

Diamond proposed a three-factor model of executive functions and stated that inhibitory control, working memory, and cognitive flexibility are the three core executive functions (EF); the three aforementioned cognitive abilities work together to influence higher-order executive functions such as reasoning, planning, and problem solving (Diamond, 2013). However, there is little longitudinal experimental evidence in the field of sports and health promotion to prove that physical activity is relevant to high-level executive functions such as decision-making and reasoning in children and adolescents. In contrast, the more such evidence appears in the context of techniques and tactics in high-level athletes (Taddei et al., 2012; Bjoern et al., 2018; Beavan et al., 2020). Therefore, this review only considers the three main executive functions of inhibitory control, working memory, and cognitive flexibility. Firstly, inhibitory control (self-control) refers to the ability to suppress irrelevant reactions, allowing children to control automatic or impulsive behaviors while performing minimal automatic reactions (Pindus et al., 2019); secondly, working memory (refreshing tasks) allows children to register information in the brain and then to perform cognitive operations on it (Keita et al., 2011); thirdly, cognitive flexibility (tasks of conversion) refers to the ability of a child to move flexibly to a new situation or another state Masley et al., 2009). When EF are impaired, children generally show abnormalities in social functions, emotions, and cognition Goodall et al., 2018; Wang et al., 2019), often accompanied by learning difficulties, conduct disorders, and maladaptive phenomena (Rocha et al., 2019). Thus, such cognitive abilities in the growth and development stage are undoubtedly crucial for children and adolescents.

Emerging evidence indicates that physical activity and exercise can influence executive functions such as inhibitory control, working memory and cognitive flexibility both acutely and chronically (Rathore and Lom, 2017; De Greeff et al., 2018; Vazou et al., 2019). Furthermore, chronic exercises as a part of healthy lifestyle behaviors are widely recognized to be associated with improved EF across different age groups (Hillman et al., 2011; Li et al., 2017), while the expanding topic on acute exercises (referring to a single bout of exercises taking 10–60 min) indicates their potential to improve these cognitive outcomes (Byun et al., 2014). However, to date, very few reviews have systematically and simultaneously evaluated the effects of both exercise types on the three key EF components in children and adolescents; the reviews on this topic either focused on healthy adults and older adults (Ludyga et al., 2016; McSween et al., 2019; Chen et al., 2020) or chronic exercises alone in the same age group (Ludyga et al., 2016; Xue et al., 2019), or presented unclear information on a selected outcome (reaction time, accuracy, or derived scores) (Li et al., 2017; De Greeff et al., 2018; Sember et al., 2020). Meanwhile, previous studies have shown that physical activity is more sensitive to reaction time than the three key cognitive components (Ellemberg and St-Louis-Deschênes, 2010; Zhu, 2015). Against this background, the primary purpose of this review was to comprehensively analyze the effects of acute and chronic exercises on the EF of children and adolescents and to further explore the effects of acute and chronic exercises on the three different tasks of inhibitory control, working memory, and cognitive flexibility. In response to these differences in the literature, this review highlighted the relationship between exercises and EF, regulated by factors such as exercise type, exercise intensity, exercise duration, individual factors, and subcomponents of executive function.

METHOD

Our research follows the requirements of the international meta-analysis writing guidelines (the PRISMA statement for reporting systematic reviews and meta-analyses of studies that evaluate health-care interventions: explanation and elaboration) for selecting and utilizing research methods (Shamseer et al., 2015).

Retrieval Strategy

The databases PubMed, Web of Science, Scopus, The Cochrane Library, China National Knowledge Infrastructure (CNKI), and

Wan Fang were searched from January 1 2009 to December 31 2019. Two reviewers independently searched articles published in Chinese and English, supplemented by a manual search, and retrospectively included references if necessary. The following two sets of search terms were used: "physical activity" or "exercises" or "physical fitness" or "physical endurance" or "motor activity" or "physical education" or "sport" or "basketball" or "football" or "running" or "cycling" or "jumping" or "dancing" or "tai chi" or "yoga" or "aerobic" and "executive function" or "inhibition" or "inhibiting ability" or "self-control" or "working memory" or "updating" or "refreshing" or "cognitive flexibility" or "task-switching" or "shifting" and "child" or "student" or "toddler" or "preschooler" or "adolescents." If an article was incomplete or unavailable, we contacted the corresponding author by email to obtain detailed information. For literature tracing, based on the retrieved literatures or related references listed in the review, we used Baidu Scholar and Google Scholar to search for them retrospectively.

Inclusion Criteria and Exclusion Criteria

Two reviewers independently screened the articles. When there was a disagreement between the two reviewers, a third reviewer evaluated the original study to reach a consensus. Any potentially relevant research needed to meet the following inclusion criteria: (1) children and adolescent participants aged 5–18 years with right-hand dominance, corrected or normal vision and a healthy body were deemed eligible; (2) the exercise group was the primary intervention measure (e.g., aerobic-based, motor skill-based, combining aerobic, muscular activity, yoga, basketball), compared with different types of control groups (i.e., no-intervention control group, waiting list, and routine care) and all the intervention measures were motor skill-based or aerobic-based and clearly defined in terms of the exercise protocol; (3) preliminary studies were randomized controlled trials, and the randomization was done either on an individual or on a group (e.g., classroom) basis; (4) outcome indicators included test data on executive function (working memory, inhibition and cognitive flexibility), with a minimum of one outcome with quantitative data for calculating the pooled effect size. Conditions for exclusion from the study included: (1) ambiguous explanations of exercises interventions; (2) irrelevant outcomes; and (3) studies for which the full text could not be obtained.

Data Extraction

Two reviewers independently extracted data according to a predefined protocol. If there were any differences or inconsistencies, they would discuss the study with a third reviewer. They gathered the following information: (1) literature information, including author name, year of publication and country; (2) sample size (male sample); (3) socioeconomic status; (4) age of subjects, mainly used to divide the type of population; (5) intensity of exercise intervention, duration of intervention, time of intervention, frequency of intervention; (6) intervention program; (7) measurements, mainly including the three dimensions of working memory, inhibition and cognitive flexibility; and (8) adverse events and follow-up.

The Methodological Quality of the Included Studies

Similar to previous studies (Zou et al., 2018, 2019), the Physiotherapy Evidence Database Scale (PEDro) was used to assess the risk of bias (Macedo et al., 2010). The assessment tool includes 10 items, as follows: eligibility criteria, randomization, concealed allocation, similar baseline, assessor blindness, subject blindness, point estimation, comparison between groups, a retention rate of 85% or above and completeness of measurement results. Notably, the use of a blinded instructor was unrealistic during exercise interventions, and so this item was not considered. A higher total score (0–10 points) represents a better methodological quality, where a PEDro score ≥ 6 is categorized as the high-quality group while a PEDro score <6 is categorized into the low-quality group (Maher et al., 2003). The methodological quality of the included studies was independently assessed by two panelists using PEDro, and any differences were resolved by a third reviewer.

Statistical Analysis

Stata 12.0 (Stata Corp, College Station, TX) was used as data processing software (Press, 2009). We used the standardized mean difference (SMD) with a 95% confidence interval (CI) to analyze the combined effect size. According to the Cochrane systematic review manual, if a study included more than one control group, the sample size of the exercise intervention should be equally assigned during pair comparison in order to avoid analysis unit errors (Handoll et al., 2002). If statistical heterogeneity was found across studies ($I^2 \geq 50\%$, $p < 0.10$), we applied the random-effects model—otherwise, the fixed-effect model was applied—and we used the Hedges' g method to reflect the magnitude of exercise intervention (Liu et al., 2019). According to the criteria for evaluating effect volumes, a small effect was between ≥ 0.2 and <0.5, a medium effect was between ≥ 0.5 and <0.8, and a large effect was ≥ 0.8 (Hanley et al., 2003). The heterogeneity of the included studies was determined with the p-value (threshold point of 0.1) and I^2 statistics (25, 50, and 75%, representing small, medium, and large heterogeneity, respectively) (Liu et al., 2019).

Given that overall effect sizes may be influenced by heterogeneity factors (age, study quality, motor skill type, composite type, intervention duration, intervention frequency, and intervention time), several regression analyses were separately performed. Additionally, subgroup analyses were also performed for age, study quality, motor-skill type, composite type, and intervention duration, frequency, and time: (1) prepubertal children (5–12 years) vs. adolescents (12–18 years) (Cardoso, 2007); (2) PEDro scores of >6 points (high-quality studies) vs. PEDro scores of <6 (low-quality studies) (Maher et al., 2003); (3) open-skilled exercises (different types of motor skills that respond to individual requirements in a dynamically changing or unpredictable external environment, where physical education, basketball, and ping-pong belong to open exercises) vs. closed-skill exercises (movements with relatively stable sports environments, such as yoga and running) (Liu et al., 2019); (4) sole-mode training (the use of a single skill) vs. multimodal training (the use of a variety of skills including yoga and running, aerobic exercises); (5) 12 weeks was used as a cutoff for chronic exercise intervention; (6) intervention time referred to the timing of intervention, where a threshold of 30 min for chronic exercise was recommended; and (7) three times a week was used as a threshold for chronic exercise intervention frequency. The selection of these moderators was principally inspired by McMinn and Rathore (Mcminn, 2012; Rathore and Lom, 2017).

Evidence Certainty Assessment

The Grading Recommendations to Assess Development and Evaluation system (GRADE) is an evidence evaluation system and is one of the international standards for evidence quality and the classification of recommendation strength (Zhang et al., 2019). We evaluated the quality of the evidence for each outcome using the GRADE classification with four possible levels: I (high), where the real effect is similar to a credible estimate; II (moderate), where the true effect is closest to the estimated effect; III (low), where the actual effect may be significantly different from the estimated effect; and IV (very low), where the actual effect is likely to be significantly different from the estimated effect. Five factors can cause the quality of the evidence to decrease: (1) risk of bias; (2) imprecision; (3) inconsistency; (4) indirectness; and (5) publication bias.

RESULTS

Literature Search Results

The latest review of electronic searches (as of December 2019) retrieved a total of 455 articles. During the preliminary screening, we excluded 353 studies based on their title and abstract for reasons including duplications ($n = 95$), language ($n = 6$), or not being related to the subject content ($n = 252$). Further screening was performed by reading the full text, and 66 records were excluded because of non-randomized controlled trials ($n = 22$), no reported data for analysis ($n = 21$), review ($n = 3$), no major exercise interventions ($n = 13$), or non-healthy participants ($n = 7$). Finally, the meta-analysis included 36 articles: 14 for acute exercises and 22 for chronic exercises (**Figure 1**).

Eligible Research Features

The 36 articles included were randomized controlled trials (14 acute exercises, 22 chronic exercises), including 4,577 healthy participants (1,308 participants of acute exercises), of which 2,227 were in the experimental group (670 participants of

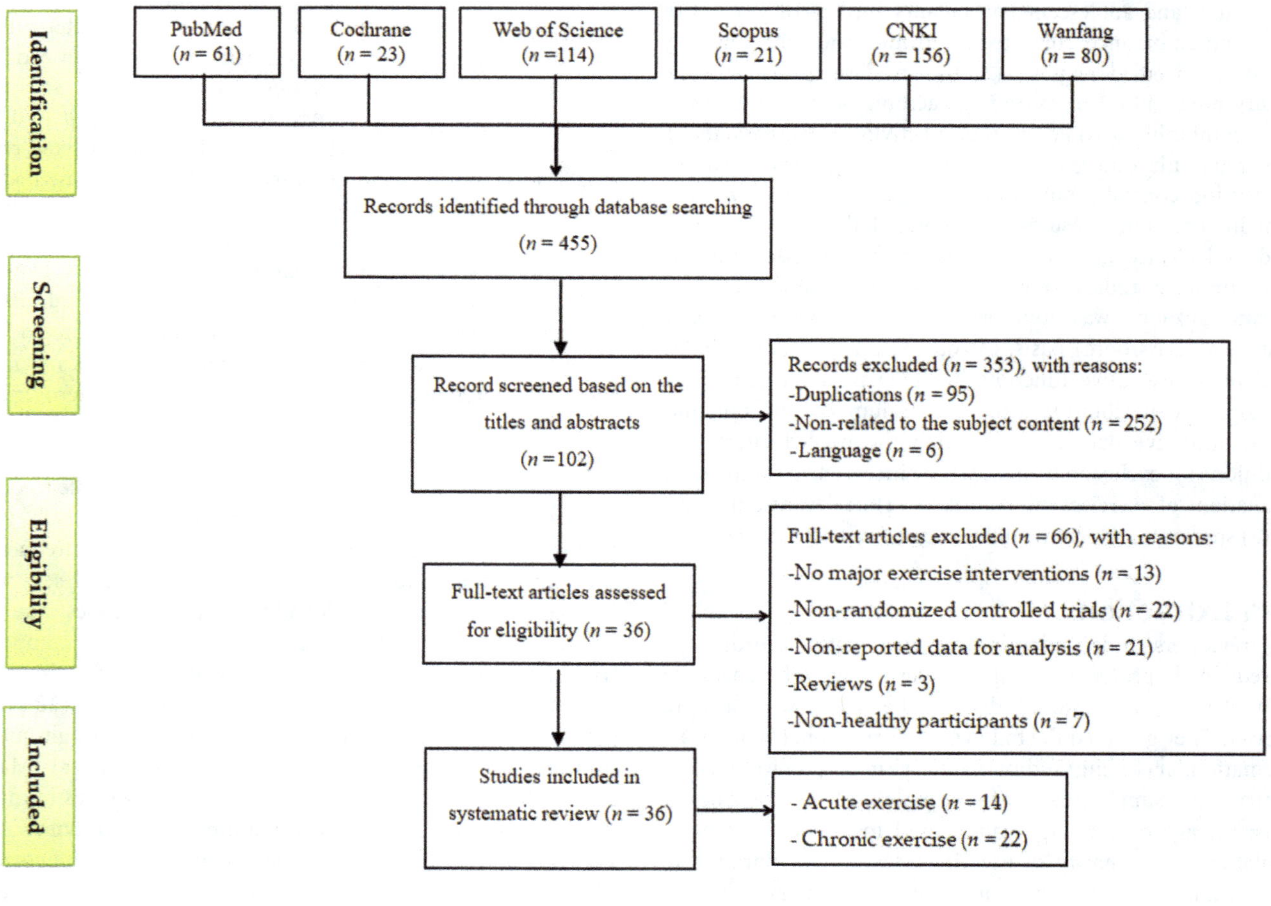

FIGURE 1 | Flow of the study selection method.

acute exercises) and 2,350 were in the control group (635 participants of acute exercises) (**Tables 1, 2**). In acute exercises and chronic exercises, the ages of the included students ranged from 5 to 18 years old, while three of the studied articles did not specify age (Chaddock-Heyman et al., 2013; Weng et al., 2014; Budde et al., 2016). In terms of interventions, 12 studies used acute exercises—short-term, medium-intensity aerobic exercises, such as jogging or power cycling, with an exercise time from 10 to 40 min—and 20 studies used chronic exercise interventions with a duration from 8 to 20 weeks, 2–5 times a week, and with 30–90 min per session. Furthermore, each study consisted of at least one dimension of the outcome indicators of inhibitory control (10 acute exercises, 15 chronic exercises), working memory (nine acute exercises, 13 chronic exercises), and cognitive flexibility (three acute exercises, eight chronic exercises) in three dimensions. In addition, only three articles in the included studies reported follow-up status (Fisher et al., 2011; Telles et al., 2013; Tarp et al., 2016), and no adverse events occurred.

Methodological Quality Evaluation

The methodological quality of the included studies is presented in **Table 3**. The mean scores for acute and chronic exercise types were 7 and 6.77, respectively, indicating a high degree of credibility. All 36 studies were randomized controlled trials, five articles described the method for hiding random allocation (Kubesch et al., 2009; Ellemberg and St-Louis-Deschênes, 2010; Telles et al., 2013; Hillman et al., 2014; Budde et al., 2016), and the rest only mentioned random allocation. Eight studies adopted the blind-reviewer method (Fisher et al., 2011; Telles et al., 2013; Hillman et al., 2014; Chun et al., 2015; Jager et al., 2015; Budde et al., 2016; Chen et al., 2016; Yin et al., 2018), and five articles used the blind-examiner method (Fisher et al., 2011; Telles et al., 2013; Yan et al., 2014; Jager et al., 2015; Chen et al., 2016); the rest were implemented without a blind method. There were 11 articles that did not describe the source of their examination.

META-ANALYSIS RESULTS

Twenty-three studies examined the effect of exercises on inhibitory control (as measured by the Stroop, Go/no-go, or Flanker tasks). The aggregated result showed a significant benefit in favor of acute exercises on the inhibitory control of children and adolescents (SMD = −0.25; 95% CI −0.40 to −0.09, $I^2 = 9.9\%$, $p = 0.002$) (**Figure 2**). The aggregated result showed that chronic exercises can significantly shorten response times (SMD = −0.30; 95% CI −0.38 to −0.22, $I^2 = 64.2\%$, $p < 0.001$) (**Figure 3**). The SMDs of acute and chronic exercises were considered as small ESs.

Twenty-two studies (27 pairwise comparisons) examined the effect of exercises on working memory (as measured by digit span backward, Tower of London, and N-back tasks). A higher negative value of the mean change score for the reaction time

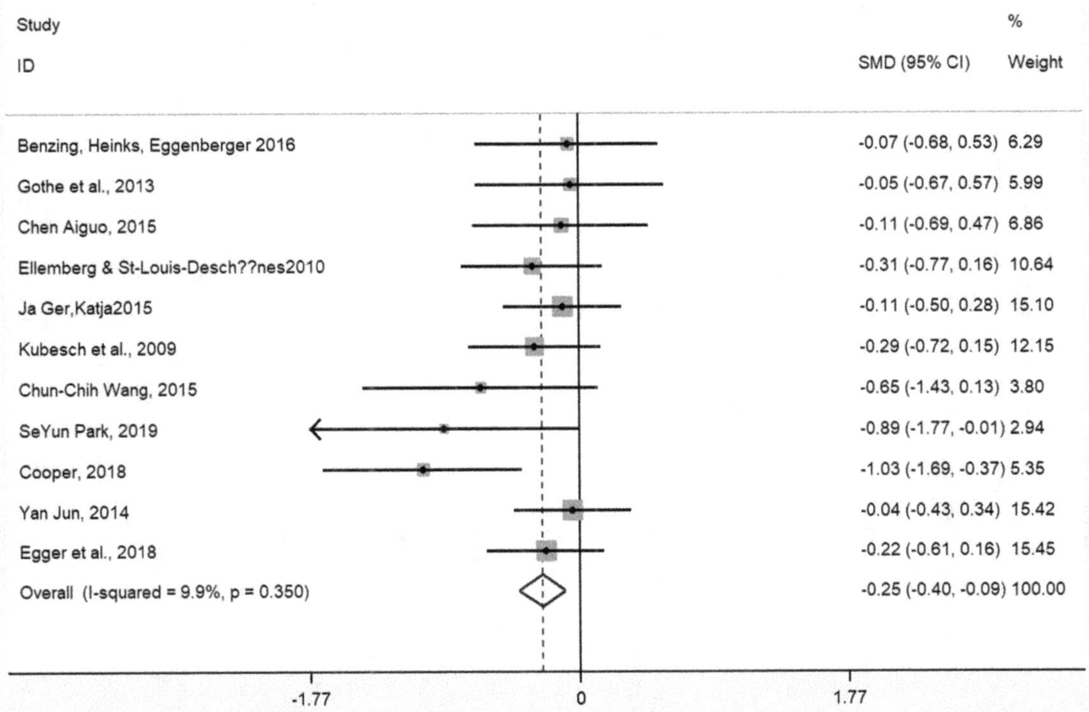

FIGURE 2 | The effect of acute exercises on inhibitory control (SMD = standardized mean difference; CI = confidence interval).

TABLE 1 | Characteristics of the studies included in the meta-analysis (acute exercises).

References	Location (Language)	Participant characteristics			Intervention program	Intervention characteristics		Outcome measured	Adverse event; Follow-up
		N (male)	SES	Mean age or Age range		Time (min)	Motion intensity		
Benzing et al. (2016)	Bern, Switzerland (English)	65 (34)	NR	14.51 ± 1.08	EG: Run + jump + resistance exercises (aerobic-based) CG: Usual care	15	60%–70%	① (Inhibition) ② (Fluency) ③ (Cognitive flexibility)	No No
Pate (2015)	Carolina, USA (English)	96 (37)	NR	10.70 ± 0.60	EG: Better ideas through exercises (aerobic-based) CG: Usual care	10–20	NR	② (Digit Recall)	No No
Gothe et al. (2013)	Urbana, USA (English)	40 (20)	NR	9.50 ± 0.50	EG: Yoga (motor skill-based) CG: Usual care	20	60%–70%	① (Stroop Test)	No No
Chen et al. (2015)	Yangzhou, China (Chinese)	130 (53)	NR	9.40 ± 0.30	EG: Basketball (motor skill-based) CG: Usual care	15–30	65%	① (Flanker task) ② (1-back) ③ (More-odd shifting)	No No
Ellemberg and St-Louis-Deschênes (2010)	Montreal, Canada (English)	72 (38)	NR	7.75 ± 0.65	EG: Basketball (motor skill-based) CG: Usual care	40	63%	① (Flanker task)	No No
Jager et al. (2015)	Bern, Switzerland (English)	219 (112)	6.90 (1.56)	11.35 ± 0.65	EG: Run + bicycle (combining aerobic and muscular activity) CG: Usual care	30	70%	① Wisconsin Card Sorting Test	No No
Kubesch et al. (2009)	Ulm, Germany (English)	81 (NR)	NR	13–14	EG: Run + resistance exercises (aerobic-based) CG: Usual care	30	NR	① (Flanker task) ② (1-back)	No No
Chun et al. (2015)	Taiwan, China (English)	22 (9)	NR	15.42 ± 1.47	EG: Bicycle (aerobic-based) CG: Usual care	30	65%	① Wisconsin Card Sorting Test	No No
Budde et al. (2010)	Berlin, Germany (English)	60 (0)	NR	14.37 ± 0.53	EG: Run (aerobic-based) CG: Usual care	12	50%-85%	② Digit Span task	No No
Yan et al. (2014)	Yangzhou, China (Chinese)	244 (113)	NR	9.50 ± 0.30	EG: Run (aerobic-based) CG: Usual care	30	60%–69%	① (Go/no-go) ② (1-back) ③ (More-odd shifting)	No No
Cooper et al. (2018)	Nottingham, UK (English)	41 (NR)	NR	12.30 ± 0. 71	EG: Basketball (motor skill-based) CG: Usual care	60	60%–70%	① (Stroop test) ② (Sternberg paradigm)	No No
Park and Etnier (2019)	Daejeon, Korea (English)	22 (NR)	NR	15.90 ± 0. 29	EG: Better ideas through exercises (aerobic-based) CG: Usual care	20	60%–70%	① (Stroop Test)	No No
Egger et al. (2018)	Bern, Switzerland (English)	216 (110)	NR	7.94 ± 0. 44	EG: Better ideas through exercises (aerobic-based) CG: Usual care	20	NR	① (Stroop Test)	No No
Vera et al. (2018)	Netherlands, Amsterdam (English)	38 (12)	NR	12.30±0.60	EG: Bicycle (aerobic-based) CG: Usual care	20-30	40%–60%	② (N-back)	No No

NR = not reported; EG = experimental group; CG = control group; SES = socioeconomic status; ① represents inhibitory control; ② represents working memory; ③ represents cognitive flexibility.

TABLE 2 | Characteristics of the studies included in the meta-analysis (chronic exercises).

Reference	Location (language)	Participant characteristics			Intervention program	Intervention characteristics			Outcome measured	Adverse event; follow-up
		N (male)	SES	Mean age or age range		Time (min)	Frequency (weekly)	Duration (week)		
Chen et al. (2016)	Yangzhou, China (Chinese)	40 (20)	NR	11.36 ± 0.57	EG: Aerobic dance CG: Usual care	40	3	8	① (Flanker task) ② (1-back) ③ (More-odd shifting)	No No
De Greeff et al. (2016)	Groninge, Netherlands (English)	499 (216)	NR	8.20 ± 0.70	EG: Aerobic exercises CG: Usual care	20–30	3	22	① Wisconsin Card Sorting Test	No No
Kval et al. (2017)	Stavanger, Norway (English)	429 (NR)	NR	10–11	EG: Jump rope + running + strength training (combining aerobic and muscular activity) CG: Usual care	45	2	10	① (Stroop Test)	No No
Jiang (2015)	Beijing, China (Chinese)	61 (25)	NR	5.56 ± 0.35	EG: Football (motor skill-based) CG: Usual care	35	2	8	① (Flexible-Item Selection)	No No
Xin (2012)	Shandong, China (Chinese)	40 (20)	NR	9.10 ± 0.32	EG: Tennis (motor skill-based) CG: Usual care	40	5	16	① (Flanker task); ② (1-back) ③ (More-odd shifting)	No No
Budde et al. (2016)	Hamburg, Germany (English)	71 (32)	NR	9.35± 0.60	EG: Run + jump + resistance exercises (aerobic-based) CG: Usual care	45	3	10	② (Letter Digit Span)	No No
Purohit and Pradhan (2016)	Bengaluru, India (English)	72 (30)	NR	12.69 ± 1.35	EG: Yoga (motor skill-based) CG: Usual care	90	4	12	① (Stroop Test) ③ (More-odd shifting)	No No
Wang (2017)	Beijing, China (Chinese)	30 (14)	NR	5–6	EG: Tennis (motor skill-based) CG: Usual care	60	2	8	① (Flanker task) ② (1-back)	No No
Yin et al. (2018)	Beijing, China (Chinese)	326 (165)	NR	7–9	EG: Run (aerobic-based) EG: Taijiquan (aerobic-based) CG: Usual care	30	3–5	20	① (Flanker task) ② (1-back) ③ (More-odd shifting)	No No
Chaddock-Heyman et al. (2013)	Urbana, USA (English)	26 (11)	2.32 (1.09)	NR	EG: Bicycle (aerobic-based) CG: Usual care	76.8	5	22	② (1-back) ③ (More-odd shifting)	No No
Stroth et al. (2009)	Ulm, Germany (English)	35 (NR)	NR	14.20 ± 0.50	EG: Aerobic exercises CG: Usual care	40	3	12	② (1-back)	No No
Lina (2017)	Yangzhou, China (Chinese)	17 (9)	NR	11.37 ± 1.53	EG: Run (aerobic-based) CG: Usual care	30	4	11	② (0-back)	No No
Yan Jun and Chen (2013)	Yangzhou, China (Chinese)	87 (42)	NR	9.50 ± 0.30	EG: Aerobic dance CG: Usual care	30	3	12	① (Flanker task) ② (1-back) ③ (More-odd shifting)	No No
Keita et al. (2011)	Illinois, USA (English)	36 (19)	NR	7–9	EG: Medicine balls + resistance exercises (combining aerobic and muscular activity) CG: Usual care	70	5	24	② (Reaction time)	No No

(Continued)

TABLE 2 | Continued

Reference	Location (language)	Participant characteristics			Intervention program	Intervention characteristics			Outcome measured	Adverse event; follow-up
		N (male)	SES	Mean age or age range		Time (min)	Frequency (weekly)	Duration (week)		
Hillman et al. (2014)	Illinois, USA (English)	221 (NR)	NR	8–9	EG: Yoga + run (aerobic-based) CG: Usual care	70	5	24	① (Flanker task) ③ (Cognitive flexibility)	No No
Telles et al. (2013)	Uttarakhand, India (English)	98 (60)	NR	10.50 ± 1.30	EG: Yoga (aerobic-based) CG: Usual care	45	5	12	① (Stroop Test)	No Yes
Fisher et al. (2011)	Glasgow, UK (English)	64 (29)	7(1)	6.10± 0.30	EG: Run (aerobic-based) CG: Usual care	120		10	② (Reaction time)	No Yes
Tarp et al. (2016)	Rotterdam, Netherlands (English)	698 (309)	NR	12.90± 0.60	EG: Whole-body movement games CG: Usual care	60	4	12	② (Reaction time)	No Yes
Ludyga et al. (2017)	Basel, Switzerland (English)	36 (18)	NR	12-15	EG: Medicine balls + relay games (combining aerobic and coordinative exercises)	5-10	5	8	① (Stroop Test)	No Yes
Nie (2019)	Nanjing, China (Chinese)	40 (19)	NR	13.81± 0.30	EG: Wuqinxi (aerobic-based) CG: Usual care	45	3	8	① (Flanker task) ② (1-back) ③ (More-odd shifting)	No Yes
Egger et al. (2019)	Bern, Switzerland (English)	142 (70)	NR	7.91± 0.40	EG: Better ideas through exercises (aerobic-based) CG: Usual care	20	5	20	① (Flanker task)	No No
Vera et al. (2019)	Netherlands, Amsterdam (English)	201 (108)	NR	10.90± 0.70	EG: Dance (aerobic-based) CG: Usual care	10	5	9	① (Stroop Test)	No No

NR = not reported; EG = experimental group; CG = control group; SES = socioeconomic status; ① represents inhibitory control; ② represents working memory; ③ represents cognitive flexibility.

TABLE 3 | Physiotherapy Evidence Database Scale (PEDro) of the included randomized controlled trials (acute exercises and chronic exercises).

Author [Reference]	Item 1	Item 2	Item 3	Item 4	Item 5	Item 6	Item 7	Item 8	Item 9	Item 10	Score
Benzing et al. (2016)	1	1	0	1	0	0	1	1	1	1	7
Pate (2015)	1	1	0	0	0	0	1	1	1	1	6
Gothe et al. (2013)	1	1	0	0	0	0	1	1	1	1	6
Chen et al. (2015)	1	1	0	1	0	0	1	1	1	1	7
Ellemberg and St-Louis-Deschênes (2010)	0	1	1	1	0	0	1	1	1	1	7
Jager et al. (2015)	1	1	0	0	1	1	1	1	1	1	8
Kubesch et al. (2009)	1	1	1	1	0	0	1	1	1	1	8
Chun et al. (2015)	1	1	0	1	1	0	1	1	1	1	8
Budde et al. (2010)	1	1	0	1	0	0	1	1	1	1	6
Yan et al. (2014)	0	1	0	1	0	1	1	1	1	1	7
Cooper et al. (2018)	1	1	0	1	0	0	1	1	1	1	7
Park and Etnier (2019)	1	1	0	1	0	0	1	1	1	1	7
Egger et al. (2018)	1	1	0	1	0	0	1	1	1	1	7
Vera et al. (2018)											
Vera et al. (2018)	1	1	0	1	0	0	1	1	1	1	7
Mean Score (acute exercises)											**7.00**
Chen et al. (2016)	1	1	0	1	1	1	1	1	1	1	9
De Greeff et al. (2016)	0	1	0	1	0	0	1	1	1	1	6
Kval et al. (2017)	1	1	0	1	0	0	1	1	1	1	7
Jiang (2015)	1	1	0	0	0	0	1	1	1	1	6
Xin (2012)	0	1	0	1	0	0	1	1	1	1	6
Budde et al. (2016)	1	1	1	1	0	0	1	1	1	1	8
Purohit and Pradhan (2016)	0	1	0	0	0	0	1	1	1	1	5
Wang (2017)	0	1	0	1	0	0	1	1	1	1	6
Yin et al. (2018)	1	1	0	1	1	0	1	1	1	1	8
Chaddock-Heyman et al. (2013)	1	1	0	1	0	0	1	1	1	1	7
Stroth et al. (2009)	1	1	0	0	0	0	1	1	1	0	5
Lina (2017)	0	1	0	1	0	0	1	1	1	1	6
Yan Jun and Chen (2013)	0	1	0	0	0	0	1	1	1	1	5
Keita et al. (2011)	0	1	0	1	0	0	1	1	1	1	6
Hillman et al. (2014)	1	1	1	1	1	0	1	1	1	1	9
Telles et al. (2013)	1	1	1	1	1	1	1	1	1	1	10
Fisher et al. (2011)	0	1	0	1	1	1	0	1	1	1	7
Tarp et al. (2016)	0	1	0	1	0	0	0	1	1	1	5
Ludyga et al. (2018)	1	1	0	1	0	0	1	1	1	1	7
Nie (2019)	1	1	0	1	0	0	1	1	1	1	7
Egger et al. (2019)	1	1	0	1	0	0	1	1	1	1	7
Vera et al. (2018)	1	1	0	1	0	0	1	1	1	1	7
Mean Score (chronic exercises)											**6.77**

Item 1 = eligibility criteria; Item 2 = randomization; Item 3 = concealed allocation; Item 4 = similar baseline; Item 5 = assessor blindness; Item 6 = subject blindness; Item 7 = a retention rate of 85% or above; Item 8 = comparison between groups; Item 9 = point measure and measures of variability; Item 10 = completeness of measurement results ("1" means that the corresponding item was explicitly described and present in details; "0" means that the corresponding item was absent, inadequately described, or unclear).

indicated less time being required for working memory. The aggregated result showed a significant benefit in favor of acute exercises on working memory (SMD = −0.72; 95% CI −0.89 to −0.56, $I^2 = 10.9\%$, $p < 0.001$) (**Figure 4**). Chronic exercises were shown to shorten the response time effectively (SMD = −0.54; 95% CI −0.74 to −0.33, $I^2 = 63.4\%$, $p < 0.001$) (**Figure 5**). The SMDs of acute and chronic exercises were considered as moderate ESs.

Thirteen studies (14 pairwise comparisons) examined the effect of exercises on cognitive flexibility (as measured by more-odd shifting and the Wisconsin card sorting test). A higher negative value of the mean change score for the reaction time indicated less time being required for cognitive flexibility. The aggregated result showed a significant benefit in favor of acute exercises on cognitive flexibility (SMD = −0.34; 95% CI −0.55 to −0.14, $I^2 = 0\%$, $p < 0.005$) (**Figure 6**). Similarly, chronic exercises also had a significant effect on cognitive flexibility (SMD = −0.34, 95 % CI −0.48 to −0.20, $I^2 = 49.3\%$, $p < 0.001$) (**Figure 7**). The SMDs of acute and chronic exercises were considered as small ESs.

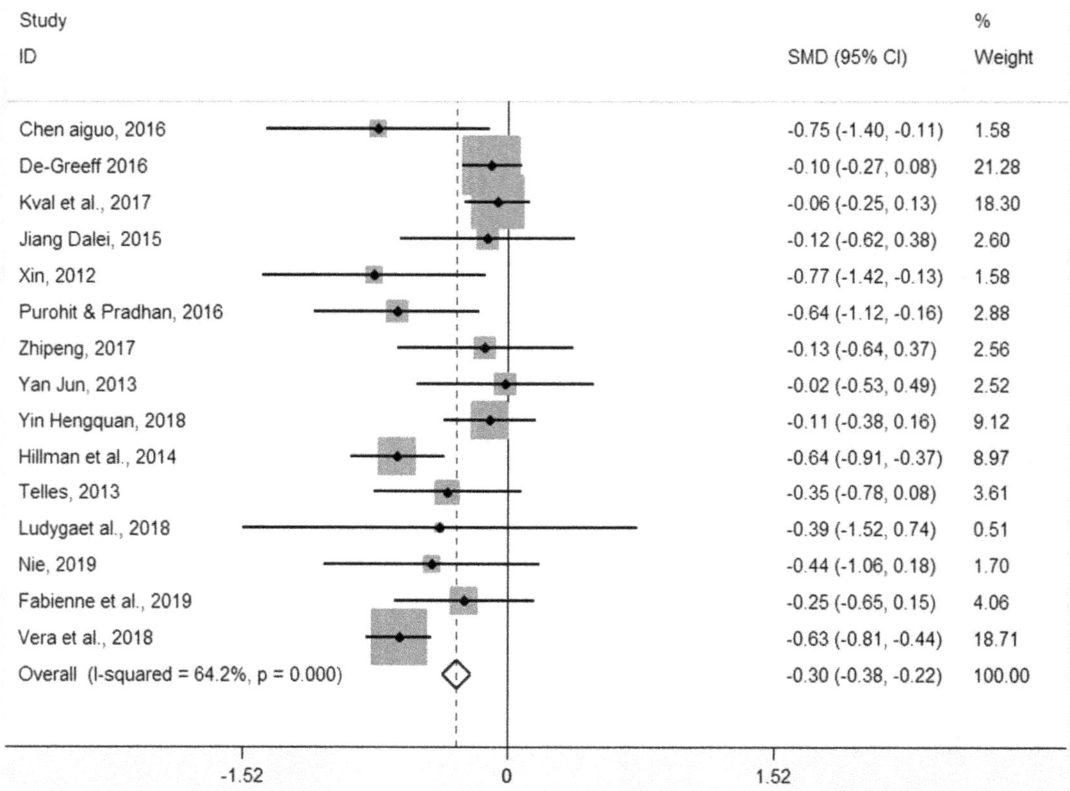

FIGURE 3 | The effect of chronic exercises on inhibitory control (SMD = standardized mean difference; CI = confidence interval).

GRADE Quality Evaluation

Based on the criteria of GRADE, the assessment of the certainty of the evidence regarding the significant impact of exercises on the subsets (inhibitory control, working memory, and cognitive flexibility) of executive functions in children and adolescents was separately evaluated (**Table 4**). Specifically, acute exercises exhibited medium-quality evidence for the working memory, inhibitory control, and cognitive flexibility of children and adolescents in their executive functions, whereas chronic exercises showed medium-quality evidence on inhibitory control and low-quality evidence on working memory and cognitive flexibility.

Moderator Analysis

For chronic exercises, variables (age, type, study quality, composite, frequency, time, and duration) are likely to be the influencing factors for children and adolescents on their inhibitory control and working memory. Moderator analysis using separate models was employed to examine potential sources of variance. All results are presented in **Table 3**.

Inhibitory Control Moderators

In terms of the composite type of intervention, either multiple exercise interventions or sole exercise interventions were employed in the original studies. There were no statistically significant differences on the ESs between the two types of interventions ($Q = 10.25$, $p = 0.001$) (**Table 5**). For chronic exercises, the sole exercise interventions had a significant improvement on inhibitory control (SMD =-0.55, 95% CI −0.83 to −0.25, $p < 0.001$) compared with the multiple exercise interventions (SMD = −0.16, 95% CI −0.27 to −0.06, $p < 0.001$). Furthermore, for intervention classification in the experimental group, open motor skills and closed motor skills were included in our current meta-analysis, showing a statistically significant difference in the ES ($Q = 14.49$, $p = 0.001$). The results showed a significant effect of open motor skills (SMD = −0.56, 95% CI −0.73 to −0.40) on inhibitory control. In terms of age, there was a statistically significant difference ($Q = 12.23$, $p = 0.01$). A large and significant reduction in the ES was attributed to children 12–18 years old (SMD = −0.81, 95% CI −1.15 to −0.48, $p < 0.001$) when compared with children 5–12 years old (SMD = −0.19, 95% CI −0.28 to −0.09, $p < 0.01$). Moreover, there were no significant differences in the duration ($Q = 0.07$, $p = 0.791$), frequency ($Q = 1.48$, $p = 0.224$), and exercise session time ($Q = 3.57$, $p = 0.110$). Similarly, the quality of studies did not produce a statistically significant difference between the two levels ($Q = 2.39$, $p = 0.124$).

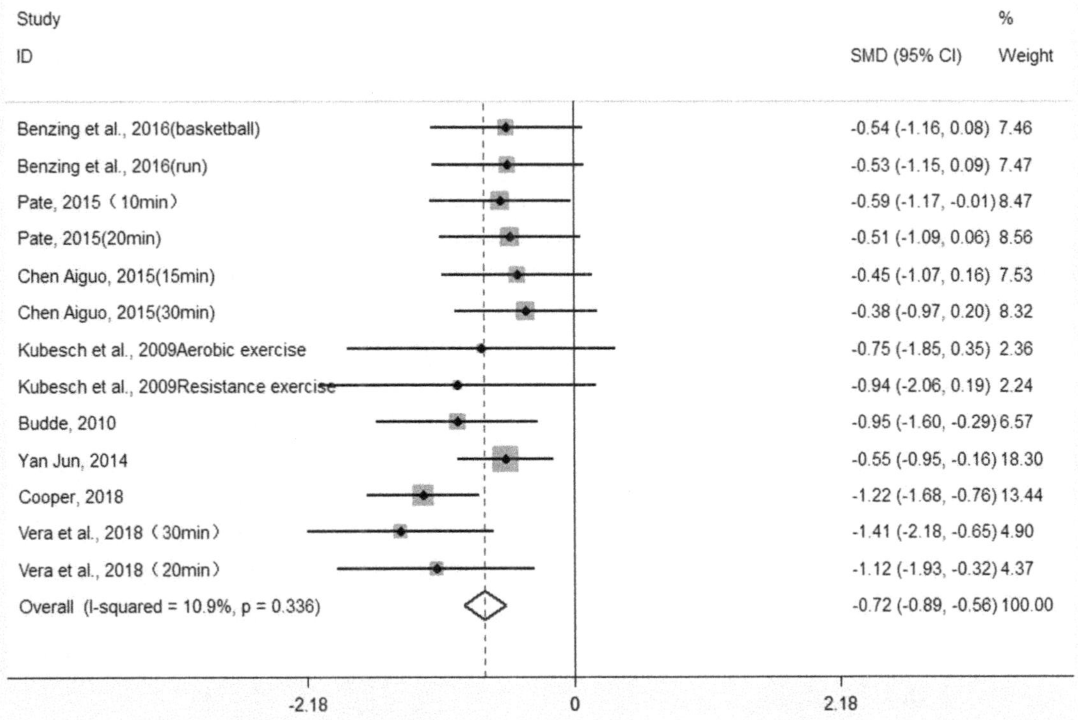

FIGURE 4 | The effect of acute exercises on working memory (SMD = standardized mean difference; CI = confidence interval).

Working Memory Moderators

In terms of intervention classification, a statistically significant difference of the evaluated ES was observed (Q = 20.53, $p = 0.001$) in open motor skills (SMD = −0.72, 95% CI −0.93 to −0.43, $p < 0.001$) and closed motor skills (SMD = −0.31, 95% CI −0.57 to −0.25, $p < 0.01$) (**Table 6**). In terms of the composite type of intervention, the two types of composite (multiple exercise interventions and sole exercise interventions) did not contribute to statistically significant differences for the ES estimate (Q = 1.47, $p = 0.257$), where both multiple exercise interventions (SMD =-0.58, 95% CI −1.15 to −0.37, $p < 0.001$) and sole exercise interventions (SMD = −0.44, 95% CI −0.83 to −0.25, $p < 0.001$) led to significant improvements in working memory. Notably, study quality produced a significant difference in working memory (Q = 27.89, $p = 0.001$). A study quality score of more than 6 had a small and significant ES (SMD = −0.33, 95% CI −0.55 to −0.21, $p < 0.01$). By contrast, a large and significant ES on working memory was found in favor of studies with a quality score of <6 (SMD = −0.86, 95% CI −1.13 to −0.39, $p < 0.01$). In addition, the factor of age contributed to statistically significant differences for the ES estimate (Q = 18.06, $p = 0.001$); children 5–12 years old had a greater improvement in working memory (SMD = −0.64, 95% CI −0.87 to −0.42, $p < 0.001$) than those 12–18 years old (SMD = −0.30, 95% CI −0.49 to −0.12, $p < 0.001$). Additionally, in terms of duration, frequency, and exercise session time, there was a statistically significant difference for exercise session time (Q = 18.92, $p = 0.001$). A moderate and significant reduction in the ES was attributed to the exercise session time (≤30 min, SMD =-0.82, 95% CI −1.01 to −0.64, $p < 0.001$) when compared with prolonged exercise (>30 min), which contributed to a small ES (SMD =0.35, 95% CI −0.47 to −0.22, $p < 0.001$). By contrast, statistically significant differences of the evaluated ESs were not observed for duration (Q = 0.16, $p = 0.694$) and frequency (Q = 0.10, $p = 0.953$).

Meta-Regression Analysis

In order to examine the effect of chronic exercises on inhibitory control and working memory, meta-regression analyses were performed to determine if the variables (age, type, study quality, composite, frequency, time, and duration) influenced the different indices in **Tables 7, 8.** Regression results showed that open motor skill interventions (β = 0.451645, Q = 1.82, df = 1, $p = 0.007$) and age (β = −0.608123, Q = 2.51, df = 1, $p = 0.029$) were significantly associated with inhibitory control. However, we found no significant relationship between composite interventions and dependent variables on inhibitory control (β = 0.406159, Q = 2.06, df = 1, $p = 0.064$).

Regarding the effects of chronic exercises on working memory, both type (β = −0.375588, Q = 3.57, df = 1, $p = 0.024$) and study quality (β =-0.555877, Q = 5.28, df = 1, $p = 0.001$) influenced the ES. Notably, we found that age could significantly moderate the ES of working memory (β = 0.293404, Q = 4.57,

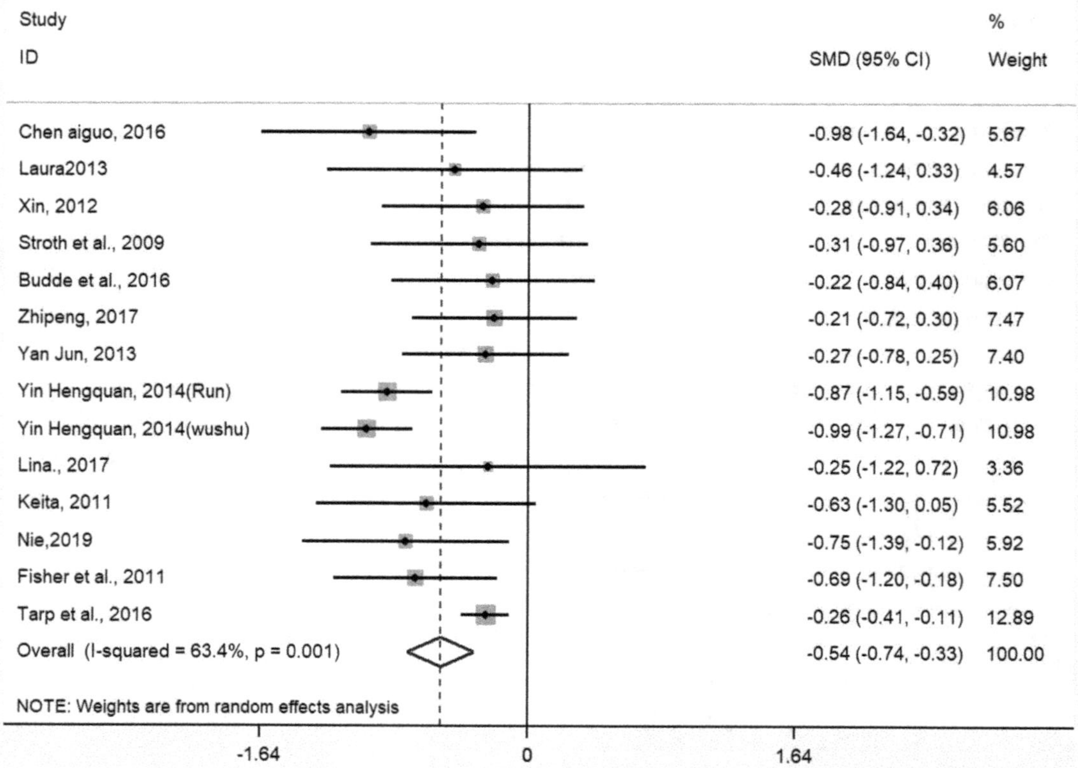

FIGURE 5 | The effect of chronic exercises on working memory (SMD = standardized mean difference; CI = confidence interval).

df = 1, p = 0.033). Additionally, there was no significant relationship between exercise session time and chronic exercises on working memory ($\beta = 0.303556$, Q = 1.71, df = 1, $p = 0.115$).

DISCUSSION

Summary of Evidence

The present meta-analysis suggests that both acute and chronic exercises may be effective for improving executive functions (e.g., inhibitory control, working memory, and cognitive flexibility) in healthy child and adolescent populations. Moreover, in chronic exercise interventions, working memory was moderated by age, exercise type, and study quality, while only two variables (age and exercise type) played a moderating role in inhibitory control.

Inhibitory Control

Inhibitory control refers to the conscious inhibition or automatic response in the cognitive process (Wright et al., 2010). The Stroop, Go/no-go, and Flanker tasks are the most commonly used tools to evaluate the performance (reaction time and/or accuracy) of inhibitory control (Chen et al., 2020). The present review suggests that both acute and chronic exercises are beneficial for inhibitory control, with small magnitudes (Xue et al., 2019; Li et al., 2020). The mechanisms of action of acute and chronic exercises on inhibitory control are unclear, but a possible explanation regarding the effects is attributed to the features of exercises; that is, whether acute or chronic exercises are used can cause an individual to need to complete more complex tasks than everyday multitasking, and this operation mode relies on the non-automatic selection of the process during exercises, which facilitates the speed of reaction of inhibition control (Li et al., 2017). Furthermore, a prior study suggested that acute exercises could significantly improve the speed of reaction of inhibitory control in children and adolescents (Ludyga et al., 2016), and a recent study suggested that chronic exercises are equal to the cumulative effect of acute exercises, while the increase in cognitive performance after chronic exercise interventions seems to be reasonable (Pesce, 2012). Therefore, further studies will be needed to identify the relationship between the influence mechanisms of acute exercises and chronic exercises on inhibitory control.

It is common that heterogeneity across studies is present in the meta-analysis, but the impact of acute exercises on the inhibitory control has a small heterogeneity, which is not in agreement with other acute exercise intervention review studies (Moreau and Chou, 2019). This may be due to the fact that our inclusion criteria only included healthy children and adolescents, and evaluation in acute exercise research is

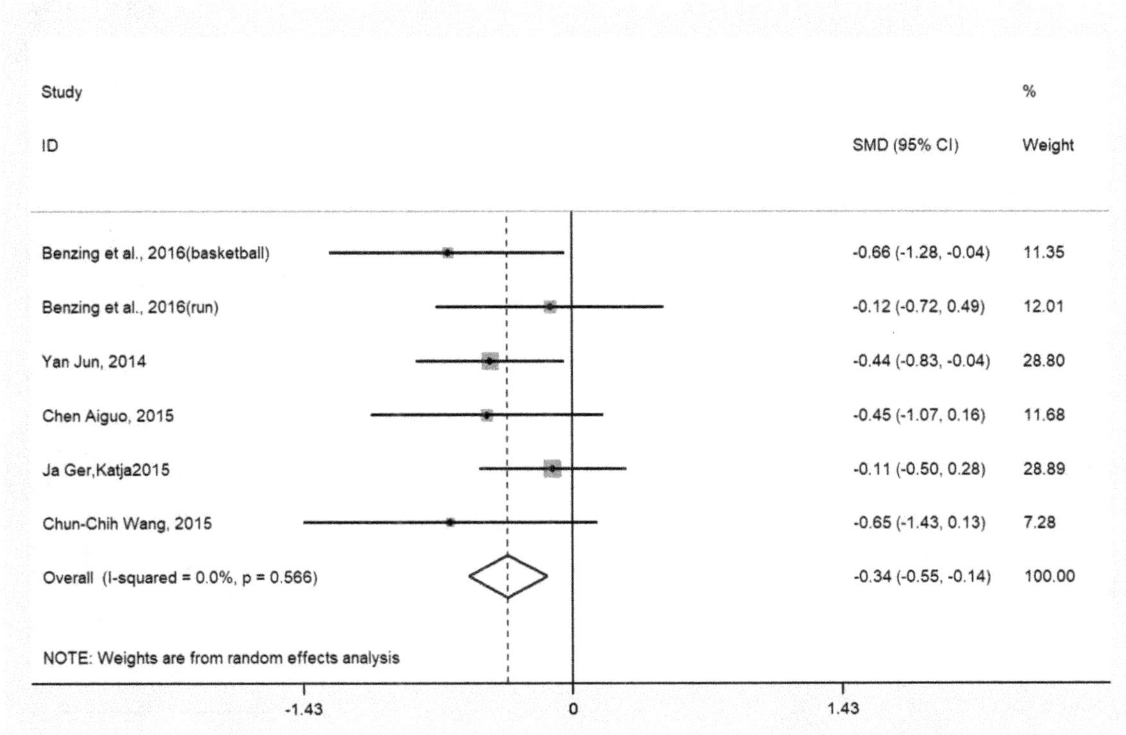

FIGURE 6 | The effect of acute exercises on cognitive flexibility (SMD = standardized mean difference; CI = confidence interval).

carried out immediately after the intervention, which leads to less heterogeneity between different studies. On the contrary, there was considerable heterogeneity regarding the effect of chronic exercises on inhibitory control ($I^2 = 68.20\%$). Meta-regression showed that age and intervention types were moderators of the effect of chronic exercises on inhibitory control, implying that the effect of chronic exercises on inhibitory control improved with age.

Furthermore, the subgroup analysis indicated that, from the age perspective, although 5–12-year-old children and 12–18-year-old adolescents showed positive effects in terms of improving inhibitory control, 5–12-year-old children showed a low inhibitory ability compared with 12–18-year-old adolescents. This finding is in agreement with a previous study (Harnishfeger, 1995) that showed that there is an obvious age trend in the development of inhibition: children between 5 and 10 years of age had a very low inhibition ability, children over 10 years of age began to approach adults, and adults had the strongest inhibition ability (Harnishfeger, 1995). In addition, from the study intervention characteristic perspective, open motor skills can improve inhibition ability significantly more than closed motor skills ($p = 0.001$). This is attributed to the fact that open skills need to respond consistently to changing circumstances. In the process of implementation, information processing methods such as perception, pattern recognition, and decision-making are more prominent than in closed skill exercises, and the level of self-regulation is higher, resulting in significant inhibitory control. A recent meta-analysis demonstrated that the strongest effects emerged from aerobic exercises (motor skills) and cognitively engaging exercises (yoga combined with meditation and stretching) (Vazou et al., 2019). Moreover, a prior study suggested that cognitively engaging physical activity and mentally enriching interventions may promote fundamental changes in the brain that benefit cognition in children (Hillman et al., 2014). These findings indicated that more advanced strategies and cognitive motor skills can contribute to improving inhibitory control for normal child and adolescent populations. Finally, our results showed that medium effect sizes emerged from chronic exercise programs focused on sole exercise interventions (i.e., football, tennis, yoga, wuqinxi). It is important to emphasize that the interpretation of the results from comparisons between sole exercises and multiple exercises of physical activity programs should be conducted with caution due to the small number of studies included in this review.

In addition, the experimental intervention characteristics involving duration, frequency, and exercise session time were not moderators of the effect of chronic exercises on inhibitory control ($p > 0.05$). However, as we found those studies had no long-term follow-up, it remains unclear whether a potential benefit will emerge after a longer period after intervention with chronic exercises on inhibitory control. Therefore, we should not make any definitive claims with respect to composite types and experimental intervention characteristics for chronic exercises in this systematic review.

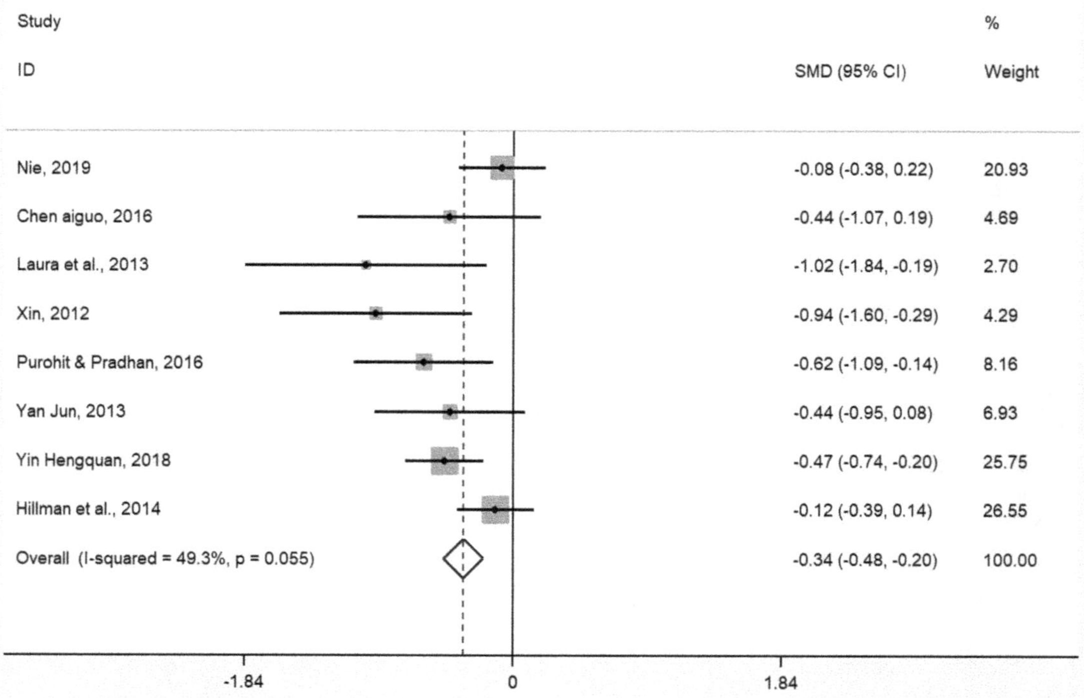

FIGURE 7 | The effect of chronic exercises on cognitive flexibility (SMD = standardized mean difference; CI = confidence interval).

Working Memory

Working memory mainly measures the preservation and update of information, and the digit span forward, digit span backward, letter digit span, Tower of London, and N-back task (1-back and 2-back) measurement tools are the most commonly used to evaluate the response time of working memory (Chen et al., 2020). The aggregated results of the present meta-analysis show that acute and chronic exercises are beneficial for working memory in children and adolescents (the magnitude of the effects were statistically significant), and the calculated ESs were −0.72 (acute exercises) and −0.54 (chronic exercises), which have similar medium efficacies for improving working memory. A prior study suggested that acute aerobic exercises have an intensity dose effect on memory in children and adolescents (Rathore and Lom, 2017). Furthermore, early meta regression analysis studies also found that acute aerobic exercises have a promoting effect on memory, and the effect size is greater than that of acute exercises affecting inhibitory control and information processing speed (Lambourne and Tomporowski, 2010). In addition, according to the international physical activity guidelines, chronic exercises are very cognitively beneficial (Schmidt et al., 2015), and a prior study suggested that the cardiorespiratory fitness level of chronic exercises is helpful for the 1-back reaction speed (Luo, 2018). However, regarding the differences between the intervention effects of chronic exercises and acute exercises, the results of a previous study (Rathore and Lom, 2017) are inconsistent with our research results due to the inclusion of older adults, while our criteria include only children and adolescents. Furthermore, some previous studies have suggested that acute exercises have no effect on working memory (Li et al., 2017; De Greeff et al., 2018). Similarly, a prior study suggested that working memory showed no improvement across a range of intervention durations (5–20 min) and intensities (Daly-Smith et al., 2018). The reason for the difference in these results is due to our working memory measurement index extraction method, which only revolved around the processing speed without considering accuracy. The current meta-analysis shows that moderate to high intensity and time (20–30 min) physical activity is effective at enhancing the response time of working memory. Although the mechanisms of action of acute and chronic exercises on working memory are unclear, the contrasting results between chronic and acute exercises offer interesting future directions to explore different mechanisms that govern both intervention types, and need further study.

In addition, our results show that acute exercises were characterized by non-significant heterogeneity ($I^2 = 24.4\%$), which indicates that the 11 studies were not significantly dissimilar from each other, adding further confidence to the result. By contrast, the meta-analysis of the 14 chronic exercise studies revealed a significant heterogeneity ($I^2 = 63.4\%$). Meta-regression showed that study quality and intervention type were

TABLE 4 | Grading Recommendations to Assess Development and Evaluation (GRADE) assessment of the evidence of certainty for exercise effects.

Outcomes		Presence of downgrading item of GRADE					Level of certainty of evidence
		Risk of bias	Inconsistency	Indirectness	Imprecision	Publication bias	
Chronic exercises	Inhibitory control	Yes	No	No	No	No	II (moderate) (1)
	Working memory	Yes	No	No	Yes	No	III (low) (1) (4)
	Cognitive flexibility	Yes	No	No	Yes	No	III (low) (1) (4)
Acute exercises	Inhibitory control	Yes	No	No	No	No	II (moderate) (1)
	Working memory	Yes	No	No	No	No	II (moderate) (1)
	Cognitive flexibility	Yes	No	No	No	No	II (moderate) (1)

(1) Risk of bias: if the risk of bias of the included studies is present in the meta-analysis, e.g., randomization, concealed allocation, or blinding of assessors/subjects; (2) Inconsistency: point estimates are concentrated, confidence intervals can overlap, and the results of the heterogeneity tests are not statistically significant; (3) Indirectness: present if the intervention studied in the meta-analysis is not directly relevant to the outcome; (4) Imprecision: present if the sum of sample sizes of all individual studies included in the meta-analysis is less than 500, and if the effect size's 95% CI is comparatively large; (5) Publication bias: present if the author only searched the Chinese database. or only one database.

TABLE 5 | Subgroup analysis of inhibitory control (chronic exercises). SMD: standardized mean difference.

Subgroup	*N*	SMD	95% conf. interval	I^2	Test for between-group heterogeneity		
					Q-value	df (Q)	*p*-value
Age							
5–12	11 (1567)	−0.20	−0.28, −0.09	50.8%	12.23	1	0.001
12–18	3 (148)	−0.81	−1.15, −0.48	72.5%			
Type							
Open motor skills	9 (859)	−0.56	−0.73, −0.40	60.1%	14.49	1	0.001
Closed motor skills	6 (856)	−0.11	−0.22, 0.00	0.0%			
Study quality							
Scores more than 6 (>6)	8 (716)	−0.32	−0.55, −0.20	25.2%	2.39	1	0.124
Scores less than 6 (≤6)	7(998)	−0.18	−0.31, −0.06	84.7%			
Duration							
More than 12 weeks	7 (545)	−0.22	−0.36, −0.09	69.6%	0.07	1	0.791
Less than 12 weeks	8(1170)	−0.25	−0.37, −0.12	72.8%			
Composite type							
Multiple exercises intervention	7 (713)	−0.16	−0.27, −0.06	64.2%	10.25	1	0.001
Sole exercises intervention	8 (1002)	−0.55	−0.83, −0.25	55.8%			
Frequency							
1–3 times/week	5(442)	−0.14	−0.25, −0.05	69.0%	1.48	1	0.224
4–7 times/week	10(1273)	−0.42	−0.58,−0.27	49.8%			
Exercise session time							
≤30	5(489)	−0.12	−0.24, 0.05	0.0%	3.57	1	0.110
>30	10(1226)	−0.47	−0.73, −0.21	70.0%			

moderators of the effect of chronic exercises on working memory. Moderator analysis suggested that a significant difference in working memory between a study quality with a score more than six and a study quality with a score <6 was observed, which implies that a less rigorous study design may consciously affect the results, thus exaggerating the effect of the intervention and resulting in a large effect size. In addition, similarly to the inhibitory control influence mechanism, open motor skills exercises may also significantly improve the reaction of working memory.

Furthermore, experimental intervention characteristics involving duration, frequency, and exercise session time are crucial to investigating the effects of chronic exercise changes in working memory. The moderator analysis indicated that each session time of ≤30 min can improve the response of large ES (−0.82) on working memory; the effect is more significant than for a session time of >30 min. A prior study suggested that the effect of aerobic exercises for 55 min is not as good as for 30 min (Fu and Fan, 2016). The possible reason for this is that an excessively long exercise time cannot induce an appropriate level of arousal and results in fatigue (Moreau and Chou, 2019). Additionally, duration (<12 weeks) and frequency (one to three times) could significantly contribute to moderate ESs on working memory; chronic exercises more than four times per week and

TABLE 6 | Subgroup analysis of working memory (chronic exercises).

Subgroup	*N*	SMD	95% conf. interval	I^2	Test for between-group heterogeneity		
					Q-value	df (Q)	*p*-value
Age							
5–12	9 (638)	−0.64	−0.87, −0.42	47.0%	18.06	1	0.001
12–18	3 (773)	−0.30	−0.49, −0.12	12.8%			
Type							
Open motor skills	5 (419)	−0.72	−0.93, −0.43	26.9%	20.53	1	0.001
Close motor skills	5 (386)	−0.31	−0.57,−0.25	12.4%			
Studies' quality							
Scores more than 6 (>6)	6 (884)	−0.33	−0.55, −0.21	6.9%	27.89	1	0.001
Scores less than 6 (≤6)	7 (593)	−0.86	−1.13, −0.39	0.0%			
Duration							
More than 12 weeks	6 (336)	−0.36	−0.79, −0.15	0.0%	0.16	1	0.694
Less than 12 weeks	7 (1141)	−0.62	−0.97,−0.26	82.8%			
Composite type							
Multiple-exercise intervention	6 (666)	−0.58	−1.15, −0.37	48.0%	1.47	1	0.257
Sole-exercise intervention	7 (811)	−0.44	−0.83, −0.25	23.2%			
Frequency							
1–3 times/week	5 (478)	−0.40	−0.65, −0.15	21.6%	0.10	1	0.953
4–7 times/week	8 (999)	−0.61	−0.61,−0.32	79.6%			
Exercise session time							
≤30	4 (295)	−0.82	−1.01, −0.64	59.5%	18.92	1	0.001
>30	9 (1182)	−0.35	−0.47, −0.22	13.1%			

TABLE 7 | Regression analysis for chronic exercises versus the control group of inhibitory control.

ES	No. of studies/ comparisons	Coef. (β)	Std. err.	95% conf. interval	Test for between-groupheterogeneity		
					Q-value	df (Q)	*p*-value
Age*	14	−0.608123	0.241830	−1.140387, −0.075859	2.51	1	0.029
Type**	15	0.451645	0.137132	0.149819, 0.753470	1.82	1	0.007
Study quality	15	−0.296366	0.229172	−0.800770, 0.208038	0.65	1	0.222
Duration	15	0.006166	0.243023	−0.528724, 0.541055	1.31	1	0.980
Frequency	15	−0.208072	0.225305	−0.703965, 0.287821	0.92	1	0.376
Time	15	−0.378365	0.222389	−1.330843, 0.923009	1.70	1	0.117
Composite	15	0.406159	0.197258	−0.028003, 0.840320	2.06	1	0.064

**shows that the data differ. *$p < 0.05$, **$p < 0.01$.*

TABLE 8 | Regression analysis for chronic exercises vs. the control group of working memory.

ES	No. of studies/ comparisons	Coef. (β)	Std. err.	95% conf. interval	Test for between-group heterogeneity		
					Q-value	df (Q)	*p*-value
Age	12	0.293404	0.263048	−0.225295, 0.683069	4.57	1	0.033
Type*	10	−0.375588	0.145919	−0.693518, −0.057659	3.57	1	0.024
Study quality**	13	−0.555877	0.105251	−0.785000, −0.326554	5.28	1	0.001
Duration	13	−0.036083	0.333311	−1.29879, −0.090172	0.11	1	0.921
Frequency	13	−0.113366	0.225896	−0.616694, 0.389962	0.50	1	0.627
Time	13	0.303556	0.177347	−0.086782, 0.693894	1.71	1	0.115
Composite	13	−0.235401	0.175217	−0.617166, 0.146365	1.34	1	0.204

**shows that the data differ. *$p < 0.05$, **$p < 0.01$.*

for more than 12 weeks did not significantly benefit working memory ($p_1 = 0.694$, $p_2 = 0.953$). The reason for this finding is not fully understood, because of the limited experimental design with no long-term follow-up. Therefore, we also should not make any definitive claim with respect to duration and frequency for chronic exercises in working memory. It is worth noting that from the age perspective, our current meta-analysis showed that the intervention effect for children aged 5–12 is greater than that for adolescents aged 12–18 ($p = 0.001$); this is the opposite of the result for the inhibitory control. This may be attributed to the fact that working memory extraction, attention distribution and focus of attention increase significantly at 6–9 years old (Wang et al., 2013), and children aged 5–12 can actively complete tasks in accordance with the teacher's requirements, which is also one of the reasons for their strong subjective initiative.

Cognitive Flexibility

Cognitive flexibility refers to the ability of individuals to constantly adjust their thoughts and behaviors in order to adapt to changing situations (Hernández et al., 2010). Specifically, when two tasks compete for the same cognitive resource, flexibility is the process of controlling the mutual conversion of these two tasks. The commonly used measurement tasks are as follows: the plus–minus task, number–letter task, more-odd shifting, the local–global task, and the Wisconsin card sorting test (WCST).

Because cognitive flexibility was present across a small number of eligible studies, the present meta-analysis only synthesized WCST and more-odd shifting. With respect to cognitive flexibility, a significant improvement in cognitive flexibility in the present meta-analysis was identified in favor of acute and chronic exercises, but the ES effects of the two types of exercises regarding cognitive flexibility were small (−0.34). It is reasonable that a significant improvement was observed for cognitive flexibility. That is because exercises intervention can change the brain's activation pattern, which specifically manifests as an increased activation of the bilateral upper frontal gyrus, bilateral middle frontal gyrus, and bilateral upper lobules, and an individual is prone to having activated pre-frontal and parietal lobes when exercising cognitive flexibility (Jamadar et al., 2010; Boucard et al., 2012). Therefore, appropriate exercises can improve cognitive flexibility. Although the positive effects of acute and chronic exercises on cognitive flexibility have been shown in the present meta-analysis, it is necessary to explore the literature evidence because of the small number of studies included.

Study Limitations

This study has a certain number of limitations and deficiencies. (1) There was a limited number of works on cognitive flexibility. Therefore, we could not obtain an accurate result regarding the effect of executive function interventions on children and adolescents. (2) The high-level executive functions, such as decision-making and reasoning, can be understood with a detailed assessment of the dynamics of EF performance, but the studies reviewed in this meta-analysis did not include this information. We believe that future studies should collect, retain, and ideally share these types of data to allow more detailed analyses. (3) Only three articles in this study explained random sequence generation in detail, and no other work mentioned the method of random allocation and hiding. (4) The intervention method in some of the included studies was aerobic exercises, which has not been explained in great detail, and thus we were unable to confirm which skills were involved in aerobic exercises. (5) Most studies had no long-term follow-up, and it remains unclear whether a potential benefit will emerge after a longer period post-intervention of chronic exercises in executive function. (6) The current meta-analysis only made relevant reports on the reaction time; in the future, we also need to report on the effect of physical activity on the accuracy of executive functions.

CONCLUSIONS

The results of the current meta-analysis demonstrate that acute and chronic exercises may have a positive effect on executive function for children and adolescents, especially in terms of working memory. To better understand the effects of acute and chronic exercises on children and adolescents, rigorous study designs are necessary. In addition, the impact of exercise training on cognitive flexibility needs to be further explored. We should explore the impact of long-term physical exercises on cognitive flexibility, which would also provide a reference for improving executive functions through exercises in the future.

AUTHOR CONTRIBUTIONS

SL, ZL, and YC: conceptualization. SL and ZL: methodology, software, and resources. PC, QY, and YZ: validation. ZK, WL, YZ, and SC: formal analysis. SL, QY, and ZL: investigation and data curation. SL, ZL, and YC: writing—original draft preparation. QY, PC, YZ, ZK, WL, SC, and YC: writing—review and editing. All authors contributed to the article and approved the submitted version.

REFERENCES

Beavan, A., Spielmann, J., Mayer, J., Skorski, S., and Fransen, J. (2020). The rise and fall of executive functions in high-level football players. *Psychol. Sport Exerc.* 49:101677. doi: 10.1016/j.psychsport.2020.101677

Benzing, V., Heinks, T., Eggenberger, N., and Schmidt, M. (2016). Acute cognitively engaging exergame-based physical activity enhances executive functions in adolescents. *PLoS ONE* 11:e0167501. doi: 10.1371/journal.pone.0167501

Berardelli, I., Corigliano, V., Hawkins, M., Comparelli, A., Erbuto, D., and Pompili, M. (2018). Lifestyle interventions and prevention of suicide. *Front. Psychiatry* 9:567. doi: 10.3389/fpsyt.2018.00567

Best, J. R. (2010). Effects of physical activity on children's executive function: contributions of experimental research on aerobic exercise. *Develop. Rev.* 30, 331–351. doi: 10.1016/j.dr.2010.08.001

Bjoern, K., Thomas, F., Sabine, W., and Günter, A. (2018). Sport type determines differences in executive functions in elite athletes. *Psychol. Sport Exerc.* 38, 72–79. doi: 10.1016/j.psychsport.2018.06.002

Boucard, G. K., Albinet, C. T., Bugaiska, A., Bouquet, C. A., Clarys, D., and

Audiffren, M. (2012). Impact of physical activity on executive functions in aging: a selective effect on inhibition among old adults. *J. Sport Exerc. Psychol.* 34, 808–27. doi: 10.1123/jsep.34.6.808

Budde, H., Niemann, C., Wegner, M., and Koutsandreou, F. (2016). Effects of motor versus cardiovascular exercise training on children's working memory. *Med. Sci. Sports Exerc.* 48, 1145–1152. doi: 10.1249/MSS.0000000000000869

Budde, H., Voelcker-Rehage, C., Pietrassyk-Kendziorra, S., Machado, S., Ribeiro, P., and Arafat, A. M. (2010). Steroid hormones in the saliva of adolescents after different exercise intensities and their influence on working memory in a school setting. *Psychoneuroendocrinology* 35, 382–391. doi: 10.1016/j.psyneuen.2009.07.015

Byun, K., Hyodo, K., Suwabe, K., Ochi, G., Sakairi, Y., Kato, M., et al. (2014). Positive effect of acute mild exercise on executive function via arousal-related prefrontal activations: an fNIRS study. *Neuroimage* 98, 336–345. doi: 10.1016/j.neuroimage.2014.04.067

Cardoso, H. F. V. (2007). Epiphyseal union at the innominate and lower limb in a modern Portuguese skeletal sample, and age estimation in adolescent and young adult male and female skeletonsandnbsp. *Am. J. Phys. Anthropol.* 135, 161–170. doi: 10.1002/ajpa.20717

Chaddock-Heyman, L., Erickson, K. I., Voss, M. W., Knecht, A. M., Pontifex, M. B., Castelli, D. M., et al. (2013). The effects of physical activity on functional MRI activation associated with cognitive control in children: a randomized controlled intervention. *Front. Hum. Neurosci.* 7:72. doi: 10.3389/fnhum.2013.00072

Chen, A., Fu, L., and Zhu, L. (2015). Effects of medium-intensity basketball with different durations on children's executive function. *J. Capital Ins. Phys. Educ.* 27, 223–227. doi: 10.14104/j.cnki.1006-2076.2017.01.015

Chen, A., Li, H., and Yan, J. (2016). Developmental characteristics of executive function and psychosomatic motor intervention in left-behind children. *China Spec. Educ.* 11, 69–74.

Chen, F.-T., Etnier, J. L., Chan, K.-H., Chiu, P.-K., Hung, T.-M., and Chang, Y.-K. (2020). Effects of exercise training interventions on executive function in older adults: a systematic review and meta-analysis. *Sports Med.* 50, 1451–1467. doi: 10.1007/s40279-020-01292-x

Chun, C. H., Caterina, P., Song, T., Tsung-Min, H., and Chang, Y.-K. (2015). Failure to identify an acute exercise effect on executive function assessed by the Wisconsin Card Sorting Test. *J. Sport Health Sci.* 1, 64–72. doi: 10.1016/j.jshs.2014.10.003

Cooper, S. B., Dring, K. J., Morris, J. G., Sunderland, C., Bandelow, S., and Nevill, M. E. (2018). High intensity intermittent games-based activity and adolescents' cognition: moderating effect of physical fitness. *BMC Public Health* 18:603. doi: 10.1186/s12889-018-5514-6

Daly-Smith, A. J., Zwolinsky, S., McKenna, J., Tomporowski, P. D., Defeyter, M. A., and Manley, A. (2018). Systematic review of acute physically active learning and classroom movement breaks on children's physical activity, cognition, academic performance and classroom behaviour: understanding critical design features. *Bmj Open Sport Exerc Med.* 4:e000341. doi: 10.1136/bmjsem-2018-000341

De Greeff, J. W., Bosker, R. J., Oosterlaan, J., Visscher, C., and Hartman, E. (2018). Effects of physical activity on executive functions, attention and academic performance in preadolescent children: a meta-analysis. *J. Sci. Med. Sport* 21, 501–507. doi: 10.1016/j.jsams.2017.09.595

De Greeff, J. W., Hartman, E., Mullender-Wijnsma, M. J., Bosker, R. J., Doolaard, S., and Visscher, C. (2016). Long-term effects of physically active academic lessons on physical fitness and executive functions in primary school children. *Health Educ. Res.* 24:102. doi: 10.1093/her/cyv102

Diamond, A. (2013). Executive functions. *Annu. Rev. Psychol.* 64, 135–168. doi: 10.1146/annurev-psych-113011-143750

Egger, F., Benzing, V., Conzelmann, A., and Schmidt, M. (2019). Boost your brain, while having a break! The effects of long-term cognitively engaging physical activity breaks on children's executive functions and academic achievement. *PLoS ONE* 14:e0212482. doi: 10.1371/journal.pone.0212482

Egger, F., Conzelmann, A., and Schmidt, M. (2018). The effect of acute cognitively engaging physical activity breaks on children's executive functions: too much of a good thing? *Psychol. Sport Exerc.* 36, 178–186. doi: 10.1016/j.psychsport.2018.02.014

Ellemberg, D., and St-Louis-Deschênes, M. (2010). The effect of acute physical exercise on cognitive function during development. *Psychol. Sport Exerc.* 11, 0–126. doi: 10.1016/j.psychsport.2009.09.006

Ferguson, G. D., Aertssen, W. F. M., Rameckers, E. A. A., Jelsma, J., and Smits-Engelsman, B. C. M. (2014). Physical fitness in children with developmental coordination disorder: measurement matters. *Res. Dev. Disabil.* 35, 1087–1097. doi: 10.1016/j.ridd.2014.01.031

Fisher, A., Boyle, J. M. E., Paton, J. Y., Tomporowski, P., and Reilly, J. J. (2011). Effects of a physical education intervention on cognitive function in young children: randomized controlled pilot study. *BMC Pediatr.* 11:97. doi: 10.1186/1471-2431-11-97

Flashner, B. M., Rifas-Shiman, S. L., Oken, E., Camargo, C. A. Jr., Platts-Mills, T. J., Workman, L., et al. (2019). Obesity, sedentary lifestyle, and exhaled nitric oxide in an early adolescent cohort. *Pediatr. Pulmonol.* 55, 503–509. doi: 10.1002/ppul.24597

Fu, J., and Fan, Y. (2016). Experimental study on the influence of moderate-intensity physical exercise on executive function and academic performance of junior high school students at different times. *Sports Sci.* 37, 110–116. doi: 10.13598/j.issn1004-4590.2016.06.016

Goodall, J., Fisher, C., Hetrick, S., Phillips, L., Parrish, E. M., and Allott, K. (2018). Neurocognitive functioning in depressed young people: a systematic review and meta-analysis. *Neuropsychol. Rev.* 28, 216–231. doi: 10.1007/s11065-018-9373-9

Gothe, N., Pontifex, M. B., Hillman, C., and Mcauley, E. (2013). The acute effects of yoga on executive function. *J. Phys. Activity Health* 10:488. doi: 10.1123/jpah.10.4.488

Handoll, H. H. G., Howe, T. E., and Madhok, R. (2002). The cochrane database of systematic reviews. *Physiotherapy* 88, 714–716. doi: 10.1016/S0031-9406(05)60709-2

Hanley, J. A., Abdissa, N., Edwardes, M. D. deB., and Forrester, J. E. (2003). Statistical analysis of correlated data using generalized estimating equations: an orientation. *Am. J. Epidemiol.* 157, 364–375. doi: 10.1093/aje/kwf215

Harnishfeger, K. K. (1995). 6–The development of cognitive inhibition: theories, definitions, and research evidence. *Interfer. Inhibiti. Cogn.* 25, 175–204. doi: 10.1016/B978-012208930-5/50007-6

Hernández, M., Costa, A., Fuentes, L. J., Vivas, A. B., and Sebastian Galles, N. (2010). The impact of bilingualism on the executive control and orienting networks of attention. *Bilingual. Lang. Cogn.* 13, 315–325. doi: 10.1017/S1366728909990010

Hillman, C. H., Kamijo, K., and Scudder, M. (2011). A review of chronic and acute physical activity participation on neuroelectric measures of brain health and cognition during childhood. *Prevent. Med.* 52, 21–28. doi: 10.1016/j.ypmed.2011.01.024

Hillman, C. H., Pontifex, M. B., Castelli, D. M., Khan, N. A., Raine, L. B., Scudder, M. R., et al. (2014). Effects of the FITKids randomized controlled trial on executive control and brain function. *Pediatrics* 134, 1063–1071. doi: 10.1542/peds.2013-3219

Jager, K., Schmidt, M., Conzelmann, A., and Roebers, C. (2015). The effects of qualitatively different acute physical activity interventions in real-world settings on executive functions in preadolescent children. *Ment. Health Phys. Act.* 9, 1–9. doi: 10.1016/j.mhpa.2015.05.002

Jamadar, S., Hughes, M., Fulham, W. R., Michie, P. T., and Karayanidis, F. (2010). The spatial and temporal dynamics of anticipatory preparation and response inhibition in task-switching. *Neuroimage* 51, 432–449. doi: 10.1016/j.neuroimage.2010.01.090

Jiang, D. (2015). Effects of 8-week moderate intensity football games on executive function development of preschool children. *China Sport Sci. Technol.* 51, 43–50. doi: 10.16470/j.csst.2015.02.007

Keita, K., Roetzheim, R., and Gualtieri, T. (2011). The effects of an afterschool physical activity program on working memory in preadolescent children. *Dev. Sci.* 14, 1046–1058. doi: 10.1111/j.1467-7687.2011.01054.x

Kong, Z., Sze, T.-M., Yu, J. J., Loprinzi, P. D., Xiao, T., Yeung, A. S., et al. (2019). Tai Chi as an alternative exercise to improve physical fitness for children and adolescents with intellectual disability. *Int. J. Environ. Res. Public Health* 16:1152. doi: 10.3390/ijerph16071152

Koolhaas, C. M., van Rooij, F. J. A., Kocevska, D., Luik, A. I., Ikram, M. A., Franco, O. H., et al. (2019). Objectively measured sedentary time and mental and cognitive health: cross-sectional and longitudinal associations in The Rotterdam Study. *Ment. Health Phys. Act.* 17, 423–482. doi: 10.1016/j.mhpa.2019.100296

Kubesch, S., Walk, L., Spitzer, M., Kammer, T., Lainburg, A., Heim, R., et al. (2009). A 30-minute physical education program improves students. *Execut Attent.* 43, 892–904. doi: 10.1111/j.1751-228X.2009.01076.x

Kval, S. E., Bru, E., Brnnick, K., and Dyrstad, S. M. (2017). Does increased physical activity in school affect childrens executive function and aerobic fitness? *Scand. J. Med. Sci. Sports* 43, 42–72. doi: 10.1111/sms.12856

Lambourne, K., and Tomporowski, P. (2010). The effect of exercise-induced arousal on cognitive task performance: a meta-regression analysis. *Brain Res.* 1341, 12–24. doi: 10.1016/j.brainres.2010.03.091

Li, J. W., O'Connor, H., O'Dwyer, N., and Orr, R. (2017). The effect of acute and chronic exercise on cognitive function and academic performance in adolescents: a systematic review. *J. Sci. Med. Sport* 20, 841–848. doi: 10.1016/j.jsams.2016.11.025

Li, L., Zhang, J., and Cao, M. (2020). The effects of chronic physical activity interventions on executive functions in children aged 3-7 years: a meta-analysis. *J. Sci. Med. Sport* 23, 949–954. doi: 10.1016/j.jsams.2020.03.007

Lina, Z. (2017). *Effects of Aerobic Exercise Intervention on Executive Function and Brain Network Function Connection in Deaf Children.* Yangzhou:Yangzhou University.

Liu, S., Xiao, T., Yang, L., and Loprinzi, P. D. (2019). Exercise as an alternative approach for treating smartphone addiction: a systematic review and meta-analysis of random controlled trials. *Int. J. Environ. Res. Public Health* 16, 489–505. doi: 10.3390/ijerph16203912

Loprinzi, P. D., Ponce, P., Zou, L., and Li, H. (2019). The counteracting effects of exercise on high-fat diet-induced memory impairment: a systematic review. *Brain Sci.* 9:145. doi: 10.3390/brainsci9060145

Ludyga, S., Gerber, M., Brand, S., Holsboer-Trachsler, E., and Puhse, U. (2016). Acute effects of moderate aerobic exercise on specific aspects of executive function in different age and fitness groups: a meta-analysis. *Psychophysiology* 53, 1611–1626. doi: 10.1111/psyp.12736

Ludyga, S., Gerber, M., Herrmann, C., Brand, S., and Pühse, U. (2017). Chronic effects of exercise implemented during school-break time on neurophysiological indices of inhibitory control in adolescents. *Trends Neuro. Educ.* 10, 1–7. doi: 10.1016/j.tine.2017.11.001

Ludyga, S., Gerber, M., Kamijo, K., Brand, S., and Pühse, U. (2018). The effects of a school-based exercise program on neurophysiological indices of working memory operations in adolescents. *J. Sci. Med. Sport* 32, 178-189. doi: 10.1016/j.jsams.2018.01.001

Luo, J. (2018). Review on the influence of physical exercise on working memory. *J. Shandong Univ. Phys. Educ.* 34, 70–77.

Macedo, L. G., Elkins, M. R., Maher, C. G., Moseley, A. M., Herbert, R. D., and Sherrington, C. (2010). There was evidence of convergent and construct validity of Physiotherapy Evidence Database quality scale for physiotherapy trials. *J. Clin. Epidemiol.* 63, 920–925. doi: 10.1016/j.jclinepi.2009.10.005

Maher, C. G., Sherrington, C., and Herbert, R. D. (2003). Reliability of the PEDro scale for rating quality of randomized controlled trials. *Phys. Ther.* 83, 713–721. doi: 10.1093/ptj/83.8.713

Masley, S., Roetzheim, R., and Gualtieri, T. (2009). Aerobic exercise enhances cognitive flexibility. *J. Clin. Psychol. Med. Sett.* 16:186. doi: 10.1007/s10880-009-9159-6

Mcminn, D. (2012). Re: Effectiveness of intervention on physical activity of children: systematic review and meta-analysis of controlled trials with objectively measured outcomes (EarlyBird 54). *BMJ Clin. Res.* 345:e5888. doi: 10.1136/bmj.e5888

McSween, M.-P., Coombes, J. S., MacKay, C. P., Rodriguez, A. D., Erickson, K. I., Copland, D. A., et al. (2019). The immediate effects of acute aerobic exercise on cognition in healthy older adults: a systematic review. *Sports Med.* 49, 67–82. doi: 10.1007/s40279-018-01039-9

Moreau, D., and Chou, E. (2019). The acute effect of high-intensity exercise on executive function: a meta-analysis. *Perspect. Psychol. Sci.* 14, 734–764. doi: 10.1177/1745691619850568

Nie, X. (2019). An experimental study on the Effect of Wuqinxi Exercise on executive function of junior high school students. *J. Shandong Normal Univ.* 3:32.

Padulo, J., Bragazzi, N. L., De Giorgio, A., Grgantov, Z., Prato, S., and Ardigò, L. P. (2019). The effect of physical activity on cognitive performance in an italian elementary school: insights from a pilot study using structural equation modeling. *Front. Physiol.* 10:202. doi: 10.3389/fphys.2019.00202

Park, S., and Etnier, J. L. (2019). Beneficial effects of acute exercise on executive function in adolescents. *J. Phys. Activ. Health.* 16, 1–7. doi: 10.1123/jpah.2018-0219

Pate, R. R. (2015). Acute effects of classroom exercise breaks on executive function and math performance: a dose–response study. *Res. Q. Exerc. Sport* 32, 212–221. doi: 10.1080/02701367.2015.1039892

Pesce, C. (2012). Shifting the focus from quantitative to qualitative exercise characteristics in exercise and cognition research. *J. Sport Exerc. Psychol.* 34, 766–786. doi: 10.1123/jsep.34.6.766

Pindus, D. M., Drollette, E. S., Raine, L. B., Kao, S.-C., Khan, N., Westfall, D. R., et al. (2019). Moving fast, thinking fast: the relations of physical activity levels and bouts to neuroelectric indices of inhibitory control in preadolescents. *J. Sport Health Sci.* 8, 301–314. doi: 10.1016/j.jshs.2019.02.003

Press, S. (2009). *Stata Longitudinal Data/Panel Data Reference Manual (Release 11).* Drive College Station, TX: Stata Press.

Purohit, S. P., and Pradhan, B. (2016). Effect of yoga program on executive functions of adolescents dwelling in an orphan home: a randomized controlled study. *J. Trad. Complem. Med.* 7, 99–105. doi: 10.1016/j.jtcme.2016.03.001

Qi, F., Kong, Z., Xiao, T., Leong, K., Zschorlich, V. R., and Zou, L. (2019). Effects of combined training on physical fitness and anthropometric measures among boys aged 8 to 12 years in the physical education setting. *Sustainability* 11:1219. doi: 10.3390/su11051219

Rathore, A., and Lom, B. (2017). The effects of chronic and acute physical activity on working memory performance in healthy participants: a systematic review with meta-analysis of randomized controlled trials. *Syst. Rev.* 6:124. doi: 10.1186/s13643-017-0514-7

Rey-Lopez, J. (2008). Sedentary behaviour and obesity development in children and adolescents. *Nutr. Metab. Cardiovasc. Dis.* 3, 718–734. doi: 10.1016/j.numecd.2007.07.008

Riquelme, I., Arnould, C., Hatem, S. M., and Bleyenheuft, Y. (2019). The two-arm coordination test: maturation of bimanual coordination in typically developing children and deficits in children with unilateral cerebral palsy. *Dev. Neurorehabil.* 22, 312–320. doi: 10.1080/17518423.2018.1498552

Rocha, M. S., Yaruss, J. S., and Rato, J. R. (2019). Temperament, executive functioning, and anxiety in school-age children who stutter. *Front. Psychol.* 10:2244. doi: 10.3389/fpsyg.2019.02244

Schmidt, M., JäGer, K., Egger, F., Roebers, C. M., and Conzelmann, A. (2015). Cognitively engaging chronic physical activity, but not aerobic exercise, affects executive functions in primary school children: a group-randomized controlled trial. *J. Sport Exerc. Psychol.* 37:575. doi: 10.1123/jsep.2015-0069

Sember, V., Jurak, G., Kovac, M., Morrison, S. A., and Starc, G. (2020). Children's physical activity, academic performance, and cognitive functioning: a systematic review and meta-analysis. *Front. Public Health* 8:307. doi: 10.3389/fpubh.2020.00307

Shamseer, L., Moher, D., Clarke, M., Ghersi, D., Liberati, A., Petticrew, M., et al. (2015). Preferred reporting items for systematic review and meta-analysis protocols (PRISMA-P) 2015: elaboration and explanation. *Bmj* 349, 489–499. doi: 10.1136/bmj.g7647

Sisson, S. B., Church, T. S., Martin, C. K., Tudor-Locke, C., Smith, S. R., Bouchard, C., et al. (2009). Profiles of sedentary behavior in children and adolescents: The US National Health and Nutrition Examination Survey, 2001–2006. *Int. J. Pediatr. Obes.* 4, 353–359. doi: 10.1080/17477160902934777

Stroth, S., Kubesch, S., Dieterle, K., Ruchsow, M., Heim, R., and Kiefer, M. (2009). Physical fitness, but not acute exercise modulates event-related potential indices for executive control in healthy adolescents. *Brain Res.* 1269, 114–124. doi: 10.1016/j.brainres.2009.02.073

Taddei, F., Bultrini, A., Spinelli, D., and Russo, F. D. (2012). Neural correlates of attentional and executive processing in middle-age fencers. *Med. Sci. Sports Exerc.* 44, 1057–1066. doi: 10.1249/MSS.0b013e31824529c2

Tarp, J., Domazet, S. L., Froberg, K., Hillman, C. H., Andersen, L. B., and Bugge, A. (2016). Effectiveness of a school-based physical activity intervention on cognitive performance in Danish Adolescents: LCoMotion—learning, cognition and motion – a cluster randomized controlled trial. *PLoS ONE* 11:e0158087. doi: 10.1371/journal.pone.0158087

Telles, S., Singh, N., Bhardwaj, A. K., Kumar, A., and Balkrishna, A. (2013). Effect of yoga or physical exercise on physical, cognitive and emotional measures in children: a randomized controlled trial. *Child Adolesc. Psychiatry Ment. Health* 7:37. doi: 10.1186/1753-2000-7-37

Thivel, D., Tremblay, A., Genin, P. M., Panahi, S., Rivière, D., and Duclos, M. (2018). Physical activity, inactivity, and sedentary behaviors: definitions and implications in occupational health. *Front. Public Health* 6:288. doi: 10.3389/fpubh.2018.00288

Torrens-Burton, A., Basoudan, N., Bayer, A. J., and Tales, A. (2017). Perception and reality of cognitive function: information processing speed, perceived memory function, and perceived task difficulty in older adults. *J. Alzheimers Dis.* 60, 1601–1609. doi: 10.3233/JAD-170599

Tremblay, M. S., LeBlanc, A. G., Janssen, I., Kho, M. E., Hicks, A., Murumets, K., et al. (2011). Canadian sedentary behaviour guidelines for children and youth. *Appl. Physiol. Nutr. Metabol.* 36, 59–64. doi: 10.1139/H11-012

Vazou, S., Pesce, C., Lakes, K., and Smiley-Oyen, A. (2019). More than one road leads to Rome: a narrative review and meta-analysis of physical activity intervention effects on cognition in youth. *Int. J. Sport Exerc. Psychol.* 17, 153–178. doi: 10.1080/1612197X.2016.1223423

Vera, V. D. B., Saliasi, E., De Groot, R. H. M., Chinapaw, M. J. M., and Singh, A. S. (2019). Improving cognitive performance of 9–12 years old children: just dance? A Randomized Controlled Trial. *Front. Psychol.* 10:174. doi: 10.3389/fpsyg.2019.00174

Vera, V. D. B., Saliasi, E., Jolles, J., De Groot, R. H. M., Chinapaw, M. J. M., and Singh, A. S. (2018). Exercise of varying durations: no acute effects on cognitive performance in adolescents. *Front. Neurosci.* 12:672. doi: 10.3389/fnins.2018.00672

Wang, X., Li, Y., and Fan, H. (2019). The associations between screen time-based sedentary behavior and depression: a systematic review and meta-analysis. *BMC Public Health* 19, 32–58. doi: 10.1186/s12889-019-7904-9

Wang, X., Ma, J., Sun, X., and Sun, Z. (2013). Development of working memory in children aged 6-9 years. *Psychol. Sci.* 36, 92–97. doi: 10.16719/j.cnki.1671-6981.2013.01.029

Wang, Z. (2017). Effect of 8-week tennis game on executive control function of preschool children. *Capital Ins. Phys Educ.* (Beijing).

Weng, T. B., Pierce, G. L., Darling, W. G., and Voss, M. W. (2014). Differential effects of acute exercise on distinct aspects of executive function. *Med. Sci. Sports Exerc.* 47, 1460–1469. doi: 10.1249/MSS.0000000000000542

Willoughby, M. T., Blair, C. B., Wirth, R. J., and Greenberg, M. (2012). The measurement of executive function at age 5: psychometric properties and relationship to academic achievement. *Psychol. Assess* 24, 226–239. doi: 10.1037/a0025361

Wright, I., Waterman, M., Prescott, H., and Murdoch-Eaton, D. (2010). A new Stroop-like measure of inhibitory function development: typical developmental trends. *J. Child Psychol. Psychiatry* 44, 561–575. doi: 10.1111/1469-7610.00145

Xin, L. (2012). *Effects of Short-Term Moderate-Intensity Aerobic Exercise on Executive Function of Female College Students.* Shanghai: East China Normal University.

Xue, Y., Yang, Y., and Huang, T. (2019). Effects of chronic exercise interventions on executive function among children and adolescents: a systematic review with meta-analysis. *Br. J. Sports Med.* 53:1397. doi: 10.1136/bjsports-2018-099825

Yan Jun, M. S., and Chen, A. (2013). Experimental study on the effect of different duration aerobics exercises on executive function of college girls. *Sport Sci.* 33, 88–91. doi: 10.13297/j.cnki.issn1005-0000.2014.04.015

Yan, J., Wu, Y., and Chen, A. (2014). Effects of short-term, medium-intensity and different types of exercise on executive function of primary school students. *Sport Sci.* 35, 94–100. doi: 10.13598/j.issn1004-4590.2012.06.016

Yin, H., Pan, J., and Lai, Y. (2018). Development and empirical study of exercise intervention programs to improve brain executive function of pupils with different types of learning difficulties. *J. Wuhan Ins. Phys. Educ.* 52, 78–89.

Zhang, Y., Alonso-Coello, P., Guyatt, G. H., Yepes-Nunez, J. J., Akl, E. A., Hazlewood, G., et al. (2019). GRADE Guidelines: 19. Assessing the certainty of evidence in the importance of outcomes or values and preferences-Risk of bias and indirectness. *J. Clin. Epidemiol.* 111, 94–104. doi: 10.1016/j.jclinepi.2018.01.013

Zhu, F. (2015). Research on the Improvement of college students' self-control ability and brain processing characteristics by Physical *exercise.* PhD, Shanghai Institute of Physical Education, Shanghai, China.

Zou, L., Loprinzi, P. D., Yeung, A. S., Zeng, N., and Huang, T. (2019). The beneficial effects of mind-body exercises for people with mild cognitive impairment: a systematic review with meta-analysis. *Arch. Phys. Med. Rehabil.* 100, 1556–1573. doi: 10.1016/j.apmr.2019.03.009

Zou, L., Sasaki, J. E., Zeng, N., Wang, C., and Sun, L. (2018). A systematic review with meta-analysis of mindful exercises on rehabilitative outcomes among poststroke patients. *Arch. Phys. Med. Rehabil.* 99, 2355–2364. doi: 10.1016/j.apmr.2018.04.010

4

Augmenting Mental Health in Primary Care: A 1-Year Study of Deploying Smartphone Apps in a Multi-site Primary Care/ Behavioral Health Integration Program

Liza Hoffman[1,2*], *Emily Benedetto*[1*], *Hsiang Huang*[3], *Ellie Grossman*[1], *Dorosella Kaluma*[1], *Ziva Mann*[3] *and John Torous*[2]

[1] *Department of Primary Care, Cambridge Health Alliance, Cambridge, MA, United States,* [2] *Division of Digital Psychiatry, Department of Psychiatry, Beth Israel Deaconess Medical Center, Boston, MA, United States,* [3] *Department of Psychiatry, Cambridge Health Alliance, Cambridge, MA, United States*

Correspondence:
Liza Hoffman
lizahoffman25@gmail.com
Emily Benedetto
eBenedetto@challiance.org

Background: Integrating behavioral health (BH) services into primary care is an evidence-based intervention that can increase access to care, improve patient outcomes, and decrease costs. Digital technology, including smartphone apps, has the potential to augment and extend the reach of these integrated behavioral health services through self-management support impacting lifestyle behaviors. To date, the feasibility and acceptability of using mental health mobile apps within an integrated primary care setting has not yet been explored as part of routine clinical care.

Objectives: The objectives of this study were to (a) test the feasibility of using mental health applications to augment integrated primary care services; (b) solicit feedback from patients and providers to guide implementation, and (c) develop a mental health apps toolkit for system-wide dissemination.

Methods: Cambridge Health Alliance (CHA) is a safety-net healthcare system that includes three community hospitals and 12 Primary Care (PC) clinics serving nearly 150,000 ethnically and socioeconomically diverse patients around Boston. To select and disseminate mental health apps, a four-phase implementation was undertaken: (1) Evaluation of mental health mobile applications (2) Development of an apps toolkit with stakeholder input, (3) Conducting initial pilot at six primary care locations, and (4) Rolling out the app toolkit across 12 primary care sites and conducting 1-year follow-up survey.

Results: Among BH providers, 24 (75%) responded to the follow-up survey and 19 (83%) indicated they use apps as part of their clinical care. Anxiety was the most common condition for which app use was recommended by providers, and 10 (42%) expressed interest in further developing their knowledge of mental health apps. Among patients, 35 (65%) of participants provided feedback; 23 (66%) reported the tools to be helpful, especially for managing stress and anxiety.

Conclusions: Our findings indicate mental health apps are applicable and relevant to patients within integrated primary care settings in safety-net health systems. Behavioral health providers perceive the clinical value of using these tools as part of patient care, but require training to increase their comfort-level and confidence applying these tools with patients. To increase provider and patient engagement, mobile apps must be accessible, simple, intuitive and directly relevant to patients' treatment needs.

Keywords: mental health, mobile apps, smartphone apps, integrated primary care, behavioral health integration, mental health integration

INTRODUCTION

Integrating behavioral health care services into primary care is an evidence-based intervention that can increase access to care, improve patient outcomes, and decrease costs (1). The need for integrated behavioral health (BH) is driven by the heavy burden of mental health conditions, including depression, which is now recognized by the World Health Organization as the leading global cause of disability (2), as well as insufficient numbers of specialized behavioral health clinicians like social workers, psychiatrists, psychologists, and case managers. Key elements of integrated care models include screening for high prevalence mental health conditions, integration of behavioral health clinicians into primary care settings, collaborative team building, and care management for patients (3). With ~40% of mental health care in the United States delivered in the primary care setting, the demand for integrated BH services has outpaced availability (4).

Like other areas of healthcare, digital technology has been proposed as a means to augment and extend the reach of BH integrated care services. These technologies can be classified into three categories: (1) patient facing, (2) primary care facing, and (3) virtual visits (5). Patient facing technologies to extend integrated care may include smartphone apps that offer self-management or guided interventions like Cognitive Behavioral Therapy. Primary care facing technologies include tools to support increased capacity and confidence to offer mental health treatment such as consultation platforms, tele-mentoring, and clinical decision support for integrated care teams. Virtual visits reflect the ability to offer telemedicine services to support integrated care. While there is a growing evidence base and clinical experience with using both virtual visits and primary care facing technologies (5) there is limited to no research or clinical evidence for using smartphone apps to support integrated care.

The lack of knowledge on incorporating mental health-related smartphone apps into integrated care systems is especially surprising considering the potential of mobile technology in mental health. Numerous survey studies have demonstrated those with mental health conditions own smartphones and are interested in using apps for their care (6–8). Meta-analysis of randomized clinical studies of smartphone apps for depressive symptoms (9) and anxiety disorders (10) have demonstrated early efficacy data. In many cases, consumers with mental health conditions are not waiting for the evidence to catch up; today over 10,000 mental health related apps are available from the iTunes and Android app stores (11). Case reports and clinical experience support that people are using these apps to learn about their mental health, track symptoms, and self-manage their condition (12, 13). However, exploring the utility of these apps outside of research studies remains largely uncharted.

Prior efforts transitioning promising mental health research apps into actual clinical care settings underscores the need for careful assessment. One substance use disorder app that showed promising evidence to reduce frequency of alcohol consumption (14) was later found to be difficult to support and maintain in actual clinical settings without the additional support and structure offered in the research setting (15). Reviews of smartphone app adoption by healthcare professionals, beyond mental health and integrated care settings, suggest that perceived barriers can include concerns about privacy, legal ramifications, cost, workload, and need for increased information technology (IT) support (16). Despite barriers, there is evidence that apps are being introduced to care. For instance, research from the United Kingdom suggests that already 30% of mental health providers recommend apps to patients (17). On the patient side, there is also concern that many commercially available mental health apps may not be designed for those with more severe symptoms (18).

In this study, we sought to provide early clinical data from both the patient and clinician perspective on the usage and integration of mental health apps in a busy integrated BH care service at Cambridge Health Alliance (CHA), a safety net healthcare system that includes three community hospitals and 12 Primary Care (PC) clinics which serve nearly 150,000 ethnically and socioeconomically diverse patients in the greater Boston area (19). The healthcare system had implemented an integrated model of care, based on the collaborative care model (20) and Screening, Brief Intervention and Referral to Treatment (SBIRT) (21), to support screening, assessment, and treatment of behavioral health conditions in primary care clinics. The integrated BH staff provide evidence-based brief clinical interventions focusing on patients primarily experiencing low to moderate anxiety, depression, and substance use disorders. Consult psychiatrists provide diagnostic clarification and management strategies for the primary care team. Integrated psychotherapists provide brief treatment (6–8 sessions) grounded in evidence-based treatment modalities including Cognitive Behavioral Therapy (CBT), Problem-Solving Therapy (PST), Behavioral Activation (BA), and Mindfulness Based Stress Reduction (MBSR). Care managers work primarily with patients experiencing low to moderate anxiety and depression; they use interventions including Motivational Interviewing (MI) and BA to support patients in reaching health and lifestyle-related goals and to bridge patients to BH providers. To answer the question of whether mental health apps can be adopted within routine BH care and serve as a helpful tool for patients, we present the results of one institution's experience evaluating, piloting, and disseminating mental health apps across an integrated primary care system.

METHODS

Step 1: Selecting Apps

The first step in introducing apps into care was to identify a series of existing apps that could be recommended to patients receiving integrated care services. Given that the vast majority of these apps fall outside of the Food and Drug Administration (FDA) regulation and there is no formal evaluation or gold standard for judging these apps, we assembled a seven-person multi-disciplinary team of integrated therapists, care managers, administrative and Informational Technology (IT) leadership, and patients to identify and evaluate mental health self-management apps over the course of 10 months. We sought apps that offered patient facing interventions, avoided direct use with a clinician, were free, and claimed to provide privacy protections for patient generated data—understanding there is no set of gold standard apps or criteria to pick apps. Thus, we focused on apps that were: (1) aligned with clinical interventions utilized in our program; (2) developed by a "trusted" source such as medical, academic, and/or research institutions, and/or companies with clinical consultants; (3) free to download, and (4) contained privacy statements at the time of our evaluation. Drawing from our workgroup's clinical knowledge and experience caring for CHA's safety-net patient population, we also considered apps' accessibility in terms of our patients' language needs, literacy levels, and alignment with treatment goals (22). In seeking such apps, we read select literature to help orient us to broader findings and challenges in the mHealth space (23), consulted with app researchers and designers, and sought feedback from our clinical teams and the patients they serve. Without validated app evaluation tools to guide our selection process, we relied on expert consensus throughout the four-stage study process to select a set of apps that best supported our clinical interventions and the needs of our patient population.

Step 2: Creating a Toolkit Around Apps

We identified an initial list of 13 applications and sought guidance from our institution's Patient Partner Lead who represents CHA's patient partners, a group of patient volunteers who serve on quality improvement teams to advise on key projects. Drawing on feedback from our Patient Partner Lead, staff member expertise, papers on app evaluation (24), and elements of the user version of the Mobile Apps Rating System (U-MARS) (25), the workgroup next narrowed the list to nine apps and drafted a process for introducing the apps through the Primary Care Behavioral Health Integration program (PCBHI) in Primary Care. In drafting the process for introducing these apps to patients, we aimed to incorporate several elements: (a) suggestions to staff as to when to introduce the apps; (b) appropriate language for staff to use in discussing the apps with patients, and (c) brief descriptions of the apps in patient-facing materials. The evaluation team and Patient Partner Lead co-designed a set of tools for introducing the BH apps, including a patient-facing summary sheet describing the risks/benefits of using smartphone applications and a mobile apps "toolkit" that contained descriptions of the purpose and main features of the nine selected apps. We then trained six care managers to identify patients who might benefit from using mobile apps and introduce the tools to patients (including clinical rationale, product demonstration, goal setting, and plan for follow-up). Care managers were given additional training around discussing app privacy/security with patients and reviewed all points detailed within the patient-facing summary sheet. As a quality improvement project to improve access to high quality self-management tools within primary care, this implementation study was not subject to formal approval by our Institutional Review Board as per Cambridge Health Alliance's ethics guidelines and national regulations. Before introducing the selected mobile apps to patients, care managers obtained informed verbal and written consent from all pilot participants and no personally identifiable information was collected during the course of the pilot.

Step 3: Initial Pilot Testing

Before disseminating the apps toolkit across our integrated care system, the team conducted pilot-testing over 2 months at the six primary care clinics where the trained care managers were located. During the pilot, patients were referred to care managers by consult psychiatrists, integrated therapists, and primary care providers through "warm handoffs" or the real-time transfer of patients from one provider to another. When demonstrating mobile applications, care managers used iPads available in the clinic or their own smartphones (with appropriate security measures in place). After ~2–4 weeks, care managers followed up with patients either in person or by phone to conduct structured interviews in which patients were asked the following questions: Did you use the app? Did you find it to be helpful? Do you have any additional comments?

Following the formal conclusion of the pilot, care managers continued to gather feedback related to patients' experience over the course of 1 year. Preliminary themes were identified through review of all available data, several group discussions leading to consensus in our multidisciplinary team, and updated with data gathered in the larger roll out as described below.

Following the pilot test, we evaluated patient and care manager feedback and adapted procedures to roll out the program to all 12 of our primary-care practices. Our final toolkit contained seven apps as we removed two apps from the list of nine used during the pilot. As smartphone apps are dynamic and always changing, during this phase of the study new information about a smoking app became available that led our team to substitute for one from the pilot—reflecting the real-world challenge of using apps in health care (see **Figure 1**).

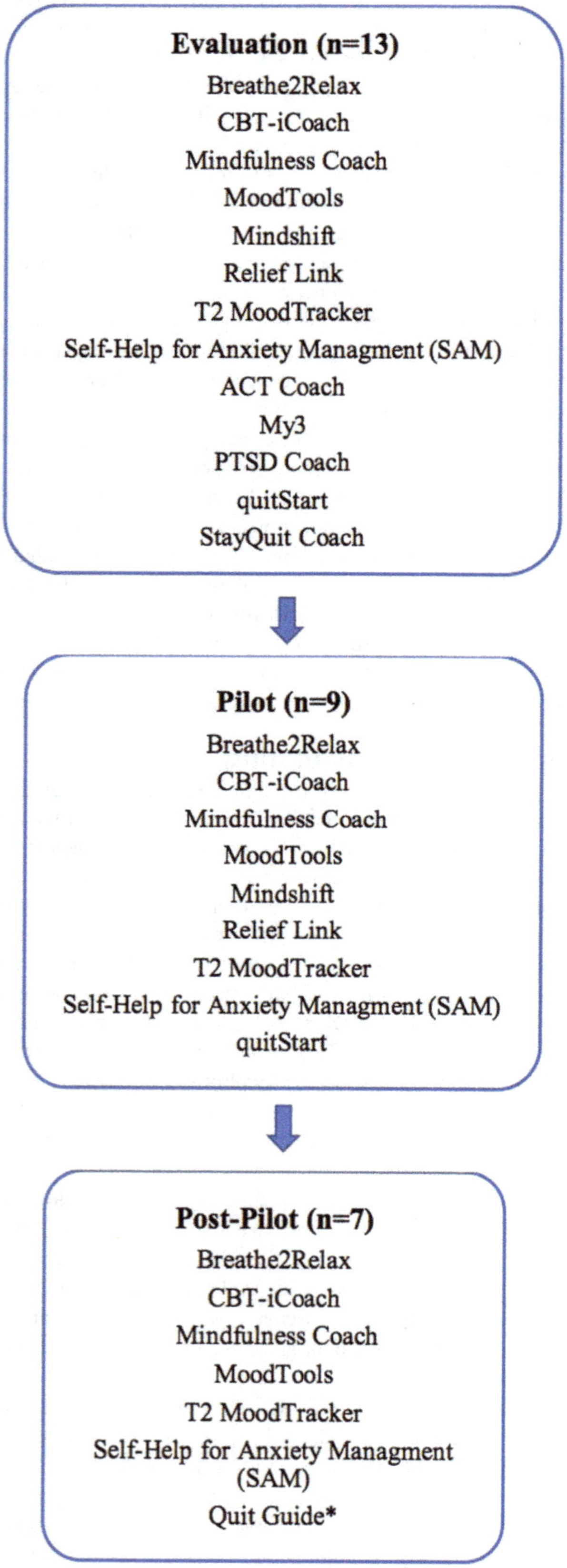

FIGURE 1 | App selection across stages of the study. *Quit guide replaced quitStart with post-pilot input from CHA's tobacco treatment team.

Step 4: Staff Training and App Dissemination

To facilitate use of apps by staff, we wrote two electronic medical record (EMR) standardized "smart phrases" which could be incorporated into patient-facing after-visit summary documents. These "smart phrases" contained the list of recommended self-management apps and the patient-facing summary sheet explaining risks/benefits of using mobile apps. Through a series of staff meetings, we trained all integrated BH staff (therapists, consult psychiatrists, care managers) on best practices for utilizing mental health apps within clinical care. Because of the pilot testing and early staff engagement in the project, many were already familiar with the basic premise of the project and supportive of its goals.

One year after staff training and dissemination of CHA's mobile apps toolkit across all 12 primary care clinics, we followed up by sending a survey to integrated BH staff. In this survey, we asked questions exploring (a) staff utilization of apps; (b) perceived clinical impact, and (c) experience introducing apps to patients.

RESULTS

Quantitative Patient Experience

Over the 2-month duration of the pilot intervention, care managers introduced mental health apps to 56 adult patients. Fifty-four (96.4%) patients agreed to use the tools while 2 (3.5%) patients declined (1 due to security concerns and 1 due to time constraints). Patients in the pilot were 18–70 years old with a mean age of 36.5 years, and 37 (66.1%) were female. English was not the language of medical care for 6 (10.7%) patients; 4 (7.1%) primarily spoke Portuguese and 2 (3.5%) primarily spoke Spanish. The tools were introduced to 35 (62.5%) patients for anxiety and stress-related issues and to 20 (35.7%) patients for depression. Eight (14.2%) patients received apps to target sleep issues and 3 (5.3%) patients were introduced to apps for other issues. Thirteen (23.2%) of the 56 patients were introduced to the tools for multiple conditions/issues.

The care managers were unable to follow-up with 19 patients during the 2-month pilot period. Of the 35 (64.8%) patients who provided feedback on usage of the tools, 7 (20%) patients were unable to use the tools (3 due to equipment limitations, 4 for other reasons). Twenty-three (65.7%) of patients who provided feedback found the apps to be helpful. Twenty-four (68.5%) of patients reported using Breathe2Relax and 24 (68.5%) reported using Self-Help for Anxiety Management (SAM). Patients used Breathe2Relax to help them sleep, to manage anxiety, and to prepare for stressful or mentally taxing situations. When using SAM, patients tended to access just a few of the features that focused on symptom relief, education about anxiety, strategies for managing strong emotions, and mood tracking. (**Figure 2**)

Qualitative Patient Experience

After the 2-month pilot and over the course of the following year, care managers collected general feedback from patients that is presented in **Table 1** as a combination of paraphrasing and direct quotes. Review of this feedback by our multidisciplinary team

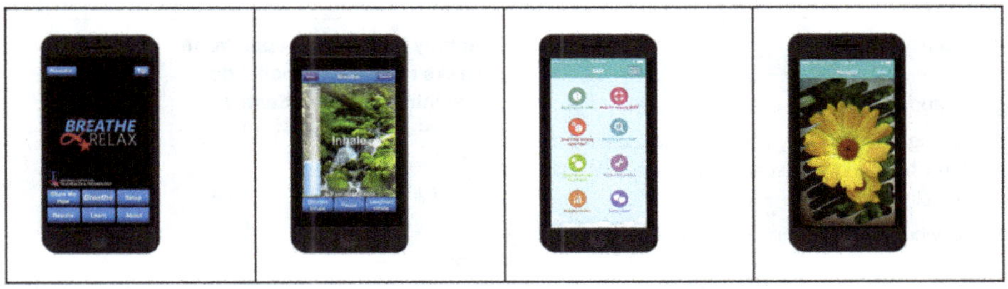

FIGURE 2 | Screenshots of Breathe2Relax (Left two) and Self-Help for Anxiety Management (Right two).

and discussion yielded consensus around 7 broad themes: ease of use, educational value, role in self-monitoring and enhancing self-awareness, relaxation/mindfulness, ability to incorporate into daily life, data and security concerns, and value of staff role in encouraging engagement with mental health apps.

Quantitative Staff Experience

After 1 year of the intervention (which involved 32 integrated BH staff), 24 (75%) completed the follow-up survey. Within the integrated BH team roles, nine (100%) care managers, 12 (75%) psychotherapists, and 3 (43%) consult psychiatrists responded. The number of responses to each survey item varied.

Twenty-three (95.8%) BH staff members answered the survey question regarding their utilization of mobile tools with patients; nineteen people (82.6%) indicated that they incorporate BH apps into their clinical work. Five (25%) BH staff members out of 20 indicated that they introduce apps to patients 25–50% of the time, and 9 (45%) introduce mobile tools <25% of the time. When using apps with patients, the condition addressed most often by BH staff was anxiety 20 (83.3%), followed by stress 18 (75%), depression 14 (58.3%), alcohol use 6 (25%), and tobacco use 6 (25%). Of the 23 (95.8%) staff members who reported on their experience using the CHA's mobile app toolkit, the apps most commonly used were Breathe2Relax, Mindfulness Coach, and Self-Help for Anxiety Management (see **Table 2** below). The survey also assessed techniques and strategies staff employed in introducing apps to patients: 19 (79.1%) reported discussing access/interest/ability, 14 (58.3%) discussed clinical basis for recommending that app and how it connects with the patient's goals, 14 (58.3%) demonstrated how to use the app, 13 (54.1%) helped the patient download the app, 13 (54.1%) followed up and discussed app use with patients at later visits, 12 (50%) set a follow up plan for app use, 9 (37.5%) discussed security and privacy risk associated with app use, and 7 (29.1%) created an action plan around app use.

BH staff found a variety of benefits and challenges to incorporating apps into clinical care (see **Table 3**) and 10 out of 24 BH staff (42%) expressed a need for more practice and training on using each tool within the CHA's mobile app toolkit.

Qualitative Staff Experience

Consult psychiatrists, therapists, and care managers were also asked to provide qualitative/free-text feedback on apps in the 1 year follow-up survey. Representative responses for the three most utilized apps are presented below in **Table 4** alongside patient feedback. Feedback concerning clinical use, accessibility, patient engagement/motivation, and other areas is presented below in **Table 5**.

DISCUSSION

Our results of piloting the use of smartphone apps in a primary care setting with integrated BH staff demonstrate the feasibility, opportunity, and challenges of introducing mobile technologies into formal care settings. Through our program of mobile app evaluation, pilot-testing, and 1 year long local dissemination into routine practice we demonstrated that mental health apps can be introduced to patients of varying ages, literacy levels, and English-language proficiency. On the patient side, our results suggest that patients found the mobile tools helpful in learning about their mental health conditions, practicing relaxation skills, and monitoring mood symptoms. Barriers to use included technical limitations (e.g., lack of smartphone, limited data), difficulty incorporating into daily life, low motivation, and limited mental health app options for non-English speaking patients. On the clinical side, members of the integrated care teams were receptive to apps but used them with patients <50% of the time—with chief barriers including lack of time to discuss apps and being unfamiliar or uncomfortable with apps.

While our study results reflect the experience at a single healthcare system in an urban environment, several lessons learned in our experience are generalizable. Reflecting on both the successes as well as areas for further improvement in our development and rollout of apps for integrated care teams offers insights for others seeking to build their own app libraries, develop app toolkits, onboard staff, and engage patients.

Selecting Apps and the Need to Update

Selecting appropriate apps to recommend for use in integrated care is a core element in a successful rollout, but also a moving target as these apps are constantly updating and evolving. Relying on websites or services that claim to curate apps and score them based on certain metrics is not helpful, as such scores do not take into account the unique needs of intended users (e.g., lower literacy levels), and do not reflect the simple reality that apps frequently update and change. We found that gathering a multidisciplinary panel to search, evaluate, and test apps was

TABLE 1 | Key themes and illustrative quotes from the 1 year study.

Theme	Illustrative quote
Ease of use	"I like that this app is simple and easy to navigate"
	"I do the breathing exercise every time I get into the car. I also shared it with my boyfriend who speaks Portuguese. We do the exercise together."
	"I use this app when I'm waiting in the car at my daughter's school"
	"I like short exercises. I can use them in different places"
	"I can do a walking meditation during my lunch break"
Education	"The TED talks were helpful"
	"I re-read the education sections as a reminder"
	"I like being told I'm not crazy"
	"It was helpful learning more about anxiety and coping thoughts"
Self-monitoring and Self-awareness	"I want to track my mood so I can show the data to my therapist. I can't always remember how I felt during the week"
	"I like data. Recording my mood every day helps me to know I'm doing ok"
	"I track my mood before and after I do an activity. The next time I think about exercising, I can look back to see how I felt afterwards"
	"The sleep diary helps me to keep track of my sleep patterns. It's easier than trying to remember later on"
	"I record how I'm feeling and also what's making me anxious"
	"I had a hard time identifying my thoughts. Maybe I could focus on this in therapy?"
	"Doing the exercise helped me to recognize how tense and anxious I can be"
	"When I use the app, it's easier for me to size up my thoughts. I can then figure out whether they're trivial or beyond my control"
Relaxation/ Mindfulness	"The progressive muscle relaxation exercise helps me to fall asleep"
	"I enjoyed the exercise focusing on one sensation. I think this app could be helpful to many patients"
	"The app was calming and relaxing"
	"I love the app and guided relaxation for mindfulness"
	"I use the guided imagery exercise with a student at my school. We do it every day during nap time. It helps him and it helps me too!"
	"It used to take me hours to fall asleep. Now it takes me 7 min"
Difficulty incorporating into daily life	"I don't always remember to use the app when I'm stressed"
	"Sometimes I forget to use it. I tell myself I'm going to do it later and then I forget"
	"I looked at the app, but I didn't use it on a regular basis"
	"Apps are overwhelming when I'm stressed. I need to get away from technology"
Data and security concerns	"I worry about my virtual image. I'd feel more comfortable using an app from CHA that is protected in the same way my EMR is protected"
	"I don't have space on my phone"
	"I'm worried about my data"
Staff support	"It was helpful learning about the different parts of the app. I downloaded it in the past, but I didn't understand the point of the exercises"
	"Having you check in with me helped to keep me on track"

TABLE 2 | Apps most frequently recommended by BH staff.

Survey Item: Which apps from CHA's mobile app toolkit do you introduce to patients?	Reponses ($N = 23$) *n* (%)
Breathe2Relax	14 (61)
Mindfulness coach	12 (52)
SAM	10 (43)
CBT-iCoach	9 (39)
Moodtools	5 (22)
T2Moodtracker	3 (13)
QuitforLife	3 (13)

TABLE 3 | Staff views on the benefits and challenges of utilizing BH apps.

Survey Item	Response ($N = 23$) *n* (%)
IN GENERAL, WHAT DO YOU THINK ARE THE BENEFITS OF INCORPORATING APPS INTO CLINICAL CARE? (SELECT ALL THAT APPLY)	
Patients have the opportunity to practice self-management skills between meetings	15 (65)
Using apps enhances care provided by therapist and primary care provider	13 (57)
Patients' ability to manage mood/anxiety/substance use improves when using apps	13 (57)
Patients are excited to try self-management tools	11 (48)
Patients feel more confident in managing their BH conditions independently	9 (38)
IN GENERAL, WHAT DO YOU THINK ARE SOME CHALLENGES TO INCORPORATING APPS INTO CLINICAL CARE? (SELECT ALL THAT APPLY)	
My patients do not have enough data on phones to use apps	6 (26)
I do not have enough time during my sessions to introduce self-help tools	5 (22)
I am unfamiliar with apps' content and functionality	5 (22)
I do not feel comfortable navigating apps and demonstrating use to patient	5 (22)
My patients are not interested in using apps	2 (8)
I do not believe they would be helpful for my patients	0 (0)
My patients are concerned about data security	0 (0)
I am unsure how to assess whether a patient could benefit from using an app	0 (0)

useful and practical. Such a panel should remain an ongoing and integral part of any app rollout and ideally meet at least quarterly to continue to update and evaluate new apps and new evidence. In terms of searching for new apps to support integrated care, we noted that apps selected in our search focused on helping patients learn more about their mental health conditions, enhance self-awareness, develop skills related to distress tolerance, and improve anxiety management. While we realize that today's mental health apps offer functionalities that can allow for real time monitoring and facilitate communication with the treatment team, such functionalities raise a number of complex questions related to risk/privacy/liability that

TABLE 4 | Top three apps utilized by staff during the 1 year study (as reported through the staff survey).

App	Developer	Description	Popular features	Patient feedback	Staff feedback
Breathe2Relax	Defense health agency connected health (formerly the National Center for Telehealth and Technology)	Developed for military personnel. Contains step-by-step instructions for diaphragmatic breathing, provides a visually engaging audio guided breathing exercise, and enables users to record their stress levels using a tracking function. http://t2health.dcoe.mil/apps/breathe2relax	Guided diaphragmatic breathing exercise	"I have been doing it every day. I feel like it is cleaning my brain. I have been suggesting it to my friends. I learned that problems we will always have, but I feel more patient now. I noticed some changes on my self-esteem I am becoming more optimistic. I used to have mind racing and not anymore"	"I like Breathe2Relax's visuals" "Breathe2Relax is more popular because it is easier - no language barrier" "Breathe2Relax is very useful as it contains education about deep breathing, a basic exercise and the option to personalize settings"
Self-Help for Anxiety Management (SAM)	The University of the West of England	Developed for college students with low to moderate anxiety. SAM is a "platform of interactive, therapeutic, and well-being exercises" meant to assist users with learning about anxiety, cognitive reframing, relaxation, distress tolerance, lifestyle change and self-monitoring of physical and emotional states related to anxiety. http://sam-app.org.uk	"Picture Peace" "Stop That Thought" "It's Only a Thought" Anxiety Tracker Anxiety Education	Picture Peace: "I slow down and think about what's bothering me" Stop That Thought: "I noticed my thoughts going from "this is annoying" to "I've made a horrible mistake taking this job". Writing my thoughts down makes me realize how absurd they are and banishing them in the app helps me to better reframe the situation and get more perspective"	"For SAM, I use the picture peace, stop that thought, and it's only a thought features most often" "Patients really like the picture peace feature; I use it too!"
Mindfulness coach	VA's National Center for PTSD and DoD's National Center for Telehealth & Technology	This app was developed to help Veterans, Service members, and others learn how to practice mindfulness. It offers exercises, information, and a tracking log so that you can optimize your practice. https://mobile.va.gov/app/mindfulness-coach	Guided mindfulness exercises	"I used to get jammed up about small things. Doing these exercises helped me to realize that burnt pizza isn't the end of the world"	"Mindfulness coach is great, but I wish it were also available for android. I like the guided mindfulness better than on moodtools especially if it is for a patient not with depression"

could not be addressed within the scope of this quality improvement project.

Building a Toolkit and the Need for More Hands-On Training or a New Digital Navigator

Although the app toolkit that we developed to help the clinical teams introduce, integrate, and support app use was critical to success, it was not sufficient in and of itself. Offering the clinical team a list of apps, core information and talking points on each app, and electronic medical record smart phrases to document app usage was key to the feasibility of the intervention. Clinical staff recommended apps that had a clear purpose, simple user-interface, and were easy to navigate and demonstrate within a brief period of time. When introducing Breathe2Relax, for example, staff were often able to review the technique of diaphragmatic breathing, help patients to personalize settings, and practice the app's guided breathing exercise in under 10 min. Mental health apps that have a clear purpose and that are easy to review during staff trainings may enhance BH staff confidence and efficiency in introducing these tools to patients and facilitate higher adoption across the primary care system.

However, we found that the clinical teams sought additional support in understanding how each app worked, in demonstrating apps to patients, and having enough time in clinical visits to discuss an app. This suggests two possible responses: either (a) further hands-on training for clinical staff or (b) the introduction of a new member of the care team in the form of a digital navigator. While there is little evidence to support optimal teaching strategies for app use, we propose that hands on training involving role playing introducing and using apps with patients may offer an effective means to help the clinical team feel more confident in using apps in care settings. Another option would be to refer patients to a new member of the care team called a digital navigator—much as we did in the initial pilot study with the care manager—who is an expert at setting up, teaching, and supporting use of apps. This is akin to

TABLE 5 | Organizing themes and illustrative quotes from staff survey.

Theme	Illustrative quote
Clinical use	"For CBT-iCoach, I use the "quiet your mind" tools that contains progressive muscle relaxation exercises and guided imagery"
	"Before the app, I tried to do sleep diaries with patients on paper. They were mostly unsuccessful since the patient would lose the paper or forget to complete it. With the app, patients have access to their phones all the time and can send reminders to themselves"
	"Great way to have patients practice exercises between sessions; both provider and patient happy to have concrete tool"
	"Apps are containing when patients feeling stressed; some are fun to use"
	"The positive is that the app is free and easy to utilize, the downside is that a patient may spend too much time engaging on their phone and not building relationships with others/community. The young adult patients enjoy the apps, while the older patients want to belong to a community, i.e., yoga, tai chi, or meditation class"
	"I don't use them very often because I do a lot of guided relaxation in session and have my patients record them on their phone. Usually I think this kind of approach is best because it allows me to make the exercise specific to their needs. That some of the apps are helpful for specific skills like breathing with the metronome (if that is what it is called I am not sure)"
	"Sometimes I think my training in behavioral medicine allows me to create a different tool with the patient that is more specific to them"
	"I like PTSD Coach and Insight Timer as well"
	"The simple practice of using the app(phone) as a way to relax and take a mindful minute"
	"I use them very often. Mostly Breathe2Relax and SAM"
Accessibility	"To me, it is very difficult to incorporate the apps because they are only in English"
	"Some apps too complicated to explain quickly; patient seems overwhelmed"
	"Sometimes it takes too long to download an app with the patient, sometimes they need to come and see me for a second time to practice together"
	"Definitely language is a barrier for some of them"
Patient engagement & motivation	"Patients are generally receptive to the idea. Most that have put it into practice have been practicing mindful breathing, some are still having trouble maintaining ongoing use in order to derive any benefit"
	"Most of them don't end up downloading it/using it"
	"Patient only used app one time to learn deep breathing exercise, but continued practicing deep breathing before bed without assistance of app"
	"Usually I do not have negative feedback but I notice a good number of patients mentions they did not continue using in home. Sometimes they say: "I forgot to use it." Maybe because this area is still new for patients? I am not sure"
	"Patients like it- they like that they have an option to do something on their own to look at after the visit"
	"Recently I had a good feedback from a patient (serious case of DV) that the breathing exercises was helping her a lot and she was even teaching her friends. I was impressed how excited she was about the exercises. Patient states feeling more calm, has been sleeping much better. She is still not completely free of nightmares but improved a lot. She used to have nightmares every day but this week had two times a week"
	"Usually I get good feedback from patients. I call them about 2 weeks after my visit and check with them but I do not have the info if they continue using for a long time"
Additional feedback	"Technology is in"
	"Re: question 7: training the PCPs about the tools; a lot of them don't know about it. They could introduce patients to tools then do a warm handoff to the care partner"
	"Instead of formal training, I think more case examples of how the apps were incorporated can be a helpful reminder about using the apps. I admit that since I see both kids and young adults, I sometimes forget about the many options available to someone 18+"

referring a patient to a pharmacist on the team to learn more about medication or dietician to craft a customized healthy eating plan.

Supporting Patients With Apps and Ensuring Apps Are Accessible

Patients in our study found apps useful and preferred those with clear purpose that had an engaging interface, were intuitive to use, and easy to navigate. The preference for simplicity aligns with findings within the field of user experience and design (26) as well as emerging research (27, 28) suggesting that apps containing a limited number of concepts and activities may be more appealing than those with a number of features. Apps containing limited text and simple/concrete language demand less from a cognitive standpoint (29) and may prove most accessible if patients are turning to apps during times of emotional distress when their cognitive abilities are compromised. Of note, the most popular feature within our mobile apps "toolkit" was "Picture Peace" a grounding exercise within Self-Help for Anxiety Management (SAM) that involves swiping across a blank screen to reveal a nature photo beneath. Patients described this feature as being "fun" and chose to use it over other exercises that were less visually pleasing and that demanded more from a cognitive standpoint.

However, the lack of apps available in multiple languages was also a limiting factor that made it impossible to use apps with some patients who may have benefited from this intervention. Several patients were also unable to run apps on their phone because of issues installing the apps or lacking sufficient memory on their smartphone to run the apps.

Connecting to Care Through Apps

Our results also suggest new clinical applications for mental health apps beyond those studied and implemented in our study. Within our integrated primary care model, care managers often serve as a "bridge" to longer-term BH care, providing education about BH conditions, teaching basic distress-tolerance skills, and focusing on brief interventions related to lifestyle behavior change. In using mental health apps, patients can begin to develop greater insight into their thoughts, feelings, and behaviors, an essential component of any therapeutic treatment intervention. Providing patients with self-management apps while they are waiting for in-person BH services may also help patients to stay connected to their care team and cultivate a sense of "emotional holding" during this bridging period (29). These apps may also spread awareness and interest in BH services, as evidenced by multiple patients who shared a recommended app with friends and family because they thought it may be useful to them as well.

These same apps may help introduce patients to BH treatment who would have otherwise not been interested or declined to engage because of stigma, discomfort or misunderstanding about the field and treatments offered. Thus, the potential of population health enabled through apps and digital technology will remain a focus of our continued research. While our study did not explore potential cost-savings associated with our intervention, we plan to investigate the financial implications of digitally augmented integrated BH care in future studies.

Limitations

Like all studies, ours has several limitations. As a real-world implementation study that sought to understand feasibility of app selection, uptake, and introduction into integrated care clinics—we were unable to control for many variables including patient severity, disease state, and clinician participation among others. In considering our patients' feedback that was not incorporated into a formal qualitative framework, we recognize that having care managers solicit feedback directly from patients may have influenced patient self-report and the subsequent interpretation of this data. Also given how often apps update and change—we realize that our results are difficult for others to replicate especially as we tailored our research to the local needs of the patients we serve. While we believe our study included a representative sample, it is difficult to quantify the number of types of patients, or clinicians, who are willing to engage and use apps as part of care. Further, we realize there are currently no gold standard apps, gold standard methods to select apps, or gold standard tools to quantify the impact of apps on care. Thus, we hope that the process and results of this present research can help guide others in taking the first steps to study the best ways to introduce digital technologies like apps into their clinical settings.

CONCLUSIONS

Although there are barriers to implementing digital technologies like smartphone apps into integrated BH settings, with careful planning and stakeholder engagement they can be useful tools in real-world clinical settings. While apps alone are not a panacea to addressing limited access to mental health care and lifestyle interventions, when deployed thoughtfully, they can help extend care to support patients with mild and moderate behavioral health conditions on a personal level and communities on a population level.

AUTHOR CONTRIBUTIONS

All authors listed have made a substantial, direct and intellectual contribution to the work, and approved it for publication.

REFERENCES

World Health Organization, World Organization of National Colleges, Academies, Academic Associations of General Practitioners/Family Physicians. *Integrating Mental Health into Primary Care: A Global Perspective.* New York, NY: World Health Organization (2008).

http://www.who.int/en/news-room/fact-sheets/detail/depression Joseph R, Kester R, O'Brien C, Huang H. The evolving practice of psychiatry in the era of integrated care. *Psychosomatics* (2017) 58:466–73. doi: 10.1016/j.psym.2017.04.003

Wang PS, Demler O, Olfson M, Pincus HA, Wells KB, Kessler RC. Changing profiles of service sectors used for mental health care in the United States American. *J Psychiatry* (2006) 163:1187–98. doi: 10.1176/ajp.2006.16 3.7.1187

Raney L, Bergman D, Torous J, Hasselberg M. Digitally driven integrated primary care and behavioral health: how technology can expand access to effective treatment. *Curr Psychiatry Rep.* (2017) 19:86. doi:10.1007/s11920-017-0838-y

Torous J, Chan SR, Tan SY, Behrens J, Mathew I, Conrad EJ, et al. Patient smartphone ownership and interest in mobile apps to monitor symptoms of mental health conditions: a survey in four geographically distinct psychiatric clinics. *JMIR Ment Health* (2014) 1:e5. doi: 10.2196/mental.4004

Chan S, Godwin H, Gonzalez A, Yellowlees PM, Hilty DM. Review of use and integration of mobile apps into psychiatric treatments. *Curr Psychiatry Rep.* (2017) 19:96. doi: 10.1007/s11920-017-0848-9

Anthes E. Pocket psychiatry: mobile mental-health apps have exploded onto the market, but few have been thoroughly tested. *Nature* (2016) 532:20–4. doi: 10.1038/532020a

Firth J, Torous J, Nicholas J, Carney R, Pratap A, Rosenbaum S, et al. (2017). The efficacy of smartphone-based mental health interventions for depressive symptoms: a meta-analysis of randomized controlled trials. *World Psychiatry* 16:287–98. doi: 10.1002/wps.20472

Firth J, Torous J, Nicholas J, Carney R, Rosenbaum S, Sarris J. Can smartphone mental health interventions reduce symptoms of anxiety? a meta- analysis of randomized controlled trials. *J Affect Disord.* (2017) 218:15–22. doi:10.1016/j.jad.2017.04.046

Torous J, Roberts LW. Needed innovation in digital health and smartphone applications for mental health: transparency and trust. *JAMA Psychiatry* (2017) 74:437–8. doi: 10.1001/jamapsychiatry.2017.0262

Sandoval LR, Torous J, Keshavan MS. Smartphones for smarter care? self-management in schizophrenia. *Am J Psychiatry* (2017) 174:725–8. doi:10.1176/appi.ajp.2017.16090990

Torous J, Roux S. Patient-driven innovation for mobile mental health technology: case report of symptom tracking in schizophrenia. *JMIR Ment Health* (2017) 4:e27. doi: 10.2196/mental.7911

Gustafson DH, McTavish FM, Chih MY, Atwood AK, Johnson RA, Boyle MG, et al. A smartphone application to support recovery from alcoholism: a randomized clinical trial. *JAMA Psychiatry* (2014) 71:566–72. doi: 10.1001/jamapsychiatry.2013.4642

Ford II JH, Alagoz E, Dinauer S, Johnson KA, Pe-Romashko K, Gustafson DH. Successful organizational strategies to sustain use of A-CHESS: a mobile intervention for individuals with alcohol use disorders. *J Med Internet Res.* (2015) 17:e201. doi: 10.2196/jmir.3965

Gagnon MP, Ngangue P, Payne-Gagnon J, Desmartis M. m-Health adoption by healthcare professionals: a systematic review. *J Am Med Informat Assoc.* (2015) 23:212–20. doi: 10.1093/jamia/ocv052

Bennion MR, Hardy G, Moore RK, Millings A. E-therapies in England for stress, anxiety or depression: what is being used in the NHS? A survey of mental health services. *BMJ Open* (2017) 7:e014844. doi: 10.1136/ bmjopen-2016-014844

Sarkar U, Gourley GI, Lyles CR, Tieu L, Clarity C, Newmark L, et al. Usability of commercially available mobile applications for diverse patients. *J Gen Int Med.* (2016) 31:1417–26. doi: 10.1007/s11606-016-3771-6

Zallman L, Joseph R, O'Brien C, Benedetto E, Grossman E, Arsenault L, et al. (2017). Does behavioral health integration improve primary care providers' perceptions of health-care system functioning and their own knowledge? *Gen Hosp Psychiatry* 46:88–93. doi: 10.1016/j.genhosppsych.2017.03.005

Archer J, Bower P, Gilbody S, Lovell K, Richards D, Gask L, et al. Collaborative care for depression and anxiety problems. *Cochrane Database Syst Rev.* (2012):10:CD006525. doi: 10.1002/14651858.CD006525.pub2

Babor TF, McRee BG, Kassebaum PA, Grimaldi PL, Ahmed K, Bray J. Screening, brief intervention, and referral to treatment (SBIRT) toward a public health approach to the management of substance abuse. *Subst Abuse* (2007) 28:7–30. doi: 10.1300/J465v28n03_03

East ML, Havard BC. Mental health mobile apps: from infusion to diffusion in the mental health social system. *JMIR Ment Health* (2015) 2:e10. doi: 10.2196/mental.3954

Torous J, Firth J, Huckvale K, Larsen ME, Cosco TD, Carney R, et al. The emerging imperative for a consensus approach toward the rating and clinical recommendation of mental health apps. *J Nerv Ment Dis.* (2018) 206:662–6 doi: 10.1097/NMD.0000000000000864

Chan S, Torous J, Hinton L, Yellowlees, P. (2015). Brief Communication: toward a framework for evaluating mobile mental health apps. *Telemed J E Health* 21:1038–41 doi: 10.1089/tmj.2015.0002

Stoyanov SR, Hides L, Kavanagh DJ, Wilson H. Development and validation of the user version of the mobile application rating scale (uMARS). *JMIR Mhealth Uhealth* (2016) 4:e72. doi: 10.2196/mhealt h.5849.

https://www.nngroup.com/articles/simplicity-vs-choice/?lm=outcomes-vs-features&pt=article Mohr DC, Tomasino KN, Lattie EG, Palac HL, Kwasny MJ, Weingardt K, et al. (2017). Intellicare: an eclectic, skills-based app suite for the treatment of depression and anxiety. *J Med Internet Res.* 19:1–14. doi: 10.2196/jmi r.6645

Bakker D, Kazantzis N, Rickwood D, Rickard N. Mental health smartphone apps: review and evidence-based recommendations for future developments. *JMIR Ment Health* (2016) 3:e7 doi: 10.2196/mental.4984

Topham P,Matthews P. *Project SAM: Developing an App to Provide Self-Help for Anxiety PART 1: REPORT* (2015). Available online at: http://eprints.uwe.ac.uk/27231

5

The Effect of Mindfulness-Based Intervention on Brain-Derived Neurotrophic Factor (BDNF)

Patama Gomutbutra[1,2*], *Nalinee Yingchankul*[1], *Nipon Chattipakorn*[3], *Siriporn Chattipakorn*[3,4] *and Manit Srisurapanont*[5]

[1] Department of Family Medicine, Faculty of Medicine, Chiang Mai University, Chiang Mai, Thailand, [2] The Northern Neuroscience Center, Faculty of Medicine Chiang Mai University, Chiang Mai, Thailand, [3] Center of Excellence in Cardiac Electrophysiology Research, Faculty of Medicine, Chiang Mai University, Chiang Mai, Thailand, [4] Department of Oral Biology and Diagnostic Sciences, Faculty of Dentistry, Chiang Mai University, Chiang Mai, Thailand, [5] Department of Psychiatry, Faculty of Medicine Chiang Mai University, Chiang Mai, Thailand

***Correspondence:**
Patama Gomutbutra
patthama.g@cmu.ac.th

Background: This systematic review aims to answer three questions. First, how much do mindfulness-based interventions (MBIs) affect peripheral brain-derived neurotrophic factor (BDNF)? Second, do mindfulness exercise–based interventions (exercise-MBIs) and mindfulness meditation–based interventions (meditation-MBIs) affect peripheral BDNF differently? Third, does the age of participants and the accumulative hours of MBI practice affect peripheral BDNF?

Methods: We included randomized controlled trials comparing MBI and no intervention in adults (age >18 years) who reported peripheral BDNF. Database searches included PubMed, CINAHL, CENTRAL, PsyInfo, and Scopus. Two reviewers independently selected the studies and assessed the trial quality. We used the standardized mean difference (SMD) as the effect size index and conducted moderator analyses.

Results: Eleven studies are included in this systematic review. Five studies applying exercise-MBI and three studies applying meditation-MBI are included in the meta-analysis ($N = 479$). The pooled effect size shows a significantly greater increase of peripheral BDNF in MBI groups compared to the control groups (k = 8, N = 479, SMD = 0.72, 95% CI 0.31–1.14, $I^2 = 78\%$). Significantly more increases of BDNF in the MBI groups are found in both subgroups of exercise-MBI and meditation-MBI. The effect sizes of both subgroups are not significantly different between subgroups ($\chi^2 = 0.02$, $p = 0.88$). We find no significant correlation between the effect sizes and the age of participants ($r = -0.0095$, $p = 0.45$) or accumulative hours of MBI practice ($r = 0.0021$, $p = 0.57$).

Conclusion: The heterogeneous data of this small sample-size meta-analysis suggests that MBI can increase peripheral BDNF. Either exercise-MBI or meditation-MBI can increase peripheral BDNF.

Keywords: brain-derived neurotrophic factor, BDNF, mindfulness, meditation, neuroplasticity

INTRODUCTION

It is well-established that brain-derived neurotrophic factor (BDNF), a neuronal growth factor, affects neuronal survival and regeneration, called "neuronal plasticity" (Lu et al., 2014). Hence, there is increasing interest in the potential therapeutic effect of interventions that increase BDNF (Bathina and Das, 2015). BDNF is produced in both the central nervous system and peripheral tissues. The BDNF measured from blood, either from serum, plasma, or saliva, is called peripheral BDNF. Previous studies show peripheral BDNF is related to numerous brain disorders. A recent meta-analysis finds that lower levels of peripheral BDNF are associated with an increased risk of depression (Brunoni et al., 2008), Alzheimer's disease (Balietti et al., 2018), Parkinson's disease (Rahmani et al., 2019), and strokes with an unfavorable outcome (Xu et al., 2018). There have been attempts to provide external BDNF, but this has not been successful (Houlton et al., 2019) due to poor blood–brain barrier permeability and short therapeutic half-life (Poduslo and Curran, 1996). Some studies claim that acetylcholinesterase inhibitors and antidepressants may increase peripheral BDNF (Ströhle et al., 2015); however, the evidence still needs to be evaluated (Zhou et al., 2017). Currently, it would be safer and more feasible to promote lifestyle modification that increases BDNF.

Mindfulness, in a focused-attention practice, has been developed to be a health intervention. Mindfulness has been defined as "paying attention in a particular way, on purpose, in the present moment, and non-judgmentally" (Kabat-Zinn, 2003). Mindfulness-based interventions (MBIs) are practices that employ a variety of techniques designed to facilitate mindfulness to affect bodily function and symptoms. Regarding this definition, MBI can be divided into (1) mindfulness-based exercise, which emphasizes body movement, such as yoga, tai chi, and qi gong, and (2) meditation and its derivatives, which emphasize mentality training, such as mindfulness breathing, compassionate body scan, and working with emotions through imagination. This latter type of MBI also includes secular therapy like mindfulness-based stress relaxation (MBSR) and mindfulness-based cognitive therapy (MBCT) (Goldberg et al., 2018).

Numerous studies show that practicing MBI affects brain structure and function. In a meta-analysis of 21 studies, Fox and colleagues applied diffuse tensor imaging and voxel-based morphology imaging MRI to 300 meditation-naïve participants. They find brain changes, namely a moderate increase in brain size, in eight regions. These brain regions are the hippocampus, anterior and midcingulate gyrus, frontopolar cortex, sensory cortices and insula, orbitofrontal cortex, superior longitudinal fasciculus, and corpus callosum (Fox et al., 2014). Another meta-analysis of 18 studies of MBSR and MBCT also finds the improvement of working memory, autobiography memory, and cognitive flexibility after practicing MBI (Lao et al., 2016).

Similar to other interventions affecting brain function, MBIs have been assessed regarding their effects on the brain using the measure of peripheral BDNF. A recent meta-analysis finds that physical exercise, including mindfulness-based exercise (e.g., yoga, tai chi) increased peripheral BDNF (Dinoff et al., 2016). Because mindfulness-based exercise comprises light-to-moderate exercise and mindfulness meditation, it is not yet known if mindfulness meditation plays any role in such an increment (Ainsworth et al., 2000). Another study examining the effect of yoga on peripheral BDNF also reports that the increased peripheral BDNF is negatively correlated with age ($r = -0.446$) (Pal et al., 2014). In addition, a meta-analysis reports that cumulative hours of physical exercise is an effect modifier of peripheral BNDF increment (Dinoff et al., 2017).

The evidence mentioned above suggests that the effect of MBIs, especially the meditation part, on peripheral BDNF remains inconclusive. This systematic review and meta-analysis aims to answer three questions. First, how much does MBI affect peripheral BDNF? Second, do mindfulness exercise-based interventions (exercise-MBIs) and mindfulness meditation-based interventions (meditation-MBIs) affect peripheral BDNF differently? Third, does the age of MBI practitioners and the accumulative hours of MBI practice affect peripheral BDNF?

MATERIALS AND METHODS

The protocol of this systematic review (CRD42018093786) is registered at PROSPERO (International Prospective Register of Systematic Reviews). This present report follows the format of the PRISMA (Preferred Reporting Items for Systematic Reviews and Meta-analyses) Statement.

Inclusion Criteria of Studies

Studies that are included meet the following criteria: (i) a parallel or crossover randomized, controlled trial (RCT) in adults (age > 18 years); (ii) the experimental group receiving any type of MBI; (iii) the comparator group receiving no treatment, treatment as usual, or being on the waitlist; and (iv) the changes in plasma or serum BDNF after receiving MBI being reported or calculable.

Our meta-analysis does not include non-controlled (single-arm) trials due to the presence of confounding factors. One of the important confounders is called the "vacation effect." This effect is reported in some studies that show the non-intervention group also had peripheral BDNF changes during follow-up (Epel et al., 2016; Kwak et al., 2019). The BDNF changes suggesting a vacation effect, refers to the temporary improvements in health and psychological well-being after taking a vacation, which soon fade after work resumption (Goldberg et al., 2018). However, improved reliability should result from the balance of confounders in the comparison groups of RCTs. For this reason, it was decided to include only RCTs in our meta-analysis.

Data Sources and Searches

Searches were conducted on PubMed, EMBASE, The Cochrane Central Register of Controlled Trials (CENTRAL), and CINAHL (nursing and allied health professions), and PsyInfo from inception (2008) up to June 2020. For all full-text articles that passed the screening, their reference lists were examined to identify additional relevant studies ("snowball" method).

Study Selection and Quality Assessment

Two reviewers (PG and NY) independently selected the searched records, extracted the data, selected the studies, and assessed the trial quality. If any discrepancy existed, other investigators would additionally review and discuss with the first two reviewers to form a consensus.

After the completion of study selection, the data was extracted as recommended by the Center for Reviews and Dissemination. Each trial was evaluated using the Cochrane Collaboration four criteria for assessing the risk of bias. Those include (i) adequate generation of allocation sequence, (ii) concealment of allocation, (iii) prevention of knowledge of the allocated intervention, (iv) dealing with an incomplete data set, (v) selective report, and (vi) other bias.

Data Extraction

Apart from demographic and clinical characteristics, the changes in peripheral BNDF are the outcome of interest. In comparison to the endpoint peripheral BDNF, the mean changes are preferred because the included studies are likely to have small sample sizes. We declined to use the endpoints of peripheral BDNF because baseline data of paired groups enrolled in a small study might not be comparable although the randomization was applied.

The mean changes and standard deviations (SDs) of peripheral BDNF were extracted. If the study in which the means and SDs of BDNF level changes were not available, the means and SDs at baseline and endpoints were used to calculate the means and SDs of BDNF level changes. To estimate the SD of mean change of BDNF level changes, the baseline and postintervention correlation coefficient (r) were needed. If such r was not available, r was defined as 0.5 for the treatment group and 0.05 for the control group. This estimation was obtained from Ledreux et al. (2019), which is the only study that clearly reports the Pearson r for mindfulness practice $= 0.439$ and Pearson $r = 0.037$ for the control group.

Meta-Analysis

Because peripheral BDNF can be measured by various laboratory kits and reported in many unit systems, the standardized mean difference (SMD) is used as the effect size index. The present SMD is defined as the difference between the mean change of peripheral BDNF obtained from the experimental group and that obtained from the control groups. This, in turn, is divided by the pooled within-group SD. This is an appropriate index when the subjects are randomly assigned to the comparison groups with the assumption that both groups are equivalent at baseline (Rubio-Aparicio et al., 2018).

Heterogeneity is estimated using the I^2 statistic. If the heterogeneity of data is significantly high ($I^2 > 50\%$), effect sizes are pooled using a random-effect model. The effect sizes are interpreted as Cohen's recommendations: 0–0.19 = negligible effect, 0.20–0.49 = small effect, 0.50–0.79 = moderate effect, 0.80 or more = large effect (Schäfer and Schwarz, 2019). The publication bias is assessed visually using the funnel plot as in **Figure 1**. The number of trials expected to be able to be included in the meta-analysis is <10. Begg's test for funnel plot symmetrical also applies (Begg and Mazumdar, 1994).

Moderator Analyses

A subgroup analysis was conducted by separating the included studies into three subgroups based on the types of MBI. These included (i) exercise-MBI (e.g., yoga, tai chi), (ii) meditation-MBI, and (iii) other MBI practices (e.g., MBI added on other programs). Two meta-regression analyses were performed by computing the correlation coefficients (rs) between (i) the effect sizes and the average ages of participants and (ii) the effect sizes and the accumulated hours of MBI practice. The accumulated hours of MBI practice of each study were computed by multiplying the practice hours per week with the number of study weeks.

Software

All analyses and most of Figures were conducted using R 4.0 (R Core Team, 2016) and Figure 2 was produced by Robvis (McGuinness and Higgins, 2020).

RESULTS

Study Characteristics and Quality

The searches retrieved 522 records in total (see **Figure 1**). After the removal of duplicated records, record screening, and assessment of full-text articles, 11 studies met the inclusion criteria and are included in this systematic review. All studies were conducted in adults with a median age of 48 (range 31–84) years, slightly predominantly female with common diagnoses of psychiatric problems and low burdens of physical health. The median accumulative intervention exposure was 28 h (range 8–158 h). **Table 1** shows other characteristics of the included studies. The included studies pose a low-to-moderate risk of bias. The common risk is that no study could blind interventions. **Figure 2** shows other issues of methodological quality in the included studies.

Of 11 included studies, five (Ikai et al., 2014; Naveen et al., 2016, Tolahunase et al., 2017; Sungkarat et al., 2018) and three (Fox et al., 2014; Gagrani et al., 2018; Nery et al., 2019) studies are parallel RCTs applying exercise-MBI and meditation-MBI, respectively. These eight studies had a follow-up duration between 8 and 36 weeks. Due to their similarities, these eight studies are included in the meta-analysis ($N = 479$).

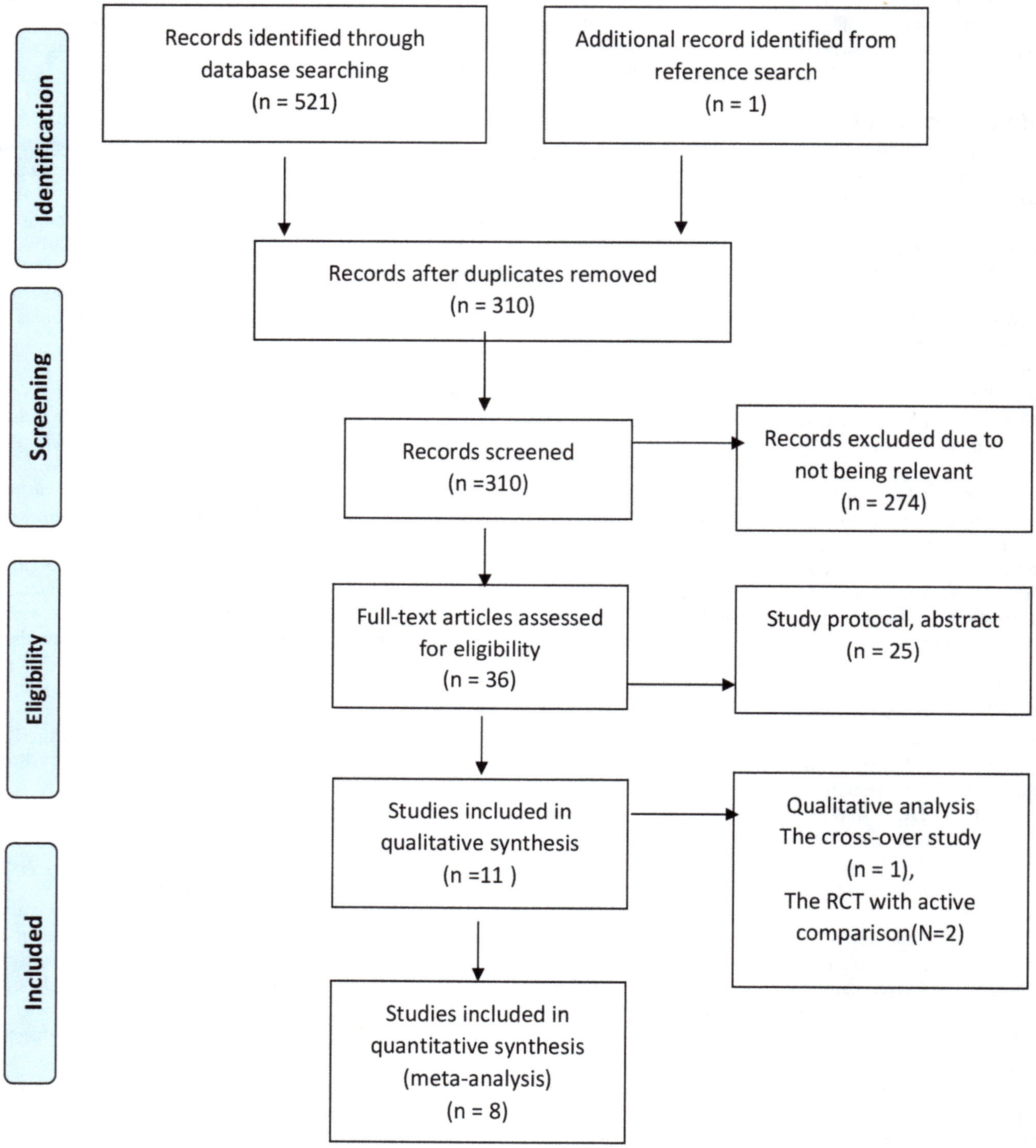

FIGURE 1 | Algorithm of study selection following PRISMA guideline.

The three following studies (Håkansson et al., 2016; Montero-Marin et al., 2019; Ng et al., 2020) are very dissimilar in character of intervention and control group to the first eight studies. They are included in the qualitative analysis only. Håkansson et al. conducts a crossover study in 19 healthy elders. However, this study was excluded because it applied only active interventions of cognitive training and physical exercise in the control arms. All participants went through different training commercial applications for 35 min each. The study measured the peripheral BDNF within 0, 20, and

TABLE 1 | The included studies for systematic review (*Not included studies in the meta-analysis).

Study	Study design	Participant condition and number	Average age of participants	Intervention	Control	Accumulative hours of mindfulness intervention practice	BDNF baseline and post-intervention	BDNF change from baseline comparing intervention and control (effect size, SE)
MINDFULNESS BASED EXERCISE								
Lee et al. (2014)	Parallel RCT	low back pain with depression $N = 25$	40.5 F 100%	Yoga	Regular lifestyle	1 h X 3 times/week X 12 weeks = 36 h	Serum, ng/ml baseline 23.97 post 30.39	1.52 (0.46) Intervention increase more than control
Ikai et al. (2014)	Parallel RCT	Schizophrenia $N = 50$	52.8 F 35%	Yoga + standard treatment	Standard treatment	1 h X 1 times/week × 8 weeks = 8 h	Plasma ng/ml baseline 0.149 post 0.190	−0.06 (0.28) intervention increase less than control
Naveen et al. (2016)	Parallel RCT	Depression $N = 44$	33.5 F 45%	Yoga + standard treatment	standard treatment	1 h X 1 times/week × 12 weeks =12 h	Plasma ng/ml baseline 0.203 post 0.214	0.74 (0.34) Intervention increase more than control
Tolahunase et al. (2018)	Parallel RCT	Depression $N = 58$	39.4 F 15%	Yoga + standard treatment	Standard treatment	120 min × 12 weeks = 168 h	Serum, ng/ml baseline 13.5 post 18.6	1.01 (0.28) Intervention increase more than control
Sungkarat et al. (2018)	Parallel RCT	Mild cognitive impairment $N = 66$	67.5 F 80%	Tai Chi	Regular lifestyle	50 min × 3 times/week × 24 weeks = 60 h	Plasma, ng/ml baseline 0.1123 post 0.385	0.12 (0.24) Intervention increase more than control
MINDFULNESS MEDITATION AND DERIVATIVES								
Gagrani et al. (2018)	Parallel RCT	primary angle glaucoma $N = 60$	57.28 F 42%	Meditation	Regular lifestyle	45 min × 7 times/week × 6 weeks = 31.5 h	Serum, ng/ml baseline 52.24 Post 63.25	0.13 (0.25) Intervention increase more than control
Ledreux et al. (Ledreux et al., 2019)	Parallel RCT	Healthy N =78	72.9 F=70%	Meditation	Regular lifestyle	3 h per weeks × 5 week = 15 h	Serum, ng/ml baseline 26.60 post 26.59	1.18 (0.69–1.16) Intervention decrease less than control
Nery et al. (2019)	Parallel RCT	Infertility with anxiety N =62	37.2 F 100%	Meditation	Regular lifestyle	2 h per week for 8 weeks = 16 h	Serum, ng/ml baseline 84.64 post 91.92	0.58 (0.21) Intervention increase more than control
(Håkansson et al., 2016)*	Crossover trial control trial	Healthy $N = 57$	70.2 F 58%	Mindfulness practice	Physical exercise, Cognitive training	35 min	Serum, ng/ml Pre-crossing 21.6 Post 21.05	−0.55 (1.27) Mindfulness and cognitive training did not change while physical exercise increase
(Montero-Marin et al., 2019)*	Parallel RCT	Fibromyalgia $N = 24$	53.05 F 100%	Attachment-based compassion therapy (ABCT)	Relaxation technique	2 h per week × 8 weeks + 2 h per month × 3 months = 32 h	Serum, ng/ml, baseline 23.03 post 16.03	−1.56 (0.4) Intervention decrease more than control
Siang Ng et al. (2020)*	Parallel RCT	Mild cognitive impairment $N = 55$	71.28 F 70%	Mindfulness Awareness Practice (MAP)	Health education Program	1 h per week × 12 weeks + 1 h per month x 6 months =18 h	Serum, log transformation adjusted mean baseline 7.238 post 6.323	−1.61 (0.31) BDNF decrease in both intervention and control group.

**Not include in met analysis.*

60 min after finishing each intervention. They find peripheral BDNF in those receiving physical exercise is significantly increased from a baseline although mindfulness and cognitive training show no significant change. There were two studies related to disease-specific mindfulness programs compared to active interventions. Montero-Martin et al. conducted a parallel RCT in patients with fibromyalgia. They compare attachment-based compassion therapy (ABCT), a fibromyalgia-specific mindfulness-based program with relaxation therapy. The study shows the ABCT group had a significantly greater improved quality of life concurrent with a greater reduction of BDNF. Siang Ng et al. conducted a parallel RCT in elders with mild cognitive impairment. The intervention was a modified MBSR program for the cognitively impaired person called mindful-awareness practice (MAP). The control arm received a lifestyle modification health education program. The study resulted in BDNF in both MAP and control groups reduced from baseline at 3 and 9 months of the program.

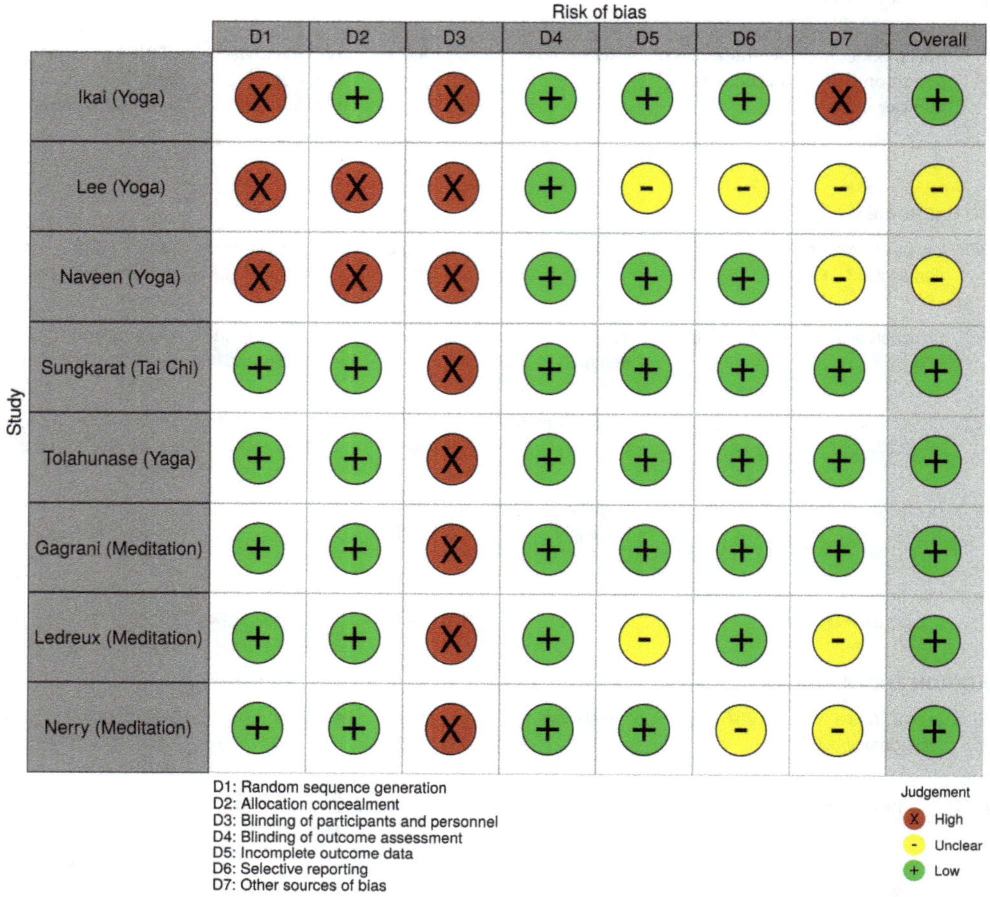

FIGURE 2 | The quality of research.

Meta-Analysis

Figure 3 shows the meta-analysis of the eight included studies using a random effect model. The pooled effect size shows a significantly greater increase of peripheral BDNF in MBI groups compared to the control groups (k = 8, N = 479, SMD = 0.72, 95% CI 0.31–1.14, I^2 =78%). Regarding the publication bias, the funnel plot of effect sizes against their standard errors shows a relative symmetry of plots. The Begg's rank test of funnel plot asymmetry indicates no significant asymmetry of effect-size plots (k = 8, z = 0.72, $p = 0.45$) in **Figure 4**.

Moderator Analyses

Figure 3 shows the subgroup analysis comparing the pooled effect sizes of BDNF changes between the exercise-MBI and control groups and between the meditation-MBI and control groups. In the MBI groups, significantly greater increases in peripheral BDNF are found in both subgroups (k = 5, N = 242, SMD = 070, 95% CI = 0.12–1.29, $I^2 = 78\%$) and meditation-MBI (k = 3, N = 237, SMD = 077, 95% CI = 0.07–1.48, $I^2 = 85\%$). The effect sizes of both subgroups are not significantly different between subgroups ($\chi^2 = 0.02, p = 0.88$).

The meta-regression analyses shows no significant correlation between the effect sizes and participants' age ($r = -0.0095, p = 0.45$) or accumulative hours of practice ($r = 0.0021, p = 0.57$) (see the bubble plot in **Figure 5**).

DISCUSSION

Our meta-analysis examines the effect of MBI on peripheral BDNF by including eight RCTs ($N = 479$). Based on the heterogeneous data, it is found that MBIs can increase peripheral BDNF. The increases in peripheral BDNF are not different between those practicing exercise-MBI and meditation-MBI.

The practitioners' age or the accumulative hours of MBI practice do not appear to be effect modifiers on peripheral BDNF affected by MBIs.

The present evidence supports previous findings and extends our knowledge in this area. The present meta-analytic results are in line with the report that mild-to-moderate exercise incorporated in MBI (e.g., yoga, tai chi) can increase peripheral BDNF. However, our subgroup analytic results extend current knowledge that not only exercise-MBI but also meditation-MBI can increase BDNF. This new knowledge suggests that, for exercise-MBI, both components of exercise and meditation contribute to the increase of peripheral BDNF.

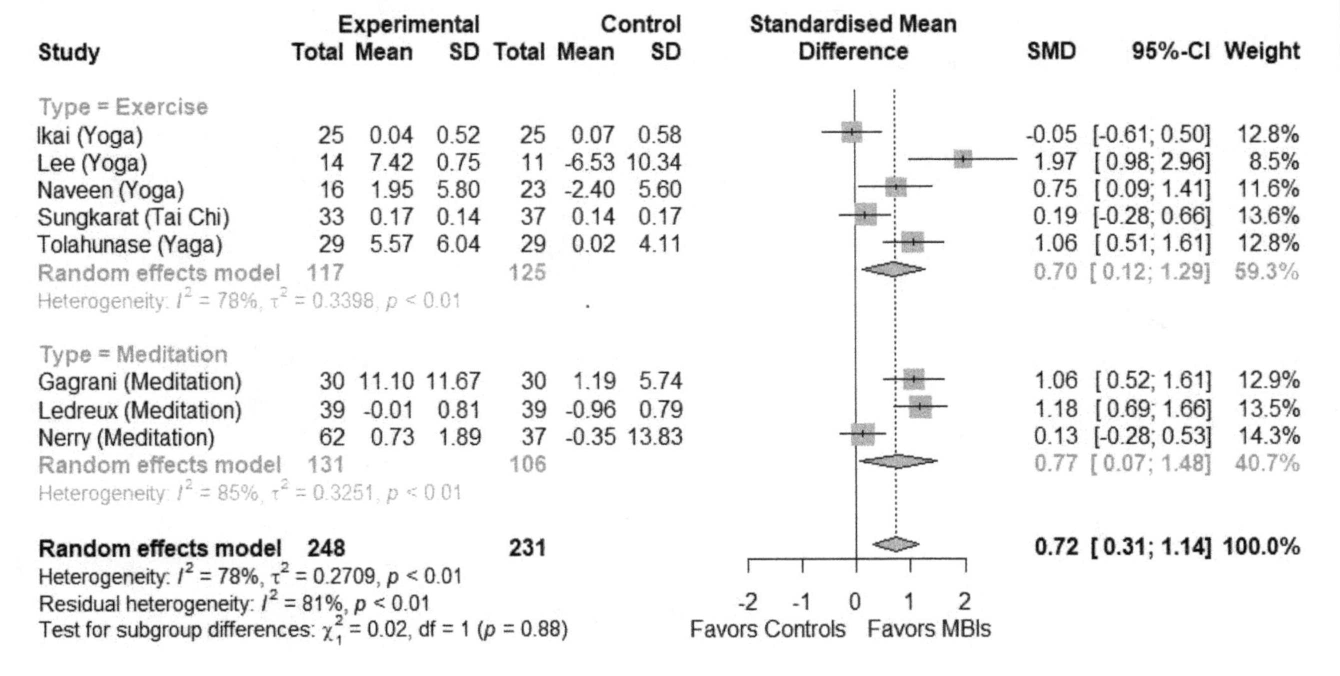

FIGURE 3 | The forest plot of included studies (K = 8).

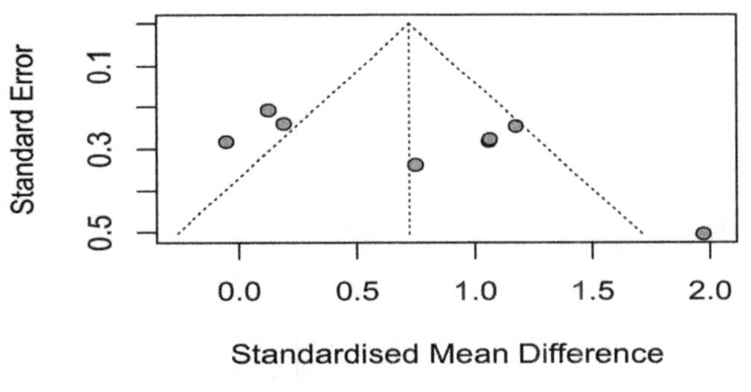

FIGURE 4 | The funnel plot. K = 8, The Egger's test for publication bias: $t = 1.7856$, df = 6, $p = 0.1244$.

Our meta-regression analytic results suggest that effect modifiers of peripheral BDNF changes affected by physical exercise may not be applicable for MBI. Previous studies report that practitioners' age and hours of practice are associated with the changes in peripheral BDNF related to yoga or exercise practice (Dinoff et al., 2016; Lao et al., 2016). However, our meta-analyses does not show the association of those effect modifiers in MBI practitioners. It is possible that the inclusion of three meditation studies, which are non-exercise-based interventions, may reduce the strength of such association. In addition, the small sample sizes of the included studies might cause a type II error, which results in the discovery of false-negative findings.

Håkansson et al. (2016) shows that a short bout of mindfulness does not change peripheral BDNF. He hypothesizes that physical exercise and mindfulness meditation may increase blood BDNF via a different mechanism. This may imply the relatively delayed effect of mindfulness on peripheral BDNF. One possibility is that blood BDNF increases from BDNF efflux from the brain. However, this hypothesis has a counter-argument; because BDNF has a relatively short half-life (around 45 min), it may disappear before getting through the blood–brain barrier (Poduslo and Curran, 1996; Pan et al., 1998). Another possible explanation is that mindfulness can reduce systemic inflammation and free radicals, which help reduce BDNF eradication (Yang et al., 2017). This is supported by a previous meta-analysis, in which MBI, both exercise-MBI and meditation-MBI, show a significant correlation with clinical improvement. Concurrently, there is also a significant correlation with reduced inflammatory biomarkers, specifically salivary levels of interleukin 6 and tumor necrosis factor-alpha in depression and generalized anxiety disorder (Hofmann et al., 2010; Sanada et al., 2020).

There might be a unique interaction between MBI and chronic pain. A study in patients with fibromyalgia (Montero-Marin et al., 2019) shows participants had decreased BDNF concurrent with improving pain symptoms after the intervention and active intervention control. The author refers to a result supported by clinical observations that, in patients with central sensitivity pain syndrome, during the active symptoms, peripheral BDNF is higher than when symptoms are improving (Deitos et al., 2015). Preclinical studies find that BDNF might be involved in maladaptive mechanisms in neuropathic pain, spasticity, and convulsive activity (Smith, 2014). Hence, more studies on the effect of MBI on BDNF in chronic pain syndrome are warranted.

The low adherence to mindfulness practice can mask the effectiveness of MBI for BDNF. Ng et al. report decreased BDNF in both intervention and control groups after 9-months follow-up. The author discusses that low compliance to homework mindfulness practice in mild cognitive impairment might influence the result. This is supported by a meta-analysis that finds adherence to home practice significantly impacts the

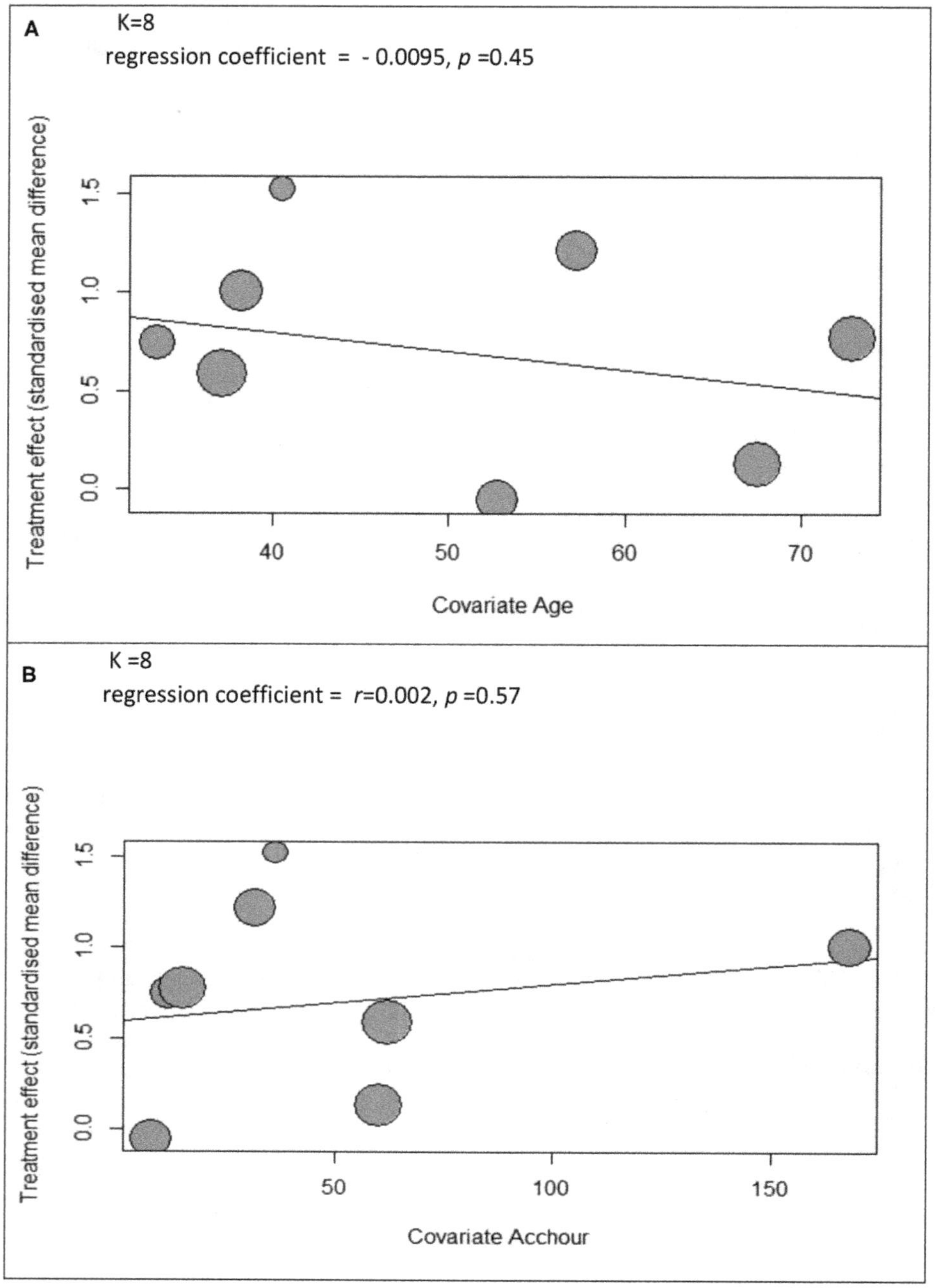

FIGURE 5 | The bubble plots of met regression analysis of **(A)** participants' age and **(B)** accumulated hours of practice.

effectiveness of MBI (Parsons et al., 2017). This lesson highlights the need to explore the optimum dose response for mindfulness practice to balance between achieving desired outcomes and being suitable for the participant's feasibility.

There are some limitations to this current systematic review. First, our review includes a smaller number of RCTs and participants compared to previous systematic reviews that include all trials examining the changes of peripheral BDNF affected by some interventions, e.g., physical exercise (Dinoff et al., 2016). This limitation may cause some type II errors in our statistical analyses, e.g., meta-regression analyses. As mentioned in the present method section, for the studies in this area, the data as well as the meta-analyses obtained from RCTs would be more reliable. However, second, the majority of participants in our meta-analysis are mentally ill and have a low burden of physical health problems. The generalizability of the present results to other groups of patients may be limited. Third, there is a lack of detailed information about factors that may affect peripheral BDNF across each study discussed before; such as the intervals between the last session of intervention and blood obtainment, the proportion of participants with chronic pain syndrome, and adherence to the mindfulness program. Last, the exclusion of non-English articles might raise the risk of publication bias.

More studies in this area remain needed. These include head-to-head RCTs comparing the effects of exercise-MBI and meditation-MBI on peripheral BDNF. Because BDNF activities are also related to physical illnesses, studies of metabolic syndrome as well as patients with chronic pain syndrome should be also carried out.

Despite the above limitations, the present findings are still helpful for clinical practice, in particular, the patients with a physical disability. Increased BNDF may decrease emotional problems. Meanwhile, more exploration is needed on the influence of chronic pain syndrome and the aging brain on the effect of MBI on BDNF. Many people may wish to increase their BDNF. For an individual without a physical disability, he/she can practice physical exercise to increase his/her BDNF. However, those who have a physical disability may choose to practice meditation-MBI to increase their BDNF.

CONCLUSIONS

The heterogeneous data of this small sample size meta-analysis suggest that MBI can increase peripheral BDNF. Either mindfulness exercise or mindfulness meditation-based intervention can increase peripheral BDNF. Patients with a physical disability may choose to practice MBI to increase their BDNF. More studies in this area are warranted.

ETHICS STATEMENT

This study meets the criteria of Chiang Mai University for ethical approval and consent exemption (Exemption number 2561-05447).

AUTHOR CONTRIBUTIONS

PG and MS designed the study. PG and NY conducted the research. PG and MS conducted the meta-analysis. PG wrote the first draft of the manuscript. NC, SC, and MS participated in the revision of the subsequent draft. All authors read and approved the final manuscript.

ACKNOWLEDGMENTS

We are gratefully acknowledge Ms. Chompunuch Saravudeecha for her searching assistance, Ms. Kamonchanok Masangta for her plagiarism check, and Dr. Elisabeth Young for her medical writing assistance.

REFERENCES

Ainsworth, B. E., Haskell, W. L., Whitt, M. C., Irwin, M. L., Swartz, A. M., Strath, S. J., et al. (2000). Compendium of physical activities: an update of activity codes and MET intensities: *Med Sci Sports Exerc.* 32 (Suppl.), S498–516. doi: 10.1097/00005768-200009001-00009

Balietti, M., Giuli, C., and Conti, F. (2018). Peripheral blood brain-derived neurotrophic factor as a biomarker of alzheimer's disease: are there methodological biases? *Mol. Neurobiol.* 55, 6661–6672. doi: 10.1007/s12035-017-0866-y

Bathina, S., and Das, U. N. (2015). Brain-derived neurotrophic factor and its clinical implications. *Arch. Med. Sci.* 6, 1164–1178. doi: 10.5114/aoms.2015.56342

Begg, C. B., and Mazumdar, M. (1994). Operating characteristics of a rank correlation test for publication bias. *Biometrics* 50, 1088–1101. doi: 10.2307/2533446

Brunoni, A. R., Lopes, M., and Fregni, F. (2008). A systematic review and meta-analysis of clinical studies on major depression and BDNF levels: implications for the role of neuroplasticity in depression. *Int. J. Neuropsychopharmacol.* 11, 1169–1180. doi: 10.1017/S14611457080 09309

Deitos, A., Dussán-Sarria, J. A., de Souza, A., Medeiros, L., da Graça Tarrag,ô M., Sehn, F., et al. (2015). Clinical value of serum neuroplasticity mediators in identifying the central sensitivity syndrome in patients with chronic pain with and without structural pathology: *Clin. J. Pain.* 31, 959–967. doi: 10.1097/AJP.0000000000000194

Dinoff, A., Herrmann, N., Swardfager, W., and Lanctôt, K. L. (2017). The effect of acute exercise on blood concentrations of brain-derived neurotrophic factor in healthy adults: a meta-analysis. *Eur. J. Neurosci.* 46, 1635–1646. doi: 10.1111/ejn.13603

Dinoff, A., Herrmann, N., Swardfager, W., Liu, C. S., Sherman, C., Chan, S., et al. (2016). The effect of exercise training on resting concentrations of peripheral brain-derived neurotrophic factor (BDNF): a meta-analysis. *PLoS ONE.* 11:e0163037. doi: 10.1371/journal.pone.0163037

Epel, E. S., Puterman, E., Lin, J., Blackburn, E. H., Lum, P. Y., Beckmann, N. D., et al. (2016). Meditation and vacation effects have an impact on disease-associated molecular phenotypes. *Transl. Psychiatry.* 6:e880. doi: 10.1038/tp.2016.164

Fox, K. C. R., Nijeboer, S., Dixon, M. L., Floman, J. L., Ellamil, M., Rumak, S. P., et al. (2014). Is meditation associated with altered brain structure? A systematic review and meta-analysis of morphometric neuroimaging in meditation practitioners. *Neurosci. Biobehav. Rev.* 43, 48–73. doi: 10.1016/j.neubiorev.2014.03.016

Gagrani, M., Faiq, M. A., Sidhu, T., Dada, R., Yadav, R. K., Sihota, R., et al. (2018). Meditation enhances brain oxygenation, upregulates BDNF and improves quality of life in patients with primary open angle glaucoma: a randomized controlled trial. *Restor. Neurol. Neurosci.* 36, 741–753. doi: 10.3233/RNN-180857

Goldberg, S. B., Tucker, R. P., Greene, P. A., Davidson, R. J., Wampold, B. E., Kearney, D. J., et al. (2018). Mindfulness-based interventions for psychiatric disorders: a systematic review and meta-analysis. *Clin. Psychol. Rev.* 59:52–60. doi: 10.1016/j.cpr.2017.10.011

Håkansson, K., Ledreux, A., Daffner, K., Terjestam, Y., Bergman, P., Carlsson, R., et al. (2016). BDNF Responses in healthy older persons to 35 minutes of physical exercise, cognitive training, and mindfulness: associations with working memory function. *J. Alzheimers Dis.* 55, 645–657. doi: 10.3233/JAD-160593

Hofmann, S. G., Sawyer, A. T., Witt, A. A., and Oh, D. (2010). The effect of mindfulness-based therapy on anxiety and depression: A meta-analytic review. *J. Consult. Clin. Psychol.* 78, 169–183. doi: 10.1037/a0018555

Houlton, J., Abumaria, N., Hinkley, S. F. R., and Clarkson, A. N. (2019). Therapeutic potential of neurotrophins for repair after brain injury: a helping hand from biomaterials. *Front. Neurosci.* (2020). 13:790. doi: 10.3389/fnins.2019.00790

Ikai, S., Suzuki, T., Uchida, H., Saruta, J., Tsukinoki, K., Fujii, Y., et al. (2014). Effects of weekly one-hour hatha yoga therapy on resilience and stress levels in patients with schizophrenia-spectrum disorders: an eight-week randomized controlled trial. *J. Altern. Complement. Med.* 20, 823–830. doi: 10.1089/acm.2014.0205

Kabat-Zinn, J. (2003). Mindfulness-based interventions in context: past, present, and future. *Clin. Psychol. Sci. Pract.* 10, 144–156. doi: 10.1093/clipsy.bpg016

Kwak, S., Lee, T. Y., Jung, W. H., Hur, J.-W., Bae, D., Hwang, W. J., et al. (2019). The immediate and sustained positive effects of meditation on resilience are mediated by changes in the resting brain. *Front. Hum. Neurosci.* 13:101. doi: 10.3389/fnhum.2019.00101

Lao, S.-A., Kissane, D., and Meadows, G. (2016). Cognitive effects of MBSR/MBCT: a systematic review of neuropsychological outcomes. *Conscious Cogn.* 45, 109–123. doi: 10.1016/j.concog.2016.08.017

Ledreux, A., Håkansson, K., Carlsson, R., Kidane, M., Columbo, L., Terjestam, Y., et al. (2019). Differential effects of physical exercise, cognitive training, and mindfulness practice on serum BDNF levels in healthy older adults: a randomized controlled intervention study. *J. Alzheimers Dis.* 71, 1245–1261. doi: 10.3233/JAD-190756

Lee, M., Moon, W., Kim, J. (2014). Effect of yoga on pain, brain-derived neurotrophic factor, and serotonin in premenopausal women with chronic low Back Pain. *Evid. Based Complement. Alternat. Med.* 2014, 1–7. doi: 10.1155/2014/203173

Lu, B., Nagappan, G., and Lu, Y. (2014). "BDNF and synaptic plasticity, cognitive function, and dysfunction," in: *Neurotrophic Factors,* eds G. R. Lewin and B. D. Carter (Berlin; Heidelberg: Springer) 223–250. doi: 10.1007/978-3-642-45106-5_9

McGuinness, LA, Higgins, JPT. (2020). Risk-of-bias VISualization (robvis): An R package and Shiny web app for visualizing risk-of-bias assessments. *Res Syn Meth.* 1–7. doi: 10.1002/jrsm.1411

Montero-Marin, J., Andrés-Rodríguez, L., Tops, M., Luciano, J. V., Navarro-Gil, M., Feliu-Soler, A., et al. (2019). Effects of attachment-based compassion therapy (ABCT) on brain-derived neurotrophic factor and low-grade inflammation among fibromyalgia patients: a randomized controlled trial. *Sci. Rep.* 9:15639. doi: 10.1038/s41598-019-52260-z

Naveen, G. H., Varambally, S., Thirthalli, J., Rao, M., Christopher, R., Gangadhar, B. N. (2016). Serum cortisol and BDNF in patients with major depression—effect of yoga. *Int. Rev. Psychiatry.* 28, 273–278. doi: 10.1080/09540261.2016.1175419

Nery, S. F., Paiva, S. P. C., Vieira, É. L., Barbosa, A. B., Sant'Anna, E. M., Casalechi, M., et al. (2019). Mindfulness-based program for stress reduction in infertile women: randomized controlled trial. *Stress Health.* 35, 49–58. doi: 10.1002/smi.2839

Ng, T. K. S., Fam, J., Feng, L., Cheah, I. K.-M., Tan, C. T.-Y., Nur, F., et al. (2020). Mindfulness improves inflammatory biomarker levels in older adults with mild cognitive impairment: a randomized controlled trial. *Transl. Psychiatry* 10:21. doi: 10.1038/s41398-020-0696-y

Pal, R., Singh, S. N., Chatterjee, A., and Saha, M. (2014). Age-related changes in cardiovascular system, autonomic functions, and levels of BDNF of healthy active males: role of yogic practice. *Age.* 36:9683. doi: 10.1007/s11357-014-9683-7

Pan, W., Banks, W. A., Fasold, M. B., Bluth, J., and Kastin, A. J. (1998). Transport of brain-derived neurotrophic factor across the blood-brain barrier. *Neuropharmacology* 37, 1553–1561. doi: 10.1016/S0028-3908(98)00141-5

Parsons, C. E., Crane, C., Parsons, L. J., Fjorback, L. O., and Kuyken, W. (2017). Home practice in mindfulness-based cognitive therapy and mindfulness-based stress reduction: a systematic review and meta-analysis of participants' mindfulness practice and its association with outcomes. *Behav. Res. Ther.* 95, 29–41. doi: 10.1016/j.brat.2017.05.004

Poduslo, J. F., and Curran, G. L. (1996). Permeability at the blood-brain and blood-nerve barriers of the neurotrophic factors: NGF, CNTF, NT-3, BDNF. *Mol. Brain Res.* 36, 280–286. doi: 10.1016/0169-328X(95)00250-V

R Core Team. (2016). R: A Language and Environment for Statistical Computing [Internet]. Vienna, Austria. Available from: https://www.R-project.org/

Rahmani, F., Saghazadeh, A., Rahmani, M., Teixeira, A. L., Rezaei, N., Aghamollaii, V., et al. (2019). Plasma levels of brain-derived neurotrophic factor in patients with parkinson disease: a systematic review and meta-analysis. *Brain Res.* 1704, 127–136. doi: 10.1016/j.brainres.2018.10.006

Rubio-Aparicio, M., Marín-Martínez, F., Sánchez-Meca, J., and López-López, J. A. (2018). A methodological review of meta-analyses of the effectiveness of clinical psychology treatments. *Behav. Res. Methods.* 50, 2057–2073. doi: 10.3758/s13428-017-0973-8

Sanada, K., Montero-Marin, J., Barceló-Soler, A., Ikuse, D., Ota, M., Hirata, A., et al. (2020). Effects of mindfulness-based interventions on biomarkers and low-grade inflammation in patients with psychiatric disorders: a meta-analytic review. *Int. J. Mol. Sci.* 21:2484. doi: 10.3390/ijms21072484

Schäfer, T., and Schwarz, M. A. (2019). The meaningfulness of effect sizes in psychological research: differences between sub-disciplines and the impact of potential biases. *Front. Psychol.* 10:813. doi: 10.3389/fpsyg.2019.00813

Smith, P. A. (2014). BDNF: no gain without pain? *Neuroscience* 283, 107–123. doi: 10.1016/j.neuroscience.2014.05.044

Ströhle, A., Schmidt, D. K., Schultz, F., Fricke, N., Staden, T., Hellweg, R., et al. (2015). Drug and exercise treatment of alzheimer disease and mild cognitive impairment: a systematic review and meta-analysis of effects on cognition in randomized controlled trials. *Am. J. Geriatr. Psychiatry.* 23, 1234–1249. doi: 10.1016/j.jagp.2015.07.007

Sungkarat, S., Boripuntakul, S., Kumfu, S., Lord, S. R., and Chattipakorn, N. (2018). Tai chi improves cognition and plasma BDNF in older adults with mild cognitive impairment: a randomized controlled trial. *Neurorehabil. Neural. Repair.* 32, 142–149. doi: 10.1177/1545968317753682

Tolahunase, M., Sagar, R., and Dada, R. (2017). Impact of yoga and meditation on cellular aging in apparently healthy individuals: a prospective, open-label single-arm exploratory study. *Oxid. Med. Cell Longev.* 2017, 1–9. doi: 10.1155/2017/7928981

Tolahunase, M. R., Sagar, R., Faiq, M., and Dada, R. (2018). Yoga- and meditation-based lifestyle intervention increases neuroplasticity and reduces severity of major depressive disorder: a randomized controlled trial. *Restor. Neurol. Neurosci.* 36, 423–442. doi: 10.3233/RNN-1 70810

Xu, H.-B., Xu, Y.-H., He, Y., Xue, F., Wei, J., Zhang, H., et al. (2018). Decreased serum brain-derived neurotrophic factor may indicate the development of poststroke depression in patients with acute ischemic stroke: a meta-analysis. *J. Stroke Cerebrovasc. Dis.* 27, 709–715. doi: 10.1016/j.jstrokecerebrovasdis.2017.10.003

Yang, B., Ren, Q., Zhang, J., Chen, Q.-X., and Hashimoto, K. (2017). Altered expression of BDNF, BDNF pro-peptide and their precursor proBDNF in brain and liver tissues from psychiatric disorders: rethinking the brain–liver axis. *Transl. Psychiatry* 7:e1128. doi: 10.1038/tp.2 017.95

Zhou, C., Zhong, J., Zou, B., Fang, L., Chen, J., Deng, X., et al. (2017). Meta-analyses of comparative efficacy of antidepressant medications on peripheral BDNF concentration in patients with depression. *PLoS ONE.* 12:e0172270. doi: 10.1371/journal.pone.0172270

6

Pilot-Testing of "Healthy Body Healthy Mind": An Integrative Lifestyle Program for Patients with a Mental Illness and Co-morbid Metabolic Syndrome

Jenifer A. Murphy[1*], *Georgina Oliver*[1], *Chee H. Ng*[1,2], *Clinton Wain*[2], *Jennifer Magennis*[2], *Rachelle S. Opie*[3], *Amy Bannatyne*[4] *and Jerome Sarris*[1,5]

[1] *Professorial Unit, The Melbourne Clinic, Department of Psychiatry, The University of Melbourne, Melbourne, VIC, Australia,* [2] *The Melbourne Clinic, Melbourne, VIC, Australia,* [3] *Institute for Physical Activity and Nutrition, School of Exercise and Nutrition Sciences, Deakin University, Geelong, VIC, Australia,* [4] *Faculty of Health Sciences and Medicine, Bond University, Gold Coast, QLD, Australia,* [5] *NICM Health Research Institute, Western Sydney University, Westmead, NSW, Australia*

***Correspondence:**
Jenifer A. Murphy
j.sarris@westernsydney.edu.au

Background: Metabolic syndrome and co-morbid physical health conditions are highly prevalent in people with a mental illness. Modifiable lifestyle factors have been targeted to improve health outcomes. Healthy Body Healthy Mind (HBHM) program was developed to provide an integrated evidence-based program incorporating practical diet and exercise instruction; alongside meditation and mindfulness strategies, and comprehensive psychoeducation, to improve the physical and mental health of those with a mental illness.

Methods: We report on two data points: (1) Qualitative data derived from the first HBHM program (version 1) exploring its utility and acceptance according to patient feedback; (2) Biometric and mental health data collected on the modified and enhanced 12-week HBHM program (version 2) involving a pilot of 10 participants. Mental and physical health outcomes, weight, abdominal circumference, fasting glucose, cholesterol, and triglycerides were measured at program entry and completion.

Results: Qualitative data from HBHM version 1 provided valuable feedback to redevelop and enhance the program. At the end of the HBHM (version 2) 12-week program, a significant mean weight loss of 2 kg was achieved, $p = 0.023$. There was also a significant reduction in abdominal circumference (mean = 2.55 cm) and a decrease in BMI of almost one point (mean = 0.96 kg/m^2), $p = 0.046$ and $p = 0.019$, respectively. There were no significant changes in mental health measures or on any other biometrics.

Conclusion: Pilot data from the HBHM program found significant reductions in weight and abdominal obesity. The HBHM program could benefit from further modifications, and study replication is required using a controlled design in a larger sample.

Keywords: healthy lifestyles, lifestyle medicine, metabolic syndrome, depression, program development

INTRODUCTION

A highly complex relationship exists between physical and mental health. The rates of physical morbidity and mortality in people with mental illness is substantially higher than the general population (1, 2). Even in countries with adequate health care systems, the mortality gap is on the rise, up to a difference of 20 years (3). Obesity and related conditions such as cardiovascular disease, hyperlipidaemia, and diabetes mellitus are highly prevalent in people with mental illness (4).

The cluster of symptoms associated with these lifestyle diseases such as, excess visceral fat, along with hypertension, glucose intolerance/insulin resistance, and/or hyperlipidaemia has been labeled Metabolic Syndrome (MetS). In mental health populations, the rate of MetS is thought to be between 41 and 67% (5). A large proportion of the physical health burden in patients with a mental illness can be linked to side effects of second generation antipsychotics, lifestyle factors (e.g., higher rates of smoking, low levels of exercise), and factors associated with socioeconomic disadvantage (e.g., poverty and lack of access to nutritious foods) (6). Weight gain can result in lowered self-esteem, impaired body-image, and reduced social interactions, which can ultimately lead to poorer mental health (7). Furthermore, it is also a common cause of medication non-adherence, which can lead to illness relapse, hospitalization, and poorer outcomes (7, 8).

There is potential to modify lifestyle factors that contribute to MetS (e.g., caloric intake, physical activity levels, sleep hygiene) to improve the health and well-being of people with a mental illness. There are calls for an integrated response involving early diagnosis, treatment and management of physical and mental health via lifestyle modification (9). Several lifestyle-based programs have been developed to modify the lifestyle factors contributing to MetS (10). These programs typically focus on exercise and nutrition for metabolic issues and result in minimal weight loss and modest effects on well-being (10). In one review of lifestyle interventions in adults with a serious mental illness at risk of MetS, few programs incorporated behavioral components such as stress management and motivation alongside exercise and/or nutrition interventions (10). Thus, programs that target both mental and physical outcomes in patients who are taking psychotropic medication have not been adequately developed. Further, previous programs often do not provide a truly "integrative" model, tending to focus on nutrition and exercise without incorporating components that may improve general health and well-being (10).

To bridge the gap and provide an evidence-based integrated health approach, we developed the "Healthy Body, Healthy Mind Program (HBHM)." The aim was to assist people with a diagnosed mental illness and metabolic syndrome to improve mental and physical well-being. We presently report on: (1) Qualitative data derived from our first version of the HBHM program in 2011, exploring its utility and acceptance according to patient and clinician feedback; (2) Biometric data and mental health data collected on the modified and enhanced 12-week, second version of HBHM program involving a pilot of 10 participants.

TABLE 1 | Metabolic syndrome clinical diagnosis guidelines*.

Measure	Categorical cut point
Elevated waist circumference (European/North American)	≥ 102 cm for men, ≥ 88 cm for women
Elevated triglyceride levels (or drug treatment for elevated triglycerides)	≥1.7 mmol/L
Reduced HDL-C (or drug treatment for reduced HDL-C)	<1.0 mmol/L in men, <1.3 mmol/L in women
Elevated blood pressure (or drug treatment for hypertension)	≥130 systolic or ≥85 diastolic
Elevated fasting glucose (or drug treatment for elevated glucose)	>5.5 mmol/L

*For a diagnosis of Metabolic Syndrome, an individual must meet three of the five specified criteria. *As per the International Diabetes Federation Task Force on Epidemiology and Prevention; National Heart Lunch and Blood Institute; American Heart Association; World Heart Federation; International Atherosclerosis Society; and International Association for the Study of Obesity (11).*

MATERIALS AND METHODS

Setting And Overview

The Melbourne Clinic in Melbourne, Australia is a private psychiatric hospital with inpatient and outpatient services. The clinic had a longstanding weight management and lifestyle program, called Healthy Body Healthy Mind (HBHM), developed and facilitated by a general practitioner (GP), exercise physiologist and dietitian. HBHM program (version 1) provided weekly nutritional support from a dietitian, psychoeducation sessions on lifestyle modification and exercise practicals with an exercise physiologist. In late 2011, ethics approval was granted by The Melbourne Clinic Research Ethics Committee (HREC project number: 209) to collect qualitative data from participants to evaluate the perceived efficacy of the program's content, barriers in implementing the components, and feedback on how it could be improved. The qualitative data collected during 2011–2012 was used to redevelop and enhance the integrated lifestyle program which was pilot-tested at The Melbourne Clinic in 2016 (HREC project number: 249). This modified second program will henceforth be labeled as HBHM program (version 2).

Recruitment

Patients attending The Melbourne Clinic outpatient services were invited to attend the program via a doctor's referral. Patients with a diagnosed mental illness (e.g., Major Depressive Disorder, Bipolar Disorder; or with multiple diagnoses) taking stable psychotropic medication (same dose for at least 4 weeks) with co-morbid diagnosed metabolic syndrome (see **Table 1**) or obesity (defined as a BMI of >30 OR abdominal circumference of >80 cm for women and >94 cm for men) were the target participants for the program. Written informed consent was obtained from all participants to evaluate the two versions of the program.

HBHM Version 2 (2016) Measures

At week 0, a range of medical and demographic information was collected including, age, gender, employment status, medication information, psychiatric diagnosis and medical co-morbidity.

At week 0 and week 12, participants also had anthropometric measurements taken by an exercise physiologist (BP, height, weight, abdominal circumference) and completed self-report questionnaires on their mental health (Depression Anxiety Stress Scales—DASS-21). In addition at week 0, participants were asked to state their goals for the program and what they hoped to achieve. They were also asked to rate their readiness to change in order to achieve their listed goals on a scale of 1–10 with 1 being "not ready" and 10 being "ready." Participants were provided with a blood test request form to have fasting cholesterol, glucose and triglycerides measured at week 0 and week 12. The blood tests were conducted by Australian Clinical Labs.

Depression Anxiety Stress Scales—DASS-21

The DASS-21 is a self-reported screening instrument used to measure depression, anxiety and stress symptomatology (12). It consists of 21-items, across three scales, which measure symptoms of depression (7 items), anxiety (7 items), and stress (7 items). Individuals are asked to respond to each item on a four-point Likert scale (0 = *not at all* to 3 = *very much or most of the time*). Higher scores on each scale are indicative of greater symptom severity. Scores above 11 (depression), 8 (anxiety), and 13 (stress) are considered severe, as indicated by the recommended cut-offs (12).

Statistics

Qualitative data assessing the 2011 HBHM Program (version 1) was analyzed from written participant feedback forms. Comments were coded and grouped in categories by theme (beneficial/useful content, barriers to implementation and program improvements) and counted to obtain a frequency of mention by the 12 participants. For the quantitative data from the 2016 HBHM program (version 2), paired *t*-tests and Pearson's r correlations were used to compare the repeated measurements of the sample (week 0 vs. week 12). All data was analyzed in SPSS 24. An alpha level of <0.05 was used to determine significance.

RESULTS

HBHM Version 1 (2011)—Qualitative Data

Written qualitative data from 12 participants (83% female; mean age 43.4 years old) who participated in the first version of the HBHM program during 2011–2012 was thematically analyzed to aid the development of the 2016 HBHM program. **Table 2** summaries the qualitative data on the early program.

The most beneficial/useful components of the program reported by the majority of participants were the cooking and exercise practicals (n = 11; 91%). One participant commented that he/she needed "*practical examples that can be implemented in day-to-day life*" and less theory in order to engage with the program. However, many participants (n = 9; 75%) commented that furthering their knowledge on how food effects the body and the harms of nutritionally poor food and no exercise on the body's functioning was useful as, "*understanding aids motivation to change, oversimplification does not.*" Poor motivation (n = 4; 33%), fear of change (n = 3; 25%) and difficulties engaging with the program due to low mood and anxiety (n = 8; 66.7%) were common among participants. Additionally, many participants found cooking for one person and/or maintaining momentum on their own difficult (n = 4; 33%). As one person stated, "*[the] desire to try a new recipe is high at time of session but then lost when at home.*" Participants requested more diagram-based notes of exercises/recipes and program content to be accessible at home due to poor recall (n = 3; 25%). Injury and co-morbid physical health problems were some of the main barriers in adding exercise to their day-to-day lives (n =8; 66.67%). At home chair-based exercises and information on how and why to vary exercise was deemed helpful (n = 4; 33.3%).

TABLE 2 | Qualitative feedback from HBHM (version 1).

Beneficial/useful content	• Cooking practicals
	  • Hands-on experience
	  • Meal planning with simple and practical recipes
	  • Templates for shopping/organizing pantry
	  • Providing alternative foods to swap out "bad" foods
	• Label reading and understanding ratios of good fats, proteins and hidden sugars
	• More understanding of the psychological underpinnings on "why I eat" and overeating
	• Exercise class
	  • Chair exercises
	  • Fresh air/park exercises
	  • Information about benefits of varying exercise
	• Further knowledge on
	  • Certain foods and their effects on the body (e.g., what sugar does to the body, proteins, good fats etc.)
	  • The harms of poor eating and no exercise on body mechanisms
	  • Cravings and how to beat them
	• Reminders of program schedule and encouragement to attend
	• Sharing experiences and "wins" with peers

Barriers	• Unable to concentrate/absorb content/participate fully because of low mood/anxiety • Injury/pain and physical health issues make exercise difficult or impossible • Poor motivation/discipline and difficulty getting started and maintaining momentum • Fear of change or not ready to make changes • Cooking for one person too hard or can't be bothered • Changing the eating patterns of the entire household
Program lessons	• Provide notes at each session rather than at the following week • Provide diagrams of exercises to do at home • Not enough practical cooking/exercise classes • Group size too big with new people coming in every week

HBHM Version 2 (2016)—Program Development

Based on the qualitative data detailed above, the HBHM program in 2016 was remodeled and refined in consultation with a team of experts in the fields of psychiatry, endocrinology/cardiology, nutrition and dietetics, and exercise physiology. The program was designed to integrate five evidence-based components: lifestyle psychoeducation (13), exercise (theory and practicals) (14), diet and nutrition (theory and practical skills e.g., cooking

TABLE 3 | Example HBHM (version 2) practical components and education sessions.

	Diet and nutrition	Exercise	Motivation and goal setting	Meditation and mindfulness	Psychoeducation
Practical components	- Cooking demonstrations - Excursion to supermarket for healthy shopping tips - Food label reading	- Chair based exercises to increase strength - Pilates - Yoga and stretching - Body weight exercises - Interval, circuit and resistance training	- Goal setting - Ongoing review of personal goals throughout the program	- Meditation to improve sleep - Mindfulness for reducing and managing stress - Mindfulness for self-compassion	N.A
Education session topics	- Why diets don't work? - Sugar—myths and realities - Exploring macronutrients in foods—protein, fats and carbohydrates	- Benefits of physical exercise - The benefits of "greenexercise" (exercising in nature) - Incidental exercise strategies for everyday life	- Ways to plan realistic and attainable goals—SMART goal setting - Finding Motivation—the motivation matrix - Dealing with setbacks and the transtheoretical model of change	- What are the benefits of mindfulness meditation? - Mindful eating for weight loss and well-being	- What is the link between mental and cardiovascular health? - The "brain-gut" connection and its influence on mental & cardiovascular health The importance of sleep and how to improve sleep quality for our health & well-being

demonstrations and label reading exercises) (15), motivation and goal setting skills (16), and mindfulness techniques (17) (see **Table 3**). Each week, for 12 weeks, participants attended a 6-h session at TMC, where content and practical exercises from each of the five modules was delivered by an exercise physiologist, dietitian and/or a GP (see **Table 3** for examples). Participants were provided with a printed booklet each week outlining content for that session (e.g., psychoeducation theory, exercise diagrams, step by step recipes, label reading guidelines) with areas to take notes and complete tasks such as goal setting activities and shopping lists. **Table 4** provides an example program day.

HBHM Version 2 (2016)—Pilot Data

Characteristics

Fifteen patients were referred to the pilot program, five patients declined to participate and ten patients were willing to take part. All participants attended the week 0 and week 12 sessions. Some of the weekly follow-up sessions were missed due to illness or other personal commitments with an average attendance rate of 80%.

Most of the sample was female (n = 8; 80%) with a mean age of 51.8 years (SD = 12.9 years) (see **Table 5**). Over half the sample were unemployed/not working or on a disability pension (n = 6; 60%). The most common primary DSM-IV psychiatric diagnosis as reported in the treating psychiatrist referral to the program was Major Depressive Disorder (MDD) (n = 6; 60%) followed by Bipolar Affective Disorder (n = 2; 20%), Generalized Anxiety Disorder (GAD) (n = 1; 10%) and Alcohol Abuse (n = 1; 10%). Psychiatric co-morbidity was common with diagnoses of Generalized Anxiety Disorder (GAD) (n =3; 30%), Binge Eating Disorder (n = 1; 10%), Borderline Personality Disorder (n = 1; 10%) and Major Depressive Disorder (n = 1; 10%).

All participants were taking psychotropic medications defined as an antidepressant, mood stabilizer, second generation antipsychotic or benzodiazepine. The participant's primary medications were agomelatine (n = 2; 25–50 mg/day), desvenlafaxine (n = 2; 50–100 mg/day), fluvoxamine (n = 2; 200–300 mg/day), paroxetine (n = 1; 20 mg), venlafaxine (n= 1; 75 mg/day); escitalopram (n = 1; 40 mg/day); lamotrigine (n = 1; 50 mg). On average participants were taking 2.4 (SD = 1.17) psychotropic medications ranging from 1 to 4 psychotropic medications. The most common psychotropic medication taken alongside a primary psychotropic medication were second generation antipsychotics (e.g., quetiapine, lurasidone; n = 6; 60%) followed by mood stabilizers (n = 4; 40) (see **Table 5**).

The most common chronic medical conditions self-reported by participants or as listed in the referral to the program were hyperlipidaemia (n = 4; 40%), hypertension (n = 3; 30%), arthritis (n = 3; 30%), Type II Diabetes (n = 3; 20%), sleep apnoea (n = 2; 20%), and chronic pain/fibromyalgia (n = 2; 20%). Other conditions such as, fatty liver disease (n = 1; 10%), pancreatitis (n = 1; 10%), ulcerative colitis (n = 1; 10%), costochondritis (n = 1; 10%), fructose malabsorption syndrome (n = 1; 10%), endometriosis (n = 1; 10%), restless leg syndrome (n = 1; 10%) and hypothyroidism (n = 1; 10%) were self-reported.

Table 6 presents the anthropometrics of the participants at week 0 and week 12. The average BMI of the cohort at week 0 was 36.18 (SD = 4.67) which, according to the World Health Organization, classes the participants as Obese Class I. As a cohort, the participants also had impaired glucose tolerance as evidenced by a fasting glucose test average > 5.5 (mean = 5.57 ± 1.19). The participants' cholesterol and BP were normal, most likely due to their use of prescribed statins and hypertensive medications. According to DASS

TABLE 4 | An example HBHM (version 2) program day.

Time	Key component
9.30–10.00 a.m.	Greeting and brief overview of the session • Includes questions about the previous week or any updates
10.00–10.45 a.m.	Exercise theory and practice with an Exercise physiologist • Education session: Yoga theory and benefits • Practical component: Yoga
10.45–11.00 a.m.	Tea break
11.00–12.15 p.m.	Lifestyle psychoeducation with dietitian/GP • Education session: Cortisol—The "good" and "bad" of stress • Brainstorming strategies to manage stress
12.15–1.00 p.m.	Lunch • Practical component: Cooking demonstration with dietitian (example recipe: stuffed capsicums, roast vegetable and grain salad)
1.00–2.00 p.m.	Nutrition theory with dietitian • The evidence, benefits and "how to" of a Mediterranean diet
2.00–2.15 p.m.	Tea break
2.15–2.45 p.m.	Mindfulness meditation • Practical session: Mindfulness based stress reduction
2.45–3.30 p.m.	Motivation and goal setting – • Identify goal for the week using SMART guidelines

measurement at week 0, participants had low to moderate levels of depression (mean = 8.30; SD = 4.69), anxiety (mean = 6.0; SD = 4.64), and stress (mean = 8.70; SD = 4.24) symptomatology (see **Table 6**).

Participant Goals

The most common goal was to increase exercise levels and fitness ($n = 5$; 50%) followed by eat healthier ($n = 4$; 40%), reduce sugar intake ($n = 3$; 30%) and lose weight ($n = 3$; 30%). On average the participants rated their readiness to change as 7.75 (SD = 2.12) with ratings ranging from 3 to 10. Thus, as a whole the participants were very ready to make change.

Outcome Data

The cohort had a significant weight loss over the 12 weeks with an average loss of 2 kg, $t_{(9)} = 2.75, p = 0.023$. Weight change ranged from a +1.4 kg weight gain to a −6 kg weight loss. Along with weight loss, there was also a significant reduction in abdominal circumference (mean = 2.55 cm) and a drop in BMI of almost one point (mean = 0.96 kg/m^2), $t_{(9)} = 2.32$, $p = 0.046$ and $t_{(9)} = 0.96$, $p = 0.019$. No significant changes in participant's blood levels or anthropometrics were found. Additionally, no significant changes in participant's mental health was found on the DASS when comparing week 0 to week 12 (see **Table 6**). Participant's readiness to change (mean = 7.75; SD = 2.12) was not correlated with change in BMI, abdominal circumference, or weight change at end of the program, $r = -0.615$, $p = 0.105$, $r = -0.205$, $p = 0.626$, and $r = -0.692$, $p = 0.057$, respectively.

TABLE 5 | HBHM (version 2) Baseline characteristics ($n = 10$).

Characteristic	Mean ± SD/ *n* (%)
Age	51.80 ± 12.93
Female	8 (80%)
Primary psychiatric diagnosis	
Major Depressive Disorder	6 (60%)
Bipolar Affective Disorder	2 (20%)
Generalized Anxiety Disorder	1 (10%)
Alcohol Dependence	1 (10%)
Primary psychotropic medication*	
Antidepressant	9 (90%)
Mood stabilizer	1 (10%)
Other psychotropic medications*	
Second generation antipsychotic	6 (60%)
Mood stabilizer	4 (40%)
Antidepressant	2 (20%)
Benzodiazepine	2 (20%)

**Participants could be taking more than one psychotropic medication (mean = 2.4; SD = 1.17).*

DISCUSSION

This pilot study found that an integrated 12-week lifestyle program was associated with significant weight loss in patients with a mental illness. We found a mean 2 kg weight loss and a drop in BMI of almost one point across the course of 12 weeks. Our findings are in line with a recent meta-analysis which found lifestyle interventions were superior to treatment-as-usual in producing weight loss in patients with a serious mental illness (18). This improvement in anthropometric measures is clinically significant when considering the challenges experienced by patients with a mental illness in maintaining physical and mental wellness.

No beneficial effect on participant's mental health was found despite incorporating meditation, goal setting, mindfulness, and motivation modules, which was a distinguishing feature of the program. This finding was surprising given mindfulness-based therapies have been consistently related to improvements in mood and anxiety in clinical populations (17). However, a recent lifestyle intervention for residential patients with a serious mental illness also found no positive changes on psychosocial outcomes (19). This suggests that it is challenging to get a beneficial effect on psychosocial outcomes while attempting to improve physical and mental health outcomes simultaneously. The addition of individual psychotherapy alongside participation in the program might be warranted and the incorporation of other evidence-based psychotherapies such as, cognitive behavioral therapy should be considered in future versions of the program. Future iterations of the program should also incorporate quality of life assessments and measures of psychosocial functioning to more accurately assess the program's potential benefit.

Alternatively, the modest effect on participant's mental health during the program could be due to the low baseline levels of depression, anxiety, and stress (as captured on the DASS), and hence had less scope for improvement. Furthermore, when

TABLE 6 | HBHM (version 2) program ($n = 10$) outcome data (week-0 to week-12).

Outcome	Week 0	Week 12	Paired *t*-test
Weight (kgs)	100.3 ± 9.79	98.3 ± 9.72	$t = 2.75$ $p = 0.023^*$
Abdominal circumference (cm)	119.95 ± 12.69	117.40 ± 12.47	$t = 2.32$ $p = 0.046^*$
BMI	36.18 ± 4.67	35.22 ± 4.73	$t = 2.86$ $p = 0.019^*$
Waist to hip ratio	0.96 ± 0.08	0.96 ± 0.07	$t = -0.362$ $p = 0.726$
Systolic blood pressure	122.67 ± 15.23	130.25 ± 14.82	$t = -1.12$ $p = 0.300$
Diastolic blood pressure	79.67 ± 11.59	80.88 ± 10.27	$t = 0.144$ $p = 0.890$
Fasting glucose[a]	5.57 ± 1.19	5.72 ± 1.03	$t = -0.44$, $p = 0.682$
HDL cholesterol[a]	1.21 ±.26	1.24 ±.21	$t = 0.500$, $p = 0.705$
LDL cholesterol[a]	2.61 ±.98	3.30 ± 1.20	$t = -2.00$, $p = 0.295$
Total fasting cholesterol[a]	5.34 ± 1.41	5.95 ± 1.20	$t = -2.61$, $p = 0.080$
Triglycerides[a]	2.30 ±.57	2.13 ±.30	$t = -0.33$, $p = 0.761$
DASS 21—Depression score	8.30 ± 4.69	9.70 ± 5.44	$t = -0.87$, $p = 0.408$
DASS 21—Anxiety score	6.00 ± 4.64	5.50 ± 5.10	$t = 0.75$, $p = 0.475$
DASS 21—Stress score	8.70 ± 4.24	8.50 ± 4.72	$t = 0.38$, $p = 0.716$

$^*p < 0.05$.
[a]Missing data on week 12 ($n = 4$).

identifying goals of the program, not one participant mentioned they would like to improve their mental health. Rather the goals reported by participants were orientated toward improving their eating habits and losing weight. The incorporation of behavioral and psychological components (such as mindful eating and goal setting) is deemed to benefit the delivery and engagement of the program contents and helped to adhere to recommendations in order to achieve the weight loss results.

A major limitation to the current study was the small sample size and that it was uncontrolled. A larger sample with an appropriate control is required to assess the program effectiveness and allow for further feedback from participants to fine-tune the program. We also recognize that more work is needed to refine the delivery and format structure in respect to determining the best application of the program given costs and time constraints. In particular, the exercise component should aim to provide at least 90 min of moderate-to-vigorous exercise per week, as this intensity has been shown to improve psychiatric symptoms in patients with a serious mental illness (20). Furthermore, closer monitoring of physical activity outside of the program should be employed in order to assess the translational impact of the program to the home environment.

While the 12-week program was comprehensive, it also has its drawback in terms of time requirements, and a 6-h once per week delivery is quite intensive for people with a mental illness. A follow-up should also be employed to determine whether weight loss results are maintained, continued, or regained following the cessation of the program.

There is the potential to restructure the program to have a blend of face-to-face delivery with online components, and even the use of a mobile phone app. This would provide flexibility, less demands on time, and less financial burden for the participants. Weight loss in this population is extremely challenging as many patients have co-morbid medical conditions, and limited social and economic resources. Thus, facilitating weight loss using strategies that can be implemented into everyday life is paramount to success. In addition, implementing and assessing strategies which prevent the all too frequent "weight regain" phenomena is crucial (21).

As 60% of the sample were taking second generation antipsychotics, the results are encouraging for metabolically vulnerable patients. However, it is important to note, that the results cannot be generalized to participants with a serious mental illness as the current pilot did not include participants with schizophrenia who are at the most risk of developing MetS. It is unclear how this particular patient population would engage with this intervention. In conclusion, the pilot data of the HBHM program found significant benefits in reducing weight and abdominal obesity, with the potential to achieve substantial health benefits for patients with a mental illness and co-morbid metabolic syndrome. Study replication is required using a controlled design in a larger sample over a longer time period.

ETHICS STATEMENT

This study was carried out in accordance with the recommendations of The National Statement on Ethical Conduct in Human Research 2007 and The Melbourne Clinic Ethics Committee. All subjects gave written informed consent in accordance with the Declaration of Helsinki. The projects were approved by the Melbourne Clinic Ethics Committee (Project 209 and 249).

AUTHOR CONTRIBUTIONS

All authors contributed to the drafting and editing of the manuscript. JAM and JS is responsible for the data analysis and manuscript preparation. JM, GO, CW, RO, and AB were involved in designing the program, running the program and collecting data. CN and JS contributed to the design of the program and provided oversight of the program.

ACKNOWLEDGMENTS

Thanks are extended to The Melbourne Clinic staff for support of this program and for the patients participating in it.

REFERENCES

Everett A, Mahler J, Biblin J, Ganguli R, Mauer B. Improving the health of mental health consumers: Effective policies and practices. *Int J Mental Health.* (2008) 37:8–48. doi: 10.2753/IMH0020-7411370201

Osborn DP, Levy G, Nazareth I, Petersen I, Islam A, King MB. Relative risk of cardiovascular and cancer mortality in people with severe mental illness from the United Kingdom's General Practice Research Database. *Arch Gen Psychiatry* (2007) 64:242–9. doi: 10.1001/archpsyc.64.2.242

Lawrence D, Hancock KJ, Kisely S. The gap in life expectancy from preventable physical illness in psychiatric patients in Western Australia: retrospective analysis of population based registers. *BMJ.* (2013) 346:f2539. doi: 10.1136/bmj.f2539

De Hert M, Correll CU, Bobes J, Cetkovich-Bakmas MA, Cohen DA, Asai I, et al. Physical illness in patients with severe mental disorders. I. Prevalence, impact of medications and disparities in health care. *World Psychiatry.* (2011) 10:52–77. doi: 10.1002/j.2051-5545.2011.tb00014.x

John AP, Koloth R, Dragovic M, Lim SC. Prevalence of metabolic syndrome among Australians with severe mental illness. *Med J Australia.* (2009) 190:176–9. doi: 10.5694/j.1326-5377.2009.tb02342.x

Stanley SH, Laugharne JD. Clinical guidelines for the physical care of mental health consumers: a comprehensive assessment and monitoring package for mental health and primary care clinicians. *Aust NZ J Psychol.* (2011) 45:824–9. doi: 10.3109/00048674.2011.614591

McCloughen A, Foster K. Weight gain associated with taking psychotropic medication: an integrative review. *Int J Mental Health Nurs.* (2011) 20:202–22. doi: 10.1111/j.1447-0349.2010.00721.x

Nihalani N, Schwartz TL, Siddiqui UA, Megna JL. Weight gain, obesity, and psychotropic prescribing. *J Obesity.* (2011) 2011:893629. doi: 10.1155/2011/893629

Lake J, Turner MS. Urgent need for improved mental health care and a more collaborative model of care. *Perm J.* (2017) 21. doi: 10.7812/TPP/17-024

Richards L, Batscha CL, McCarthy VL. Lifestyle and behavioral interventions to reduce the risk of metabolic syndrome in community-dwelling adults with serious mental illness: implications for nursing practice. *J Psychosoc Nurs Mental Health Serv.* (2015) 54:46–55. doi: 10.3928/02793695-20151109-02

Alberti KG, Eckel RH, Grundy SM, Zimmet PZ, Cleeman JI, Donato KA, et al. Harmonishing the metabolic syndrome: a joint interim statement of the International Diabetes Federation Task Force on Epidemiology and Prevention; National Heart Lunch and Blood Institute; American Heart Association; World Heart Federation; International Atherosclerosis Society; and International Association for the Study of Obesity. *Circulation.* (2009) 120:1640–45. doi: 10.1161/CIRCULATIONAHA.109.192644

Lovibond PF, Lovibond SH. The structure of negative emotional states: Comparison of the Depression Anxiety Stress Scales (DASS) with the Beck Depression and Anxiety Inventories. *Behav Res Ther.* (1995) 33:335–43. doi: 10.1016/0005-7967(94)00075-U

Naslund JA, Whiteman KL, McHugo GJ, Aschbrenner KA, Marsch LA, Bartels SJ. Lifestyle interventions for weight loss among overweight and obese adults with serious mental illness: a systematic review and meta-analysis. *Gen Hosp Psychiatry.* (2017) 47:83–102. doi: 10.1016/j.genhosppsych.2017. 04.003

Rosenbaum S, Tiedemann A, Ward PB. Meta-analysis physical activity interventions for people with mental illness: a systematic review and meta- analysis. *J Clin Psychiatry.* (2014) 75:1–11. doi: 10.1016/j.jsams.2014.11.161

Teasdale SB, Ward PB, Rosenbaum S, Samaras K, Stubbs B. Solving a weighty problem: systematic review and meta-analysis of nutrition interventions in severe mental illness. *Brit J Psychiatry.* (2017) 210:110–8. doi: 10.1192/bjp.bp.115.177139

Rodriguez-Cristobal JJ, Alonso-Villaverde C, Panisello JM, Travé- Mercade P, Rodriguez-Cortés F, Marsal JR, et al. Effectiveness of a motivational intervention on overweight/obese patients in the primary healthcare: a cluster randomized trial. *BMC Fam Pract.* (2017) 18:74. doi: 10.1186/s12875-017-0644-y

Rodrigues MF, Nardi AE, Levitan M. Mindfulness in mood and anxiety disorders: a review of the literature. *Trends Psychiatry Psychother.* (2017) 39:207–15. doi: 10.1590/2237-6089-2016-0051

Singh VK, Karmani S, Malo PK, Virupaksha HG, Muralidhar D, Venkatasubramanian G, Muralidharan K. Impact of lifestyle modification on some components of metabolic syndrome in persons with severe mental disorders: a meta-analysis. *Schizophr Res.* (2018) 202: 17–25. doi: 10.1016/j.schres.2018.06.066

Stiekema AP, Looijmans A, van der Meer L, Bruggeman R, Schoevers RA, Corpeleijn E, et al. Effects of a lifestyle intervention on psychosocial well-being of severe mentally ill residential patients: ELIPS, a cluster randomized controlled pragmatic trial. *Schizophr Res.* (2018) 199: 407–13. doi: 10.1016/j.schres.2018.02.053

Firth J, Cotter J, Elliott R, French P, Yung AR. A systematic review and meta-analysis of exercise interventions in schizophrenia patients. *Psychol Med.* (2015) 45:1343–61. doi: 10.1017/S0033291714003110

Stelmach-Mardas M, Mardas M, Walkowiak J, Boeing H. Long-term weight status in regainers after weight loss by lifestyle intervention: status and challenges. *Proc Nutr Soc.* (2014) 73:509–18. doi: 10.1017/S0029665114 000718

7

Altered Brain Functional Connectivity Density in Fast-Ball Sports Athletes with Early Stage of Motor Training

Chengbo Yang[1†], Ning Luo[2†], Minfeng Liang[2], Sihong Zhou[2], Qian Yu[3], Jiabao Zhang[2], Mu Zhang[4], Jingpu Guo[1], Hu Wang[1], Jiali Yu[2], Qian Cui[5], Huafu Chen[6,7] and Qing Gao[2]*

[1] The Third Department of Physical Education and Training, Chengdu Sport University, Chengdu, China, [2] School of Mathematical Sciences, University of Electronic Science and Technology of China, Chengdu, China, [3] Exercise and Mental Health Laboratory, School of Psychology, Shenzhen University, Shenzhen, China, [4] Information Technology Center, Chengdu Sport University, Chengdu, China, [5] School of Public Affairs and Administration, University of Electronic Science and Technology of China, Chengdu, China, [6] Ministry of Education Key Lab for Neuroinformation, High-Field Magnetic Resonance Brain Imaging Key Laboratory of Sichuan Province, University of Electronic Science and Technology of China, Chengdu, China, [7] The Clinical Hospital of Chengdu Brain Science Institute, School of Life Sciences and Technology, University of Electronic Science and Technology of China, Chengdu, China

Correspondence:
Qing Gao
gaoqing@uestc.edu.cn

† These authors have contributed equally to this work

The human brain shows neuroplastic adaptations caused by motor skill training. Of note, there is little known about the plastic architecture of the whole-brain network in resting state. The purpose of the present study was to detect how motor training affected the density distribution of whole-brain resting-state functional connectivity (FC). Resting-state functional magnetic resonance imaging data was assessed based on a comparison of fast-ball student athletes (SA) and non-athlete healthy controls (NC). The voxel-wise data-driven graph theory approach, global functional connectivity density (gFCD) mapping, was applied. Results showed that the SA group exhibited significantly decreased gFCD in brain regions centered at the left triangular part of the inferior frontal gyrus (IFG), extending to the opercular part of the left IFG and middle frontal gyrus compared to the NC group. In addition, findings suggested the idea of an increased neural efficiency of athletes' brain regions associated with attentional–motor modulation and executive control. Furthermore, behavioral results showed that in the SA group, faster executive control reaction time relates to smaller gFCD values in the left IFG. These findings suggested that the motor training would decrease the numbers of FC in IFG to accelerate the executive control with high attentional demands and enable SA to rapidly focus the attention to detect the intriguing target.

Keywords: athlete training, global functional connectivity density, resting-state functional magnetic resonance imaging, attention, neuroplasticity

INTRODUCTION

The brain of skilled elite athletes who have improved sport performance reveals neuroplastic adaptations caused by motor skill training (Gao et al., 2019; Chen et al., 2020; Jung et al., 2020). It has attracted special attention from researchers exploring how and where the structural and functional plasticity of the brain occurs in the course of motor skill training using imaging techniques [e.g., functional magnetic resonance imaging (fMRI) and functional near infrared spectroscopy (fNIRs)] (Crawford et al., 2019; Yu et al., 2020; Yue et al., 2020a,b). In particular, fMRI is widely accepted as an effective method to help researchers to understand the physiological mechanisms of brain plasticity via motor training; furthermore, findings might be practically meaningful for improving athletic performance (Gao et al., 2019; Zhang et al., 2019). However, it is largely unknown how brain functions change in the process of motor training (Lappi, 2015). Some researchers attempted to investigate the difference in brain activity between athletes and non-athlete controls (NC) during certain tasks (Gao et al., 2019), with different regions of task-induced activation between the two groups that are being reported. For instance, in the visual smooth pursuit task, football players showed greater activation in the oculomotor region of the cerebellar vermis and areas of the frontal eye fields than NC, suggesting visual motor skill is required for elite football players to successfully execute complex movement during games (Kellar et al., 2018). In addition, enhanced inferior parietal/frontal gyrus activity has been proposed in basketball players anticipating a free-throw task (Wu et al., 2013). Previous research suggested that when familiar sports environmental sounds surrounded, elite athletes tend to have greater activation in somatosensory regions but less activation in brain regions, which associated with perception and motor planning and processing (Woods et al., 2014). Except for the aforementioned results, a decreased brain activation in athletes (e.g., archery and table tennis) was reported across various cognitive tasks (e.g., mental rehearsal and visual–spatial task) compared to non-experts (Chang et al., 2011; Guo et al., 2017).

Resting-state fMRI (rsfMRI) is the commonly used method in the human brain map to evaluate intrinsic spontaneous fluctuations in the blood oxygen level-dependent (BOLD) signal in the resting or task-free state (Gao et al., 2013). This innovative and effective method was widely used in previous studies to investigate intrinsic brain plasticity or regional interaction induced by motor training. A study which implemented seed-based functional connectivity (FC) in distance runners shows increased connectivity between the fronto-parietal network and brain regions for execution functions compared to non-expert runners (Raichlen et al., 2016). These functional alterations in fronto-parietal connectivity were also found in badminton athletes (Di et al., 2012; Xu et al., 2016). In addition, similar results are found in elite karate players, suggesting brain areas associated with movement planning and visual perception having increased connectivity (Duru and Balcioglu, 2018). Our recent study using seed-based stepwise FC showed that fast-ball athletes were reported with a significantly smaller optimal connectivity distance from seed regions to the dorsal attention network (DAN) and larger optimal connectivity distance to the default mode network (DMN; Gao et al., 2019). Given the evidences above, changes in resting-state-FC brain plasticity occur in different brain areas across various sport events.

However, seed-based methods involved with the *a priori* selection of appropriate seed regions are unable to fully characterize the brain functional connectome as well as get a whole picture on the plastic architecture of the whole-brain network (Joel et al., 2011). Recently, functional connectivity density (FCD) mapping, a voxel-wise data-driven graph theory approach, has been established to determine the density distribution of whole-brain resting-state FC (Tomasi and Volkow, 2011; Huang et al., 2018). It measures the number of functional connections of a given voxel with the remaining voxels in the whole brain. The brain regions with high FCD values are considered as functional hubs of the human brain, which play a very important role in brain function (Tomasi and Volkow, 2011). Thus, this approach is a reliable and effective method and has been increasingly accepted in research detecting biomarkers of neuropsychiatric disorders through resting-state functional network alterations, including schizophrenia (Huang et al., 2018), major depressive disorder (Zhang et al., 2016; Zou et al., 2016), migraine (Gao et al., 2016), and aging brain (Li et al., 2019).

Here, we aimed to explore the neuroplasticity on brain functional organization induced by motor training using the global FCD (gFCD) approach. Fast-ball student athletes (SA) who play badminton, tennis, and table tennis were recruited. In fast-ball sports like badminton, tennis, and table tennis, the players require well-refined hand–eye coordination and visuospatial ability to achieve improved sports-related cognitions such as perception, focus, anticipation, planning, and fast responses (Di et al., 2012; Wolf et al., 2014). We started with an assumption that the fast-ball athletes would show changes in FC architecture in brain regions related to the visual attention and visual–motor coordination. To test whether the brain gFCD values relate to attentional processes, all subjects were asked to perform a revised attention network test (ANT) processing. The relationships between gFCD and reaction time of each attention subnetwork of alerting, orienting, and executive control were also investigated.

MATERIALS AND METHODS

Participants

Forty-two SA majoring in fast-ball sports (badminton, tennis, and table tennis) were recruited from Chengdu Sport University. All SA were required to pass the college entrance examination for sports majors in Sichuan province of China before entering Chengdu Sport University. The examination consisted of 40 points of the sport-specific test and 20 points of three physical fitness events, including 100-m run, standing triple jump, and standing shot put. The full mark of all test items is based on or slightly higher than the Standard of Technical Grade of Athletes issued by the General Administration of Sport of China. For example, the full mark of 100 m is 11.54 s, and the total score of all four test items has to exceed 85 points. After entering Chengdu Sport University, SA have been engaged in the fast ball-specific training. The training duration was less than 3 years, and the training frequency was less than 25 h per week. Thirty-nine NC with matched age, gender, and education level were also recruited. Except the sports-required course in the university, the NC group spent no more time on physical activity. All participants were tested handedness using the Chinese version of the Edinburgh-Handedness Questionnaire (coefficients > 50) (Oldfield, 1971), and all showed right-handedness. Participants had no history of neurological or psychiatric diseases or concussions. The study protocol was approved by the research ethical committee of School of Life Sciences and Technology, University of Electronic Science and Technology of China. Participants were provided written informed consent prior to any assessment.

Data Acquisition

Magnetic resonance imaging (MRI) images were acquired on a 3.0 T GE Signa MR750 system (GE Healthcare, Milwaukee) with an 8-channel phased array head coil. High-resolution 3D T1-weighted anatomical images were obtained in axial orientation using a 3D spoiled gradient-recalled (SPGR) sequence. The acquisition parameters were as follows: TR = 5.97 ms, TE = 1.96 ms, field of view (FOV) = 240 mm × 240 mm, flip angle = 12°, matrix size = 512 × 512, 156 slices, and voxel size = 1 mm × 1 mm × 1 mm. Resting-state fMRI images were acquired using a gradient-recalled echo planar imaging (EPI) sequence. The parameters were TR = 2000 ms, TE = 30 ms, FOV = 220 mm × 220 mm, flip angle = 90°, matrix size = 64 × 64, 43 transverse slices without a slice gap, voxel size = 3.75 mm × 3.75 mm × 3.2 mm, and a total of 266 volumes for each subject. During the scan, the subjects were instructed to lie down with their eyes closed, not to think of anything in particular, and not to fall asleep. Padded foams were used to restrict head motion, and earplugs were used to attenuate scanner noise.

Data Preprocessing

Conventional fMRI data preprocessing was performed using Data Processing Assistant for Resting-State fMRI software (DPARSF, Advanced Edition, V4.5).[1] The first 10 volumes of each subject were discarded to ensure steady-state longitudinal magnetization. The remaining 256 resting-state fMRI images were first corrected for the acquisition time delay between different slices and then realigned to the first volume to correct for head motion. We required that the transient movement during the scanning was no more than 1.0 mm of translation and 1.0° of rotation. The images were further spatially normalized into a standard stereotaxic space at 3 mm × 3 mm × 3 mm, using the EPI template in the Statistical Parametric Mapping software (SPM8). The images were not smoothed to avoid introducing artificial local spatial correlations. Images were then linearly detrended and were corrected using linear regression to remove the possible spurious variances including 24 head-motion parameters, averaged signals from cerebrospinal fluid, and white matter. The residuals of these regressions were temporally band-pass filtered ($0.01 < f < 0.08$ Hz) to reduce low-frequency drifts and physiological high-frequency respiratory and cardiac noises. Finally, scrubbing with the interpolation method was used to remove the bad points of the data. Since FC analysis is sensitive to gross head motion effects (Power et al., 2012), the mean frame-wise displacement (FD) was calculated to further determine the comparability of head movement across groups. The largest FD obtained from the subjects was less than 0.2 mm (which was 0.178 mm).

[1] http://www.restfmri.net/forum/

Global Functional Connectivity Density Analysis

Global functional connectivity density is defined as the number of statistically significant FCs between a given voxel and the rest of voxels across the whole brain in a binary network (Tomasi and Volkow, 2010). It is capable of quantifying the importance/centrality of a given voxel within the whole-brain network (Tomasi and Volkow, 2010). The voxel-wise gFCD maps were computed by an in-house program coded in MATLAB (The MathWorks, Natick, MA) according to the approach introduced by Tomasi and Volkow (2010). Briefly, we calculated the Pearson's correlation (r) between brain voxels that limited in a gray matter mask based on the automated anatomical labeling (AAL) atlas to obtain a whole-brain FC map at the voxel level. Two voxels were considered to be connected if their Pearson's correlation coefficient of the two voxels was greater than a given correlation threshold $Tc = 0.6$ according to the significant level of $p < 0.01$ (Bonferroni multiple correction), in order to eliminate the weak correlation which may be caused by noise (Tomasi and Volkow, 2010; Huang et al., 2018). Here, the significant level was set for testing the hypothesis of no functional connection against the alternative that there is a functional connection (non-zero correlation). The value of gFCD was defined of the global number of functional connections n_i, between voxel i and all other voxels in the brain. For each participant, gFCD maps were further standardized by the total number of edges in the whole brain (Li et al., 2018) and were spatially smoothed with full-width at half-maximum (FWHM) = 8 mm to minimize the individual overall differences of gFCD values (Tomasi and Volkow, 2011).

The Attention Network Test

To test whether the altered FC network architecture relates to attentional processes, all subjects were asked to perform a revised ANT (Wang et al., 2016), as shown in **Figure 1**. Briefly, the stimuli were presented via E-Prime 2.0 (Psychology Software Tools,

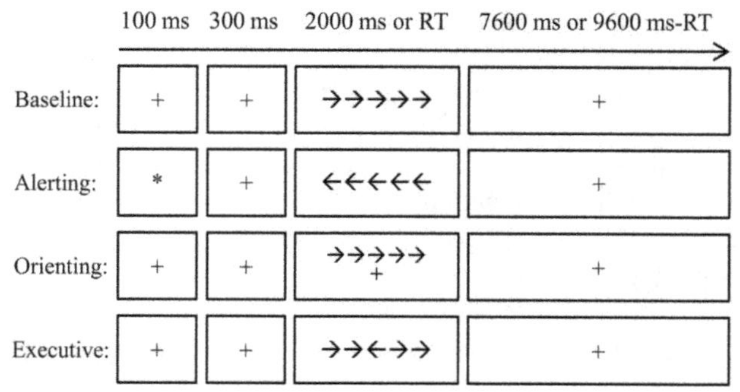

FIGURE 1 | The diagram for the attention network test (ANT) procedure. The four conditions, i.e., baseline, alerting, orienting, and executive control, were arranged in separated blocks. Each trial started with a cue (the alerting condition) or a fixation with 100 ms. After a 300-ms interval, the target was presented for 2,000 ms or disappeared after one key was pressed. A fixation was then presented until the end of that trial. Each trial lasted for 10 s. RT, reaction time.

Inc[2]) on a Lenovo PC. Responses were collected via Q (for left targets) and P (for right targets) on the keyboard. All participants completed four blocks (alerting block, orienting block, executive control block, and baseline block) of the ANT. The order of the four blocks was counterbalanced across subjects. Each block took 424 s, which contained a buffer time of 4 s, two practice trials of 10 s, and 40 experimental trials of 10 s. As shown in **Figure 1**, each trial began with a fixation or cue for 100 ms which was followed by a 300-ms fixation. After that, a target (congruent or incongruent, central, or spatial) appeared for 2000 ms or until the participant pressed a key. Lastly, another fixation was presented to ensure that the overall time of one trial was 10,000 ms (0.1 Hz). The subjects were asked to judge the direction of the third arrow (the central one) by pressing Q if it points to the left and P if it points to the right. The attention network scores (ANSs) were computed to measure the reaction time of each attention subnetwork of alerting, orienting, and executive control compared to the baseline (Wang et al., 2016).

Statistical Analysis

We used two-sample t-test analysis to compare the group differences of gFCD between the two groups. Age, gender, and education were considered as covariate variables. The statistically significant threshold of the gFCD was set for multiple comparisons at the cluster level with $p < 0.05$ (AlphaSim corrected). This correction was conducted using the DPARSF software.

To investigate whether the altered gFCD was associated with the behavioral reaction time of each attention subnetwork of alerting, orienting, and executive control, relationships between gFCD values in regions showing significant group differences and the reaction time of the three attention subnetworks were further detected by partial correlation analysis. The partial correlation analysis was performed for the SA group and the NC group, separately, with age and gender as confounding factors.

RESULTS

Demographic Data

The demographic data of the recruited subjects are shown in **Table 1**. The athlete group and the control group did not differ significantly in age (Mann–Whitney U-test, $p = 0.17$), gender (Pearson χ^2 test, $p = 0.35$), education (Mann–Whitney U-test, $p = 0.58$), or mean FD (Mann–Whitney U-test, $p = 0.94$).

gFCD in Athletes and Controls

Figure 2 shows the spatial distribution maps of the average gFCD in the SA group and the NC group, respectively. In both the SA and NC groups, the prefrontal cortex, posterior cingulate cortex, precuneus, and occipital cortex had relatively high gFCD values, as reported in previous studies (Tomasi and Volkow, 2010; Luo et al., 2014; Huang et al., 2018). **Figure 3** (left) shows the significantly different gFCD between the groups ($p < 0.05$, AlphaSim corrected). The SA group exhibited significantly decreased gFCD in brain regions centered at the left triangular part of the inferior frontal gyrus (IFG), extending to the left opercular part of the IFG and middle frontal gyrus (MFG) compared to the NC group. **Table 2** presented the Montreal Neurological Institute (MNI) coordinates of peak voxels and statistical t-values of the brain regions with significantly different gFCD between the two groups. The positive t-values represented that the NC group had higher gFCD values than the SA group. No significantly increased gFCD in the SA group compared with the NC group was found.

ANT Scores and Relationships With gFCD

Figure 3 (right) shows the significant correlations between the gFCD values and the reaction time of executive control in the SA group. In the SA group, the gFCD values in the left triangular part of IFG showed significant positive correlations with the executive control reaction time. In the NC group, subjects had relatively low values in reaction time, and the within-group dispersion of the reaction time was relatively small. The significant correlation between the gFCD values and the reaction time was not detected in the NC group.

DISCUSSION

The frontal cortex is one of the most crucial areas related to high-level functional integration (Woods et al., 2014). The inferior and middle frontal cortex especially contributed to the visual attention modulation and executive functions (Woods et al., 2014; Guo et al., 2017). In the task research in athletes, expert athletes had less activation in IFG and MFG when listening to familiar sports environmental sounds, suggesting the neural efficiency in these brain regions associated with perception and motor planning and processing (Woods et al., 2014). During the motor reaction and the visuo-spatial tasks, formula racing-car drivers recruited distributed networks including the middle and inferior frontal cortices, which devoted to executive functions (Bernardi et al., 2013). However, professional drivers recruited these regions to a significantly smaller extent as compared to naïve subjects (Bernardi et al., 2013). As support, table tennis athletes perform the visuo-spatial task with less brain activation in bilateral MFG than non-athletes (Guo et al., 2017). A similar finding was also observed in expert hockey players, suggesting neural efficiency in these brain regions for action decision as they were presented videos for shooting a puck toward a hockey goal (Olsson and Lundstrom, 2013). However, there were controversial results in some tasks. For instance, an increased activity in the inferior parietal lobule and IFG was detected in basketball athletes performing a free-throw task (Wu et al., 2013). Therefore, the task-related results demonstrated IFG and MFG as functional hubs of visual motor integration, motor control, and executive functions. In addition, the results suggested their functional plasticity induced by motor skill training.

The rsfMRI results are independent of task. The task-free approach can explore the intrinsic neural plasticity induced by

[2]http://www.pstnet.com

TABLE 1 | Demographics of the subjects.

	Age (years)	Gender (female/male)	Education (years)	Training time (h/week)	Duration (years)	Mean FD (mm)
SA (n = 42)	20.43 ± 0.59	12/30	14.57 ± 0.67	17.17 ± 0.83	1.95 ± 0.08	0.08 ± 0.02
NC (n = 39)	20.33 ± 1.33	15/24	15.05 ± 1.43	–	–	0.08 ± 0.03
P value	0.1736[a]	0.3454[b]	0.5803[a]	–	–	0.9363[a]

Data are presented as mean ± SD. SD, standard deviation; FD, frame-wise displacement; NC, non-athlete controls; SA, student athlete. [a]Obtained using Mann–Whitney U-test. [b]Obtained using the Pearson χ^2 test.

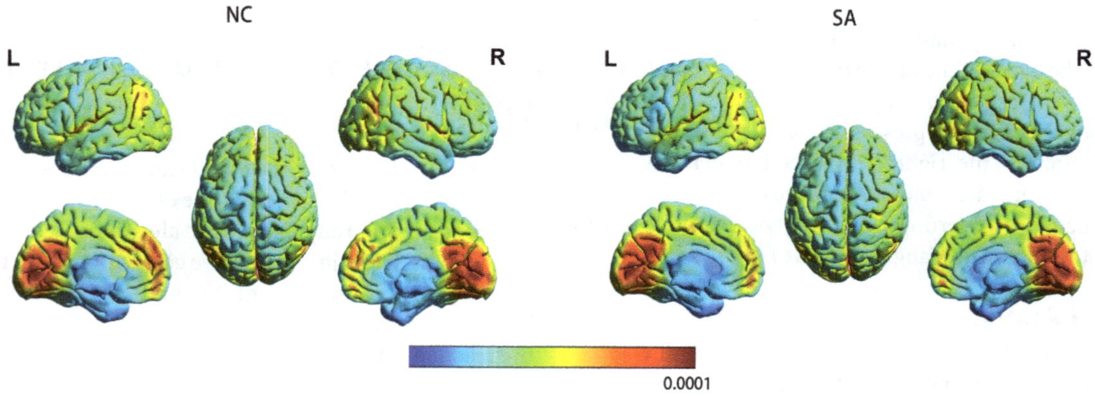

FIGURE 2 | The spatial distribution maps of the average gFCD maps for the SA group and the NC group. For each participant, the gFCD value of each voxel was standardized by the total number of edges in the whole brain. L, left; NC, non-athlete control; R, right; SA, student athlete.

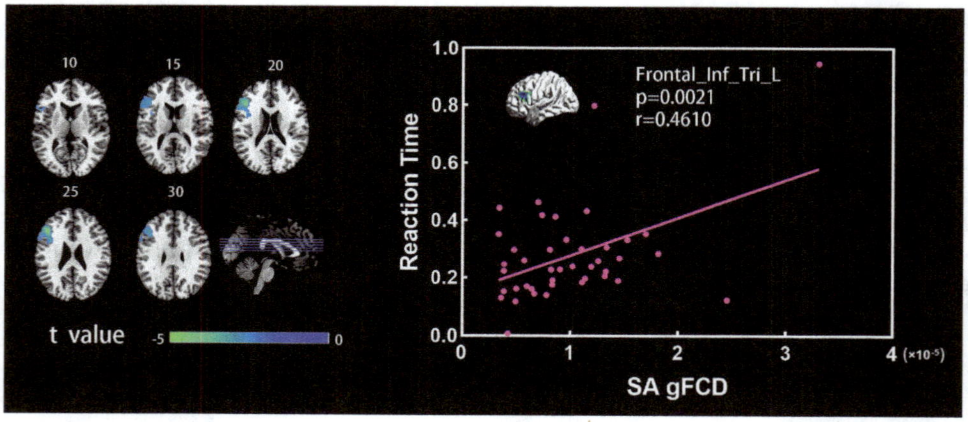

FIGURE 3 | **(Left)** Brain regions showing significant differences between the SA and NC groups in the gFCD analysis (two sample t-test, $p < 0.05$, GRF corrected). Numbers above each image refer to the z-plane coordinates of the MNI space. **(Right)** Significant correlation between reaction time and gFCD values in the SA group. Frontal_Inf_Tri_L, left triangular part of inferior frontal gyrus.

TABLE 2 | Brain regions showed significantly different gFCD between the athlete group and the control group.

Brain regions	Hem	Peak coordinates	Cluster size	T-value
Inferior frontal gyrus, triangular	L	(–39,27,24)	328	5.63
Inferior frontal gyrus, opercular	L	(–57,27,18)	68	3.83
Middle frontal gyrus	L	(–54,36,21)	144	3.72

motor skill training. There has been local seed-based FC analysis, which showed altered FC between the athlete group and controls within the left frontoparietal network (Di et al., 2012). In the athlete group, an enhanced FC between the left superior parietal lobule and left MFG (BA6) was detected, whereas a lower FC between the left superior parietal lobule and the left MFG (BA9) was observed compared to the control group (Di et al., 2012). In addition, previous research was found that distance runners exhibited enhanced connectivity between the right parietal cortex and MFG (Raichlen et al., 2016).

Global functional connectivity density is a powerful framework to characterize the FC architecture within the whole-brain network without any prior hypothesis (Tomasi and Volkow, 2011). From the point of view of the whole-brain resting-state FC, our results showed decreased gFCD values in the left IFG and MFG in the fast-ball SA group compared to the NC group. This is a distinct but complementary information on the brain plasticity caused by motor skill training in fast-ball SA. Such results demonstrated reduced connections between these brain regions and the remaining brain voxels in the SA group. The findings were consistent with the previous research, regardless of skilled groups, such as racing-car drivers (Bernardi et al., 2013), table tennis players (Guo et al., 2017), basketball players (Pi et al., 2019), golfers (Milton et al., 2007), and musicians (Haslinger et al., 2004; Meister et al., 2005). The possible explanation could be that athletes' brain might exhibit an improved neural efficiency in the brain regions associated with attentional-motor modulation and executive control along with a reduced "resource consumption" (Rypma and Prabhakaran, 2009; Bernardi et al., 2013; Guo et al., 2017; Sommer et al., 2018; Zhang et al., 2019).

Importantly, we further detected a positive correlation between gFCD values in the left triangular part of IFG and reaction time of the executive control in the SA group. Of the three attention subnetworks, the executive control network is very useful for producing top-down regulation and thus is related to executive control (Petersen and Posner, 2012). This system was presented under the heading of target detection (Petersen and Posner, 2012). It is related to the limited capacity of the attention system, and to awareness itself, and has often been called focal attention (Petersen and Posner, 2012). Fast-ball sport events require athletes to execute actions in a short time (Ermutlu et al., 2015), in terms of well-refined hand–eye coordination and visuospatial ability to achieve enhanced perception, concentration, anticipation, planning, and fast response requirements (Di et al., 2012; Gao et al., 2019). Our results suggested that faster executive control reaction time was associated with smaller gFCD values in the left triangular part of IFG. The behavioral results further supported that in the SA group, shorter reaction time of executive control was associated with smaller gFCD values, which referred to the numbers of FC between a given voxel and the rest of voxels across the whole brain. The findings implied that motor skill training results in a decrease in the number of FC in the left triangular part of IFG, which athletes are interested in developing reaction capacity, movement planning, and execution with high attentional demands, and focus the attention to the target detection (Wolf et al., 2014). Of note, sample size was relatively low in the present study, and only the student-athletes who were trained in fast ball of badminton, tennis, and table tennis were recruited. Our findings only limited to the fast-ball sports athletes with early stage of motor training.

CONCLUSION

Using resting-state functional imaging techniques and graph theory approach, the present study revealed that compared with the NC group, the SA group exhibited significantly decreased gFCD in IFG and MFG. As supportive of the behavioral data, faster executive control reaction time was associated with smaller gFCD values in the left triangular part of IFG in the SA group. The findings supported the idea of an increased neural efficiency of athletes' brain in the brain regions associated with attentional-motor modulation and executive control and implied the training-induced neuroplasticity occurring in these brain regions. In addition, our findings were based on the resting-state brain functional network, which was independent of specific tasks. The neural mechanisms of functional adaptations in the athletes' brain that made their exceptional performance possible might have potential applications in designing optimal sports coaching methods, in overcoming learning disabilities, and in neurological rehabilitation (Lappi, 2015).

ETHICS STATEMENT

The study protocol was approved by the research ethical committee of School of Life Sciences and Technology, University of Electronic Science and Technology of China. The patients/participants provided their written informed consent to participate in this study. Written informed consent was obtained from the individual(s) for the publication of any potentially identifiable images or data included in this article.

AUTHOR CONTRIBUTIONS

CY, NL, and QG contributed to the conception and design of the research. MZ, JG, HW, and ML collected the data. ML, SZ, and JZ applied the statistical analysis. NL and CY analyzed and interpreted the data. CY, NL, and QG wrote the manuscript. QG and HC edited the manuscript. QG was responsible for the overall project. QY edited and modified the manuscript. All authors contributed to the article and approved the submitted version.

REFERENCES

Bernardi, G., Ricciardi, E., Sani, L., Gaglianese, A., Papasogli, A., Ceccarelli, R., et al. (2013). How skill expertise shapes the brain functional architecture: an fMRI study of visuo-spatial and motor processing in professional racing-car and naive drivers. *PLoS One* 8:e77764. doi: 10.1371/journal.pone.0077764

Chang, Y., Lee, J. J., Seo, J. H., Song, H. J., Kim, Y. T., Lee, H. J., et al. (2011). Neural correlates of motor imagery for elite archers. *NMR Biomed.* 24, 366–372.

Chen, L. Z., Yuan, X., Zhang, Y., Zhang, S., Zou, L., Yang, L., et al. (2020). Brain functional specialization is enhanced among tai chi chuan practitioners. *Arch. Phys. Med. Rehabil.* 101, 1176–1182.

Crawford, L., Zou, L., and Loprinzi, P. D. (2019). Oxygenation of the prefrontal cortex during memory interference. *J. Clin. Med.* 8:2055. doi: 10.3390/jcm8122055

Di, X., Zhu, S., Jin, H., Wang, P., Ye, Z., Zhou, K., et al. (2012). Altered resting brain function and structure in professional badminton players. *Brain Connect.* 2, 225–233.

Duru, A. D., and Balcioglu, T. H. (2018). Functional and structural plasticity of brain in elite karate athletes. *J. Healthc. Eng.* 2018:8310975. doi: 10.1155/2018/8310975

Ermutlu, N., Yücesir, I., Eskikurt, G., Temel, T., and Ý??oǑlu-Alkaç, Ü (2015). Brain electrical activities of dancers and fast ball sports athletes are different. *Cogn. Neurodyn.* 9, 257–263. doi: 10.1007/s11571-014-9320-2

Gao, Q., Xu, F., Jiang, C., Chen, Z., Chen, H., Liao, H., et al. (2016). Decreased functional connectivity density in pain-related brain regions of female migraine patients without aura. *Brain Res.* 1632, 73–81. doi: 10.1016/j.brainres.2015.12.007

Gao, Q., Xu, Q., Duan, X., Liao, W., Ding, J., Zhang, Z., et al. (2013). Extraversion and neuroticism relate to topological properties of resting-state brain networks. *Front. Hum. Neurosci.* 7:257. doi: 10.3389/fnhum.2013.00257

Gao, Q., Yu, Y., Su, X., Tao, Z., Zhang, M., Wang, Y., et al. (2019). Adaptation of brain functional stream architecture in athletes with fast demands of sensorimotor integration. *Hum. Brain Mapp.* 40, 420–431.

Guo, Z., Li, A., and Yu, L. (2017). "Neural efficiency" of athletes' brain during visuo-spatial task: an fMRI study on table tennis players. *Front. Behav. Neurosci.* 11:72. doi: 10.3389/fnbeh.2017.00072

Haslinger, B., Erhard, P., Altenmüller, E., Hennenlotter, A., Schwaiger, M., Gräfin von Einsiedel, H., et al. (2004). Reduced recruitment of motor association areas during bimanual coordination in concert pianists. *Hum. Brain Mapp.* 22, 206–215. doi: 10.1002/hbm.20028

Huang, H., Jiang, Y., Xia, M., Tang, Y., Zhang, T., Cui, H., et al. (2018). Increased resting-state global functional connectivity density of default mode network in schizophrenia subjects treated with electroconvulsive therapy. *Schizophr. Res.* 197, 192–199. doi: 10.1016/j.schres.2017.10.044

Joel, S. E., Caffo, B. S., van Zijl, P. C., and Pekar, J. J. (2011). On the relationship between seed-based and ICA-based measures of functional connectivity. *Magn. Reson. Med.* 66, 644–657. doi: 10.1002/mrm.22818

Jung, M., Zou, L., Yu, J. J., Ryu, S., Kong, Z., Yang, L., et al. (2020). Does exercise have a protective effect on cognitive function under hypoxia? A systematic review with meta-analysis. *J. Sport Health Sci.* [Epub ahead of print]. doi: 10.1016/j.jshs.2020.04.004

Kellar, D., Newman, S., Pestilli, F., Cheng, H., and Port, N. L. (2018). Comparing fMRI activation during smooth pursuit eye movements among contact sport athletes, non-contact sport athletes, and non-athletes. *Neuroimage Clin.* 18, 413–424. doi: 10.1016/j.nicl.2018.01.025

Lappi, O. (2015). The racer's brain - how domain expertise is reflected in the neural substrates of driving. *Front. Hum. Neurosci.* 9:635. doi: 10.3389/fnhum.2015.00635

Li, H., Zhang, X., Sun, B., Jiang, S., Li, J., Liu, C., et al. (2019). BOLD-fMRI reveals the association between renal oxygenation and functional connectivity in the aging brain. *Neuroimage* 186, 510–517. doi: 10.1016/j.neuroimage.2018.11.030

Li, R., Wang, L., Chen, H., Guo, X., Liao, W., Tang, Y. L., et al. (2018). Abnormal dynamics of functional connectivity density in children with benign epilepsy with centrotemporal spikes. *Brain Imaging Behav.* 13, 985–994. doi: 10.1007/s11682-018-9914-0

Luo, C., Tu, S., Peng, Y., Gao, S., Li, J., Dong, L., et al. (2014). Long-term effects of musical training and functional plasticity in salience system. *Neural. Plast.* 2014:180138.

Meister, I., Krings, T., Foltys, H., Boroojerdi, B., Müller, M., Töpper, R., et al. (2005). Effects of long-term practice and task complexity in musicians and nonmusicians performing simple and complex motor tasks: implications for cortical motor organization. *Hum. Brain Mapp.* 25, 345–352. doi: 10.1002/hbm.20112

Milton, J., Solodkin, A., Hlustík, P., and Small, S. L. (2007). The mind of expert motor performance is cool and focused. *Neuroimage* 35, 804–813. doi: 10.1016/j.neuroimage.2007.01.003

Oldfield, R. C. (1971). The assessment and analysis of handedness: the Edinburgh inventory. *Neuropsychologia* 9, 97–113. doi: 10.1016/0028-3932(71)90067-4

Olsson, C. J., and Lundstrom, P. (2013). Using action observation to study superior motor performance: a pilot fMRI study. *Front. Hum. Neurosci.* 7:819. doi: 10.3389/fnhum.2013.00819

Petersen, S. E., and Posner, M. I. (2012). The attention system of the human brain: 20 years after. *Annu. Rev. Neurosci.* 35, 73–89. doi: 10.1146/annurev-neuro-062111-150525

Pi, Y. L., Wu, X.-H., Wang, F.-J., Liu, K., Wu, Y., Zhu, H., et al. (2019). Motor skill learning induces brain network plasticity: a diffusion-tensor imaging study. *PLoS One* 14:e0210015. doi: 10.1371/journal.pone.0210015

Power, J. D., Barnes, K. A., Snyder, A. Z., Schlaggar, B. L., and Petersen, S. E. (2012). Spurious but systematic correlations in functional connectivity MRI networks arise from subject motion. *Neuroimage* 59, 2142–2154. doi: 10.1016/j.neuroimage.2011.10.018

Raichlen, D. A., Bharadwaj, P. K., Fitzhugh, M. C., Haws, K. A., Torre, G. A., Trouard, T. P., et al. (2016). Differences in resting state functional connectivity between young adult endurance athletes and healthy controls. *Front. Hum. Neurosci.* 10:610. doi: 10.3389/fnhum.2016.00610

Rypma, B., and Prabhakaran, V. (2009). When less is more and when more is more: the mediating roles of capacity and speed in brain-behavior efficiency. *Intelligence* 37, 207–222. doi: 10.1016/j.intell.2008.12.004

Sommer, M., Häger, C. K., Boraxbekk, C. J., and Rönnqvist, L. (2018). Timing Training in female soccer players: effects on skilled movement performance and brain responses. *Front. Hum. Neurosci.* 12:311. doi: 10.3389/fnhum.2018.00311

Tomasi, D., and Volkow, N. D. (2010). Functional connectivity density mapping. *Proc. Natl. Acad. Sci. U.S.A.* 107, 9885–9890. doi: 10.1073/pnas.1001414107

Tomasi, D., and Volkow, N. D. (2011). Association between functional connectivity hubs and brain networks. *Cereb. Cortex* 21, 2003–2013. doi: 10.1093/cercor/bhq268

Wang, Y. F., Long, Z., Cui, Q., Liu, F., Jing, X. J., Chen, H., et al. (2016). Low frequency steady-state brain responses modulate large scale functional networks in a frequency-specific means. *Hum. Brain Mapp.* 37, 381–394. doi: 10.1002/hbm.23037

Wolf, S., Brölz, E., Scholz, D., Ramos-Murguialday, A., Keune, P. M., Hautzinger, M., et al. (2014). Winning the game: brain processes in expert, young elite and amateur table tennis players. *Front. Behav. Neurosci.* 8:370. doi: 10.3389/fnbeh.2014.00370

Woods, E. A., Hernandez, A. E., Wagner, V. E., and Beilock, S. L. (2014). Expert athletes activate somatosensory and motor planning regions of the brain when passively listening to familiar sports sounds. *Brain Cogn.* 87, 122–133. doi: 10.1016/j.bandc.2014.03.007

Wu, Y., Zeng, Y., Zhang, L., Wang, S., Wang, D., Tan, X., et al. (2013). The role of visual perception in action anticipation in basketball athletes. *Neuroscience* 237, 29–41. doi: 10.1016/j.neuroscience.2013.01.048

Xu, H., Wang, P., Ye, Z., Di, X., Xu, G., Mo, L., et al. (2016). The role of medial frontal cortex in action anticipation in professional badminton players. *Front. Psychol.* 7:1817. doi: 10.3389/fpsyg.2016.01817

Yu, Q., Herold, F., Becker, B., KluGah-Brown, B., Zhang, Y., Perrey, S., et al. (2020). Cognitive benefits of exercise interventions: an fMRI activation likelihood estimation meta-analysis. *bioRxiv* [Preprint]. doi: 10.1101/2020.07.04.187401

Yue, C., Zhang, Y., Jian, M., Herold, F., Yu, Q., Mueller, P., et al. (2020a). Differential effects of tai chi chuan (motor-cognitive training) and walking on brain networks: a resting-state fMRI study in chinese women aged 60. *Healthcare* 8:67. doi: 10.3390/healthcare8010067

Yue, C., Zou, L., Mei, J., Moore, D., Herold, F., Müller, P., et al. (2020b). Tai chi training evokes significant changes in brain white matter network in older women. *Healthcare* 8:57. doi: 10.3390/healthcare8010057

Zhang, B., Li, M., Qin, W., Demenescu, L. R., Metzger, C. D., Bogerts, B., et al. (2016). Altered functional connectivity density in major depressive disorder at rest. *Eur. Arch. Psychiatry Clin. Neurosci.* 266, 239–248. doi: 10.1007/s00406-015-0614-0

Zhang, L., Qiu, F., Zhu, H., Xiang, M., and Zhou, L. (2019). Neural efficiency and acquired motor skills: an fMRI study of expert athletes. *Front. Psychol.* 10:2752. doi: 10.3389/fpsyg.2019.02752

Zou, K., Gao, Q., Long, Z., Xu, F., Sun, X., Chen, H., et al. (2016). Abnormal functional connectivity density in first-episode, drug-naive adult patients with major depressive disorder. *J. Affect. Disord.* 194, 153–158. doi: 10.1016/j.jad.2015.12.081

8

Less Medication use in Inpatients with Severe Mental Illness Receiving a Multidisciplinary Lifestyle Enhancing Treatment

Jeroen Deenik[1,2]*, Diederik E. Tenback[1], Harold F. van Driel[1], Erwin C. P. M. Tak[3], Ingrid J. M. Hendriksen[4] and Peter N. van Harten[1,2]

[1] GGz Centraal, Amersfoort, Netherlands, [2] School for Mental Health and Neuroscience, Maastricht University, Maastricht, Netherlands, [3] Tak Advies en Onderzoek, Leiden, Netherlands, [4] Living Active, Santpoort-Zuid, Netherlands

***Correspondence:**
Jeroen Deenik
j.deenik@ggzcentraal.nl

Besides having an unhealthy lifestyle contributing to premature mortality, inpatients with severe mental illness (SMI) use high dosages of medication. Previous research has shown improved health after lifestyle improvements in SMI. In addition, we aimed to retrospectively study whether a multidisciplinary lifestyle enhancing treatment (MULTI) was associated with changes in medication use after 18 months, as compared with patients that continued treatment as usual (TAU) and explored mediation by a change in physical activity. We conducted an observational study within a cohort of inpatients with SMI, who received MULTI (N = 65) or continued TAU (N = 49). Data on their somatic and psychotropic medications were collected, converted into defined daily dose (DDD), and analyzed using linear multilevel regression, correcting for baseline value and differences between groups in age, diagnosis, and illness severity. Compared with TAU, the DDD for psychotropic medication significantly decreased with MULTI (B = −0.55, P = 0.02). Changes in total activity did not mediate this association, suggesting that multiple components of MULTI contributed. Corrected between-group analyses for subgroups of medication were not possible due to lack of power and skewed distributions. Within-group data showed a decreased proportion of users as well as median DDD in both groups for almost all medications. In addition to previously reported health improvements after 18 months of MULTI, we observed a significant decrease in dose of psychotropic medication in MULTI compared to TAU. This first study evaluating a wide range of medications indicates a possible effect of lifestyle improvements on medication use in inpatients with SMI. Findings need to be confirmed in future controlled studies, however.

Keywords: medication, antipsychotics, physical activity, hospitalization, severe mental illness, schizophrenia, lifestyle, side effects

INTRODUCTION

In patients with severe mental illness (SMI), a high prevalence of metabolic risk factors (1–3) contribute to their poor cardiovascular health, largely contributing to a reduced life expectancy of at least 7–20 years compared to the general population (4–6). Besides a sedentary lifestyle (7–10), side effects of psychotropic medication (such as weight gain, dyslipidemia, diabetes mellitus, and direct and indirect harm to the vascular system) are associated with these cardiovascular health issues (11–14). Polypharmacy, higher dosages, and longer-term use are associated with higher risk for most of these side effects and somatic diseases (11, 12, 15). A study in people diagnosed with schizophrenia showed that both no exposure as well as high exposure to antipsychotics were associated with higher cardiovascular mortality than either low or moderate exposure (16). Unfortunately, polypharmacy is very prevalent among people with SMI (15, 17) and the dosage of antipsychotic medication has only increased during the last decades for long-term hospitalized patients (18, 19). Alongside this psychotropic medication, patients use antihypertensive, lipid-lowering, antihyperglycemic and other additional drugs if cardiovascular health issues (whether or not caused by psychotropic medication) are too severe (20–24).

Nowadays, there is more focus on the lowest effective dose, on the avoidance of inappropriate polypharmacy to minimize the side effect of antipsychotics (25–28), and on supporting a healthy lifestyle (29–32). Despite an increased number of studies showing benefits of lifestyle interventions in people with SMI, there is a lack of evidence to support the long-term effectiveness of such interventions in hospitalized patients (33, 34). Moreover, to the best of our knowledge, studies evaluating lifestyle interventions in inpatients did not analyze changes in medication use. Recently, improved physical activity and metabolic health were shown after 18 months in this group of patients receiving a multidisciplinary lifestyle enhancing treatment for inpatients with SMI (MULTI) (35). MULTI was pragmatically implemented in a group of inpatients whose psychotropic medication was already critically reviewed prior to its implementation; hence, dose reduction was not a specific goal. The treatment focused on decreasing sedentary behavior, increasing physical activity, and improving dietary habits in the context of daily treatment.

Because the (side) effects of medications are associated with cardiometabolic health issues, we hypothesized that we might observe changes in medication use after lifestyle changes, in addition to improvements in physical health. Therefore, the present study aimed to retrospectively study whether 18 months of MULTI was associated with changes in medication use, as compared with patients that continued treatment as usual (TAU) and to explore whether changes were mediated by increased physical activity as an essential component of MULTI.

MATERIALS AND METHODS

Study Design

This observational cohort study was conducted at wards for long-term inpatient mental healthcare in a psychiatric hospital of GGz Centraal (The Netherlands). The current study is part of a comprehensive evaluation of MULTI, a treatment that was implemented pragmatically in February 2014 in three wards. MULTI was developed because of the identified need to address the comorbidity (e.g., sleep apnea and cardiovascular morbidity) in this population, in part due to a lack of physical activity, obesity, and dietary risks). The implementation of MULTI (described in the next paragraph) was conducted by psychiatrists, nurses and team leaders in collaboration with activity coordinators and a dietitian. During a previous MULTI study (35), data of baseline (Aug.–Dec. 2013) and one follow-up (Aug.–Dec. 2015) were collected from 114 patients (65 received MULTI and 49 continued TAU). Data on types and dose of medication were extracted from electronic patient records and compared between patients receiving MULTI and those receiving TAU. Because of the observational nature of this study, whereby MULTI was already implemented pragmatically in three wards before the start of this study, no randomization took place. Therefore, we analyzed potential differences between groups at baseline and, if significant, corrected for these differences in analyses as potential confounders. The study protocol was approved by the Medical Ethical Committee of the Isala Academy (case 14.0678). All subjects gave written informed consent in accordance with the Declaration of Helsinki.

Study Population

The cohort consisted of patients with SMI who had been hospitalized for at least 1 year. Patients were included in the MULTI study if they had not received any other intervention related to lifestyle within 18 months since the start of MULTI and if baseline accelerometer data was available. Exclusion criterion was a lack of data after 18 months due to being either discharged or deceased. Patients included for follow-up were dropped out for further analyses if they had insufficient accelerometer data (see Physical Activity below) or refused the repeated accelerometer measurement.

MULTI

The purpose of MULTI was a holistic lifestyle change with a focus on decreasing sedentary behavior, increasing physical activity, and improving dietary habits. Improving the daily structure formed the base of the treatment, by starting each day with getting up on time, having three joint meals per day, and an active day program consisting of sports-related activities (e.g., walking, running, yoga, biking, indoor team sports), work-related activities (e.g., gardening and helping out with daily jobs), psycho-education (e.g., about side effects, dietary habits), and skills training (e.g., making a grocery list, shopping, cooking). Also, existing policies were reviewed critically—e.g., the use of personal transport within walking distance around the hospital area for every patient was reduced to its use for immobile patients and in case of extreme weather only. Because of heterogeneity in illness severity and different capabilities and interests, the content and intensity of the day-to-day program were tailored to the particular ward and individual patients by the nurses and specific disciplines (see below). Therefore, the actual frequency, intensity, kind of activities and format (e.g., group or alone) could vary between patients and wards. However, it was intended that all patients were doing some of the activities in the morning and afternoon, to prevent prolonged periods lying in bed or sitting at the ward. Also, the participation of nurses in the day-to-day program was an essential element, which contributed to the culture change within the institution and in the provision of support to patients. MULTI was based on a "change from within-principle" developed by current staff (psychiatrists, nurses, and team leader in collaboration with activity coordinators and a dietitian), working with regular context and resources in daily routine care. It was supervised and disseminated per ward by the head practitioner (a psychiatrist) as an innovative treatment method. Nurses received support from the psychiatrists (psycho-education), activity coordinators, and the dietitian. Adherence to and compliance with the treatment was discussed in the weekly multidisciplinary consultation. If a patient could not get along in the day-to-day program (e.g., getting out of bed or attending selected activities), it was agreed upon that specific action was to be taken to physically activate a particular patient, using extra individual motivational interviewing by their mentor (one of the nurses) or psychiatrist, who were trained in this, and by consulting an activity coordinator or dietitian if needed.

Patients who received TAU continued their treatment, which mainly concerned pharmacological treatment and a less structured day program and did not include any supported lifestyle interventions or adjustments.

Measurements

Medication

Medication use was classified by type of medication in the main groups and by converting doses to daily defined doses (DDD) according to the Anatomical Therapeutic Chemical (ATC) Classification System of the World Health Organization (36). Somatic medications included medications for the alimentary tract and metabolism (A), blood and blood-forming organs (B), cardiovascular system (C), and respiratory system (R). Psychotropic medications included the medications for the nervous system (N). Due to the differences in specific purpose, efficacy, and side effects of psycholeptics (N05), we distinguished antipsychotics (N05A) from anxiolytics, hypnotics, and sedatives (N05B & N05C). Likewise, we distinguished the category antipsychotics into three groups: (i) typical and (ii) atypical antipsychotics (occurring in different subgroups) and (iii) lithium (N05AN). For this study, we only used fixed prescriptions (i.e., not including medication to be given as needed). Physical activity.

Physical Activity

To test for potential mediation by a change in physical activity, we used accelerometer data (ActiGraph GT3X+) that was collected within the MULTI study. Detailed procedures and settings used in the baseline and follow-up measurement were described elsewhere (9, 35). Accelerometers were worn on the right hip; wear time of $\geq$6 h/day for $\geq$3 days was used as the criterion for sufficient measurement, and the same timeframe (9:00 a.m–10:00 p.m) was used for each dataset to be able to compare individual data. These were analyzed using the ActiGraph (*ActiGraph Corp., Pensacola FL, USA*) software ActiLife 6.8.0 and calculated into average total activity counts per hour (TAC/h) as a continuous and detailed outcome variable, where more counts indicate a higher level of activity. The GT3X+ showed a high inter- and intra-instrumental reliability and validity in healthy adults. Inter-instrument reliability in free-living conditions (hip worn) was high for overall activity (ICC = 0.97 and a 95% limit of agreement of $\pm$81.3 counts per minute for vector magnitude) (37, 38) and moderate-to-vigorous activity (ICC = 0.99) (39). The GT3X+ showed acceptable agreement between step counts observed in a laboratory setting (ICC = 0.61–0.99) and free-living situations (ICC = 0.90) (40).

Statistical Analysis

Data analyses were performed using SPSS 22.0 and interpreted at a two-tailed significance level of $p < 0.05$. Differences in patient and disease characteristics between patients who received MULTI and those receiving TAU were analyzed using independent t-test and chi-square statistics. Continuous variables were examined for linearity, normality, and homogeneity as assumptions for linear analysis by comparing means with medians and analyzing frequency histograms, normality plots, and plots of residuals vs. predicted values. If variables were not distributed linearly toward the dependent variables, they were added as tertiles in the analysis, with the first tertile as the reference category. If data was not distributed normally, analyses were performed using non-parametric tests.

Sum scores of changes in DDDs of somatic and psychotropic medications were distributed normally, after excluding two outliers ($z < -3$) from the DDD of somatic medication. We used linear multilevel regression to evaluate changes in these outcomes between MULTI and TAU, whereby possible clustering of data within wards was taken into account using a two-level structure, with the wards as the first level and the patients as the second. The change scores of the outcome variables were regressed on the treatment variable and adjusted for the baseline value to prevent potential regression to the mean (crude, model 1). We added patient and disease characteristics that significantly differed between patients receiving MULTI and TAU as covariates in models 2 and 3, respectively. We were not able to properly run corrected between-group analyses on subgroups of medication due to skewed distributions and insufficient power for non-parametric between-group analyses. Therefore, we analyzed the change in DDDs within subgroups of medication separately within MULTI and TAU, using Wilcoxon signed-rank tests.

Additionally, final significant models were analyzed for possible mediation by a change in total activity counts per hour (TAC/h), using the PROCESS tool in SPSS (41) (**Figure 1**). The mediation effect was calculated as the product of those coefficients (ab, not shown within the model) and was considered significant if the bias-corrected and accelerated (BCa) bootstrapped confidence intervals did not include zero.

RESULTS

Table 1 shows the baseline characteristics of patients receiving MULTI and TAU. None of the included 114 patients dropped out.

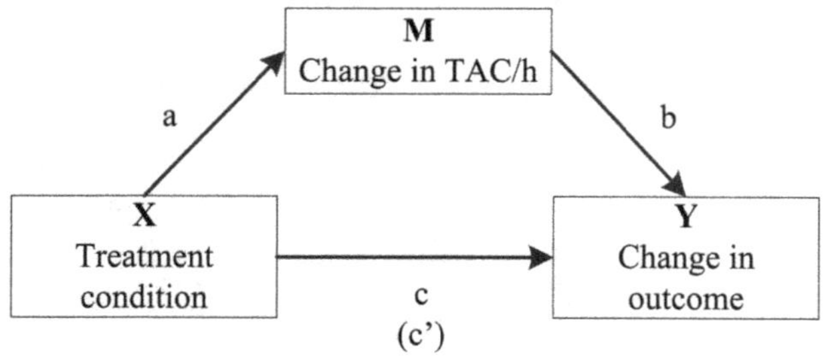

FIGURE 1 | Model summarizing how the role of change in average total activity counts per hour (TAC/h) as a potential mediator (M) in the association between treatment condition (X) and significant change in medication use (Y) is quantified in mediation analysis. It includes the associations between treatment condition and TAC/h (a), TAC/h and the particular outcome variable (b) and treatment condition on the particular outcome variable (c). The coefficient between the latter two, controlling for change in TAC/h, is in parentheses (c′).

TABLE 1 | Baseline characteristics of patients (*N* = 114).

Outcome (scale)	MULTI (*n* = 65)	TAU (*n* = 49)
Sex, *n* (%) male	43 (66.2)	27 (55.1)
Age, years, mean (*SD*)	**52.2(8.9)**	**58.7 (11.6)**
Diagnosis, *n* (%)		
Schizophrenia and other psychotic disorders	**61[a](93.8)**	**28[b](57.1)**
Other disorders	**4[c] (6.2)**	**21[d] (42.9)**
Illness severity, CGI-S scale 1-7, mean (*SD*)	**5.0 (1.2)**	**4.3(1.2)**
Years of hospitalization, mean (*SD*)	14.4 (10.9)	13.2 (12.7)

Significant differences between groups are shown in bold.
MULTI, MUltidisciplinary Lifestyle enhancing Treatment for Inpatients with severe mental illness; TAU, Treatment As Usual; CGI-S, Clinical Global Impression–Severity scale.
[a]*other: schizoaffective disorder (n = 4) and a psychotic disorder not otherwise specified (n = 1).*
[b]*other: schizoaffective disorder (n = 4) and psychotic disorder not otherwise specified (n =2).*
[c]*mood disorders (n = 2): a pervasive disorder not otherwise specified (n = 1) and an anxiety disorder (n = 1).*
[d]*mood disorders (n = 8): personality disorders (n = 4), alcohol-related disorders (n = 4), somatoform disorders (n = 2), delirium, dementia, and amnestic and other cognitive disorders (n = 2) and a pervasive disorder not otherwise specified (n = 1).*

On average, patients receiving MULTI were younger ($M = -6.45$ years, 95% CI: −10.27 to −2.64), had a higher baseline illness severity ($M = 0.63$, 95% CI: 0.17 to 1.08) and were more frequently diagnosed with schizophrenia or other psychotic disorders ($X^2 = 21.98, p < 0.001$) than patients receiving TAU.

Total Use of Somatic and Psychotropic Medication

Table 2 shows the number of patients using ≥1 medicine within the relevant groups at baseline and follow-up, including their median DDD and the result of analyzing dose changes within both groups. In both MULTI and TAU, there were fewer patients using somatic medication after 18 months, and their median DDD significantly decreased. The same was observed in the totals for psychotropic medication. **Table 3** shows the linear regression estimating the effect of MULTI on the change in DDD sum scores for both somatic and psychotropic medication. After adjusting for baseline sum scores, age, diagnosis, and baseline illness severity, the association with the change in the dose of psychotropic medication remained significant in favor of MULTI. This association was not mediated by a change in TAC/h, as no indirect effect was found (ab = 0.06, 95% BCa CI: −0.01–0.26).

Analyses on Medication Subgroups

The results of analyses of changes in subgroups of medication are shown in **Table 2**. For almost all somatic medications, a reduction in the percentage of users was shown in both MULTI and TAU, the largest being in the subgroup regarding the cardiovascular system. The DDD concerning the alimentary tract and metabolism significantly decreased within both groups. For MULTI and TAU this concerned significantly decreased doses of drugs for acid-related disorders (A02; $z = -4.22$, $p < 0.001$), constipation (A06; $z = -4.68$, $p < 0.001$), and diabetes (A10; $z = -2.97$, $p = 0.003$). For TAU, decreases in this main group were also reflected in dose reductions in drugs for acid-related disorders (A02; $z = -4.0$, $p < 0.001$) and constipation (A06; $z = -4.11$, $p < 0.001$), but not for diabetes. Although the median dose of cardiovascular system drugs increased within TAU, the percentage of users decreased. A significant decrease in dose was observed in beta-blocking agents in both MULTI (C07; $z = -4.00$, $p < 0.001$) and TAU (C07; $z = -3.54$, $p < 0.001$). Patients receiving MULTI also used a lower dose for disorders of the respiratory system, as shown by a significant decrease of medication for obstructive airway diseases (R03; $z = -2.56$, $p = 0.01$), while TAU showed a decreased use of medication of blood and blood-forming organs, as reflected by lower use of antithrombotic agents (B01; $z = -2.06$, $p = 0.04$).

For psychotropic medication, a reduction in the percentage of users was shown for almost all subgroups as well, the highest decrease being 40% in users of anxiolytics, hypnotics, and sedatives within MULTI. Both groups showed significant reductions in dose of medications such as antiepileptics, anti-Parkinson drugs, atypical antipsychotics, anxiolytics, hypnotics and sedatives, and psychoanaleptics. In contrast to TAU, MULTI also showed a decrease in the dose of typical antipsychotics.

DISCUSSION

In the current study, we observed a significant dose reduction in psychotropic medications after 18 months of MULTI, compared to TAU. Although the dose reduction in somatic medication was in favor of MULTI too, it was not significant. When these main groups were split into subgroups, there was a lack of power for corrected between-group analyses. However, the first steps in gaining more detailed insight into dose reductions by using within-group analyses showed interesting leads, for example, in the reduction of medication for diabetes and the respiratory system, which is in line with previously reported physical health improvements within MULTI (35). It also showed clearly the remarkable dose reductions in TAU. It is not likely that this is a time effect, as there was no change of policy in the organization regarding the dosage of medication during these 18 months. The reductions might, however, be a disruptive effect caused by

TABLE 2 | Number of patients using at least one medicine within main groups of medication at baseline and follow-up, their median daily defined dose, physical activity scores and the results of analyzing changes in dose and physical activity within both MULTI and TAU ($N = 114$).

Outcome	MULTI ($n = 65$)									TAU ($n = 49$)								
	Baseline				Follow-up					Baseline				Follow-up				
	n	(%)			*n*	(%)			*p*	*n*	(%)			*n*	(%)			*p*
Somatic medication[a]	60	(92)	**2.65**	**(1.51–5.13)**	54	(83)	**0.58**	**(0.50-1.69)**	**<0.01**	48	(98)	**2.35**	**(0.84–3.90)**	42	(86)	**1.00**	**(0.50–2.37)**	**<0.01**
Alimentary tract and metabolism (A)	53	(82)	**2.33**	**(1.38–3.61)**	53	(82)	**0.50**	**(0.50–1.05)**	**<0.01**	46	(94)	**1.83**	**(0.50–3.05)**	40	(82)	**0.50**	**(0.50–1.19)**	**<0.01**
Blood and blood forming organs (B)	2	(3)	3.00	(2.00–*)	2	(3)	1.62	(1.00–*)	0.72	10	(20)	**1.25**	**(1.00–2.25)**	6	(12)	**0.67**	**(0.30–1.20)**	**0.04**
Cardiovascular system (C)	34	(52)	**0.85**	**(0.36–1.67)**	13	(20)	**0.73**	**(0.33–1.17)**	**<0.01**	24	(49)	**0.42**	**(0.19–1.25)**	12	(25)	**0.83**	**(0.42–1.13)**	**0.02**
Respiratory system (R)	15	(23)	**1.00**	**(1.00–1.50)**	5	(8)	**0.50**	**(0.25–0.75)**	**<0.01**	6	(12)	1.10	(0.92–3.03)	5	(10)	1.00	(0.25–1.35)	0.16
Psychotropic medication[a]	65	(100)	**3.74**	**(2.32–5.87)**	49	(75)	**0.79**	**(0.43–1.50)**	**<0.01**	45	(92)	**2.61**	**(1.92–4.49)**	39	(80)	**0.95**	**(0.42–1.83)**	**<0.01**
Antiepileptics (N03)	20	(31)	**0.82**	**(0.38–1.30)**	9	(14)	**0.17**	**(0.08–0.33)**	**<0.01**	7	(14)	**1.00**	**(0.60–1.67)**	5	(10)	**0.20**	**(0.11–0.30)**	**0.02**
Anti-Parkinson (N04)	20	(31)	**0.40**	**(0.40–0.60)**	5	(8)	**0.20†**	**†**	**<0.01**	10	(20)	**0.40**	**(0.20–0.53)**	4	(8)	**0.20†**	**†**	**0.01**
Typical antipsychotics (N05A)	30	(46)	**1.25**	**(0.72–2.33)**	17	(26)	**0.83**	**(0.23–1.79)**	**<0.01**	20	(41)	0.73	(0.48–1.13)	13	(27)	0.36	(0.13–1.21)	0.07
Atypical antipsychotics (N05A)	53	(82)	**1.25**	**(1.00–1.85)**	37	(57)	**1.17**	**(0.88–1.70)**	**<0.01**	28	(57)	**1.27**	**(0.88–2.00)**	24	(49)	**1.00**	**(0.14–1.88)**	**<0.01**
Lithium (N05AN)	5	(8)	0.90	(0.56–0.90)	3	(5)	0.68	(0.45–*)	0.21	3	(6)	0.45	(0.45–*)	2	(4)	0.23†	†	0.10
Anxiolytics, hypnotics & sedatives (N05B+C)	39	(60)	**1.20**	**(0.70–1.80)**	13	(20)	**0.40**	**(0.40–0.80)**	**<0.01**	31	(63)	**1.20**	**(0.50–2.40)**	20	(41)	**0.40**	**(0.20–1.00)**	**<0.01**
Psychoanaleptics (N06)	28	(43)	**1.50**	**(1.00–2.00)**	9	(14)	**0.38**	**(0.29–0.75)**	**<0.01**	23	(47)	**1.00**	**(1.00–1.50)**	9	(18)	**1.00**	**(0.29–1.00)**	**<0.01**
Other nervous system drugs (N07)	2	(3)	0.88	(0.69–*)	2	(3)	0.71	(0.18–*)	1.00	1	(2)	0.36†	†	1	(2)	0.18†	†	0.32
Physical activity[b]																		
Wear time during measurement (hours)			55.9	(7.8)			53.6	(9.1)	0.07			55.1	(10.2)			53.3	(10.0)	0.29
Average total activity counts per hour			**29102**	**(12371)**			**33020**	**(14453)**	**0.01**			24636	(14210)			23793	(13151)	0.62

Significant differences within groups are shown in bold.
MULTI, MUltidisciplinary Lifestyle enhancing Treatment for Inpatients with severe mental illness; TAU, Treatment As Usual.
[a] *Median (IQR)*
[b] *Mean (SD)*
[*] *not available due to a low number of users and therefore a lack of dispersion.*
[†] *the daily dosages are constant.*

TABLE 3 | Linear regression estimating treatment effects of MULTI compared to treatment as usual on mean daily defined dose ($N = 114$).

Outcome (ATC code)	B	(95% CI)	*p*
Somatic medications (A, B, C, R)*			
Model 1	**−0.48**	**(−0.90– −0.06)**	**0.025**
Model 2	−0.44	(−0.88–0.01)	0.054
Model 3	−0.38	(−0.87–0.11)	0.130
Psychotropic medications (N)			
Model 1	**−0.47**	**(−0.86– −0.07)**	**0.022**
Model 2	**−0.48**	**(−0.90– −0.07)**	**0.023**
Model 3	**−0.55**	**(−1.00– −0.09)**	**0.020**

Significant results are shown in bold. MULTI, MUltidisciplinary Lifestyle enhancing Treatment for Inpatients with severe mental illness; ATC code, Anatomical Therapeutic Chemical code; A, Alimentary tract and metabolism; B, Blood and blood-forming organs; C, Cardiovascular system; R, Respiratory system; N, Nervous system.
Model 1: crude model, corrected for baseline measurement.
Model 2: adjusted model, corrected for baseline measurement and age.
Model 3: adjusted model, corrected for baseline measurement, age, diagnosis (schizophrenia and other psychotic disorders, yes/no) and illness severity at baseline.
**n = 112, as two outliers were excluded.*

a change in medical staff during the 18 months of this study. The psychiatrist responsible for the majority of the patients within TAU retired and was replaced by a younger colleague, who critically reviewed medication policies. Nevertheless, such a critical review had already been done on the wards receiving MULTI prior to its implementation, so dose reduction was not a specific goal within MULTI. Therefore, the significant decrease in the dose of psychotropic medication is even more striking. One explanation could be that this may be caused partly by decreased psychotic symptoms, but earlier results of the MULTI study showed no significant changes in these symptoms, as compared with TAU, after 18 months (35). Another explanation may be that the psychiatrists reduced the dose of medication based on observed improvements in psychosocial functioning in people who received MULTI (42). It is, however, challenging to clarify specific mechanisms with regard to dose reduction, as there are many variables involved (e.g., interactions between different medications; changes in and preferences of the staff; etc.).

Our findings are somewhat in line with the only other study known to us that evaluated medication use after a lifestyle focused program in patients with SMI (43). In that naturalistic study, Højlund et al. found a decrease in the use of antipsychotics in patients, although they found no specific association between these changes and the degree of participation in the intervention they delivered. However, their reported proportions of patients who used psychotropic co-medication (N categories except for N05) showed little change at follow-up, which is not in line with our observations. Differences may be caused by a different population, as their study was conducted in outpatients with a substantially shorter history of illness, who were relatively young and of whom only a minority used psychotropic co-medication. Also, the absence of a comparison group without lifestyle support makes it difficult to compare results. Indicating decreases in medication use after lifestyle improvement is however very relevant for clinical practice. The ideal situation would be to have medication that addresses the symptoms of psychosis with minimal side effects. However, due to a lack of fundamental innovation in psychopharmacology during recent decades, we still have to work with antipsychotics with a range of motor, metabolic, and cognitive side effects (28, 44). Moreover, as there is still an overall favorable benefit-to-risk ratio for the use of antipsychotics (45), addressing lifestyle is of importance to help minimize such side effects. Besides previously reported improvements in physical health (35), current results show that an integrated multidisciplinary approach is associated with a decrease in the dose of medication. Thereby, it potentially reduces (the risk for) those side effects, which are partly dose-dependent (11, 46). Additionally, because many but not all side effects are reversible, it suggests that lifestyle improvements could contribute to the prevention of irreversible effects, e.g., motor side effects. The reductions found are also promising from the patient's point of view, as side effects and negative attitudes toward medication use are associated with non-adherence, distress, and life impact (47–50).

Our explorative mediation analysis showed that the increase in physical activity observed in patients receiving MULTI after 18 months (35) did not mediate the association between MULTI and change in psychotropic medication use in this same period of time. This indicates that the decrease of psychotropic mediation was not a result of just increasing physical activity. We hypothesize that, with an organizational culture change as a base, multiple components that complement physical activity contribute to improvements, including focus on dietary habits, psycho-education, personal tailoring, and support by peers and qualified participating staff, in line with recent studies advocating the use of such elements (29, 30, 51–53). Such a holistic approach, in which patients are encouraged to do any activities instead of none (i.e., decreasing sedentary behavior), may be more feasible and beneficial in the longer term for inpatients with SMI. While previous studies have shown that structured exercise is feasible in those with SMI in general (31), sedentary behavior (as distinct from physical inactivity) is highly prevalent and associated with cardiometabolic risks that are largely independent of time spent in structured exercise (7, 8). Thus, controlled trials are needed to examine further the feasibility and effects of interventions targeting sedentary behavior.

Limitations in this study mainly arise from the naturalistic and observational design. In this design, we were not able to randomize patients (e.g., the TAU wards treated fewer patients with psychotic disorders) and control for treatment settings in advance (e.g., the continuity of psychiatrists). In addition, although dose reduction was not a specific goal of MULTI, psychiatrists were not blinded for patients' treatment condition (i.e., receiving MULTI or not), which might have affected observed dose reductions. Although this observational study seems the first indicating a possible effect of lifestyle improvements on medication use in inpatients with SMI, future well-designed trials are needed to study the efficacy of lifestyle changes on medication use. Regarding the participation of patients in MULTI, we have no specific data on (the degree of) their adherence. It was intended that all patients were doing some activities in the morning and afternoon, tailored to the particular ward and patients' abilities and interests. However, data on adherence to these individualized day-to-day programs including more detailed data on participation (e.g., frequency and intensity of activities) would make it possible to study the association between the (degree of) adherence and treatment outcomes. Also, our analyses depended on the availability of data within the cohort. Nevertheless, by using multilevel analyses adjusting for differences between MULTI and TAU, we aimed for robust results. However, more data will be needed to have sufficient power for adequate between-group analyses within subgroups of medication, whereby we could gain more detailed insight into specific reductions as indicated by within-group analyses (e.g., drugs for diabetes or obstructive airway diseases). This would provide the opportunity to control for possible differences between groups such as age, which can affect the prescribed dosages of medication (54–56). Furthermore, we used a simple mediation model to explore the influence of a change in physical activity, as an essential element of MULTI, on the association between MULTI and change in medication use. However, the main limitation of this is that by measuring all variables within the mediation analyses nearly simultaneously, we assumed that the association between change in total activity and change in medication use between our pre (T1) and post measurement (T2) would be the same as we would have measured between T2 and a (theoretical) third time point. To study if physical activity mediates associations between lifestyle interventions and medication use, in general, it would be the best to measure physical activity as a middle time-point to study the effect of a change in physical activity over time. Finally, we did not include pro necessitate medication (i.e., to be given as needed) because we cannot specify if and to what extent patients took these medications. The strength of this study is that it is the first study to report detailed dose-specific data on changes in both somatic and psychotropic medication use in inpatients with SMI after lifestyle changes. Despite the limitations, first steps were taken to analyze associations between lifestyle improvements and medication use in these patients, who are suffering from severe physical health problems and receive high dosages of medication. The naturalistic setting of the study improves the generalizability of the results and meets the need for observational studies to supplement randomized controlled trials in order to improve the external validity, such that clinicians treating patients in real-world settings have relevant evidence on which to base their clinical decisions (57). Regarding the impact of critically reviewing medication use that was most likely observed in TAU, it is a strength in favor of MULTI that medication was already critically reviewed on these wards before its implementation, so dose reduction was not a specific goal within MULTI. This suggests that lifestyle improvement has added value with regard to decreasing the dose of medication in inpatients with SMI. Above all, this strengthens the fact that we compared it with TAU. Otherwise, we would only have observed the improvements in MULTI without any context. Moreover, by analyzing possible mediation by total activity, we took a first step to gaining more insight into the contribution of different elements of MULTI to the observed improvements. Finally, by including baseline measures in this analysis, our mediation analysis is mathematically in line with a covariance approach, which was the recommended method for mediation analyses (58, 59).

In summary, in addition to previously reported improvements in physical activity and metabolic health after 18 months of MULTI, we observed a significant decrease in dose of psychotropic medication as compared with TAU. We encourage further longitudinal controlled research to gain more insight into the relationship between lifestyle changes and possible dose reductions to improve health outcomes in inpatients with SMI.

AUTHOR CONTRIBUTIONS

JD: obtaining funding, study design, retrieving, processing and analyzing data, drafting the manuscript; DT: study design, supporting retrieving, processing and analyzing data; HvD: retrieving, processing and supporting analyzing data; IH: supporting analyzing data; DT and PvH: supporting grant applications; All authors critically revised the manuscript and approved the final version.

ACKNOWLEDGMENTS

The authors would like to acknowledge, with thanks, all patients and staff of GGz Centraal who have made efforts to collect the data on which this study was based.

REFERENCES

Vancampfort D, Stubbs B, Mitchell AJ, De Hert M, Wampers M, Ward PB, et al. Risk of metabolic syndrome and its components in people with schizophrenia and related psychotic disorders, bipolar disorder and major depressive disorder: a systematic review and meta-analysis. *World Psychiatry* (2015) 14:339–47. doi: 10.1002/wps.20252

Stubbs B, Vancampfort D, De Hert M, Mitchell AJ. The prevalence and predictors of type two diabetes mellitus in people with schizophrenia: a systematic review and comparative meta-analysis. *Acta Psychiatr Scand.* (2015) 132:144–57. doi: 10.1111/acps. 12439

Correll CU, Solmi M, Veronese N, Bortolato B, Rosson S, Santonastaso P, et al. Prevalence, incidence and mortality from cardiovascular disease in patients with pooled and specific severe mental illness: a large-scale meta- analysis of 3,211,768 patients and 113,383,368 controls. *World Psychiatry* (2017) 16:163–80. doi: 10.1002/wps.20420

Piotrowski P, Gondek TM, Krolicka-Deregowska A, Misiak B, Adamowski T, Kiejna A. Causes of mortality in schizophrenia: An updated review of European studies. *Psychiatr Danub.* (2017) 29:108–20.

Hjorthøj C, Sturup AE, McGrath JJ, Nordentoft M. Years of potential life lost and life expectancy in schizophrenia: a systematic review and meta-analysis. *Lancet Psychiatry* (2017) 4:295–301. doi: 10.1016/s2215-0366(17)30078-0

Tanskanen A, Tiihonen J, Taipale H. Mortality in schizophrenia: 30-year nationwide follow-up study. *Acta Psychiatr Scand.* 138:492–99. (2018). doi: 10.1111/acps.12913

Biswas A, Oh PI, Faulkner GE, Bajaj RR, Silver MA, Mitchell MS, et al. Sedentary Time and Its Association With Risk for Disease incidence, mortality, and hospitalization in adults a systematic review and meta-analysis. *Ann Intern Med.* (2015) 162:123-32. doi: 10.7326/m14-1651

Brocklebank LA, Falconer CL, Page AS, Perry R, Cooper AR. Accelerometer-measured sedentary time and cardiometabolic biomarkers: a systematic review. *Prev Med.* (2015) 76:92–102. doi: 10.1016/j.ypmed.2015.04.013

Kruisdijk F, Deenik J, Tenback D, Tak E, Beekman A, van Harten P, et al. Accelerometer-measured sedentary behaviour and physical activity of inpatients with severe mental illness. *Psychiatry Res.* (2017) 254:67–74. doi: 10.1016/j.psychres.2017.04.035

Stubbs B, Firth J, Berry A, Schuch FB, Rosenbaum S, Gaughran F, et al. How much physical activity do people with schizophrenia engage in? A systematic review, comparative meta-analysis and meta-regression. *Schizophr Res.* (2016) 176:431–40. doi: 10.1016/j.schres.2016.05.017

Correll CU, Detraux J, De Lepeleire J, De Hert M. Effects of antipsychotics, antidepressants and mood stabilizers on risk for physical diseases in people with schizophrenia, depression and bipolar disorder. *World Psychiatry* (2015) 14:119–36. doi: 10.1002/wps.20204

Kahl KG, Westhoff-Bleck M, Kruger THC. Effects of psychopharmacological treatment with antipsychotic drugs on the vascular system. *Vascul Pharmacol.* (2017). 100:20–5. doi: 10.1016/j.vph.2017.09.001

Solmi M, Murru A, Pacchiarotti I, Undurraga J, Veronese N, Fornaro M, et al. Safety, tolerability, and risks associated with first- and second-generation antipsychotics: a state-of-the-art clinical review. *Ther Clin Risk Manag.* (2017) 13:757–77. doi: 10.2147/tcrm.s117321

Verhaegen AA, Van Gaal LF. Drug-induced obesity and its metabolic consequences: a review with a focus on mechanisms and possible therapeutic options. *J Endocrinol Invest.* (2017) 40:1165–74. doi: 10.1007/s40618-017- 0719-6

Westaway K, Sluggett JK, Alderman C, Procter N, Roughead E. Prevalence of multiple antipsychotic use and associated adverse effects in Australians with mental illness. *Int J Evid Based Health.* (2016) 14:104–12. doi: 10.1097/xeb.0000000000000082

Torniainen M, Mittendorfer-Rutz E, Tanskanen A, Bjorkenstam C, Suvisaari J, Alexanderson K, et al. Antipsychotic treatment and mortality in schizophrenia. *Schizophr Bull.* (2015) 41:656–63. doi: 10.1093/schbul/sbu164

Brett J, Daniels B, Karanges EA, Buckley NA, Schneider C, Nassir A, et al. Psychotropic polypharmacy in Australia, 2006 to 2015: a descriptive cohort study. *Br J Clin Pharmacol.* (2017) 83:2581–8. doi: 10.1111/bcp. 13369

Bakker PR, de Groot IW, van Os J, van Harten PN. Long- Stay psychiatric patients: a prospective study revealing persistent Antipsychotic-Induced movement disorder. *PLoS ONE* (2011) 6:e25588. doi: 10.1371/journal. pone.0025588

Mentzel CL, Bakker PR, Van Os J, Drukker M, Matroos GE, Hoek HW, et al. Effect of Antipsychotic type and dose changes on tardive dyskinesia and parkinsonism severity in patients with a serious mental illness: the curacao extrapyramidal syndromes study XII. *J Clin Psychiatry* (2017) 78:E279–85. doi: 10.4088/JCP.16m11049

Catapano AL, Graham I, De Backer G, Wiklund O, Chapman MJ, Drexel H, et al. 2016 ESC/EAS guidelines for the management of dyslipidaemias. *Eur Heart J.* (2016) 37:2999–3058. doi: 10.1093/eurheartj/ehw272

Grundy SM, Cleeman JI, Daniels SR, Donato KA, Eckel RH, Franklin BA, et al. Diagnosis and Management of the Metabolic Syndrome. An American Heart Association/National Heart, Lung, and Blood Institute Scientific Statement. *Circulation* (2005) 112:2735–52. doi: 10.1161/circulationaha.105.169404

Maayan L, Correll CU. Management of antipsychotic-related weight gain. *Expert Rev Neurother.* (2010) 10:1175–200. doi: 10.1586/ern.10.85

Mancia G, Fagard R, Narkiewicz K, Redon J, Zanchetti A, Bohm M, et al. 2013 ESH/ESC Guidelines for the management of arterial hypertension: the Task Force for the management of arterial hypertension of the European Society of Hypertension (ESH) and of the European Society of Cardiology (ESC). *J Hypertens.* (2013) 31:1281–357. doi: 10.1097/01.hjh.0000431740.32696.cc

Ryden L, Grant PJ, Anker SD, Berne C, Cosentino F, Danchin N, et al. ESC Guidelines on diabetes, pre-diabetes, and cardiovascular diseases developed in collaboration with the EASD: the Task Force on diabetes, pre- diabetes, and cardiovascular diseases of the European Society of Cardiology (ESC) and developed in collaboration with the European Association for the Study of Diabetes (EASD). *Eur Heart J.* (2013) 34:3035–87. doi: 10.1093/eurheartj/eht108

Barnes TR. Evidence-based guidelines for the pharmacological treatment of schizophrenia: recommendations from the British Association for Psychopharmacology. *J Psychopharmacol.* (2011) 25:567–620. doi: 10.1177/0269881110391123

Bhugra D, Howes O. *Handbook for Psychiatric Trainees.* London: Royal College of Psychiatrists (2008).

Emsley R. On discontinuing treatment in schizophrenia: a clinical conundrum. *NPJ Schizophr.* (2017) 3:4. doi: 10.1038/s41537-016-0004-2

Lally J, MacCabe JH. Antipsychotic medication in schizophrenia: a review. *Br Med Bull.* (2015) 114:169–79. doi: 10.1093/bmb/ldv017

Teasdale SB, Ward PB, Rosenbaum S, Samaras K, Stubbs B. Solving a weighty problem: systematic review and meta-analysis of nutrition interventions in severe mental illness. *Br J Psychiatry* (2017) 210:110–8. doi: 10.1192/bjp.bp.115.177139

Ward MC, White DT, Druss BG. A meta-review of lifestyle interventions for cardiovascular risk factors in the general medical population: lessons for individuals with serious mental illness. *J Clin Psychiatry* (2015) 76:e477–86. doi: 10.4088/JCP.13r08657

Stubbs B, Vancampfort D, Hallgren M, Firth J, Veronese N, Solmi M, et al. EPA guidance on physical activity as a treatment for severe mental illness: a meta-review of the evidence and Position Statement from the European Psychiatric Association (EPA), supported by the International Organization of Physical Therapists in Mental Health (IOPTMH). *Eur Psychiatry* (2018) 54:124–44. doi: 10.1016/j.eurpsy.2018.07.004

Liu NH, Daumit GL, Dua T, Aquila R, Charlson F, Cuijpers P, et al. Excess mortality in persons with severe mental disorders: a multilevel intervention framework and priorities for clinical practice, policy and research agendas. *World Psychiatry* (2017) 16:30–40. doi: 10.1002/wps.20384

Levitt GA, Shinault K, Patterson S, Otaluka O. Weight Gain in Psychiatric Inpatients: Are Interventions Making a Positive Impact? *Prim Care Companion CNS Disord.* (2017) 19:17m02111. doi: 10.4088/PCC.17m02111

Looijmans A, Stiekema A, Bruggeman R, van der Meer L, Stolk RP, Schoevers RA, et al. Changing the obesogenic environment to improve cardiometabolic health in residential patients with a severe mental Illness: ELIPS, a randomized controlled trial. *Br J Psychiatry* (2017) 211:296–303. doi: 10.1186/s12888-014-0293-9

Deenik J, Tenback DE, Tak ECPM, Rutters F, Hendriksen IJM, van Harten PN. Changes in physical and psychiatric health after a multidisciplinary lifestyle enhancing treatment for inpatients with severe mental illness: the MULTI study I. *Schizophr Res.* (2018). doi: 10.1016/j.schres.2018.07.033. [Epub ahead of print].

WHO Collaborating Centre for Drug Statistics Methodology. *ATC classification index with DDDs, 2017.* Oslo: World Health Organisation (2016).

Ozemek C, Kirschner MM, Wilkerson BS, Byun W, Kaminsky LA. Intermonitor reliability of the GT3X+ accelerometer at hip, wrist and ankle sites during activities of daily living. *Physiol Meas.* (2014) 35:129–38. doi: 10.1088/0967-3334/35/2/12

Aadland E, Ylvisaker E. Reliability of the actigraph GT3X+ accelerometer in adults under free-living conditions. *PLoS ONE* (2015) 10:e0134606. doi: 10.1371/journal.pone.0134606

Jarrett H, Fitzgerald L, Routen AC. Interinstrument reliability of the ActiGraph GT3X+ambulatory activity monitor during free-living conditions in adults. *J Phys Activity Health* (2015) 12:382–7. doi: 10.1123/jpah.2013-0070

Lee JA, Williams SM, Brown DD, Laurson KR. Concurrent validation of the Actigraph gt3x+, Polar Active accelerometer, Omron HJ-720 and Yamax Digiwalker SW-701 pedometer step counts in lab-based and free-living settings. *J Sports Sci.* (2015) 33:991–1000. doi: 10.1080/02640414.2014.981848

Hayes AF. *Introduction to Mediation, Moderation, and Conditional Process Analysis, Second Edition: A Regression-Based Approach.* New York, NY: Guilford Publications (2018).

Deenik J, Tenback DE, Tak ECPM, Hendriksen IJM, van Harten PN. Improved quality of life and psychosocial functioning in inpatients with severe mental illness receiving a multidisciplinary lifestyle enhancing treatment. The MULTI study II. *Mental Health Phys Activity* (2018) 15:145–52. doi: 10.1016/j.mhpa.2018.10.004

Højlund M, Elliott AF, Madsen NJ, Viuff AG, Munk-Jørgensen P, Hjorth P. Changes in antipsychotics and other psychotropic drugs during a 30- month lifestyle intervention among outpatients with schizophrenia. *Nordic J Psychiatry* (2017) 71:598–604. doi: 10.1080/08039488.2017.1365379

Dimitrelis K, Shankar R. Pharmacological treatment of schizophrenia – a review of progress. *Prog Neurol Psychiatry* (2016) 20:28–35. doi: 10.1002/pnp.430

Correll CU, Rubio JM, Kane JM. What is the risk-benefit ratio of long- term antipsychotic treatment in people with schizophrenia? *World Psychiatry* (2018) 17:149–60. doi: 10.1002/wps.20516

Leucht S, Corves C, Arbter D, Engel RR, Li C, Davis JM. Second-generation versus first-generation antipsychotic drugs for schizophrenia: a meta-analysis. *Lancet* (2009) 373:31–41. doi: 10.1016/s0140-6736(08)61764-x

Ashoorian D, Davidson R, Rock D, Dragovic M, Clifford R. A clinical communication tool for the assessment of psychotropic medication side effects. *Psychiatry Res.* (2015) 230:643–57. doi: 10.1016/j.psychres.2015.10.022

Velligan DI, Sajatovic M, Hatch A, Kramata P, Docherty JP. Why do psychiatric patients stop antipsychotic medication? A systematic review of reasons for nonadherence to medication in patients with serious mental illness. *Patient Prefer Adher.* (2017) 11:449–68. doi: 10.2147/ppa.s124658

Wykes T, Evans J, Paton C, Barnes TRE, Taylor D, Bentall R, et al. What side effects are problematic for patients prescribed antipsychotic medication? The Maudsley Side Effects (MSE) measure for antipsychotic medication. *Psychol Med.* (2017) 47:2369–78. doi: 10.1017/s0033291717000903

Hui CL, Poon VW, Ko WT, Miao HY, Chang WC, Lee EH, et al. Risk factors for antipsychotic medication non-adherence behaviors and attitudes in adult-onset psychosis. *Schizophr Res.* (2016) 174:144–9. doi: 10.1016/j.schres.2016.03.026

Long C, Rowell A, Rigg S, Livesey F, McAllister P. What is effective in promoting a healthy lifestyle in secure psychiatric settings? A review of the evidence for an integrated programme that targets modifiable health risk behaviours. *J Forensic Pract.* (2016) 18:204–15. doi: 10.1108/jfp-12-2015-0055

Roberts SH, Bailey JE. Incentives and barriers to lifestyle interventions for people with severe mental illness: a narrative synthesis of quantitative, qualitative and mixed methods studies. *J Adv Nurs.* (2011) 67:690–708. doi: 10.1111/j.1365-2648.2010.05546.x

Vancampfort D, Rosenbaum S, Schuch F, Ward PB, Richards J, Mugisha J, et al. Cardiorespiratory fitness in severe mental illness: a systematic review and meta-analysis. *Sports Med.* (2017) 47:343–52. doi: 10.1007/s40279-016- 0574-1

Rej S, Beaulieu S, Segal M, Low NC, Mucsi I, Holcroft C, et al. Lithium dosing and serum concentrations across the age spectrum: from early adulthood to the tenth decade of life. *Drugs Aging* (2014) 31:911–6. doi: 10.1007/s40266-014-0221-1

de Mendonca Lima CA, Baumann P, Brawand-Amey M, Brogli C, Jacquet S, Cochard N, et al. Effect of age and gender on citalopram and desmethylcitalopram steady-state plasma concentrations in adults and elderly depressed patients. *Prog Neuropsychopharmacol Biol Psychiatry* (2005) 29:952–6. doi: 10.1016/j.pnpbp.2005.06.001

Beyth RJ, Shorr RI. Principles of drug therapy in older patients: rational drug prescribing. *Clin Geriatr Med.* (2002) 18:577–92. doi: 10.1016/S0749-0690(02)00017-4

Kennedy-Martin T, Curtis S, Faries D, Robinson S, Johnston J. A literature review on the representativeness of randomized controlled trial samples and implications for the external validity of trial results. *Trials* (2015) 16:495. doi: 10.1186/s13063-015-1023-4

Landau S, Emsley R, Dunn G. Beyond total treatment effects in randomised controlled trials: Baseline measurement of intermediate outcomes needed to reduce confounding in mediation investigations. *Clin Trials* (2018) 15:247–56. doi: 10.1177/1740774518760300

Twisk J, Bosman L, Hoekstra T, Rijnhart J, Welten M, Heymans M. Different ways to estimate treatment effects in randomised controlled trials. *Contemp Clin Trial Commun.* (2018) 10:80–5. doi: 10.1016/j.conctc.2018.03.008

9

The Relationship among Trait Mindfulness, Attention and Working Memory in Junior School Students under Different Stressful Situations

Yuntao Li[1†], Ningxi Yang[2†], Yan Zhang[2], Wei Xu[3] and Li Cai[2]*

[1] Psychological Education and Counselling Centre, Southwest University of Science and Technology, Mianyang, China, [2] Department of Applied Psychology, College of Humanities and Social Sciences, Harbin Engineering University, Harbin, China, [3] Faculty of Psychology, Beijing Normal University, Beijing, China

***Correspondence:**
Yan Zhang
happyzhang666@163.com

†These authors have contributed equally to this work

Attention and working memory are important cognitive functions that affect junior school students' learning ability and academic performance. This study aimed to explore the relationships among trait mindfulness, attention, and working memory and to explore differences in performance between a high trait mindfulness group and a low one in attention and working memory under different stressful situations. In study 1, 216 junior school students completed the Five Facet Mindfulness Questionnaire (FFMQ), and their attention and working memory were tested in a non-pressure situation. The results showed that attention had a partial mediating effect between mindfulness and working memory. In study 2, the high trait mindfulness group and the low one were tested for attention and working memory under situations with single and multiple pressures. One notable result was that the attention and working memory performances of the high mindfulness group were all significantly higher than those of the low mindfulness group in every stress situation (no stress, single stress, and multiple stresses). Other important results were that trait mindfulness moderates the relationship between stress and attention and between stress and working memory. These results suggest that trait mindfulness has a protective effect in the process by which various stresses affect attention and working memory. These findings indicate that trait mindfulness is an important psychological quality that affects the attention and working memory of junior school students, and it is also an important psychological resource for effectively coping with the impact of stress on attention and working memory. Therefore, it is possible that improving trait mindfulness may help to improve junior school students' attention and working memory and enable them to cope better with stress, thereby helping to improve academic performance. This research is of great significance for understanding the association between key psychological qualities and cognitive functions in different stressful situations. These findings also provide insight for future studies in educational psychology.

Keywords: stress, trait mindfulness, attention, working memory, junior school student

INTRODUCTION

Attention and working memory are two important and closely related cognitive functions. Attention refers to the ability to focus one's psychological activities on something. Working memory is a system that temporarily stores and processes current information with limited capacity. As a cognitive resource, attention helps to deal with various tasks in the working memory system (Soto et al., 2005; Kumar et al., 2009; Dunning and Holmes, 2014). Previous studies have shown that both attention and working memory are closely related to students' learning ability and performance (Durbrow et al., 2000; Ayres and Sweller, 2014). Issues surrounding students' attention and working memory are currently attracting more and more attention as topics of research (Rebok et al., 2014; Rode et al., 2017; Wimmer et al., 2020). The question of which psychological or external factors affect attention and working memory has also become a topic of discussion.

In recent years, mindfulness has attracted more and more attention in psychological research (Davidson, 2010; Brown et al., 2015; Lindsay and Creswell, 2017). Mindfulness can be viewed as both a state and as a special characteristic. State mindfulness describes the non-judgmental, present-focused awareness experienced in any given moment (Medvedev et al., 2017). Trait mindfulness or dispositional mindfulness involves stable individual differences in average frequency and intensity of mindful states over time (Brown and Ryan, 2013; Jamieson and Tuckey, 2017; Mesmer-Magnus et al., 2017). It has been shown that trait mindfulness can be improved by practice, which includes mindfulness meditation as well as some mindfulness-based interventions (Cavanagh et al., 2014; Kiken et al., 2015; Quaglia et al., 2016). Mindfulness practice also has positive effects on attention and working memory. Some studies have found that mindfulness training can improve children's sustained attention (Tarrasch, 2018), protect working memory capacity (Bailey et al., 2020), and significantly improve working memory performance (Chambers et al., 2008). It can thus be inferred that high trait mindfulness may also have positive impacts on attention and working memory.

People face pressures from different aspects of modern society. According to the Yerkes–Dodson law, moderate pressure will make individuals concentrate more energy to achieve better learning and to work efficiently (Yerkes and Dodson, 1908). However, when an individual is faced with stressful situations beyond their psychological capacity, it is difficult to make effective adjustment, resulting in negative emotions such as anxiety and depression. These in turn have adverse effects on cognitive functions such as attention and hinder the completion of tasks (Myhr et al., 2019). Working memory, as a cognitive resource with limited capacity, is more vulnerable to such effects (Matthews and Campbell, 2010; Lukasik et al., 2019).

In recent years, some studies have found that trait mindfulness is a positive psychological trait that can reduce stress sensitivity (Allen et al., 2015; Lomas et al., 2017) and the impairment of cognitive function by stress. Mindfulness meditation and high levels of mindfulness can significantly reduce the damage done to the memory of college students under stressful situations and can enable the subjects to complete the corresponding tasks more stably (Limaree, 2007). Another study was conducted on soldiers who were going to be sent to the battlefield in Iraq. The results showed that among these soldiers facing great pressure, those without psychological intervention showed a decrease in working memory capacity as the departure time approached. However, among the soldiers who received an 8-week mindfulness training, the working memory capacity of those who spent more time in self-training after class did not decrease significantly. This suggests that a certain intensity of mindfulness practice can to an extent protect working memory in the face of high-stress situations (Jha et al., 2010, 2015).

In China, junior school students are generally faced with heavy academic tasks and the pressure of gaining entry to high school. What are the effects of different stress levels on the attention and working memory of junior school students? Does trait mindfulness, as a positive psychological factor, regulate the effect of stress on junior school students' attention and working memory? These problems are of great practical significance for junior school students and other groups facing high pressure. However, so far, studies on the moderating effect of trait mindfulness on attention and working memory in stressful situations and the relationships among trait mindfulness, attention, and working memory have still been extremely rare, especially in the context of junior school students, for which no relevant research reports have been found. Therefore, this research was divided into two parts to explore these issues. In study 1, the relationship among trait mindfulness, attention, and the working memory of junior school students and the internal mechanism of that relationship were explored. In study 2, stressful situations were created in an attempt to explore whether trait mindfulness has consistently positive effects on attention and working memory across a range of stressful situations, and in particular, whether trait mindfulness has moderating effects on attention and working memory in stressful situations.

The following three hypotheses were thus proposed:

H1: Trait mindfulness can predict working memory through the mediating effect of attention.

H2: In a given stress situation (no stress, single stress, or multiple stresses), there is a significant difference in the junior school students' attention and working memory performance between the high trait mindfulness group and the low one.

H3: Trait mindfulness has a moderating effect on the influence of different intensities of stress on attention and working memory.

This research enriched the theoretical research on the influencing factors of attention and working memory. From the perspective of key psychological traits, it provides important clues toward, and a scientific basis for, improving the level of attention and working memory of individuals in stressful situations and thereby improving academic performance, and it has practical significance for carrying out effective education in schools.

STUDY 1

This research was approved by the Harbin Engineering University Ethics Committee. All subjects were informed before the test of the purpose and method of the research and their right to participate. It was explained that participation was voluntary and anonymous and that there would be no penalty for withdrawing from the study at any stage without notice. The written informed consent of the subjects was obtained for all studies.

In study 1, a cross-sectional study was conducted to investigate the correlation among mindfulness, attention, and working memory in junior school students and to explore the mediating role of attention in the influence of mindfulness on working memory.

4 8 6 1 5 6 4 6 6 8 5 3 5 6 4 8 1 5 6 5 5 6 7 6 5
7 8 1 8 5 7 6 5 2 6 7 5 3 1 6 2 5 7 8 6 2 5 7 6 3
5 6 8 2 3 5 6 7 6 2 5 4 5 3 6 5 3 4 6 6 7 9 7 5 6
6 8 5 2 1 6 7 5 2 6 7 5 4 9 5 6 5 7 9 4 6 5 8 7 6
4 6 9 5 7 6 5 1 6 5 7 4 2 4 5 8 6 7 5 6 5 9 7 6 2
5 6 4 5 5 1 6 5 8 4 6 0 5 5 4 6 4 0 7 6 8 4 6 8 7

FIGURE 1 | Schematic diagram of the digital cancelation test.

Methods

Participants and Procedures

Two hundred and seventeen junior school students who voluntarily participated in the study were studied by the convenience sampling method, and 216 valid data were finally obtained. The age range of the subjects was 9–15 years old (M = 11.88, SD = 1.20). The distribution of gender and grades was as follows: 131 boys (60.65%), 85 girls (39.35%); 106 in grade 1 (49.07%), 71 in grade 2 (32.87%), and 39 in grade 3 (18.06%). All subjects had normal intelligence and normal or corrected vision.

All studies were conducted in a quiet environment without interference or stress. The examiner used uniform instructional language to explain the purpose and specific requirements of the test. After ensuring that the subject understood the instructions, they were tested in groups for the mindfulness trait. Then individual tests of attention were performed, and 3 days later, individual tests of working memory were performed to avoid fatigue effects.

Measures

Trait mindfulness test

The Five Facet Mindfulness Questionnaire (FFMQ) is an established questionnaire that is used to assess trait mindfulness (Baer et al., 2006). In the current study, the Chinese version of the FFMQ, as revised by Deng et al. (2011), was used. It consists of 39 items rated on a five-point Likert scale from 1 = *never or very rarely true* to 5 = *very often or always true* The FFMQ is composed of five subscales, including "observe," "describe," "actaware," "non-judge," and "non-react." Item scores are summed to form a mindfulness score, with higher scores indicating higher levels of trait mindfulness. In this study, the Cronbach's alpha value for this scale was 0.744.

Attention test

A traditional cancelation test is often used to test for attention ability (Schweizer et al., 2005). In this study, a paper-and-pen, designated digital cancelation test (**Figure 1**) was used to test the directivity and concentration of attention. The study material consisted of 1,000 Arabic digits (zero to nine). Subjects were asked to cross out the designated number 6 as quickly and accurately as possible. The ratio of the number of instances of the digit to be crossed out to the number of non-delimited digits was 1:4. The sorting distribution was uniform but not regular. The cancelation time (T) was recorded, and the cancelation accuracy was calculated as $A = (c - w) / (c + o)$, where c represents the number of digits which were crossed out, o represents the number of digits which were missed, and w represents the number of digits which were crossed out incorrectly. The attention concentration index ($E = e \times A/T$, where e represents the number of digits actually checked) was used as the final score indicator to measure attention. In this study, all the subjects completed the examination of 1,000 numbers, and thus, e = 1,000.

Working memory test

The level of visual working memory was evaluated by a classical, visual graphic working memory paradigm (**Figure 2**). The test task followed the definition of working memory given by Baddeley et al. (1996), that is, information needs to be processed and stored at the same time. The test was carried out on a computer with a screen size of 33.6 cm × 27 cm and a resolution of 1,280 × 1,024. The method was to present six groups of geometric graphics successively. From the first group to the sixth group, the number of target graphics gradually increased from one to six, and the graphics gradually changed from simple to complex. Each of the graphics was presented for 4 s, and the subjects were asked to observe and remember them quickly. When a "+" appeared on the screen, it meant that the presentation of the group of graphics was completed, and there would be a pause for 4 s. Next, the subjects were asked to judge whether the direction, shape, and size of each figure in the subsequent figure group were exactly the same as in the target figure just presented. Each correct answer counted for one point, and the total score was used as the visual working memory score.

Statistical Analysis

Descriptive statistical analysis was conducted on the mean value and standard deviation of attention, working memory, and the total score and facet scores of trait mindfulness for all subjects, and Pearson correlation coefficients were calculated to analyze the correlation between variables. In addition, based on controlling the influence of age on attention and working memory, the mediating effect model of attention on mindfulness and working memory was established by using the path analysis method. Descriptive statistics and correlation analysis were performed using SPSS 22.0 (IBM Corp., Armonk, NY, United States). AMOS 21.0 (IBM Corp., Armonk, NY, United States) was used for mediating effect analysis. Significance was established at $p < 0.05$.

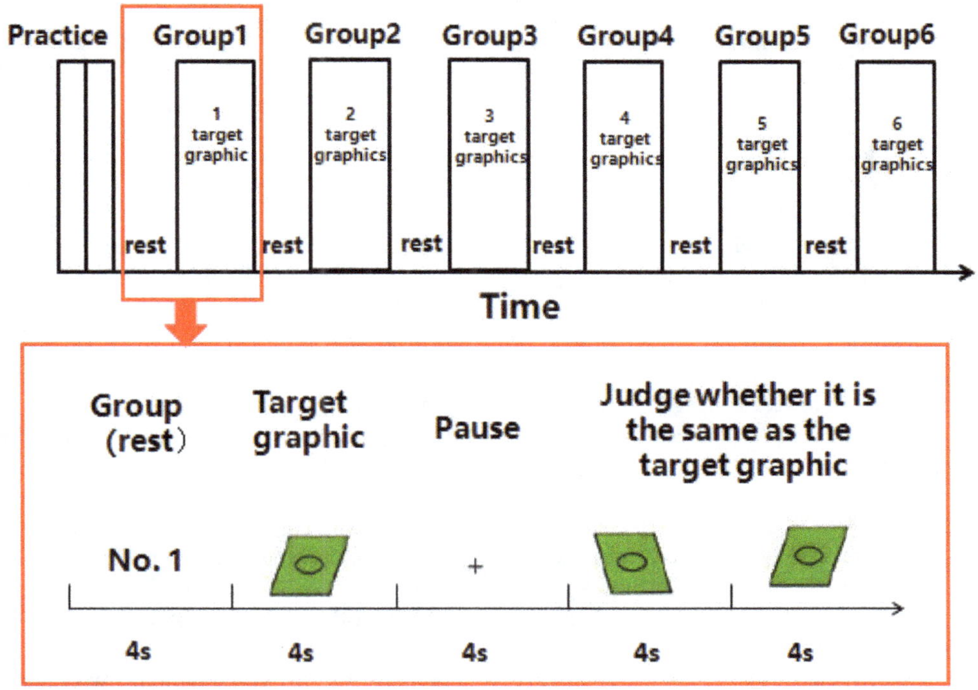

FIGURE 2 | Schematic diagram of working memory test method (take the first group of tests as an example).

Results

Descriptive Statistics and Correlation Analysis of Each Variable

The average value, standard deviation, and correlation coefficient of trait mindfulness (including total score and five facet score), attention, and working memory are shown in **Table 1**. There was a significant positive correlation between total mindfulness score, attention, and working memory. The two mindfulness facets of "observe" and "actaware" were positively correlated with attention performance, and the three mindfulness facets of "observe," "describe," and "actaware" were positively correlated with work memory performance.

Analysis of the Mediating Effect of Attention

Path analysis was used to explore the mediating effect of attention on the relationship between mindfulness and working memory, by controlling the effect of age on attention and working memory. Because the "non-judge" and "non-react" facets had no significant correlation with attention and working memory, only the sum of the other three mindfulness facets was taken as a mindfulness score when constructing the mediating effect model.

The results of the mediating effect model are shown in **Figure 3**. As the influence of age on attention and working memory was not significant ($p < 0.05$), the age is not indicated in **Figure 3**. The fitting index of this model was as follows: χ^2/df = 2.976, GFI = 0.993, AGFI = 0.932, IFI = 0.990, TLI = 0.939, NFI = 0.985, CFI = 0.990. Therefore, the goodness of fit of this model was good. The non-parametric percentile bootstrap method of deviation correction was used to test the intermediate effect and estimate the confidence interval. The number of bootstrap repeated samplings was set to 5,000 and the confidence interval was set to 95%. The results showed that the confidence intervals of the mediating effects of this model do not contain zero, and the mediating effects were statistically significant (**Table 2**).

Table 2 shows the action path, effect value, and proportion of all independent variables to dependent variables in this model. Among these, the effect value for the direct effect of mindfulness on working memory was 0.40, accounting for 68.40% of the total effect. The mediating effect of attention between mindfulness and working memory was 0.18, accounting for 31.60% of the total effect.

STUDY 2

In this study, different stress situations were established to explore the effect of the interaction between stress and mindfulness on attention and working memory as well as further simple effects. A 2 (mindfulness level: low, high) × 3 (stress situation: none, single stress, multiple stresses) mixed experimental design was used. Among these, the level of mindfulness was the intersubject variable, and the stress situation was the intrasubject variable.

Methods

Participants and Procedures

According to the total score of the FFMQ scale in study 1, participants were divided into high and low mindfulness groups. Among the test subjects, the highest scoring 27% was in the

TABLE 1 | Descriptive statistics and correlation analysis of mindfulness level, attention, and working memory of junior school students (*r*).

	M	SD	1	2	3	4	5	6	7	8
1. Observe	24.22	6.22	1							
2. Describe	22.20	4.36	0.15*	1						
3. Actaware	27.00	6.09	0.15*	0.23**	1					
4. Non-judge	22.57	4.82	0.37***	0.14*	0.10	1				
5. Non-react	19.52	4.04	0.47***	0.04	0.06	0.37***	1			
6. Total score of mindfulness	115.52	14.97	0.76***	0.50***	0.49***	0.57***	0.57***	1		
7. Attention	3.34	1.07	0.42***	0.10	0.52***	0.08	0.11	0.48***	1	
8. Working memory	36.64	11.86	0.41***	0.21**	0.51***	0.05	0.08	0.48***	0.55***	1

*$p < 0.05$, **$p < 0.01$, ***$p < 0.001$.

high mindfulness group, and the lowest scoring 27% was in the low mindfulness group. One hundred and sixteen junior school students participated in all the tests of study 2.

The test situation of study 1 was regarded as the stress-free situation, and the test results of study 1 were thus used as the attention and working memory performance scores of the subjects in the stress-free situation. Furthermore, each subject's attention and working memory under single and multiple stresses were measured individually. All tests were conducted in a quiet environment. The examiner uniformly adopted the new instructional language to explain the purpose and specific requirements of the test. After ensuring that the subjects understood, the attention test was performed first and then the working memory test. To avoid the fatigue effect, subjects were given a 3-day interval between the attention test and the working memory test in the same stressful environment. In order to avoid the memory effect, for the same kind of test across different stress situations, subjects took parallel-form tests. In order to avoid the practice effect, the interval between the two similar tests was about 1 month.

Measures

Single stress situation

Time pressure was applied to the subjects in the single stress situation, in order to make individuals feel that it was challenging to complete the experimental task within a short time. The attention test required the subjects to complete the test within 1 min, and each picture in the working memory test was only presented for 2 s. When the examiner explained the instructions, they emphasized that the time constraints of the tests were significantly shorter than that of study 1, thereby giving the participants a sense of stress.

A copy of the number cancelation test was used as the experimental material to test attention in this situation. Compared with study 1, the completion time for the single stress situation was shortened to 1 min, the designated erasure number was adjusted from six to five, and all the number sorting was readjusted; other settings were unchanged.

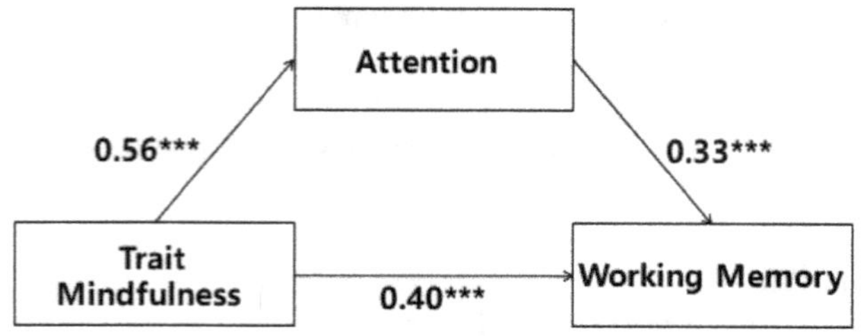

FIGURE 3 | The relationship model of trait mindfulness, attention, and working memory. ***$p < 0.001$.

A copy of the visual graphic working memory test was used as the experimental material to test working memory in this situation. Compared with study 1, the rendering time of the replica was shortened to 2 s, and the size, direction, or order of the target and alternative graphics were adjusted; other settings were unchanged.

Multiple stress situation

The premise of the multiple stress situation was to add situational pressure on top of time pressure, so that the subjects would feel the combined effect of more types of pressure. The time pressure was established in the same manner as described above. In China, learning ability and whether they are valued by teachers are important factors that affect the self-evaluation of junior school students. Therefore, when the examiner explained the instructions, it was emphasized that the participant's teacher would be informed of the results of the attention and working memory test as an indicator to evaluate their learning ability, and the teacher would focus on training the top students in the follow-up teaching. At the end of all the experiments, the students were informed of the real situation, i.e., the test results were actually confidential and would not be disclosed to the teachers, nor would they influence the teachers' evaluation and subsequent training of the students, so as to avoid any negative impact of the test on the students' psychological state.

The interval between this test and the single stress situation test was 1 month, while the interval between this test and the study 1 test was 2 months. In order to avoid a memory effect of the test materials in the single stress situation, the attention and working memory experimental materials from study 1 were reused, but the time setting was the same as that in the single stress situation.

Statistical Analysis

Descriptive analysis of attention and working memory scores under different stress situations and at different

TABLE 2 | Action path, effect size, and proportion of each variable in the model to working memory.

Path	Standardized effect value	Effect ratio	95% CI
Direct effect: mindfulness → working memory	0.40	68.40%	[0.28, 0.52]
Indirect: mindfulness → attention → working memory	0.56 × 0.33 = 0.18	31.60%	[0.12, 0.26]
Total effect	0.58		[0.49, 0.66]

TABLE 3 | Attention scores under different stress situations and mindfulness levels (M ± SD).

		Stress situation		
		Stress-free situation	Single stress situation	Multiple stress situation
Mindfulness level	High mindfulness group (n = 58)	4.04 ± 1.22	5.64 ± 1.39	4.69 ± 1.15
	Low mindfulness group (n = 58)	2.68 ± 0.69	1.29 ± 0.78	1.20 ± 0.76

levels of mindfulness was performed, with data expressed as mean ± standard deviation. The 2 × 3 mixed variance analysis was used to analyze the interaction effect and simple effect of the data. The independent variables were trait mindfulness and stress situation, and the outcome variables were attention and working memory. SPSS 22.0 (IBM Corp., Armonk, NY, United States) was used for analysis. The significance threshold was set at the $p < 0.05$ level.

Results

The Influence of Stress Situation and Mindfulness Level on Achievement at the Attention Task

The attention scores for different stress situations and mindfulness levels are shown in **Table 3**. The results of ANOVA showed that the interaction between mindfulness level and stress situation was significant [$F(2,114) = 207.94$, $p < 0.001$, $\eta^2_p = 0.646$]. These results are presented in **Figure 4**. Further simple effect analysis showed that (1) there was a significant difference in the attention performance of the high mindfulness group under different stress situations [$F(2,56) = 81.81$, $p < 0.001$]. Further results showed that the attention performance of the high mindfulness group was significantly better in the single stress situation than in the multiple stress situation, and the attention performance in the multiple stress situation was also significantly higher than that in the stress-free situation. The attention level of the low mindfulness group decreased with the increase in stress, but the difference was not significant [$F(2,56) = 26.51$, $p > 0.05$]. (2) The attention scores of the high mindfulness group and the low one were significantly different in each stress situation. In a stress-free situation, $F(2,56) = 54.61$, $p < 0.001$. In the single stress situation, $F(2,56) = 434.05$, $p < 0.001$. Under the multiple stress situation, $F(2,56) = 373.06$, $p < 0.001$. These results show that in all three different stress situations, the attention performance of the high mindfulness group was significantly higher than that of the low mindfulness group.

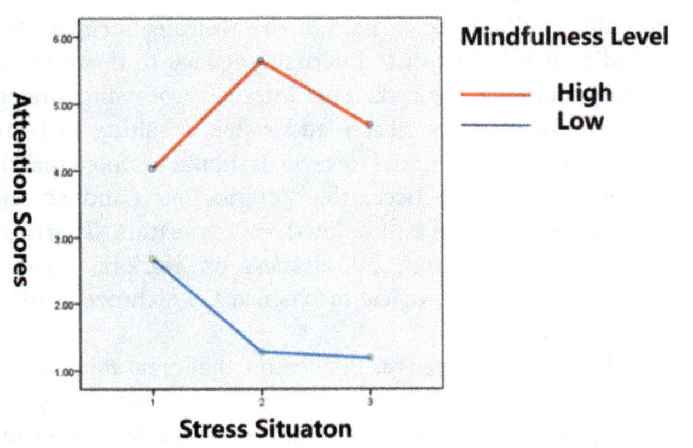

FIGURE 4 | Interaction between stress situations and mindfulness levels on attention scores. 1 is stress-free situation, 2 is single stress situation, and 3 is a multiple stress situation.

Effect of Stress Situation and Mindfulness Level on Working Memory Performance

The results of working memory under different stress situations and different mindfulness levels are shown in **Table 4**. The results of ANOVA showed that the interaction between mindfulness level and stress situation is significant (**Figure 5**), and $F(2,114) = 72.31$, $p < 0.001$, $\eta^2_p = 0.388$. Further simple effect analysis showed that the working memory performance of the low mindfulness group was significantly different under different stress situations [$F(2,56) = 258.28$, $p < 0.001$]. Further results showed that the working memory performance of the low mindfulness group in the stress-free situation was significantly better than that in the single stress situation, and their working memory performance in the single stress situation was significantly higher than that in the multiple stress situation. There was no significant difference in the working memory scores of the high mindfulness group under different stress situations [$F(2,56) = 2.21$, $p > 0.05$]. The difference in working memory performance between the high mindfulness group and the low one in each stress situation was significant. In the stress-free situation, $F(2,56) = 247.1$, $p < 0.001$. In the single stress situation, $F(2,56) = 247.1$, $p < 0.001$. Under the multiple stress situation, $F(2,56) = 550.21$, $p < 0.001$. This shows that the working memory performance of the high mindfulness group was significantly higher than that of the low mindfulness group in all three different stress situations.

TABLE 4 | Working memory performance under different stress situations and mindfulness levels ($M \pm SD$).

		Stress situation		
		Stress-free situation	Single stress situation	Multiple stress situation
Mindfulness level	High mindfulness group (n = 58)	43.59 ± 1.47	41.16 ± 0.75	42.64 ± 1.01
	Low mindfulness group (n = 58)	30.00 ± 1.05	20.90 ± 1.05	12.33 ± 0.81

DISCUSSION

The results of study 1 showed that there were positive correlations among trait mindfulness, attention, and working memory and that attention had a partial mediating effect between trait mindfulness and working memory, verifying Hypothesis 1. It can be seen that, on the one hand, the higher the level of trait mindfulness, the more concentrated and stable the individual's attention can be when completing the task, thus better promoting working memory. On the other hand, trait mindfulness can also directly affect working memory levels.

The close relationship between trait mindfulness and attention was consistent with the results from prior studies. It has been found that the human mind wanders for nearly half of its waking time (Killingsworth and Gilbert, 2010), and trait mindfulness and mindfulness training are associated with reduced mind wandering (Mrazek et al., 2012, 2013). Mindfulness controls attention by reducing habitual distribution of attention and attention to distracting information (Wadlinger and Isaacowitz, 2011). It is worth noting that the two mindfulness facets of "observe" and "actaware" were positively correlated with performance on the attention test in study 1, suggesting that these two facets may be the important factors of trait mindfulness affecting attention. The higher the level of trait mindfulness, the more consciously the individual can observe and pay attention to all kinds of experiences, pay more attention to and be aware of their current actions, and then have better performance when completing the attention task test.

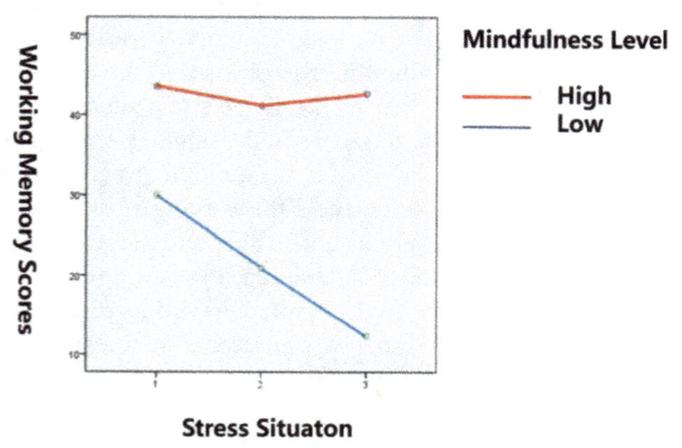

FIGURE 5 | Interaction between stress situations and mindfulness levels on working memory scores.

In this study, trait mindfulness was found to be related to working memory and positively influenced working memory performance. This is consistent with the results of previous studies (Phillipot and Segal, 2009; Satish et al., 2018). In the process of the influence of trait mindfulness on working memory, 31.60% were realized through the mediation of attention. This is because attention plays a fundamental role in cognitive processes, and this is very important in working memory. It is the first step of information processing by which external information enters the current processing range through attentional selection. On this basis, the further processing of information can be completed by working memory (Cowan et al., 2006). The results of this study also showed that the two mindfulness facets of "observe" and "actaware" are positively correlated with working memory. As mentioned before, these two facets are also positively correlated with attention. In conclusion, these two mindfulness facets can influence working memory through the mediation of attention.

Our results showed that the direct effect of trait mindfulness on working memory was 0.40, accounting for 68.40% of the total effect. This result indicates that apart from attention, trait mindfulness may directly or indirectly affect working memory through other mediating factors and that these effects were greater than those of attention. However, so far, the direct psychological mechanism of mindfulness affecting working memory is still unclear. This study showed that the "describe" facet of trait mindfulness is positively correlated with working memory, but not with attention, suggesting that the "describe" facet may be one of the internal mechanisms by which trait mindfulness directly affects working memory. The higher the "describe" facet score, the more likely the individual is to describe and mark internal experiences with language in daily life (Baer et al., 2006). When taking part in the working memory test, such individuals tend to use internal language to describe and mark the figures in the task. This internal processing strategy helps to make memory clearer and stable, resulting in better working memory test scores. However, it should be noted that the correlation coefficient between the "describe" facet and working memory performance is 0.21, a low-level correlation. Therefore, the direct impact of trait mindfulness on working memory must have other psychological mechanisms, which need further study in the future.

In addition to the above, the reason that trait mindfulness can positively predict attention and working memory may also be related to brain function and brain structure. Most previous research has focused on the impact of mindfulness training on the brain, and only several limited studies evaluating the neural basis of trait mindfulness have shown that trait mindfulness may be related to brain regions involved in attention and working memory, such as the hippocampus (Taren et al., 2013), the double lateral anterior cingulate cortex (ACC) (Lu et al., 2014), etc., and that brain function, neuroelectric activity, and even the structure of these brain areas and other areas related to attention and working memory can be changed through mindfulness practice (Cahn et al., 2010; Wang and Huang, 2011). Therefore, it can be speculated that mindfulness traits may be one of the important psychological factors in understanding the effects of mindfulness exercises on attention and working memory. That is to say, the positive influence of mindfulness exercise on attention and working memory may be achieved by improving the level of trait mindfulness and inducing changes in the corresponding brain structures and functions.

The experimental results of study 2 showed that the attention and working memory scores of the high trait mindfulness group were higher than those of the low trait mindfulness group across all three stress situations (no stress, single stress, and multiple stresses), verifying Hypothesis 4. These results also further deepened the results of study 1. They showed that the positive correlation and influence of trait mindfulness on attention and working memory were consistent across contexts; i.e., whether the stress intensity was great or not, the performance of attention and working memory from those with high trait mindfulness was always better than that from those with low trait mindfulness. These results showed that the level of trait mindfulness can be used to predict the performance of attention and working memory in different stress situations.

In study 2, we also found that stress situations and trait mindfulness interact in the process of influencing attention and working memory. Further simple effect analysis showed that the effects of different stress situations on attention and working memory are regulated by trait mindfulness, verifying Hypothesis 5. To be specific, based on the attention test scores under different stress situations, the relative performance of the high trait mindfulness group on the attention test were as follows: single stress > multiple stresses > no stress. However, for the low trait mindfulness group, although no statistical difference was found in attention under the different stress conditions, it can be seen in **Table 3** and **Figure 4** that attention had a downward trend in the process from no stress to single stress and multiple stresses. There was no significant change in the test results for working memory across the different stress situations for the high mindfulness group. The working memory performance of the low mindfulness group decreased significantly with the increase of stress intensity.

According to the Yerkes-Dodson law, stress and task performance show an inverted U-shaped curve. When the pressure is moderate, the task performance is the highest. Excessive stress will lead to a decline in task performance. However, whether a stress situation constitutes excessive pressure and how much influence it will have are affected by many factors. According to the interaction theory of stress coping, the influence of stress on individuals is related not only to changes in the stimulating environment or events but also to psychological factors such as individual cognition and coping style (Lazarus and Folkman, 1984). The results of this study showed that trait mindfulness is an important psychological factor that regulates the influence of stress on individual attention and working memory.

For the low trait mindfulness group, working memory decreased significantly with the increase in stress intensity. Although the performance of attention did not show a significant difference, there was a downward trend. This shows that for such individuals, the single stress and multiple stress levels established in this experiment exceed the highest stress level that the participants could bear, resulting in a decline of working memory and attention. Therefore, it is suggested that for such individuals, the degree of stress tolerance is very limited, and a small increase in stress may have a strong negative impact on them. Therefore, in normal learning tasks, time pressure and other factors that could readily cause stress should be reduced, to avoid damaging working memory and attention.

It has been found that increased trait mindfulness can reduce stress sensitivity (Greeson and Gabrielle, 2018). Individuals with high trait mindfulness have less stress sensitivity and better adaptability than those with low trait mindfulness (Grover et al., 2016; Lomas et al., 2017). For high trait mindfulness individuals, the single time stress situation used in this study is close to the appropriate range of stress (the highest point of the inverted U curve). This may enable individuals to reach or approach the best level of arousal, stimulate individual potential, and fully mobilize attention. This helps the individual to complete the attention test quickly and accurately and to make the score on the attention test reach or approach the best possible level. Under the multiple stress condition, the stress intensity exceeds the individual's ability to bear properly, and so, test scores decline. However, when the individual is in a stress-free situation, the potential of the individual, including attention and other cognitive resources, is not effectively mobilized, yielding the lowest score for all three conditions. Therefore, for the high trait mindfulness group, in the normal learning tasks, increasing the stress intensity appropriately, such as increasing the time pressure properly, will be more conducive to the individual's concentration and to faster and better completion of the task. In the working memory test, with the increase in stress intensity, the performance of working memory in the high trait mindfulness group was not damaged, indicating that high trait mindfulness had a protective effect on the working memory of individuals coping with stress.

This study yielded another interesting and noteworthy result. Regardless of whether the participant was in the low trait mindfulness group or the high trait mindfulness group, as the stress situation changed, the changes in individual working memory were not synchronized with changes in attention. For example, in the low trait mindfulness group, as the stress increased, working memory decreased significantly, but the performance of attention did not change significantly. In the high trait mindfulness group, the relative scores on the attention test, across all three stress conditions, were as follows: single stress > multiple stresses > no stress, but there were no significant differences in scores for working memory. This may be due to the fact that, although attention is an important factor affecting working memory (Oberauer, 2019), working memory may also be affected by other factors such as emotions

(Eysenck et al., 2005) and expectation-driven changes in cortical functional connectivity (Bollinger et al., 2010). Moreover, these factors may have different effects on working memory in different stressful situations, which may lead to the observed asynchrony of the attention and working memory test results.

In conclusion, this study suggests that a good way to improve attention and working memory in different stress situations would be to improve the level of trait mindfulness. Therefore, this study provides a strong theoretical basis and practical guidance for improving attention and working memory.

Limitations and Future Research

Although this study produced some important findings, it nonetheless has some limitations. First, with regard to research methods, study 1 adopted a cross-sectional design, and thus, it could not draw any conclusions regarding causality; this should be borne in mind when interpreting the results from study 1. Second, with regard to the research group, the subjects selected in this study were all junior school students, from a single sample source. The research conclusions may not be applicable to other groups, raising potential concerns about external validity. Third, with regard to the research content, although this study discussed the possible role of the brain in the process by which trait mindfulness affects attention and working memory, that was only a deduction and no substantive research on that specific topic was conducted.

Therefore, the following aspects need to be further explored in the future. First, a longitudinal study or combined mindfulness interventions should be considered to explore the dynamic relationship among trait mindfulness, attention, and working memory, so as to further verify the causal relationship among them. Second, attention and working memory are very important not only for junior school students but also for other groups. Therefore, one could further expand the scope of the subjects and thereby yield meaningful knowledge for promoting the attention and working memory performance of other groups. Finally, studies on the relationship between brain function and structure and trait mindfulness are still rare, and this aspect should be studied to further clarify the effective mechanisms by which trait mindfulness affects attention and working memory.

ETHICS STATEMENT

The studies involving human participants were reviewed and approved by the Harbin Engineering University Ethics Committee. Written informed consent to participate in this study was provided by the participants' legal guardian/next of kin.

AUTHOR CONTRIBUTIONS

YL was responsible for writing the manuscript and analyzing the data. NY was responsible for designing the research and collecting the data. YZ conducted the experiment and reviewed and revised the manuscript. WX took part in designing the research and collecting the data. LC took part in collecting the data. All authors approved the above version to be published.

REFERENCES

Allen, T. D., Eby, L. T., Conley, K. M., Williamson, R. L., Mancini, V. S., and Mitchell, M. E. (2015). What do we really know about the effects of mindfulness-based training in the workplace? *Ind. Organ. Psychol.* 8, 652–661. doi: 10.1017/iop.2015.95

Ayres, P., and Sweller, J. (2014). "The split-attention principle in multimedia learning," in *The Cambridge handbook of multimedia learning, 2nd edn,* ed. R. E. Mayer (New York, NY: Cambridge University Press), 206–226. doi: 10.1017/CBO9781139547369.011

Baddeley, A., Sala, S. D., Robbins, T. W., and Baddeley, A. (1996). Working memory and executive control [and discussion]. *Philos. Trans. R. Soc. B Biol. Sci.* 351, 1397–1404.

Baer, R. A., Smith, G. T., Hopkins, J., Krietemeyer, J., and Toney, L. (2006). Using self-reporassessment methods to explore facets of mindfulness. *Assessment* 13, 27–45. doi: 10.1177/1073191105283504

Bailey, N. W., Freedman, G., Raj, K., Spierings, K. N., and Fitzgerald, P. B. (2020). Mindfulness meditators show enhanced accuracy and different neural activity during working memory. *Mindfulness* 11, 1762–1781. doi: 10.1007/s12671-020-01393-8

Bollinger, J., Rubens, M. T., Zanto, T. P., and Gazzaley, A. (2010). Expectation-driven changes in cortical functional connectivity influence working memory and long-term memory performance. *J. Neurosci.* 30, 14399–14410. doi: 10.1523/JNEUROSCI.1547-10.2010

Brown, D. B., Bravo, A. J., Roos, C. R., and Pearson, M. R. (2015). Five facets of mindfulness and psychological health: evaluating a psychological model of the mechanisms of mindfulness. *Mindfulness* 6, 1021–1032. doi: 10.1007/s12671-014-0349-4

Brown, K. W., and Ryan, R. M. (2013). The benefits of being present: mindfulness and its role in psychological well-being. *J. Pers. Soc. Psychol.* 84, 822–848. doi: 10.1037/0022-3514.84.4.822

Cahn, B. R., Delorme, A., and Polich, J. (2010). Occipital gamma activation during Vipassana meditation. *Cogn. Process.* 11, 39–56. doi: 10.1007/s10339-009-0352-1

Cavanagh, K., Strauss, C., Forder, L., and Jones, F. (2014). Can mindfulness and acceptance be learnt by self-help? a systematic review and meta-analysis of mindfulness and acceptance-based self-help interventions. *Clin. Psychol. Rev.* 34, 118–129. doi: 10.1016/j.c-pr.2014.01.001

Chambers, R., Lo, B. C. Y., and Allen, N. B. (2008). The impact of intensive mindfulness training on attentional control, cognitive style, and affect. *Cogn. Ther. Res.* 32, 303–322. doi: 10.1007/s10608-007-9119-0

Cowan, N., Fristoe, N. M., Elliott, E. M., Brunner, R. P., and Saults, J. S. (2006). Scope of attention, control of attention, and intelligence in children and adults. *Mem. Cogn.* 34, 1754–1768. doi: 10.3758/BF03195936

Davidson, R. J. (2010). Empirical explorations of mindfulness: conceptual and methodological conundrums. *Emotion* 10, 8–11. doi: 10.1037/a0018480

Deng, Y. Q., Liu, X. H., Rodriguez, M. A., and Xia, C. Y. (2011). The five facet mindfulness questionnaire: psychometric properties of the chinese version. *Mindfulness* 2, 123–128. doi: 10.1007/s12671-011-0050-9

Dunning, D. L., and Holmes, J. (2014). Does working memory training promote the use of strategies on untrained working memory tasks? *Mem. Cogn.* 42, 854–862. doi: 10.3758/s13421-014-0410-5

Durbrow, E. H., Schaefer, B. A., and Jimerson, S. R. (2000). Learning behaviours, attention and anxiety in caribbean children: beyond the \"usual suspects\" in explaining academic performance. *Sch. Psychol. Int.* 21, 242–251. doi: 10.1177/0143034300213002

Eysenck, M., Payne, S., and Derakshan, N. (2005). Trait anxiety, visuospatial processing, and working memory. *Cogn. Emot.* 19, 1214–1228. doi: 10.1080/

02699930500260245

Greeson, J. M., and Gabrielle, R. (2018). Mindfulness and physical disease: a concise review. *Curr. Opin. Psychol.* 28, 204–210. doi: 10.1016/j.copsyc.2018.12.014

Grover, S. L., Teo, S. T. T., Pick, D., and Roche, M. (2016). Mindfulness as a personal resource to reduce work stress in the job demands-resources model. *Stress Health* 33, 426–436. doi: 10.1002/smi.2726

Jamieson, S. D., and Tuckey, M. R. (2017). Mindfulness interventions in the workplace: a critique of the current state of the literature. *J. Occup. Health Psychol.* 22, 180–193. doi: 10.1037/ocp0000048

Jha, A. P., Morrison, A. B., Dainer-Best, J., Parker, S., Rostrup, N., and Stanley, E. A. (2015). Minds "at attention": mindfulness training curbs attentional lapses in military cohorts. *PLoS One* 10:e0116889. doi: 10.1371/journal.pone.0116889

Jha, A. P., Stanley, E. A., Kiyonaga, A., Wong, L., and Gelfand, L. (2010). Examining the protective effects of mindfulness training on working memory capacity and affective experience. *Emotion* 10, 54–64. doi: 10.1037/a0018438

Kiken, L. G., Garland, E. L., Bluth, K., Palsson, O. S., and Gaylord, S. A. (2015). From a state to a trait: trajectories of state mindfulness in meditation during intervention predict changes in trait mindfulness. *Pers. Indiv. Differ.* 81, 41–46. doi: 10.1016/j.paid.2014.12.044

Killingsworth, M. A., and Gilbert, D. T. (2010). A wandering mind is an unhpppy mind. *Science* 330:932. doi: 10.1126/science.1192439

Kumar, S., Soto, D., and Humphreys, G. W. (2009). Electrophysiological evidence for attentional guidance by the contents of working memory. *Eur. J. Neurosci.* 30, 307–317. doi: 10.1111/j.1460-9568.2009.06805.x

Lazarus, R. S., and Folkman, S. (1984). *Stress, Appraisal and Coping*. New York, NY: Springer Publishing Company, doi: 10.1007/978-1-4419-1005-9_215

Limaree, S. (2007). "Meditation and Emotional Quotient," in *Proceedings of the 1st International Conference on Educational Reform*, (Talat: Mahasarakham University), 402–407.

Lindsay, E. K., and Creswell, J. D. (2017). Mechanisms of mindfulness training: monitor and acceptance theory (mat). clinical psychology review. *Clin. Psychol. Rev.* 51, 48–59. doi: 10.1016/j.cpr.2016.10.011

Lomas, T., Medina, J. C., Ivtzan, I., Rupprecht, S., Hart, R., and Eiroa-Orosa, F. J. (2017). The impact of mindfulness on well-being and performance in the workplace: an inclusive systematic review of the empirical literature. *Eur. J. Work Organ. Psychol.* 26, 492–513. doi: 10.1080/1359432X.2017.1308924

Lu, H., Song, Y., Xu, M., Wang, X., Li, X., and Liu, J. (2014). The brain structure correlates of individual differences in trait mindfulness: a voxel-based morphometry study. *Neuroscience* 272, 21–28. doi: 10.1016/j.neuroscience.2014.04.051

Lukasik, K. M., Waris, O., Soveri, A., Lehtonen, M., and Laine, M. (2019). The relationship of anxiety and stress with working memory performance in a large non-depressed sample. *Front. Psychol.* 10:4. doi: 10.3389/fpsyg.2019.00004

Matthews, G., and Campbell, S. E. (2010). Dynamic relationships between stress states and working memory. *Cogn. Emot.* 24, 357–373. doi: 10.1080/02699930903378719

Medvedev, O. N., Krageloh, C. U., Narayanan, A., and Siegert, R. J. (2017). Measuring mindfulness applying generalizability theory to distinguish between state and trait. *Mindfulness* 8, 1036–1046. doi: 10.1007/s12671-017-0679-0

Mesmer-Magnus, J., Manapragada, A., Viswesvaran, C., and Allen, J. W. (2017). Trait mindfulness at work: a meta-analysis of the personal and professional correlates of trait mindfulness. *Hum. Perform.* 30, 79–98. doi: 10.1080/08959285.2017.1307842

Mrazek, M. D., Franklin, M. S., Phillips, D. T., Baird, B., and Schooler, J. W. (2013). Mindfulness training improves working memory capacity and gre performance while reducing mind wandering. *Psychol. Sci.* 24, 776–781. doi: 10.1177/0956797612459659

Mrazek, M. D., Smallwood, J., and Schooler, J. W. (2012). Mindfulness and mind wanderi-ng: finding convergence through opposing constructs. *Emotion* 12, 442–448. doi: 10.1037/a0026678

Myhr, P., Hursti, T., Emanuelsson, K., Lfgren, E., and Hjemdal, O. (2019). Can the attention training technique reduce stress in students? a controlled study of stress appraisals and meta-worry. *Front. Psychol.* 10:1532. doi: 10.3389/fpsyg.2019.01532

Oberauer, K. (2019). Working memory and attention a conceptual analysis and review. *J. Cogn.* 2:36. doi: 10.5334/joc.58

Phillipot, P., and Segal, Z. (2009). Mindfulness based psychological interventions: developing emotional awareness for better being. *J. Conscious. Stud.* 16, 285–306. doi: 10.1007/s10806-009-9172-7

Quaglia, J. T., Braun, S. E., Freeman, S. P., McDaniel, M. A., and Brown, K. W. (2016). Meta-analytic evidence for effects of mindfulness training on dimensions of self-reported dispositional mindfulness. *Psychol. Assess.* 28, 803–818. doi: 10.1037/pas0000268

Rebok, G. W., Ball, K., Guey, L. T., Jones, R. N., Kim, H. Y., King, J. W., et al. (2014). Ten-year effects of the advanced cognitive training for independent and vital elderly cognitive training trial on cognition and everyday functioning in older adults. *J. Am. Geriatr. Soc.* 62, 16–24. doi: 10.1111/jgs.12607

Rode, C., Robson, R., Purviance, A., and Mayr, U. (2017). Is working memory training effective? A study in a school setting. *PLoS One* 9:e104796. doi: 10.1371/journal.pone.0104796

Satish, J., Shao-Yang, T., Chi-Hung, J., Wei-Kuang, L., and Muggleton, N. G. (2018). Better cognitive performance is associated with the combination of high trait mindfulness and low trait anxiety. *Front. Psychol.* 9:627. doi: 10.3389/fpsyg.2018.00627

Schweizer, K., Moosbrugger, H., and Goldhammer, F. (2005). The structure of the relationship between attention and intelligence. *Intelligence* 33, 589–611. doi: 10.1016/j.intell.2005.07.001

Soto, D., Heinke, D., Humphreys, G. W., and Blanco, M. J. (2005). Early, involuntary top-down guidance of attention from working memory. *J. Exp. Psychol.* 31, 248–261. doi: 10.1037/0096-1523.31.2.248

Taren, A. A., David, C. J., Gianaros, P. J., and Allan, S. (2013). Dispositional mindfulness co-varies with smaller amygdala and caudate volumes in community adults. *PLoS One* 8:e64574. doi: 10.1371/journal.pone.0064574

Tarrasch, R. (2018). The effects of mindfulness practice on attentional functions among primary school children. *J. Child Fam. Stud.* 27, 2632–2642. doi: 10.1007/s10826-018-1073-9

Wadlinger, H. A., and Isaacowitz, D. M. (2011). Fixing our focus: training attention to regulate emotion. *Pers. Soc. Psychol. Rev.* 15, 75–102. doi: 10.1177/1088868310365565

Wang, F., and Huang, Y. X. (2011). Psychological and neural mechanisms of mindfulness. *Adv. Psychol. Sci.* 19, 1635–1644.

Wimmer, L., Bellingrathand, S., and von Stockhausen, L. (2020). Mindfulness training for improving attention regulation in university students: is it effective? And do yoga and homework matter? *Front. Psychol.* 11:719. doi: 10.3389/fpsyg.2020.00719

Yerkes, R. M., and Dodson, J. D. (1908). The relation of strength of stimulus to rapidity of habit-formation. *J. Comp. Neurol. Psychol.* 18, 459–482. doi: 10.1002/cne.920180503

10

Moderating Effect of Mindfulness on the Relationships between Perceived Stress and Mental Health Outcomes among Chinese Intensive Care Nurses

*Fang Lu[1,2], Yuanyuan Xu[1], Yongju Yu[3], Li Peng[1], Tong Wu[1], Tao Wang[1], Botao Liu[1], Junpeng Xie[1], Song Xu[1] and Min Li[1]**

[1] School of Psychology, Army Medical University, Chongqing, China, [2] School of Nursing, Army Medical University, Chongqing, China, [3] Department of Sociology, Sichuan International Studies University, Chongqing, China

Correspondence:
Min Li
limin52267@tmmu.edu.cn

This study aimed to explore the potential moderating effect of mindfulness and its facets on the relationships among perceived stress and mental health outcomes (burnout, depression, anxiety, and subjective well-being) among Chinese intensive care nurses. A total of 500 Chinese intensive care nurses completed self-report measures of mindfulness, burnout syndromes, perceived stress, depression, anxiety, and subjective well-being. Correlation and hierarchical multiple regressions were applied for data analysis. Mindfulness moderated the effects of perceived stress on emotional exhaustion (the core component of burnout syndrome), depression, anxiety, positive affect, and negative affect but not on the other two dimensions of burnout and life satisfaction. Further analyses indicated that the ability to act with awareness was particularly crucial in improving the effects of perceived stress on depression. These results further broaden our understanding of the relationships between perceived stress and burnout, depression, anxiety, and subjective well-being by demonstrating that mindfulness may serve as a protective factor that alleviates or eliminates the negative effects of perceived stress on depression, anxiety, burnout syndrome, and subjective well-being and may instigate further research into targeted mindfulness interventions for Chinese intensive care nurses.

Keywords: mindfulness, perceived stress, burnout syndrome, depressive symptom, anxiety symptom, subjective well-being, intensive care nurses

INTRODUCTION

The intensive care unit (ICU) is a fast-paced, demanding, and tension-charged environment. Nurses working in the ICU are predisposed to workplace stress owing to direct and indirect exposure to traumatic and critical events, excessive workload (1), high patient care demands (2), long shift work, close contact with death and severe illness (3), and even medical violence (4); however, nurses working in the ICU have limited authority (2). Highly stressful daily events may lead to a heightened stress response combined with negative emotions (5). A growing number of studies have examined mental health among intensive care nursing, but studies on this topic are still rare. Previous studies have produced concordant results demonstrating that ICU nurses show high rates of stress that have resulted in epidemic levels of some work-related mental health problems (6).

The most commonly explored outcome of high-level work-related stress in health care providers is burnout syndrome (7, 8). An increasing number of studies have shown that ICU nurses have an increased prevalence of burnout syndrome (9–11). Burnout is often described as a three-dimensional syndrome that is characterized by emotional exhaustion (EE), depersonalization (DP), and lack of personal accomplishment (PA) (12), which are experienced by 73%, 48%, and 60% of critical care nurses, respectively (10). Compared to nurses in other units, nurses in the ICU treat patients with specific characteristics. Triggers of stress that are different from those experienced in other units include high patient mortality and morbidity, a challenging work environment, and frequent encounters with the critical and traumatic events mentioned above.

The current data show that the prevalence of burnout among critical care staff in different countries has reached alarming levels of approximately 30% in France (11), 16% of nursing staff and 10% of nursing assistants in Spain (13), 56% in a group of pediatric intensive care unit (PICU) staff in Spain (80.9% of nurses and nursing assistants), 84.4% in Argentina (14), and from 25% to 33% in the United States, with up to 86% of the critical care staff experiencing at least one of the three dimensions of burnout. In China, one study indicated that the prevalence of burnout was 83.7% among nurses in the ICU and emergency department (15). Burnout syndrome has been reported to have many negative consequences. It was found that burnout reduces the quality of care (16), lowers patient satisfaction, increases medical error, and leads to interpersonal conflicts, negative emotions, physical symptoms, compulsive behaviors, intention to leave, a higher turnover rate, and absenteeism (9, 10, 12, 17–19).

Perceived stress, depression, and anxiety are strongly and positively related, suggesting a close link between stress and psychopathological symptoms and well-being (20). According to the WHO, over the past two decades, the number of people suffering from anxiety and/or depression worldwide has increased by nearly 50%. Mental illnesses are common among nurses from different countries. Studies have shown that 61.7% of nurses working in the Northeast China Hospital have depressive symptoms (21). The influencing factors and effects of anxiety and/or depression in nurses have been studied. Depressive symptoms among nurses have been linked to stressful work environments, job demand, effort–reward imbalance, etc., which may adversely result in sickness-related absences and affect quality of life and quality of care (21). Well-being is essential for quality of care and productivity. However, prolonged or excessive stress places increasing strain on individuals and has deleterious effects on well-being (22).

Since it is apparent that nursing in the ICU is associated with unique sets of stressors, it is imperative to study the influencing factors and strategies to prevent burnout syndrome, depression, and anxiety, and to promote well-being, and it is crucial for ICU nurses to find ways to manage their stress and prevent the development of these mental health outcomes. According to Folkman et al.'s stress and coping theory (23), stress occurs when one appraises the stressor as exceeding his or her coping resources. The theory suggests that whether perceived stress can predict negative psychological outcomes may depend on the characteristics of the stressors, as well as the individual's assessment of these stressors and his or her access to coping resources.

Mindfulness may be a potential coping strategy that moderates the negative effects of appraised stress. Mindfulness can be conceptualized as both a trait-like quality (a psychological trait that refers to the tendency to be mindful in everyday life) and a state-like quality (a receptive attention to internal and external experiences) (24). Research of mindfulness interventions in nursing staff has revealed that mindfulness was associated with lower levels of reported stress (25, 26), improved coping with stress and diminished burnout (27–29), decreased EE and anxiety (30), and increased life satisfaction (31). According to Baer et al., mindfulness has five components—observation, description, acting with awareness, nonjudgment of inner experience, and nonreactivity to inner experience (32)—and each facet of mindfulness has specific effects. For example, mindfulness provides individuals the ability to detect the signs of stress by improving awareness (33). Research showed that high dispositional mindfulness may increase awareness of low-level stress symptoms, which, in turn, increases access to coping resources and helps alleviate the negative effects of stress (34). In addition, the ability to observe the effect of the buffer against stress on reduced life satisfaction and depression has been proposed (35). Therefore, it has been suggested that mindful individuals have greater abilities to handle with a set of stressors, which could help moderate the relationship between stress and adverse mental health outcomes (34, 36).

Recently, researchers have shown increasing interest in the stress buffering role of mindfulness. Bergin and Pakenham studied a sample of 481 Australian law school students and found that dispositional mindfulness moderated the effect of perceived stress on anxiety and depression (35). In another student sample, Bodenlos et al. (37) found that the mindfulness facet of nonjudgment acted as a buffer of well-being. By studying 292 patients with gastrointestinal cancer, Zhong et al. (38) concluded that the relationship between psychological symptoms and perceived stress was notable in patients with low dispositional mindfulness. Ciesla et al. (36) conducted a prospective study of 78 high school students and found that nonjudgment and nonreactivity mitigated the effects of daily stress on the daily changes in dysphoric affect. In a sample of 382 Swedish adults, Bränström et al. (34) found that dispositional mindfulness buffered the negative impact of perceived stress on mental health. However, most of the studies mentioned above were carried out in Western societies, and whether mindfulness also constitutes a health resource for ICU nurses working in Chinese societies is insufficiently explored.

Given the high rate of stress in ICU professionals found in previous studies combined with the lack of information focused on both the negative and positive indicators of mental health outcomes, this study pursues two specific goals: first, to test how stress, mindfulness, depressive and anxiety symptoms, and subjective well-being (SWB) are interrelated in Chinese ICU nurses and, second, to detect whether mindfulness moderates the relationship between perceived stress and the related mental health outcomes mentioned previously. Moreover, out of the studies on the moderating role of mindfulness, there have been few studies examining the stress-moderating role of all five mindfulness facets illustrated by Baer et al. (39). Therefore, this study will explore the moderating effects of observation, description, acting with awareness, nonjudgment of inner experience, and nonreactivity to inner experience on perceived stress and other variables. We hypothesized that

1) High levels of mindfulness would be associated with better mental health outcomes for ICU nurses, and mindfulness would moderate the relationship between perceived stress and mental health outcomes.
2) Compared to ICU nurses with lower levels of mindfulness, the association between higher perceived stress and worse mental health outcomes would be weaker and better health outcomes would be more prevalent in nurses with higher levels of mindfulness.

MATERIALS AND METHODS

Participants and Procedure

From March 2016 to April 2017, a total of 500 intensive care nurses were recruited from hospitals in Xinjiang, Ningxia, Beijing, Shandong, Heilongjiang, Fujian, Chongqing, Sichuan, Guizhou, Yunnan, and Hubei provinces through purposive sampling methods. The nurses were recruited from local hospitals, military hospitals, first-class hospitals, and second-senior class hospitals in the northwestern, northern, northeastern, southeastern, southwestern, and central regions of China. The ages of the 500 participants ranged from 20 to 52 years (mean = 27.68 years, SD = 4.275). Among the participants, 41 were male and 459 were female, and 246 were unmarried and 256 were married. None of the participants had meditation experience or practiced meditation before.

The research design of this cross-sectional study was previously approved by the Ethics Committee of Army Medical University. Informed consent forms were obtained from participants who completed questionnaires, including the Five Facet Mindfulness Questionnaire (FFMQ), the Positive and Negative Affect Schedule (PANAS), the Perceived Stress Scale (PSS), the Maslach Burnout Inventory–Human Services Survey (MBI-HSS), the Satisfaction with Life Scale (SWSL), the Center for Epidemiological Studies Depression Scale (CES-D), and the Self-Rating Anxiety Scale (SAS). The uniform instructions were used for the test.

Measures

Demographic information. Participants provided demographic information including age, gender, marital status, and meditation experience.

Burnout. The Maslach Burnout Inventory–Human Services Survey (MBI-HSS) was used to assess the burnout syndrome of the human service professionals. The MBI-HSS includes 22 items in three job-related dimensions: emotional exhaustion (EE), depersonalization (DP), and personal accomplishment (PA), and the 22 items were rated on a seven-point Likert scale, ranging from 0 = "never" to 6 = "every day" (40). Samantha Mei-Che Peng from The Hong Kong Polytechnic University translated the Chinese version of the MBI-HSS, which demonstrated good validity and reliability in China (41). There were nine items in the EE dimension, five items in the DP dimension, and eight items in the PA dimension. The Cronbach's alpha values were 0.86 for EE, 0.76 for DP, and 0.76 for PA. Based on previous studies, medical professionals with scores >26 on the EE subscale, >9 on the DP subscale, or <34 on the PA subscale are defined as having high burnout in that field.

Mindfulness. Translated from the FFMQ (39), the Chinese version of the Five Facet Mindfulness Questionnaire (Ch-FFMQ) is a questionnaire that measures dispositional mindfulness with 39 items (42). These items are rated on a five-point Likert scale ranging from 1 (never or very rarely true) to 5 (very often or always true), focusing on five facets of mindfulness: Observation, Description, Acting with awareness, Nonjudgment of inner experience, and Nonreactivity to inner experience (32). The Observation facet evaluates a tendency to observe or focus on external and internal experiences, such as emotions, thoughts, and sensations. Description assesses the propensity to describe and categorize these experiences with words. The Acting with awareness facet measures a sense of bringing full awareness and constant attention to the present experience or activity. The Nonjudging of inner experience facet measures a nonevaluative perspective toward inner experiences and cognition. Nonreactivity to inner experience assesses the tendency to allow feelings and thoughts to surface then leave, without becoming stuck on them or becoming overwhelmed by them. It has been shown that the FFMQ has good internal consistency (39), and the Cronbach's alpha values for the Ch-FFMQ are acceptable (42).

Depression. The Chinese version of the Center for Epidemiological Studies Depression Scale (CES-D) (43) was used to assess depressive symptoms. The CES-D consists of 20 items and is widely used to measure the epidemiology of depressive symptoms, with a focus on emotional components and depression. Participants in this study rated the frequency of occurrence of depressive symptoms on a four-point Likert scale: 0 = "never," 1 = "sometimes," 2 = "frequently," or 3 = "always." The Chinese version of the CES-D has good reliability and validity ($\alpha = 0.89$) (44). Individuals with a total CES-D score 16 or higher were defined as having "depressive symptoms" (45), which was further defined as mild for CES-D scores between 16 and 26 or moderate to severe for scores 27 or higher, which was based on the established criteria (46, 47).

Anxiety. Zung's Self-Rating Anxiety Scale (SAS) (48) served as an assessment tool to reflect the severity of anxiety symptoms reported by participants during the 7 days prior to completing the questionnaire. The SAS contains 20 items rated on a four-point Likert scale from 1 = "never" to 4 = "always," with a total raw score ranging from 20 to 80 and index score ranging from 25–100,respectively. The SAS and the cutoff point defined have been used extensively in studies of anxiety in China, and the Chinese translation of the survey has been previously validated

(49). In terms of an investigation of Chinese National Normative Scores, Chinese researchers defined SAS scores >50 as the cutoff point for symptom severity associated with anxiety disorders (50). The score is positively related to the severity of anxiety. Cronbach's alpha coefficient for the scale was 0.849 in the present study.

Perceived stress. The Perceived Stress Scale (PSS) is extensively used to measure the extent to which an individual considers his or her life to be stressful and to assess how controllable and unpredictable the stress has been over the past month (51). This scale has 14 items, with 7 items negatively stated and 7 items positively stated, which are rated on a five-point Likert scale from 1 = "not at all" to 5 = "always." Higher scores indicated a higher level of perceived stress. The total score for all 14 items ranges from 14 to 70. The Chinese version of the Perceived Stress Scale (CPSS) was developed by Yang and Huang (52) to assess perceived stress with good reliability and validity. The alpha coefficient values for the positive and negative subscales were 0.86 and 0.77, respectively (53).

Subjective well-being. Subjective well-being (SWB) is a composite concept that includes a high level of satisfaction with life, more positive emotions, and fewer negative emotions (54). Greater life satisfaction, high positive affect, and low negative affect are often considered as indices of greater SWB (55). Thus, the measure of SWB was shown to be consistent with the Positive Affect and Negative Affect Schedule (PANAS) (56) and with the Satisfaction with Life Scale (SWLS) (57). The PANAS are 20 adjectives that indicate positive affect, such as enthusiasm and activity, and negative affect, such as hatred, contempt, and feelings of guilt. Participants are asked to rate each mood state listed on a five-point Likert scale ranging from 1 = "very lightly or not at all" to 5 = "very much." The internal consistency coefficients in our sample for the positive and negative affect subscales were 0.86 and 0.83, respectively. The SWLS is a five-item scale used to measure global life satisfaction. Participants were asked to describe the extent to which they agree or disagree with each item on a seven-point Likert scale from 1 = "totally disagree" to 7 = "totally agree." Higher scores indicate greater perceived life satisfaction. The internal consistency coefficient of SWLS in the present study was 0.89.

Analyses

Descriptive analyses were based on the mean (M), standard deviation (SD), and range. Preliminary analyses were carried out to test the relationships between demographic variables (age, gender, and marital status), predictors, and outcome variables to identify demographic variables that must be controlled for in further analyses. Through independent-samples *T* test, we found that unmarried ICU nurses perceived more stress and reported higher DP than married ICU nurses. Therefore, age and marital status were controlled for in further analyses.

Hierarchical multiple regression analyses were performed to determine whether stress interacts with mindfulness, as well as the five facets individually, in the prediction of burnout (including three dimensions), depression, anxiety, and SWB (including three components). To increase the interpretability of the moderation model and to control for multicollinearity, all continuous variables were centered, and then the product terms were calculated, which represent the two-way interactions among stress, depression, anxiety, well-being, and mindfulness (58). The variables were entered in the following steps: a) the controlled demographic variables, b) the total perceived stress by ICU nurses, c) the total mindfulness, and d) the interaction term of stress × total mindfulness. Mindfulness was entered after perceived stress to explore the unique differences in mindfulness in the test results. **Table 1** shows a summary of all the separate hierarchical multiple regression models. To explore the potential main and moderate effects of the five mindfulness facets, regression analyses were conducted repeatedly using the five facets to replace total mindfulness at step 3a, and five interactions between each facet and the total perceived stress were input in step 4b. Simple slope analyses were conducted to illustrate the significant interactions among all the moderating models. According to Jaccard et al. (59), the unstandardized regression coefficients (B) of the regression lines for ICU nurses for low (1 SD below mean) and high (1 SD above mean) effects of the moderating variable were adopted. SPSS 19.0 was applied for data analyses.

RESULTS

Descriptive Statistics

The descriptive statistics and internal reliability coefficients for each measure are shown in **Table 2.**

According to the cutoff of dimensions of burnout, depression, and anxiety mentioned in measures, the prevalence of these psychological symptoms was common. Of the 500 Chinese ICU nurses, 56% (280/500) were positive for symptoms of depression and 35.2% (176/500) were positive for symptoms of anxiety. There is a prevalence of burnout syndrome, with 84% (420/500) of nurses having positive symptoms in at least one of the three individual dimensions: 23% (115/500) were positive for EE, 27% (135/500) were positive for DP, and 77.8% (389/500) were positive for lack of PA.

Table 3 confirms that perceived stress was significantly positively associated with EE, DP (two negative dimensions of burnout), depressive and anxiety symptoms, and negative affect and was negatively associated with personal achievements (the positive dimension of burnout) and SWB. On the other hand, total mindfulness was negatively correlated with EE, DP, depression, and anxiety and was positively correlated with personal achievements and SWB (all $p < 0.01$). The mindfulness facets of description and acting with awareness were significantly negatively associated with EE, DP, anxiety, and depression and were significantly positively correlated with personal achievements and SWB. Observation was significantly positively correlated with DP, personal achievement, and depression; nonjudgment was significantly negatively correlated with EE, DP, personal achievement, and depression; and nonreactivity was significantly positively correlated with DP and personal achievement.

As hypothesized, after controlling for the demographic variables of age and marital status, the entry of perceived stress

TABLE 1 | Hierarchical multiple regression analyses of perceived stress and mindfulness on burnout, depression, anxiety, and subjective well-being.

Steps and independent variables	Dependent variables											
	Emotional exhaustion			Depersonalization			Personal achievement			Depression		
	β	Total R^2	ΔR^2	β	Total R^2	ΔR^2	β	Total R^2	ΔR^2	β	Total R^2	ΔR^2
Step 1												
Age	0.05			–0.01			0.08			–0.03		
Marital status	–0.05	0.01	0.01	–0.10	0.01	0.01	0.03	0.01	0.01	0.07	0.01	0.01
Step 2												
Stress	0.42***	0.18	0.17***	0.28***	0.01	0.08***	–0.38***	0.14	0.14***	0.55***	0.31	0.30***
Step 3a												
Total FFMQ	–0.78***	0.64	0.46***	–0.41***	0.21	0.12***	0.02	0.14	0.00	–0.23***	0.34	0.04***
Step 4a												
Stress × Total FFMQ	–0.09**	0.65	0.01**	–0.01	0.21	0.00	–0.01	0.13	0.00	–0.13**	0.36	0.02**
Step 3b												
Observing	–0.04			0.04			–0.00			0.05		
Describing	–0.09			–0.02			0.14**			–0.04		
Awareness	–0.25***			–0.25***			0.09			–0.31***		
Nonjudging	–0.06			0.06			–0.11*			–0.02		
Nonreactivity	–0.08	0.23	0.05***	0.11*	0.17	0.09***	0. 07	0.19	0.05***	–0.07	0.38	0.08***
Step 4b												
Stress × Observing	0.08			0.09			–0.03			0.02		
Stress × Describing	–0.05			–0.03			–0.02			0.03		
Stress × Awareness	0.01			0.02			0.04			–0.14**		
Stress × Nonjudging	0.06			0.07			–0.03			–0.03		
Stress × Nonreactivity	–0.01	0.24	0.01	0.10	0.19	0.02	0.08	0.20	0.01	–0.06	0.40	0.02*

Steps and independent variables	Dependent variables											
	Life satisfaction			Positive affect			Negative affect			Anxiety		
	β	Total R^2	ΔR^2	β	Total R^2	ΔR^2	β	Total R^2	ΔR^2	β	Total R^2	ΔR^2
Step 1												
Age	0.02			0.06			0.07			0.09		
Marital status	–0.20***	0.05	0.05***	–0.01	0.00	0.00	0.03	0.00	0.00	–0.01	0.01	0.01
Step 2												
Stress	–0.43***	0.22	0.18***	–0.37***	0.14	0.13***	0.49***	0.24	0.23***	0.50***	0.26	0.25***
Step 3a												
Total FFMQ	0.13**	0.24	0.01**	0.16**	0.16	0.00**	–0.25***	0.28	0.05***	–0.65***	0.57	0.32***
Step 4a												
Stress × Total FFMQ	0.01	0.24	0.00	–0.11**	0.16	0.01**	–0.08*	0.29	0.01*	–0.10**	0.58	0.01**
Step 3b												
Observing	0.12*			0.19***			0.02			–0.01		
Describing	0.07			0.15**			–0.03			–0.08		
Awareness	0.02			0.03			–0.25***			–0.22***		
Nonjudging	–0.03			–0.01			–0.00			0.03		
Nonreactivity	0.09	0.27	0.05***	0.12*	0.24	0.10***	–0.04	0.28	0.05***	–0.07	0.30	0.04***
Step 4b												
Stress × Observing	0.02			–0.01			–0.08			0.03		
Stress × Describing	–0.02			–0.01			0.07			0.00		
Stress × Awareness	0.03			–0.07			–0.06			–0.01		
Stress × Nonjudging	–0.02			–0.04			–0.08			0.01		
Stress × Nonreactivity	0.05	0.27	0.00	–0.02	0.25	0.01	–0.06	0.28	0.01	–0.04	0.30	0.00

TABLE 2 | Descriptive statistics and psychometric properties of the major study variables (n = 500).

Main study variables	M	SD	Internal reliability α	Range
Total perceived stress (PSS)	40.33	6.10	0.762	19–61
Total mindfulness (FFMQ)	117.98	10.21	0.890	77–160
Observing (O)	21.72	4.68	0.727	8–37
Describing (D)	24.51	4.34	0.768	8–40
Acting with awareness (AWA)	28.42	4.83	0.828	8–40
Nonjudging (NJ)	24.44	4.57	0.780	9–39
Nonreactivity (NR)	18.96	3.19	0.605	10–30
Emotional exhaustion (MBI_EE)	20.87	9.89	0.853	0–53
Depersonalization (MBI_DP)	7.88	5.33	0.803	0–30
Personal achievement (MBI_PA)	26.96	8.46	0.819	3–48
Depressive symptoms (CES-D)	19. 90	6.49	0.945	9–46
Anxiety symptoms (SAS)	46.82	11.20	0.849	25–85
Life satisfaction (SWLS)	19.69	6.23	0.885	5–35
Positive affect (PA)	27.39	6.07	0.873	11–45
Negative affect (NA)	21.12	6.70	0.902	10–50

PSS, Perceived Stress Scale; FFMQ, Five Facet Mindfulness Questionnaire; CES-D, The Center for Epidemiological Studies Depression Scale; SAS, Self-Rating Anxiety Scale; MBI, Maslach Burnout Inventory–Human Service; SWB, PA + SWLS-NA.

in step 2 indicated that perceived stress was positively associated with all negative outcome variables, such as EE, DP, depressive and anxiety symptoms, and negative affect. Moreover, as expected, perceived stress was negatively associated with all positive outcome variables, such as personal achievements, life satisfaction, and positive affect. After the entry of total mindfulness in step 3a, the results revealed a unique variance in all outcomes, except personal achievement, after controlling for perceived stress, age, and marital status. The entry of the five mindfulness facets in step 3b showed a set of significant effects on all outcome variables after controlling for perceived stress, age, and marital status. Observation was positively correlated with life satisfaction and positive affect; description was positively associated with personal achievement and positive affect; awareness was significantly correlated with all negative outcome variables and none of the positive outcome variables; nonjudgment was negatively correlated with personal achievement, which contrasted with our expectation; and nonreactivity had a positive main effect on positive affect and on DP.

The entry of the interaction term stress × total mindfulness in step 4a resulted in significant results related to EE, depression, anxiety, positive affect, and negative affect. This indicated that mindfulness alleviated the effect of perceived stress on EE, depression, anxiety, positive affect, and negative affect. A simple slopes analysis showed that perceived stress predicted EE at both low ($B = 0.20$, $t = 1.51$, $p < 0.05$) and high levels of mindfulness ($B = 0.15$, $t = 0.57$, $p < 0.05$), but the association between perceived stress and EE was weaker when the mindfulness level was high (see **Figure 1A**). As shown in **Figure 1B** through E, similar results were observed for depression (low level of mindfulness: $B = 0.52$, $t = 3.12$, $p < 0.01$; high level of mindfulness: $B = 0.42$, $t = 5.60$, $p < 0.01$), anxiety (low level of mindfulness: $B = 0.36$, $t = 1.38$, $p < 0.01$; high level of mindfulness: $B = 0.29$, $t = 2.54$, $p < 0.01$), positive affect (low level of mindfulness: $B = -0.19$, $t = -1.45$, $p < 0.01$; high level of mindfulness: $B = -0.39$, $t = -3.89$, $p < 0.01$), and negative affect (low level of mindfulness: $B = 0.47$, $t = 4.67$, $p < 0.01$; high level of mindfulness: $B = 0.33$, $t = 2.32$, $p < 0.05$). While the overall mitigating effect of mindfulness on EE, depression, anxiety, and negative affect and the promoting effect of total mindfulness on positive emotion existed at both high and low levels of perceived stress, the effects were more significant when perceived stress levels were high.

After the entry of the five two-way interactions between perceived stress and mindfulness facets in step 4b, only one moderating effect was found. Acting with awareness moderated the relationship between perceived stress and depression. The simple slopes analysis indicated that ICU nurses with higher levels of acting with awareness had a weaker positive effect of perceived stress on depression ($B = 0.71$, $t = 4.97$, $p < 0.01$) than nurses with lower levels of acting with awareness ($B = 0.34$, $t = 5.40$, $p < 0.01$), and the mitigating effect of acting with awareness was pronounced when perceived stress levels were high (see **Figure 2**).

DISCUSSION

This study aimed to explore the potential moderating effect of mindfulness on the relationships among perceived stress and both positive and negative mental health indicators in Chinese intensive care nurses. This study found that the prevalence of psychological disorders such as burnout syndrome, anxiety, and depressive symptoms is common in Chinese ICU nurses, which is consistent with the previous studies (10, 18), and there was a higher prevalence of job-related burnout syndrome among ICU nurses than among general medical/surgical nurses (10). Although several studies have reported the effects of mindfulness on nurses (31, 60, 61), to our knowledge, no published studies have examined the moderating effect of mindfulness on stress-related mental health outcomes, especially burnout syndrome, in ICU nurses. After controlling for the effects of perceived stress and demographic variables of age and marital status, the present research confirmed that a higher level of mindfulness was associated with better psychological indicators in all outcome variables, except for personal achievement. These findings are in accordance with existing literature showing that higher levels of mindfulness may serve as a buffer for negative stress responses and consequently negative emotions such as burnout (28), depression (62, 63), and anxiety (62) and may also serve as a promoter for SWB (32, 64, 65).

The facet of observation could positively predict two positive indicators: life satisfaction and positive affect. Individuals who have a higher observation ability may be attuned to internal and external positive experiences and may be associated with the absence of ruminating thoughts during periods of high stress (35). Moreover, description was also significantly positively associated with two positive indicators, positive affect and personal achievement. Higher description ability may be important for effective communication and self-control (66), which may enable individuals to receive social support or facilitate successful task completion, thereby promoting positive affect and personal achievement. The facet of acting with awareness was significantly

TABLE 3 | Summary of bivariate correlations among the main study variables (n = 500).

Main study variables	1	2	3	4	5	6	7	8	9	10	11	12	13	14	15
1. Total stress	–														
2. Total mindfulness	−0.49**	–													
3. Observing	−0.04	0.17**	–												
4. Describing	−0.46**	0.52**	0.24**	–											
5. Acting with awareness	−0.45**	0.45**	−0.33**	0.29**	–										
6. Non-judging	−0.16**	0.12**	−0.49**	−0.17**	0.34**	–									
7. Non-reactivity	0.01	0.09*	0.45**	0.10*	−0.38**	−0.52**	–								
8. Emotional exhaustion	0.40**	−0.80**	−0.01	−0.29**	−0.35**	−0.10*	0.02	–							
9. Depersonalization	0.26**	−0.48**	0.13**	−0.16**	−0.36**	−0.13**	0.19**	0.61**	–						
10. Personal achievement	−0.37**	0.20**	0.01*	0.32**	0.20**	−0.09*	0.10*	−0.17**	−0.18**	–					
11. Depressive	0.55**	−0.44**	0.01*	−0.30**	−0.49**	−0.16**	0.08	0.45**	0.35**	−0.27**	–				
12. Anxiety	0.48**	−0.74**	−0.02	−0.32**	−0.36**	−0.05	−0.01	0.82**	0.54**	−0.24**	0.55**	–			
13. Subjective well-being	−0.56**	0.80**	0.09	0.41**	0.36**	0.02	0.07	−0.82**	−0.51**	0.29**	−0.53**	−0.82**	–		
14. Life satisfaction	−0.44**	0.30**	0.20**	0.30**	0.14**	−0.08	0.15**	−0.26**	−0.10*	0.27**	−0.33**	−0.28**	0.52**	–	
15. Positive affect	−0.37**	0.30**	0.29**	0.35**	0.09	−0.14**	0.22**	−0.24**	−0.13**	0.39**	−0.20**	−0.25**	0.44**	0.36**	–
16. Negative affect	0.47**	−0.43**	0.06	−0.26**	−0.41**	−0.13**	0.07	0.43**	0.42**	−0.20**	0.54**	0.54**	−0.56**	−0.19**	0.05

*$p < 0.05$; **$p < 0.01$.

inversely correlated with all the negative indicators, including EE, DP, depression, anxiety, and negative affect. Several studies provide support for this prediction. Awareness is associated with a set of psychological benefits, such as reduced anxiety and depressive symptoms (24) and reduced EE (67). Using a single-item measure adapted from the facet of the acting with awareness subscale of the FFMQ (68), Donald et al. found that higher levels of awareness predicted greater perceived self-efficacy in dealing with stressful daily events, as increased awareness widens the range of available response options. Moreover, awareness exists independently of an individual's level of perceived threat associated with the stressor and the degree of general negative affect the person experiences on a given day, thus facilitating more effective coping with daily stressors (68). Awareness was also proposed to improve an individual's executive control (69), therefore mitigating the effect of perceived stress on mental health. Interestingly, in contrast to our predictions, non-judgment was negatively associated with personal achievement. Moreover, although non-reactivity to inner experience was positively correlated with positive affect, it was also positively correlated with DP. Only two studies were found to directly examine the interaction effects of facets of mindfulness and dimensions of burnout. Using a sample of 381 employees, Taylor et al. (70) found that all five facets of mindfulness were significantly and inversely correlated with the three components of burnout tested by the Maslach Burnout Inventory–General Survey (MBI-GS), with the exception of observation and EE. In a longitudinal cohort study of 27 clinicians who were offered a Mindfulness-Based Stress Reduction (MBSR) course, Dobkin et al. (71) found that the decrease in EE was correlated with acting with awareness and less-judgmental attitudes. Based on these results, we could posit that nonreactivity to inner experience refers to allowing thoughts and feelings to come and go without fixating on them, which may tend to detach ICU nurses' responses to workplace stressors. Nonjudgment of inner experience refers to the ability to take a nonevaluative stance toward thoughts, which may reduce the motivation to pursue personal achievement. In their most recent research, Hafenbrack and Vohs (72) found that participants in the mindfulness group reported less motivation than did the participants in the comparison group. Another possible explanation for these findings is that different individuals interpret the meaning of the items in different ways, which might be due to different cultural values. As Maslach et al. (73) noted, the concept and measures of MBI had been established based on the culture in the United States. In China, sentiments of group solidarity play a more significant role, whereas individualism plays a major role in the North American society. Therefore, public expression of some dimensions of burnout syndrome, notably cynicism or DP, may be more widely acceptable in the United States than in China. As Rudkin et al. (74) found in their most recent reliable and valid research, the absence of certain items in the FFMQ may explain the novel function of some facets of FFMQ. The author then noted that their findings have implications for the development of multidimensional measures for mindfulness assessment. It has also been proposed that a bifactor structure might provide a better assessment than the existing five facets (75). Nevertheless,

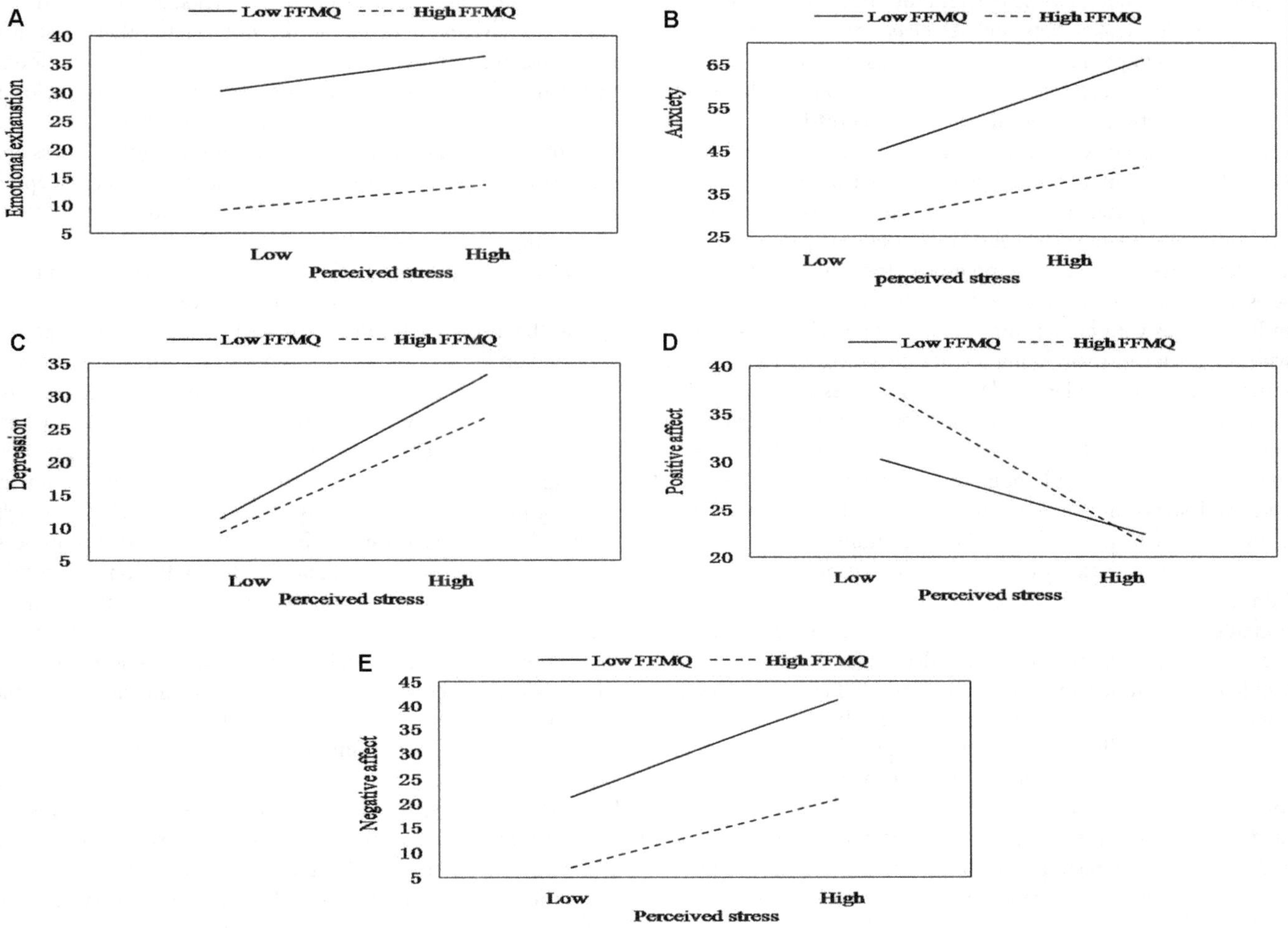

FIGURE 1 | The moderating effect of mindfulness on the relation between stress and emotional exhaustion **(A)**, depression **(B)**, anxiety **(C)**, positive affect **(D)**, and negative affect **(E)**.

these novel findings may be interpreted to mean a number of things that are potentially important for the future research and understanding of mindfulness–burnout relations.

According to the results, the total level of mindfulness moderated the relationships among perceived stress and EE, depression, anxiety, positive affect, and negative affect. Feelings of EE are generally viewed as having the strongest correlation with the burnout variable (76); thus, EE is considered a core symptom of the burnout syndrome (77). The regression model results indicated that for ICU nurses with higher levels of mindfulness, the positive relationship between perceived stress and EE was weakened. However, for those with lower mindfulness levels, the relationship between perceived stress and EE was augmented. Therefore, we conclude that mindfulness may serve as a minimizer between perceived stress and EE. This finding is in accordance with a study conducted in Italy, which also suggested that dispositional mindfulness is important for protecting against the onset of burnout in healthcare professionals (78). Mindfulness might facilitate better self-regulation of emotional and cognitive activities and reduce reactions to potentially emotional and stressful stimuli (79). These improvements in appraising and reacting to potentially stressful events in ICU working environments help ICU nurses avoid EE (67).

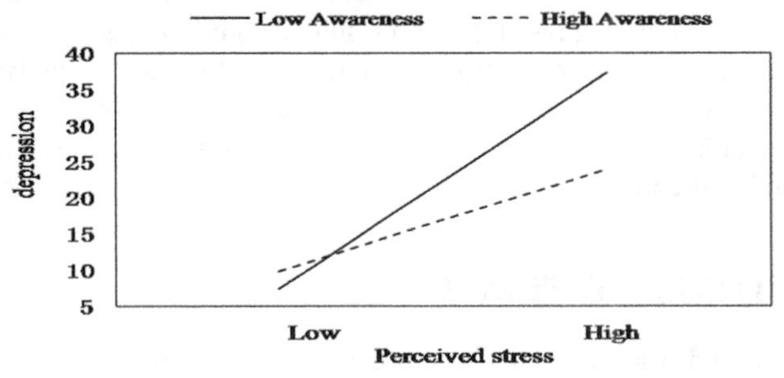

FIGURE 2 | The moderating effect of acting with awareness on the relation between stress and depression.

Moreover, higher mindfulness levels are significantly correlated with lower perceived stress and lower rates of depression and anxiety. For ICU nurses with higher mindfulness levels, the positive relationship is weaker between perceived stress and depressive and anxiety symptoms. Within individuals with lower levels of mindfulness, this relationship is exactly the opposite. That is, the relationship between perceived stress and depressive and anxiety symptoms is weaker when levels of mindfulness are higher and vice versa. Therefore, mindfulness can be used as a buffer to reduce the tendency to experience more anxiety and depressive symptoms. Mindfulness moderated the relationship between perceived stress and depressive and anxiety symptoms in the sense that perceived stress was associated with fewer depressive and anxiety symptoms in ICU nurses with higher mindfulness scores. This is consistent with the results of many other studies including a large range of samples. In a group of law students, previous research found that total levels of mindfulness buffer the effects of perceived stress on depression and anxiety (35). A Swedish study tested the buffering role of mindfulness and found that the relationship between perceived stress and depression was attenuated for those with a higher level of mindfulness (34). Mindfulness has also been shown to improve anxiety and depression in cancer patients (80). Mindfulness, which focuses on being in the very present with a nonjudgmental and nonreactive mindset, may thereby alleviate the suffering that often accompanies depression and anxiety. This highlights the importance of taking a mindful approach toward internal cues to decrease depressive and anxiety symptoms.

Although mindfulness did not moderate the negative effects of stress on overall SWB or the component of life satisfaction, the results showed that mindfulness moderated the relationships of stress with positive affect and negative affect. These findings are particularly interesting, and somewhat ironic, as mindfulness is nonjudgmental, nonpreferential (neither toward or away from positive affect or negative affect), and nondisputational (81) but may, nevertheless, paradoxically strengthen the experience of positive affect or negative affect. An alternative explanation for our research result might be that the development of dispositional mindfulness may act as a buffer against stressors that result in reduced levels of positive affect across time and contexts (82). A very recent study also verified that mindfulness predicts greater improvements in positive affect and greater reductions in negative affect (83). ICU nurses who are naturally more mindful may have a decentered perspective of the mind or self and experience greater improvements in positive affect. Moreover, ICU nurses with higher, not lower, levels of mindfulness would be mindfully aware of and accept their internal experience, which may result in more benefits in light of negative affect reductions.

Further analyses focusing on particular mindfulness skills indicated that acting with awareness moderated the relationship between perceived stress and depression. This is the only facet of mindfulness buffering effect that emerged. This finding is consistent with the results of several other studies. By studying a sample of 520 Spanish adolescents and a subsample of 461 adolescents, Royuela-Colomer and Calvete (63) found that acting with awareness correlated negatively with depressive symptoms and predicted a reduction in depression over time. Pereira et al. (84) reported that acting with awareness had a protective effect against antenatal depressive symptoms in 427 pregnant women. In an exploratory factor analysis, Rudkin et al. (74) found that all meditator and nonmeditator participants identified the emotional awareness factor as the only factor that correlated with psychological symptoms. Caluyong et al. (85) also found that acting with awareness was a significant predictor of lower depression scores. This may be because the acting with awareness facet of mindfulness enables the detection of signs of stress and increases the ability of self-regulation and facilitates adaptive reactivity to negative and distressing situations. Thus, those with a higher ability to act with awareness have more potential to increase the awareness of low-level stress-related symptoms, which may potentiate access to coping resources and buffer against the negative effects of stress, such as depressive symptoms.

Based on these findings, interventions designed to encourage adaptive stress management, improve mindfulness levels, and provide the necessary skills to deal with stressful situations are likely to reduce or eliminate burnout syndromes and depressive and anxiety symptoms and improve the well-being of nurses working in the ICU. The results of the present study may help explain the relationships among perceived stress and mindfulness, burnout, anxiety, depression, and SWB. In addition, our results verified that mindfulness was a protective factor for alleviating or eliminating the negative effects of perceived stress on burnout, depression, anxiety, and SWB. In addition to its strengths, this study also has several limitations. First, we acknowledge that the data are based on ICU nurses' self-reports. Current self-reported measurements of mindfulness may not accurately capture the constructs of the variables. A semistructured interview or longitudinal study may produce different results from those of the self-reported questionnaire used in our study. Second, as a cross-sectional study, this study failed to draw conclusions about the cause and effect relationships among the variables. For instance, whereas it seems that ICU nurses perceive less stress when they are more mindful, it might be possible that exposure to daily stressors results in decreased levels of mindfulness. Further longitudinal studies must be conducted.

CONCLUSION

The high prevalence of prolonged stress, burnout syndromes, and depressive and anxiety symptoms in Chinese ICU nurses deserves immediate attention. The findings of the present study show that mindfulness is associated with lower levels of stress and fewer mental health complaints among Chinese ICU nurses. This study also indicates that mindfulness has the potential to act as a stress-coping resource. As a result, our findings suggest that mindfulness may be a target variable for health interventionists working with ICU nurses. Given the popularity of mindfulness, it might be a useful component of preventive health interventions and may allow for more targeted interventions.

ETHICS STATEMENT

This study was carried out in accordance with the recommendations of the Ethics Committee of Army Medical University with written informed consent from all subjects. All subjects gave written informed consent in accordance with the Declaration of Helsinki.

The protocol was approved by the Ethics Committee of Army Medical University.

AUTHOR CONTRIBUTIONS

FL, YX, and ML designed the research. FL, TWa, JX, BL, and SX recruited the participants and conducted the assessments. FL, YY, and TWu analyzed the data. FL wrote the manuscript, and YX and YY assisted with the statistical interpretations. YX, YY, LP, and TWa critically reviewed the manuscript. All of the authors contributed to the revision of the initial manuscript and approved the submission.

ACKNOWLEDGMENTS

We would like to thank all the participants for their cooperation. We would especially like to thank the following people for their assistance with communication, scheduling, and facilitating the survey: Cai-zhong Zhu, Ting Chen, Wen-jing Ling, Fei Xie, Shuang Zheng, Yan Dong, Tian-tian Yang, Yuan Yuan, Xia Xu, Ping Pu, Qing-ling Zhang, Chang-Qing Sun, Jie Deng, Bei-jing Chen, Wen-qun Yang, Ze-ping Liang, Ji-shu Xian, Ning Li, Chun-mei Luo, Bin-bin Tan, and Ling-na Kong.

REFERENCES

Tummers GER, Van Merode GG, Landeweerd JA. The diversity of work: differences, similarities and relationships concerning characteristics of the organisation, the work and psychological work reactions in intensive care and non-intensive care nursing. *Int J Nurs Stud* (2002) 39(8):841. doi: 10.1016/S0020-7489(02)00020-2

Bakker AB, Le Blanc PM, Schaufeli WB. Burnout contagion among intensive care nurses. *J Adv Nurs* (2005) 51(3):276–87. doi: 10.1111/j.1365-2648.2005. 03494.x

Mallett K, Price JH, Jurs SG, Slenker S. Relationships among burnout, death anxiety, and social support in hospice and critical care nurses. *Psychol Rep* (1991) 68(3 Pt 2):1347–59. doi: 10.2466/pr0.1991.68.3c.1347

Xiong P, Hu SX, Hall BJ. Violence against nurses in China undermines task-shifting implementation. *Lancet Psychiatry* (2016) 3(6):501. doi: 10.1016/ S2215-0366(16)30046-3

Hammen C. Stress sensitivity in psychopathology: mechanisms and consequences. *J Abnorm Psychol* (2015) 124(1):152–4. doi: 10.1037/abn0000040

Rask-Andersen A, Tarlo SM. Is there an epidemic of burnout and post- traumatic stress in critical care clinicians. *Am J Respir Crit Care Med* (2007) 175(7):633–4. doi: 10.1164/rccm.200701-061ED

Bakker AB, Demerouti E. The job demands-resources model: state of the art. *Manage Psychol* (2007) 22(3):309–28. doi: 10.1108/02683940710733115

Guthrie R, Ciccarelli M, Babic A. Work-related stress in Australia: the effects of legislative interventions and the cost of treatment. *Int J Law Psychiatry* (2010) 33(2):101. doi: 10.1016/j.ijlp.2009.12.003

Embriaco N, Papazian L, Kentishbarnes N, Pochard F, Azoulay E. Burnout syndrome among critical care healthcare workers. *Curr Opin Crit Care* (2007) 13(5):482–8. doi: 10.1097/MCC.0b013e3282efd28a

Mealer M, Burnham EL, Goode CJ, Rothbaum B, Moss M. The prevalence and impact of posttraumatic stress disorder and burnout syndrome in nurses. *Depress Anxiety* (2009) 26(12):1118–26. doi: 10.1002/da.20631

Poncet MC, Toullic P, Papazian L, Kentish-Barnes N, Timsit JF, Pochard F, et al. Burnout syndrome in critical care nursing staff. *Am J Respir Crit Care Med* (2007) 175(7):698–704. doi: 10.1164/rccm.200606-806OC J

Cohen-Katz J, Wiley SD, Capuano T, Baker DM, Kimmel S, Shapiro S. The effects of mindfulness-based stress reduction on nurse stress and burnout, Part II: a quantitative and qualitative study. *Holist Nurs Pract* (2005) 19(1):26–35. doi: 10.1097/00004650-200501000-00008

Rodriguez-Rey R, Palacios A, Alonso-Tapia J, Perez E, Alvarez E, Coca A, et al. Burnout and posttraumatic stress in paediatric critical care personnel: prediction from resilience and coping styles. *Aust Crit Care* (2019) 32(1):46– 53. doi: 10.1016/j.aucc.2018.02.003

Torre M, Santos Popper MC, Bergesio A. Burnout prevalence in intensive care nurses in Argentina. *Enferm Intensiva* (2018). doi: 10.1016/j.enfi.2018.04.005

D-YL, WJ. Correlation among personality, coping style and job burnout of nurses in emergency department and ICU in Xinjiang. *J Nurs (China)* (2011) 18(9A):4–7. doi: 10.16460/j.issn 1008-9969.2011.17.005.

Shanafelt TD, Bradley KA, Wipf JE, Back AL. Burnout and self-reported patient care in an internal medicine residency program. *Ann Intern Med* (2002) 136(5):358–67. doi: 10.7326/0003-4819-136-5-200203050-00008

Kelley MA, Angus D, Chalfin DB, Crandall ED, Ingbar D, Johanson W, et al. The critical care crisis in the United States: a report from the profession. *Chest* (2004) 125(4):1514. doi: 10.1378/chest.125.4.1514

Mealer M, Jones J, Newman J, McFann KK, Rothbaum B, Moss M. The presence of resilience is associated with a healthier psychological profile in intensive care unit (ICU) nurses: results of a national survey. *Int J Nurs Stud* (2012) 49(3):292–9. doi: 10.1016/j.ijnurstu.2011.09.015

Regan A, Howard RA, Oyebode JR. Emotional exhaustion and defense mechanisms in intensive therapy unit nurses. *J Nerv Ment Dis* (2009) 197(5):330. doi: 10.1097/NMD.0b013e3181a20807

Grant KE, Compas BE, Thurm AE, McMahon SD, Gipson PY, Campbell AJ, et al. Stressors and child and adolescent psychopathology: evidence of moderating and mediating effects. *Clin Psychol Rev* (2006) 26(3):257–83. doi: 10.1016/j.cpr.2005.06.011

Gao YQ, Pan BC, Sun W, Wu H, Wang JN, Wang L. Depressive symptoms among Chinese nurses: prevalence and the associated factors. *J Adv Nurs* (2012) 68(5):1166–75. doi: 10.1111/j.1365-2648.2011.05832.x

Gatchel RJ, Kishino ND. Conceptual approaches to occupational health and wellness: an overview. In: *Handbook of occupational health and wellness*. New York: Springer (2012). doi: 10.1007/978-1-4614-4839-6_1

Folkman S, Lazarus RS, Dunkel-Schetter C, DeLongis A, Gruen RJ. Dynamics of a stressful encounter: cognitive appraisal, coping, and encounter outcomes. *J Pers Soc Psychol* (1986) 50(5):992–1003. doi: 10.1037/0022-3514.50.5.992

Brown KW, Ryan RM, Creswell JD. Mindfulness: theoretical foundations and evidence for its salutary effects. *Psychol Inq* (2007) 18(4):211–37. doi: 10.1080/10478400701598298

Bao X, Xue S, Kong F. Dispositional mindfulness and perceived stress: the role of emotional intelligence. *Pers Individ Dif* (2015) 78:48–52. doi: 10.1016/j.paid.2015.01.007

Weinstein N, Brown KW, Ryan RM. A multi-method examination of the effects of mindfulness on stress attribution, coping, and emotional well- being. *J Res Pers* (2009) 43(3):374–85. doi: 10.1016/j.jrp.2008.12.008

Heard PL, Hartman S, Bushardt SC. Rekindling the flame: using mindfulness to end nursing burnout. *Nurs Manage* (2013) 44(11):24–9. doi: 10.1097/01.NUMA.0000436366.99397.10

Cohen-Katz J, Wiley S, Capuano T, Baker DM, Deitrick L, Shapiro S. The effects of mindfulness-based stress reduction on nurse stress and burnout: a qualitative and quantitative study, part III. *Holist Nurs Pract* (2005) 19(2):78– 86. doi: 10.1097/00004650-200503000-00009

Cohen-Katz J, Wiley SD, Capuano T, Baker DM, Shapiro S. The effects of mindfulness-based stress reduction on nurse stress and burnout: a quantitative and qualitative study. *Holist Nurs Pract* (2004) 18(6):302–8. doi: 10.1097/00004650-200411000-00006

Chen Y, Yang X, Wang L, Zhang X. A randomized controlled trial of the effects of brief mindfulness meditation on anxiety symptoms and systolic blood pressure in Chinese nursing students. *Nurse Educ Today* (2013) 33(10):1166–72. doi: 10.1016/j.nedt.2012.11.014

Mackenzie CS, Poulin PA, Seidman-Carlson R. A brief mindfulness-based stress reduction intervention for nurses and nurse aides. *Appl Nurs Res* (2006) 19(2):105–9. doi: 10.1016/j.apnr.2005.08.002

Baer RA, Smith GT, Lykins E, Button D, Krietemeyer J, Sauer S, et al. Construct validity of the five facet mindfulness questionnaire in meditating and nonmeditating samples. *Assessment* (2008) 15(3):329–42. doi: 10.1177/1073191107313003

Salmon P, Sephton S, Weissbecker I, Hoover K, Ulmer C, Studts JL. Mindfulness meditation in clinical practice. *Cogn Behav Pract* (2004) 11(4):434–46. doi: 10.1016/S1077-7229(04)80060-9

Bränström R, Duncan LG, Moskowitz JT. The association between dispositional mindfulness, psychological well-being, and perceived health in a Swedish population-based sample. *Br J Health Psychol* (2011) 16(Pt 2):300– 16. doi: 10.1348/135910710X501683

Bergin AJ, Pakenham KI. The stress-buffering role of mindfulness in the relationship between perceived stress and psychological adjustment. *Mindfulness* (2016) 7(4):928–39. doi: 10.1007/s12671-016-0532-x

Ciesla JA, Reilly LC, Dickson KS, Emanuel AS, Updegraff JA. Dispositional mindfulness moderates the effects of stress among adolescents: rumination as a mediator. *J Clin Child Adolesc Psychol* (2012) 41(6):760–70. doi: 10.1080/15374416.2012.698724

Bodenlos JS, Wells SY, Noonan M, Mayrsohn A. Facets of dispositional mindfulness and health among college students. *J Altern Complement Med* (2015) 21(10):645–52. doi: 10.1089/acm.2014.0302

Zhong M, Goh PH, Li D, Bao J, Xu W. Dispositional mindfulness as a moderator between perceived stress and psychological symptoms in Chinese digestive tract cancer patients. *J Health Psychol* (2017) 10:1–9. doi: 10.1177/1359105317736576

Baer RA, Smith GT, Hopkins J, Krietemeyer J, Toney L. Using self-report assessment methods to explore facets of mindfulness. *Assessment* (2006) 13(1):27–45. doi: 10.1177/1073191105283504

Maslach C, Jackson SE. The measurement of experienced burnout. *J Organ Behav* (1981) 2(2):99–113. doi: 10.1002/job.4030020205

YE ZH, L. H, AL J. Diagnostic standard and norms of maslach burnout inventory for nurses in hangzhou. *Chin J Nurs* (2008) 43(3):207–9.

Deng Y-Q, Liu X-H, Rodriguez MA, Xia C-Y. The five facet mindfulness questionnaire: psychometric properties of the chinese version. *Mindfulness* (2011) 2(2):123–8. doi: 10.1007/s12671-011-0050-9

Rankin SH, Galbraith ME, Johnson S. Reliability and validity data for a chinese translation of the center for epidemiological studies-depression. *Psychol Rep* (1993) 73(3 Pt 2):1291. doi: 10.2466/pr0.1993.73.3f.1291

Li HC, Chung OK, Ho KY. Center for epidemiologic studies depression scale for children: psychometric testing of the chinese version. *J Adv Nurs* (2010) 66(11):2582–91. doi: 10.1111/j.1365-2648.2010.05440.x

Kohout FJ, Berkman LF, Evans DA, Cornonihuntley J. Two shorter forms of the CES-D (Center for Epidemiological Studies Depression) depression symptoms index. *JAging Health* (1993) 5(2):179–93. doi: 10.1177/0898264393 00500202

Blumenthal JA, Lett HS, Babyak MA, White W, Smith PK, Mark DB, et al. Depression as a risk factor for mortality after coronary artery bypass surgery. *Lancet* (2003) 362(9384):604. doi: 10.1016/S0140-6736(03)14190-6

Schrader G, Cheok F, Hordacre AL, Marker J, Wade V. Effect of psychiatry liaison with general practitioners on depression severity in recently hospitalised cardiac patients: a randomised controlled trial. *Med J Aust* (2005) 182(6). doi: 10.5694/j.1326-5377.2005tb06699.x.

Zung WW. A rating instrument for anxiety disorders. *Psychosomatics* (1971) 12(6):371–9. doi: 10.1016/S0033-3182(71)71479-0

Wu WY. A self-rating anxiety scale. *Chin Ment Health J* (1999) 13:235–8.

Zhang MY. *Psychiatric rating scale assessment manual [M].The second version.* Changsha: Hunan Science and Technical Publishing House (2003) p. 25–43.

Cohen S, Kamarck T, Mermelstein R. A global measure of perceived stress. *J Health Soc Behav* (1983) 24(4):385–96. doi: 10.2307/2136404

Yang TZ, Huang HT. An epidemiological study on stress among urban residents in social transition period. *Zhonghua Liu Xing Bing Xue Za Zhi* (2003) 24(9):760–4.

Leung DY, Lam TH, Chan SS. Three versions of Perceived Stress Scale: validation in a sample of Chinese cardiac patients who smoke. *BMC Public Health* (2010) 10:513. doi: 10.1186/1471-2458-10-513

Diener E. Subjective well-being. *Psychol Bull* (1984) 95(3):542–75. doi: 10.1037/0033-2909.95.3.542

Lyubomirsky S, King L, Diener E. The benefits of frequent positive affect: does happiness lead to success? *Psychol Bull* (2005) 131(6):803–55. doi: 10.1037/0033-2909.131.6.803

Lin Q, XZ, Yanfei W. Revision of the positive affect and negative affect scale. *Chin J Applied Psychology* (2008) 14(3):249–54.

Xiong C, XY. Reliability and validity of the satisfaction with life scale for Chinese demos. *China J Health Psychol* (2009) 17(8):948–9.

Kraemer HC, Blasey CM. Centring in regression analyses: a strategy to prevent errors in statistical inference. *Int J Methods Psychiatr Res* (2004) 13(3):141–51. doi: 10.1002/mpr.170

Jaccard J, Turrisi R, Wan CK. *Interaction eff cts in multiple regression* Vol. 40. Newbury Park California: Sage Publications (2003). p. 461. doi: 10.4135/9781412984522

Duarte J, Pinto-Gouveia J. Effectiveness of a mindfulness-based intervention on oncology nurses' burnout and compassion fatigue symptoms: a non- randomized study. *Int J Nurs Stud* (2016) 64:98–107. doi: 10.1016/j. ijnurstu.2016.10.002

Wang SC, Wang LY, Shih SM, Chang SC, Fan SY, Hu WY. The effects of mindfulness-based stress reduction on hospital nursing staff. *Appl Nurs Res* (2017) 38:124–8. doi: 10.1016/j.apnr.2017.09.014

Kantrowitz-Gordon I. Factor structure and external validity of the five facet mindfulness questionnaire in pregnancy. *Mindfulness* (2017) 9(1):243–57. doi: 10.1007/s12671-017-0768-0

Royuela-Colomer E, Calvete E. Mindfulness facets and depression in adolescents: rumination as a mediator. *Mindfulness* (2016) 7(5):1092–102. doi: 10.1007/s12671-016-0547-3

Brown KW, Kasser T, Ryan RM, Linley PA, Orzech K. When what one has is enough: mindfulness, financial desire discrepancy, and subjective well- being. *J Res Pers* (2009) 43(5):727–36. doi: 10.1016/j.jrp.2009.07.002

Falkenström F. Studying mindfulness in experienced meditators: a quasi-experimental approach. *Pers Individ Dif* (2010) 48(3):305–10. doi: 10.1016/j.paid.2009.10.022

Linehan MM. *Skills training manual for treating borderline personality disorder.* New York: Guilford Press (1993).

Hulsheger UR, Alberts HJ, Feinholdt A, Lang JW. Benefits of mindfulness at work: the role of mindfulness in emotion regulation, emotional exhaustion, and job satisfaction. *J Appl Psychol* (2013) 98(2):310–25. doi: 10.1037/ a0031313

Donald JN, Atkins PWB, Parker PD, Christie AM, Ryan RM. Daily stress and the benefits of mindfulness: examining the daily and longitudinal relations between present-moment awareness and stress responses. *J Res Pers* (2016) 65:30–7. doi: 10.1016/j.jrp.2016.09.002

Teper R, Segal ZV, Inzlicht M. Inside the mindful mind: how mindfulness enhances emotion regulation through improvements in executive control. *Curr Dir Psychol Sci* (2013) 22(6):449–54. doi: 10.1177/ 0963721413495869

Taylor NZ, Millear PMR. The contribution of mindfulness to predicting burnout in the workplace. *Pers Individ Dif* (2016) 89:123–8. doi: 10.1016/j. paid.2015.10.005

Dobkin PL, Bernardi NF, Bagnis CI. Enhancing clinicians' well-being and patient-centered care through mindfulness. *J Contin Educ Health Prof* (2016) 36(1):11–6. doi: 10.1097/CEH.0000000000000021

Hafenbrack AC, Vohs KD. Mindfulness meditation impairs task motivation but not performance. *Organ Behav Hum Decis Process* (2018) 147:1–15. doi: 10.1016/j.obhdp.2018.05.001

Maslach C, Schaufeli WB, Leiter MP. Job burnout. *Annu Rev Psychol* (2001) 52(1):397–422. doi: 10.1146/annurev.psych.52.1.397

Rudkin E, Medvedev ON, Siegert RJ. The five-facet mindfulness questionnaire: why the observing subscale does not predict psychological symptoms. *Mindfulness* (2017) 9(1):230–42. doi: 10.1007/ s12671-017-0766-2

Aguado J, Luciano JV, Cebolla A, Serrano-Blanco A, Soler J, Garcia-Campayo J. Corrigendum: bifactor analysis and construct validity of the Five Facet Mindfulness Questionnaire (FFMQ) in non-clinical Spanish samples. *Front Psychol* (2016) 7:706. doi: 10.3389/fpsyg.2016.00706

Maslach C, Leiter MP. *The truth about burnout.* California: Jossey-Bass Publishers (1997).

Shirom A, Ezrachi Y. On the discriminant validity of burnout, depression and anxiety: a re-examination of the burnout measure. *Anxiety Stress Coping* (2003) 16(1):83–97. doi: 10.1080/1061580021000057059

Alberto Voci, CAVMM. Affective organizational commitment and dispositionalmindfulnessascorrelatesofburnoutinhealthcareprofessionals. *J Workplace Behav health* (2016) 31(2):63–70. doi: 10.1080/15555240.2015.1047500

Arch JJ, Craske MG. Laboratory stressors in clinically anxious and non- anxious individuals: the moderating role of mindfulness. *Behav Res Ther* (2010) 48(6):495–505. doi: 10.1016/j.brat.2010.02.005

Reich RR, Lengacher CA, Alinat CB, Kip KE, Paterson C, Ramesar S, et al. Mindfulness-based stress reduction in post-treatment breast cancer patients: immediate and sustained effects across multiple symptom clusters. *J Pain Symptom Manage* (2016) 53(1):85–95. doi: 10.1016/j.jpainsymman.2016.08. 005

Kabat-Zinn J. Mindfulness-based interventions in context: past, present, and future. *Clin Psychol Sci Pract* (2003) 10(2):144–56. doi: 10.1093/clipsy.bpg016

Jislin-Goldberg T, Tanay G, Bernstein A. Mindfulness and positive affect: cross-sectional, prospective intervention, and real-time relations. *J Posit Psychol* (2012) 7(5):349–61. doi: 10.1080/17439760.2012.700724

Gawrysiak MJ, Grassetti SN, Greeson JM, Shorey RC, Pohlig R, Baime MJ. The many facets of mindfulness and the prediction of change following mindfulness-based stress reduction (MBSR). *J Clin Psychol* (2018) 74(4):523–35. doi: 10.1002/jclp.22521

Pereira AT, Xavier S, Bento E, Azevedo J, Marques M, Soares MJ, et al. Mindfulness, self-compassion and depressive symptoms in pregnant women. *Eur Psychiatry* (2016) 33:S420. doi: 10.1016/j.eurpsy.2016.01.1517

Caluyong MB, Zambrana AF, Romanow HC, Nathan HJ, Nahas R, Poulin PA. The relationship between mindfulness, depression, diabetes self-care, and health-related quality of life in patients with type 2 diabetes. *Mindfulness* (2015) 6(6):1313–21. doi: 10.1007/s12671-015-0401-z

11

Acute High-Intensity Interval Exercise Improves Inhibitory Control among Young Adult Males with Obesity

Chun Xie[1], Brandon L. Alderman[2], Fanying Meng[3], Jingyi Ai[4], Yu-Kai Chang[4,5] and Anmin Li[1]**

[1] School of Psychology, Shanghai University of Sport, Shanghai, China, [2] Department of Kinesiology and Health, Center of Alcohol and Substance Use Studies, Rutgers, The State University of New Jersey, New Brunswick, NJ, United States, [3] Institute of Physical Education, Huzhou University, Huzhou, China, [4] Department of Physical Education, National Taiwan Normal University, Taipei, Taiwan, [5] Institute for Research Excellence in Learning Science, National Taiwan Normal University, Taipei, Taiwan

***Correspondence:**
Yu-Kai Chang
yukaichangnew@gmail.com
Anmin Li
anminli@sus.edu.cn

Objective: The aim of the present study was to examine the influence of acute high-intensity interval exercise (HIIE) on neural and behavioral measures of inhibitory control in young male adults with obesity.

Design: The present study employed a within-subjects design.

Methods: Sixteen male adults with obesity [body mass index (BMI) > 28 kg/m^2] were recruited. Reaction time and response accuracy of the Flanker task as well as P3 and late positive potential (LPP) components of the event-related potential (ERP) were measured following HIIE and a sedentary control, in counterbalanced order. The HIIE session consisted of 30 min of stationary cycle exercise (5-min warm-up, 20-min HIIE, and a 5-min cool-down), whereas the control condition consisted of a time and attention-matched sedentary resting session.

Results: Faster response times were observed following HIIE regardless of Flanker task condition. Faster and more accurate responses were also observed for congruent relative to incongruent conditions across both sessions. Relative to the neuroelectric data, acute HIIE resulted in increased LPP amplitude but did not affect P3 amplitude.

Conclusion: Collectively, a single bout of HIIE has a general beneficial effect on basic information processing and inhibitory control among young adult males with obesity. Acute HIIE was found to impact LPP amplitude, but not the P3, which may suggest a modulation in the ability to successfully maintain attention and filter irrelevant information to achieve successful cognitive inhibition. Future research is warranted to extend these findings to a larger sample size that includes both genders, other cognitive functions, and a comparison of different modes of exercise.

Keywords: HIIE, executive function, inhibitory control, obesity, P3, LPP

INTRODUCTION

Obesity is a global public health concern that is associated with an increased risk of adverse health conditions including cardiovascular disease and diabetes (Ng et al., 2014) as well as impaired cognition, including executive function, attention, decision making, and memory (Smith et al., 2011; Prickett et al., 2015; Yang et al., 2018). Obesity has also been associated with impairments in inhibitory control. Inhibitory control, a core domain of the executive function, reflects as the ability to suppress inappropriate actions or override the processing of task-irrelevant or distracting information (Bari and Robbins, 2013). Inhibitory control is supported and regulated by multiple bidirectional neural connections, and has been shown to play a crucial role in the ability to inhibit excessive eating behaviors to maintain a healthy weight (Hwang et al., 2010). For instance, individuals with obesity performed worse (slower and less accurately) across several inhibitory control tasks (e.g., Flanker and Stroop inhibitory control tasks), suggesting an impaired ability to override interference information among individuals with obesity relative to their normal-weight counterparts (Kamijo et al., 2012; Gameiro et al., 2017). A recent meta-analysis also reported a moderate inverse effect size for inhibitory control deficits among overweight and obese individuals (Yang et al., 2018). Atrophy of prefrontal cortical regions implicated in cognitive control has been found in individuals with obesity, providing evidence of obesity-impaired cognitive inhibition through both structural and functional brain imaging data (García-García et al., 2015).

Robust and consistent evidence has shown that acute exercise that represents a single bout of exercise elicits beneficial effects on cognitive function (Etnier et al., 1997; Ferris et al., 2007; Chang et al., 2012b; Etnier and Chang, 2019; Wilke et al., 2019) and the beneficial effects from acute exercise have also extended to inhibitory cognitive control (Themanson and Hillman, 2006; Drollette et al., 2014; Chu et al., 2015; Hsieh et al., 2018). However, studies that have investigated acute exercise and inhibitory control have almost exclusively relied on traditional aerobic or resistance modes of exercise (Harveson et al., 2016; Hsieh et al., 2016; Ludyga et al., 2017) and the acute effect of other modes of exercise, particularly those that are engaged in by an increasing number of adults, require consideration to advance our knowledge regarding both efficacy and mechanisms of action (Chang et al., 2019).

High-Intensity Interval Training (HIIT) is a popular and emerging exercise mode that has been shown to elicit beneficial health effects in an efficient manner compared to more long-duration continuous exercise. HIIT generally involves repeated bouts of short to moderate duration high-intensity interval exercise (HIIE) with a larger than anaerobic threshold intensity and interspersed with recovery periods or light exercise (Laursen and Jenkins, 2002; Weston et al., 2014). The HIIE has been linked to improved physical fitness including cardiorespiratory fitness (O'Donovan et al., 2005), skeletal muscle metabolism (Rognmo et al., 2004), and body composition in adults with obesity (Wewege et al., 2017). HIIE has also been shown to positively impact cognitive function. For example, adults exhibited faster overall reaction times and improved accuracy in the Flanker task following 9 min of HIIE compared to a control condition (Kao et al., 2017) and adult males have demonstrated an improvement in inhibitory control (i.e., Stroop test performance) during the post-exercise recovery period after a 28 min bout of cycling HIIE (Tsukamoto et al., 2016). Yet, these studies have only been targets on healthy adults with normal weight, and whether the positive effects of HIIE on cognitive function extend to an adult population with obesity remains unclear. Though only a few studies have examined the effects of exercise on cognition in obese populations, Russo et al. (2017) found that aerobic exercise may improve cognition in obese adults. Previous studies have also demonstrated that HIIE may be more effective than continuous aerobic exercise at improving cognition among normal-weight adults (Tsukamoto et al., 2016; Kao et al., 2017, 2018); therefore, it is possible that HIIE may be an effective mode of exercise for improving cognition in individuals with obesity. One previous study was conducted to examine the impact of HIIE on cognition in obese adults, and showed an improvement in cognitive function, particularly in inhibitory control (Stroop test) after HIIE (Drigny et al., 2014). However, this study was a long-term intervention with HIIE that included only six participants and lacked a control group. Additionally, Quintero et al. (2018) conducted an acute HIIE study on cognitive function in overweight male adults and found positive effects on cognitive inhibition. However, the sample size of their study was relatively small (six participants in HIIE group) and the population was overweight rather than obese. Therefore, the effects of acute HIIE on cognitive function among obese adults is still preliminary, and further investigation is warranted.

Event-related brain potentials (ERPs) from the ongoing electroencephalographam (EEG) represents a sensitive, high temporal resolution of underlying neurocognitive mechanisms between the presentation of a stimulus to beyond response execution processes, and have been commonly utilized to examine the relation between acute exercise and inhibition aspect of executive function (Kamijo et al., 2007; Chu et al., 2015; Wang et al., 2015; Kao et al., 2017). Notably, the majority of studies to date have focused on the P3 (P300 or P3b) component of the ERP, and the acute exercise effect on other components (e.g., late positive potential, LPP) require further examination. The LPP is an ERP component with a more extended latency, which reflects high-order attention processes (Schupp et al., 2003; Carbine et al., 2018) and the influence of cognitive conflict on the later phase of processing (Ligeza and Wyczesany, 2017). Increased LPP amplitude to a stimulus is associated with the increased conscious allocation of attention (Schupp et al., 2003; Carbine et al., 2018) and cognitive control (Watson and Garvey, 2013; Carbine et al., 2018), reflecting a linkage between LPP and inhibitory control.

There has been limited research conducted to examine the influence of HIIE on cognitive function among normal weight adults (Tsukamoto et al., 2016; Kao et al., 2017, 2018) or among overweight or obese adults (Drigny et al., 2014; Quintero et al., 2018). Therefore, it remains important to investigate the effects of acute HIIE on cognitive function among obese adults. It is also unknown how HIIE may affect cognitive function among obese individuals – that is, the precise underlying mechanisms involved. Therefore, the aim of current study was to examine the effects of acute HIIE on cognitive function in young adults with obesity. Specifically, the inhibitory control domain of executive function was assessed via both behavioral and electrophysiological measures using the P3 and LPP components following HIIE. It was hypothesized that an acute HIIE session would facilitate inhibitory control performance among young adults with obesity, and this improvement would be demonstrated by increased P3 and LPP component amplitudes.

MATERIALS AND METHODS

Participants

Sixteen male adults between the age of 18 and 35 years were recruited from the Fengxian district of Shanghai. Eligible participants were screened by the following requirements: (a) obesity status: body mass index (BMI) > 28 kg/m^2 (the value represents the cutoff point obesity on the Asia weight categories); (b) right-handed dominance, (c) no history or presence of endocrine and cardiovascular diseases; (d) no history or presence of neurological disorders or head injury with loss of consciousness; (e) no current use of medication that could affect blood glucose and insulin levels, or any weight loss supplement; (f) "No" answer in any questions of Physical Activity Readiness Questionnaire; and (g) normal or corrected-to-normal vision. All participants provided written informed consent in accordance with the Institutional Review Board at the Shanghai University of Sport (#102772019RT005). The data of the demographic characteristics are provided in **Table 1**.

Cardiovascular Fitness Assessment

The YMCA submaximal ergometer exercise test (MONARK 894E, Sweden) was conducted to assess participants' cardiorespiratory fitness (i.e., maximum oxygen consumption, VO_{2max}). The protocol comprises several consecutive 3-min stages. During the test, a Polar heart rate (HR) monitor was continuously worn to monitor HRs. In the first stage, participants were instructed to cycle at a cadence of 50 rpm at a workload of 25 W (150 kg/min, 0.5 kp). The workloads of the following stages were calibrated according to the HRs of the last 15–30 s (i.e., the steady-state HRs) of the first stage. For instance, the subsequent workloads of the second and third stages were set to 100 W (600 kg/min, 2 kp) and 125 W (750 kg/min, 2.5 kp), respectively, if participant's HRs were lower than 86 bpm. If the steady-state HRs were between 86 and 100 bpm, the workloads of the second and third stages were set to 75 W (450 kg/min, 1.5 kp) and 100 W (600 kg/min, 2 kp), respectively. Lastly, if HR was higher than 100 bpm, the second and third stages were set to 50 W (300 kg/min, 1 kp) and 75 W (450 kg/min, 1.5 kp), respectively. If HR did not achieve steady state in each stage, an additional 1-min cycling was added. The original 6–20 rating of perceived exertion (RPE) (Borg, 1982) was documented every 2 min throughout the test.

TABLE 1 | Demographic characteristics of study participants (means ± SD).

Age (years)	24.50 ± 5.09
Height (m)	1.77 ± 0.06
Weight (kg)	108.11 ± 16.72
BMI (kg/m^2)	34.34 ± 4.39
Digital span	
Forward	14.44 ± 2.28
Backward	9.69 ± 3.63
Education level	
High school	2
College	11
Post-Graduate	2
VO_{2peak} (ml/kg/min)	29.74 ± 12.38
Basal metabolic rate (kJ/m^2/h)	2072.29 ± 191.84
DEBQ	
Restrained eating	3.07 ± 0.37
External eating	3.37 ± 0.62
Emotional eating	2.16 ± 0.74

BMI, body mass index; DEBQ, Dutch Eating Behavior Questionnaire.

Flanker Task

The computerized Flanker task was utilized to assess several aspects of cognitive function (e.g., basic information processing and the inhibitory control aspect of the executive function) implemented on E-Prime software (version 2.0, Psychological Software Tools, Pittsburgh, PA, United States). Each stimulus was composed of five arrows (i.e., one central target and four surrounding flankers) and was presented on the center of the 27-inch LCD screen with a gray background at a distance of 90 cm from participants. The direction of the center target was either the same as the flankers (e.g., →→→→→ or ←←←←←; the congruent condition) or opposite to the flankers (e.g., →→←→→ or ←←→←←; the incongruent condition). A black cross was flashed for 500 ms as a cue to signal the beginning of the trial, followed by the presentation of stimuli for 1000 ms. Once a response was made, a blank intertrial interval with a various time interval (i.e., 600–800 ms) was presented. Participants were asked to put their right index fingers on the number "5" key but not press it, then press the key on the keyboard (number "4" key for left directions and number "6" key for the right directions of the central target, respectively) as fast and accurate as possible. After the key was pressed, the participants were instructed to place their right index fingers back to the "5" key to await the next stimuli. Incorrect responses, responses made beyond 1000 ms after the stimulus onset, or reaction time more than ±3 standard deviations (SD) of each participant's mean reaction time, were discarded from the further analysis. The task contained one practice block and two formal blocks of trials. In the practice block, there were 12 trials with an equal number of congruent and incongruent trial conditions. Participants were required to pass the practice block of trials with an accuracy rate higher than 80%. Each of the formal blocks contained 100 trials, and each of the four stimulus trial types occupied 1/4 of the whole block of trials. The reaction time of accepted response and accuracy for the congruent and incongruent conditions were recorded as the indices of behavioral performance.

Electrophysiological Recording and Analysis

The activity of continuous EEG was recorded from a 64 Ag/AgCl cap with electrodes located at the standard International 10–20 positions using a 1000 Hz sampling rate (Brain Products GmbH, Munich, Germany) throughout the Flanker task. The reference electrode was placed over FCz, and the ground electrode was the AFz. The vertical electrooculogram (VEOG) and the horizontal electrooculogram (HEOG) were recorded through the electrodes placed below the left eye, and the electrodes at lateral-orbitally of the right eye, respectively. All electrodes impedances were kept below 10 kΩ.

All EEG offline processing was conducted using Brain Vision Analyzer 2. The offline EEG data were initially re-referenced according to the average of the left and right mastoids, and the ocular correction was performed (Gratton et al., 1983). Artifact rejection was based on the exclusion of all epochs that exceeded ±100 V. The baseline was corrected (−200 to 0 ms pre-stimulus onset). The continuous EEG data were epoched into 1700-ms time windows (from 200 ms before to 1500 ms after the stimulus onset) for correct trials and then filtered with an IIR filter (low cutoff: 0.1 Hz, high cutoff: 30 Hz, slope: 48 dB/oct). The mean number of analyzable segments of congruent and incongruent conditions were 94.41 ± 7.67 (range 70–100) and 90.84 ± 9.63 (range 60–100), respectively. P3 and LPP component amplitudes were quantified as the area-averaged amplitude within 300–400 ms and 600–1100 ms after the stimulus onset from the Fz electrode (Luijten et al., 2016; Kao et al., 2018), respectively, for both the congruent and incongruent conditions.

Experimental Procedure

Participants were invited to the laboratory on two separate occasions, with the HIIE and control sessions performed in a randomized order across participants. The written informed consent, the physical activity readiness questionnaire (Thomas et al., 1992), and a demographics survey were completed in the participant's first visit. Intelligence indexed by the Digit Span Forward and Backward tests from the Wechsler Adult Intelligence Scale-Third Edition (WAIS-III) (Wechsler, 1997) and socioeconomic status were also measured. Weight and height were measured using an electrical scale (Yaohua Weighing System Co., Shanghai, China) and a wall-mounted stadiometer (TANITA, Tokyo, Japan), respectively. The index of BMI was calculated using the standard formula as weight (kg)/height (m)^2. Participants also completed the Dutch Eating Behavior Questionnaire (DEBQ), which is used to examine eating styles and contains 33 items to specifically explore restrained eating, external eating, and emotional eating (Van Strien et al., 1986). Previous research has demonstrated strong internal consistency of this measure in both genders and among both obese and normal-weight individuals (Cronbach's alphas > 0.79) (Wardle, 1987).

For the experimental sessions (i.e., HIIE and control sessions), the HIIE session lasted approximately 30 min and involved 5 min of warm-up, a 10 × 1 min of 80–90% maximal HR (HR_{max}) interspersed by 1 min of 50–65% HR_{max} active relax (for a total for 20 min), and 5 min of cool-down. The exercise was conducted via stationary cycle exercise because of biomechanical loads and knee safety concerns that may present among obese adults (Salih and Sutton, 2013). HRs and RPE were recorded every 1 min during the 20-min formal HIIE exercise bout. In the control session, participants sat silently with their eyes opened for 30 min, and HR was recorded throughout (**Figure 1**).

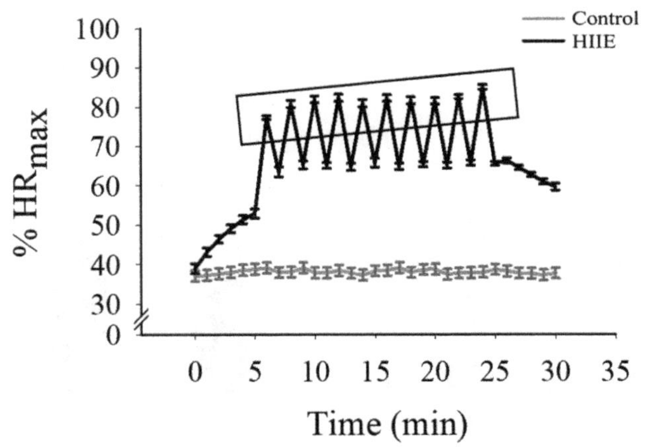

FIGURE 1 | The alteration of the percentage of HR_{max} (%HR_{max}) through both experimental conditions. The *x*-axis (1 min and 30 min) indicates %HR_{max} of the start and end of each condition, which is shown on the *y*-axis. The rectangle indicates %HR_{max} immediately following each HIIE interval.

Within 15 min following the HIIE or control session, participants were seated comfortably in a chair while EEG was prepped. Then, the cognitive task was performed, and EEG was recorded throughout the task period. The cognitive task included three blocks, with one practice and two formal blocks. The total duration for each experimental session was roughly 50 min, and participants were debriefed following the final experimental session.

Statistical Analysis

The study is a within-subject design, with session and stimuli conditions as within-subject factors. For the behavioral data, a 2 (session: HIIE vs. control) × 2 (congruency: congruent vs. incongruent) repeated-measures analysis of variance (ANOVA) was conducted for reaction time and response accuracy, respectively. For the ERP data, a 2 (session) × 2 (congruency) ANOVA was separately conducted for P3 and LPP component amplitudes at site Fz. Pairwise comparisons with Bonferroni adjustments were conducted as follow-up analyses. All statistical values were conducted with $\alpha = 0.05$, where the Greenhouse–Geisser corrections and partial eta-squared (η_p^2) values are reported for significant statistics were observed.

RESULTS

Behavioral Performance

The ANOVA analysis of reaction time revealed a significant main effect of session [$F(1,15) = 7.61$, $p < 0.05$, $\eta_p^2 = 0.34$],

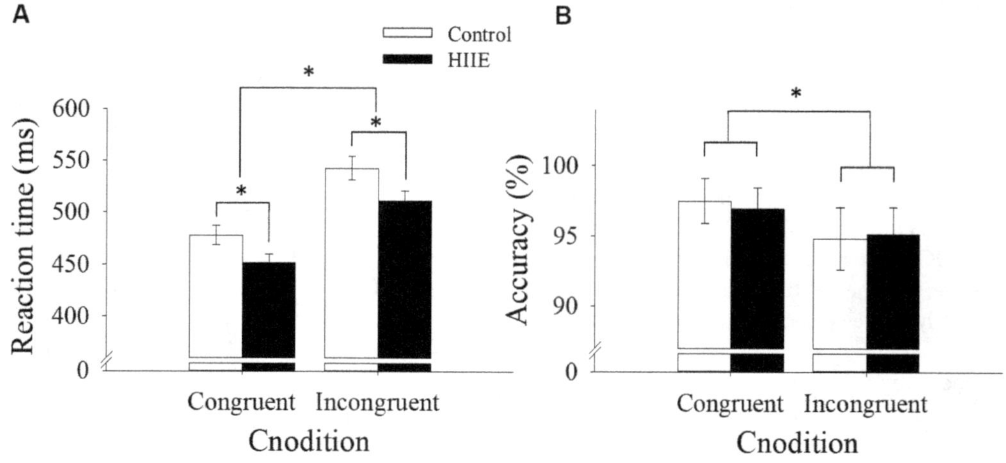

FIGURE 2 | Behavioral reaction time **(A)** and accuracy data **(B)** for the Flanker task by session and congruency. $^*p < 0.05$.

with faster reaction time observed following the HIIE condition (481.28 ± 8.69 ms) compared with the control condition (510.29 ± 10.10 ms). The analysis also revealed a significant main effect of congruency [$F(1,15) = 266.44$, $p < 0.001$, $\eta_p^2 = 0.95$], with faster reaction time for congruent (464.69 ± 7.29 ms) compared with incongruent (526.87 ± 8.73 ms) trials. There was no significant interaction between session and congruency ($p > 0.05$). The behavioral reaction time data for the Flanker task are shown in **Figure 2A**.

The analysis of response accuracy revealed a significant main effect of congruency [$F(1,15) = 14.64$, $p < 0.01$, $\eta_p^2 = 0.49$], with more accurate responses observed for congruent ($97.20 \pm 1.5\%$) than incongruent ($95.00 \pm 2.00\%$) trials. However, no significant differences in response accuracy were observed between HIIE and the control session ($p > 0.05$), nor was there a significant interaction between session and congruency ($p > 0.05$). Response accuracy data are shown in **Figure 2B**.

EEG Data

Figure 3 illustrates the mean stimulus-locked ERP waveform showing P3 and LPP component amplitudes for each session and stimulus condition.

P3 Component Amplitude

Analysis of P3 amplitude revealed no significant main effect for session or congruency (*ps* > 0.05). There was also no interaction between the experimental session and congruency for P3 amplitude ($p > 0.05$).

LPP Component Amplitude

Analysis of LPP component amplitude revealed a significant main effect of session [$F(1,15) = 6.91$, $p < 0.05$, $\eta_p^2 = 0.32$], with larger LPP amplitude observed following the HIIE (13.73 ± 1.86 μV) compared with the control condition (9.64 ± 1.43 μV) at Fz. There is also a significant main effect of congruency [$F(1,15) = 6.69$, $p < 0.05$, $\eta_p^2 = 0.31$], with larger LPP amplitude for congruent (12.27 ± 1.56 μV) compared with incongruent (11.10 ± 1.40 μV) task conditions. No significant interaction between session and congruency was found (*ps* > 0.05). In addition to the grand averaged ERPs, topographic scalp distribution of neuroelectric activity within the time frame of the LPP at site Fz has been shown in **Figure 3**.

DISCUSSION

The study examines the effect of an increasing popular mode of exercise, acute HIIE, on both behavioral and neural indices of inhibition control. Along with the few studies that have been conducted to determine the effects of a single bout of HIIE on inhibitory control, this is the first to examine the influence of this form of exercise on the P3 wave and LPP component among young adult males with obesity. The findings indicate that acute HIIE elicits faster reaction times, but no change in response accuracy, regardless of Flanker task congruency compared to a no-exercise control session. Additionally, while no acute exercise-related enhancements were observed for P3 amplitude, acute HIIE increased LPP component amplitude regardless of Flanker task conditions. Overall, these findings support previous research demonstrating that a single bout of moderate-intensity aerobic exercise increases inhibitory cognitive control (Pontifex et al., 2019) and extends these beneficial findings to HIIE and to young adult males with obesity.

Previous studies have shown that a single bout of HIIE improves inhibitory control performance among normal-weight adults (Alves et al., 2014; Tsukamoto et al., 2016; Kao et al., 2017, 2018) and the present study exhibited faster reaction time following acute HIIE that extends to male adults with obesity. The previous study also indicated decreased flanker task reaction time (Kamijo et al., 2007; Kao et al., 2017) and decreased Stroop reaction time following similar exercise protocols (Alves et al., 2014; Tsukamoto et al., 2016). Given that both of these two tasks are associated with the inhibitory domain of executive function or cognitive control (Harnishfeger and Bjorklund, 1993), the more efficient reaction times observed in these tasks suggest that acute HIIE enhances response speed (Kao et al., 2017) and improved

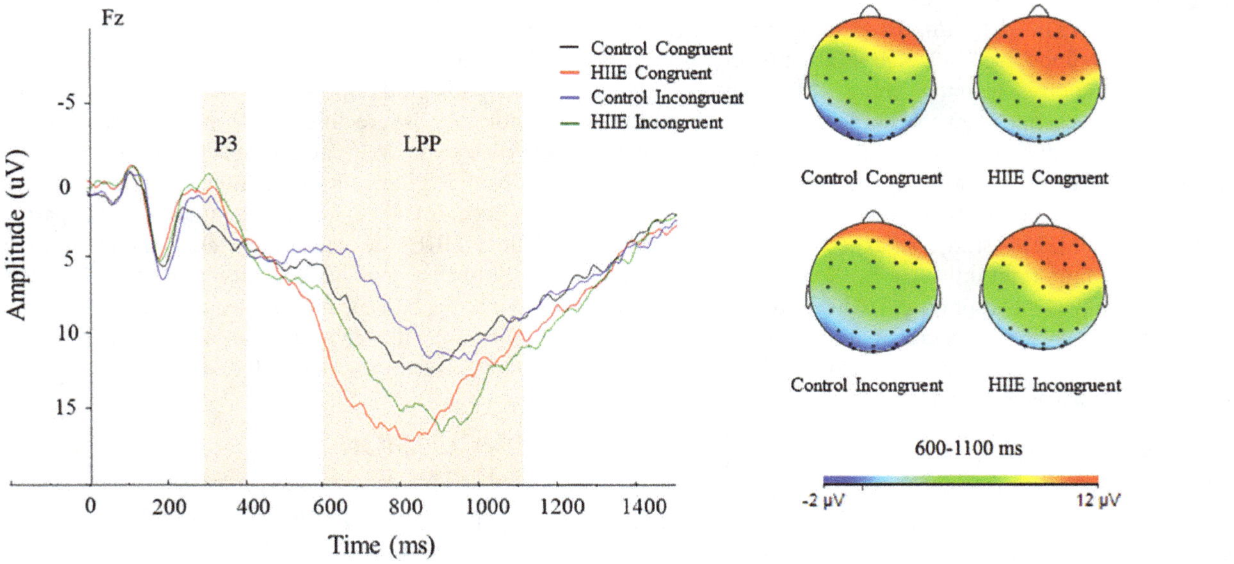

FIGURE 3 | Grand-mean stimulus-locked ERP waveforms for each session and task condition. Stimulus-locked waveforms are shown for both congruency conditions at the midline electrode sites at Fz. Topographic maps of scalp neuroelectric activity for each session and task condition for LPP amplitude (right). The average area of P3 and LPP component amplitudes are shown in shaded regions. LPP component revealed larger amplitude observed following the HIIE (green and red) compared with the control condition (black and blue) at the Fz site. Topographic scalp distribution of the LPP revealed larger activation following the HIIE condition compared with the control condition at Fz regardless of congruency condition.

efficiency in cognitive inhibition (Harnishfeger and Bjorklund, 1993; Kamijo et al., 2012), reflecting a facilitation in inhibitory control following acute HIIE. That this effect is observed in young males with obesity is also provocative since the exercise stimulus is likely to be more difficult relative to normal-weight counterparts performing similar overall workloads.

Behavioral performance of reaction time and accuracy was impaired in the more difficult incongruent relative to congruent task condition of the Flanker task, an effect that is consistently found in the literature (Alderman et al., 2016). These results have often been interpreted as a "conflict effect," suggesting an increase in the task difficulty during incongruent task trials (Eriksen and Eriksen, 1974). In the incongruent task condition, a greater amount of interference control is involved, resulting in response delays, which is due to the fact that flanking stimuli provoked by the activation of the incorrect response compete with the correct response produced by the central target stimulus (Spencer and Coles, 1999; Larson et al., 2014). Notably, the improvement in cognition observed following the acute HIIE not only occurred for congruent but also for incongruent task conditions. Given that the congruent condition reflects relative basic information processing, whereas the incongruent condition reflects high-order inhibition, our results suggest that acute HIIE may have an overall general facilitating effect on cognitive function. These results are somewhat in contrast with studies that have demonstrated a selective improvement (e.g., faster cognitive processing speed) in the incongruent condition but not in congruent or neutral conditions after acute HIIE (Kamijo et al., 2007; Kao et al., 2017). Drollette et al. (2014) found that participants with lower inhibitory capacity may be among those who benefit the most from single bouts of exercise. Therefore, it is possible that the obese individuals from this study have a less flexible cognitive function, particularly within the domain of inhibitory control, relative to their normal-weight counterparts, and acute HIIE may generally enhance both their basic cognitive functioning and high-order cognitive functions such as inhibitory control. This speculation of individual differences in acute exercise–cognition relationship warrants future investigation, particularly given the rise of obesity in nearly all developed countries around the world.

In opposition to our hypothesis, we did not observe an effect of HIIE on P3 amplitude, suggesting that the allocation of attentional resources or cognitive processes that may be indexed by the P3 is not influenced following HIIE among young obese male adults. These results contrast with many previously published studies that have observed an increased P3 amplitude following the acute exercise (Drollette et al., 2014; Chu et al., 2015; Hsieh et al., 2018); yet, it should be noted that these increased P3 amplitudes following acute exercise have only been shown following continuous moderate-intensity aerobic exercise. Indeed, Kao et al. (2018) led a recent study to investigate the short-term neurocognitive effects of acute HIIE and did not find any significant change in P3 component amplitude compared to a sedentary control condition, findings similar to those shown in this study. Collectively, the findings from these two studies suggest that the type or mode of exercise might be a significant moderator of the acute exercise-related enhancement in cognitive function. In addition, the duration of exercise might also be a critical modulator of any acute exercise effects. Kao et al. (2017) found a decrease in P3 amplitude and latency following a 9-min session of HIIE compared to seated rest. They reasoned that such decreases in P3 amplitude following HIIE could be regarded as greater neural efficiency because of less recruitment of neural resources accompanied by improved inhibitory control (Voss et al., 2011; Malinowski, 2013; Kao et al., 2017). However, the results were in contrast with their study in 2018 (Kao et al., 2018), which found no change in P3 amplitude after a 16-min session of acute HIIE, and thus one consideration for the difference may have been due to the duration of the exercise. Given that the exercise duration used in this study was similar to that used in the Kao et al. (2018) study, we expect that exercise duration might have an important influence on P3 component amplitude, particularly when incorporating HIIE protocols. Specifically, HIIE with longer durations might lead to limited effects on P3 amplitude, and the extent to which this influences overall behavioral performance remains to be examined. Lastly, previous studies have mostly examined normal-weight individuals and very few studies to date have focused on the acute HIIE effects on behavioral and neural exponents of inhibitory control among obese adults; therefore, the results from this study relative to behavioral performance outcomes of the P3 may be specific to this population.

Our findings that HIIE improved LPP amplitude is novel for several reasons. LPP reflects higher-order attentional processes (Schupp et al., 2003; Carbine et al., 2018) and the influence of cognitive conflict on the late phase of processing (Ligeza and Wyczesany, 2017). In addition, although we did not use an emotional stimulus in this study, LPP amplitude has also been interpreted as a global inhibition of activity within the visual cortex, reflecting a more adaptive emotional processing (Brown et al., 2012). Our findings demonstrate that following acute HIIE, LPP amplitude increases, suggesting a modulation in the ability to successfully maintain attention and filter irrelevant information to achieve successful cognitive inhibition involved in the Flanker task.

The major strengths of the study include the investigations of the acute HIIE effects on multiple aspects of cognitive function as well as its neuroelectric response in obese individuals; however, potential limitations should be proposed. Our study only included obese male adults in order to avoid the potential moderating role of sex (males vs. females). Along with the relatively small sample size, these findings should not be broadly generalized and future studies employing larger sample size with a specified recruitment of both genders are recommended to further examine the influence of HIIE on select aspects of cognitive function. Additionally, while inhibitory control is a core component of executive function, other distinguishable components including shifting and updating (Miyake et al., 2000) as well as planning (Chang et al., 2012a) should be studied. These distinct components might be differentially influenced by various features of acute HIIE and should be examined to provide a more complete picture of acute HIIE-related modulations of executive function. Furthermore, previous studies have indicated the physiological response to HIIE and more traditional forms of aerobic exercise are different for normal-weight adults. However, the effects and brain mechanisms involved in the acute effects of HIIE on cognition in obese individuals were unclear and thus it is recommended for future studies to compare the impact of both HIIE and aerobic exercise among obese individuals. Lastly, further investigation is also warranted to explore the dose–response relationship between acute HIIE and cognitive function, in terms of intensity, duration, and volume, to advance more precise exercise prescription for cognition.

CONCLUSION

Collectively, a single bout of HIIE has a general beneficial effect on basic information processing and inhibitory control among young adult males with obesity. Acute HIIE was shown to impact LPP component amplitude, but not P3 component amplitudes, which may suggest a modulation in the ability to successfully maintain attention and filter irrelevant information to achieve successful cognitive inhibition. Future study is suggested to extend the examination to a larger sample size that includes both genders, other cognitive functions, and a comparison of varied exercise modes.

ETHICS STATEMENT

The studies involving human participants were reviewed and approved by the Institutional Review Board at the Shanghai University of Sport (#102772019RT005). The patients/participants provided their written informed consent to participate in this study.

AUTHOR CONTRIBUTIONS

CX, Y-KC, and AL: conceptualization. CX, FM, and JA: methodology. BA, FM, and JA: formal analysis. CX, BA, Y-KC, and AL: investigation. All authors: writing – original draft preparation and review and editing.

ACKNOWLEDGMENTS

We thank FM, Junkai Chu, Xin He, Jiameng He, Zhizu Wang, Guoju Chen, and Johan Wikman for their assistance with the experiment.

REFERENCES

Alderman, B. L., Olson, R. L., and Brush, C. J. (2016). Using event-related potentials to study the effects of chronic exercise on cognitive function. *Int. J. Sport Exerc. Psychol.* 17, 106–116. doi: 10.1080/1612197x.2016.1223419

Alves, C. R. R., Tessaro, V. H., Teixeira, L. A. C., Murakava, K., and Takito, M. Y. (2014). Influence of acute high-intensity aerobic interval exercise bout on selective attention and short-term memory tasks. *Percept. Mot. Skills* 118, 63–72. doi: 10.2466/22.06.pms.118k10w4

Bari, A., and Robbins, T. W. (2013). Inhibition and impulsivity: behavioral and neural basis of response control. *Prog. Neurobiol.* 108, 44–79. doi: 10.1016/j.pneurobio.2013.06.005

Borg, G. A. (1982). Psychophysical bases of perceived exertion. *Med. Sci. Sports Exerc.* 14, 377–381.

Brown, S. B. R. E., Van Steenbergen, H., Band, G. P. H., De Rover, M., and Nieuwenhuis, S. (2012). Functional significance of the emotion-related late positive potential. *Front. Hum. Neurosci.* 6:33. doi: 10.3389/fnhum.2012.00033

Carbine, K. A., Rodeback, R., Modersitzki, E., Miner, M., Lecheminant, J. D., and Larson, M. J. (2018). The utility of event-related potentials (ERPs) in understanding food-related cognition: a systematic review and recommendations. *Appetite* 128, 58–78. doi: 10.1016/j.appet.2018.05.135

Chang, Y. K., Erickson, K. I., Stamatakis, E., and Hung, T. M. (2019). How the 2018 US physical activity guidelines are a call to promote and better understand acute physical activity for cognitive function gains. *Sports Med.* 49, 1625–1627. doi: 10.1007/s40279-019-01190-x

Chang, Y. K., Ku, P. W., Tomporowski, P. D., Chen, F. T., and Huang, C. C. (2012a). Effects of acute resistance exercise on late-middle-age adults' goal planning. *Med. Sci. Sports Exerc.* 44, 1773–1779. doi: 10.1249/mss.0b013e3182574e0b

Chang, Y. K., Labban, J. D., Gapin, J. I., and Etnier, J. L. (2012b). The effects of acute exercise on cognitive performance: a meta-analysis. *Brain Res.* 1453, 87–101. doi: 10.1016/j.brainres.2012.02.068

Chu, C. H., Alderman, B. L., Wei, G. X., and Chang, Y. K. (2015). Effects of acute aerobic exercise on motor response inhibition: an ERP study using the stop-signal task. *J. Sport Health Sci.* 4, 73–81. doi: 10.1016/j.jshs.2014.12.002

Drigny, J., Gremeaux, V., Dupuy, O., Gayda, M., Bherer, L., Juneau, M., et al. (2014). Effect of interval training on cognitive functioning and cerebral oxygenation in obese patients: a pilot study. *J. Rehabil. Med.* 46, 1050–1054. doi: 10.2340/16501977-1905

Drollette, E. S., Scudder, M. R., Raine, L. B., Moore, R. D., Saliba, B. J., Pontifex, M. B., et al. (2014). Acute exercise facilitates brain function and cognition in children who need it most: an ERP study of individual differences in inhibitory control capacity. *Dev. Cogn. Neurosci.* 7, 53–64. doi: 10.1016/j.dcn.2013.11.001

Eriksen, B. A., and Eriksen, C. W. (1974). Effects of noise letters upon the identification of a target letter in a nonsearch task. *Percept. Psychophys.* 16, 143–149. doi: 10.3758/bf03203267

Etnier, J. L., and Chang, Y. K. (2019). Exercise, cognitive function, and the brain: advancing our understanding of complex relationships. *J. Sport Health Sci.* 8, 299–300. doi: 10.1016/j.jshs.2019.03.008

Etnier, J. L., Salazar, W., Landers, D. M., Petruzzello, S. J., Han, M., and Nowell, P. (1997). The influence of physical fitness and exercise upon cognitive functioning: a meta-analysis. *J. Sport Exerc. Psychol.* 19, 249–277. doi: 10.1123/jsep.19.3.249

Ferris, L. T., Williams, J. S., and Shen, C. L. (2007). The effect of acute exercise on serum brain-derived neurotrophic factor levels and cognitive function. *Med. Sci. Sports Exerc.* 39, 728–734. doi: 10.1249/mss.0b013e31802f04c7

Gameiro, F., Perea, M. V. V., Ladera, V., Rosa, B., and García, R. (2017). Executive functioning in obese individuals waiting for clinical treatment. *Psicothema* 29, 61–66.

García-García, I., Jurado, M. Á, Garolera, M., Marqués-Iturria, I., Horstmann, A., Segura, B., et al. (2015). Functional network centrality in obesity: a resting-state and task fMRI study. *Psychiatry Res. Neuroimaging* 233, 331–338. doi: 10.1016/j.pscychresns.2015.05.017

Gratton, G., Coles, M. G. H., and Donchin, E. (1983). A new method for off-line removal of ocular artifact. *Electroencephalogr. Clin. Neurophysiol.* 55, 468–484. doi: 10.1016/0013-4694(83)90135-9

Harnishfeger, K. K., and Bjorklund, D. F. (1993). *The Ontogeny of Inhibition Mechanisms: A Renewed Approach to Cognitive Development.* New York, NY: Springer.

Harveson, A. T., Hannon, J. C., Brusseau, T. A., Podlog, L., Papadopoulos, C., Durrant, L. H., et al. (2016). Acute effects of 30 minutes resistance and aerobic exercise on cognition in a high school sample. *Res. Q. Exerc. Sport* 87, 214–220. doi: 10.1080/02701367.2016.1146943

Hsieh, S. S., Chang, Y. K., Fang, C. L., and Hung, T. M. (2016). Acute resistance exercise facilitates attention control in adult males without an age-moderating effect. *J. Sport Exerc. Psychol.* 38, 247–254. doi: 10.1123/jsep.2015-0282

Hsieh, S. S., Huang, C. J., Wu, C. T., Chang, Y. K., and Hung, T. M. (2018). Acute exercise facilitates the N450 inhibition marker and P3 attention marker during stroop test in young and older adults. *J. Clin. Med.* 7:391. doi: 10.3390/jcm7110391

Hwang, K., Velanova, K., and Luna, B. (2010). Strengthening of top-down frontal cognitive control networks underlying the development of inhibitory control: a functional magnetic resonance imaging effective connectivity study. *J. Neurosci.* 30, 15535–15545. doi: 10.1523/jneurosci.2825-10.2010

Kamijo, K., Nishihira, Y., Higashiura, T., and Kuroiwa, K. (2007). The interactive effect of exercise intensity and task difficulty on human cognitive processing. *Int. J. Psychophysiol.* 65, 114–121. doi: 10.1016/j.ijpsycho.2007.04.001

Kamijo, K., Pontifex, M. B., Khan, N. A., Raine, L. B., Scudder, M. R., Drollette, E. S., et al. (2012). The negative association of childhood obesity to cognitive control of action monitoring. *Cereb. Cortex* 24, 654–662. doi: 10.1093/cercor/bhs349

Kao, S. C., Drollette, E. S., Ritondale, J. P., Khan, N., and Hillman, C. H. (2018). The acute effects of high-intensity interval training and moderate-intensity continuous exercise on declarative memory and inhibitory control. *Psychol. Sport Exerc.* 38, 90–99. doi: 10.1016/j.psychsport.2018.05.011

Kao, S. C., Westfall, D. R., Soneson, J., Gurd, B., and Hillman, C. H. (2017). Comparison of the acute effects of high-intensity interval training and continuous aerobic walking on inhibitory control. *Psychophysiology* 54, 1335–1345. doi: 10.1111/psyp.12889

Larson, M. J., Clayson, P. E., and Clawson, A. (2014). Making sense of all the conflict: a theoretical review and critique of conflict-related ERPs. *Int. J. Psychophysiol.* 93, 283–297. doi: 10.1016/j.ijpsycho.2014.06.007

Laursen, P. B., and Jenkins, D. G. (2002). The scientific basis for high-intensity interval training. *Sports Med.* 32, 53–73. doi: 10.2165/00007256-200232010-00003

Ligeza, T. S., and Wyczesany, M. (2017). Cognitive conflict increases processing of negative, task-irrelevant stimuli. *Int. J. Psychophysiol.* 120, 126–135. doi: 10.1016/j.ijpsycho.2017.07.013

Ludyga, S., Brand, S., Gerber, M., Weber, P., Brotzmann, M., Habibifar, F., et al. (2017). An event-related potential investigation of the acute effects of aerobic and coordinative exercise on inhibitory control in children with ADHD. *Dev. Cogn. Neurosci.* 28, 21–28. doi: 10.1016/j.dcn.2017.10.007

Luijten, M., Kleinjan, M., and Franken, I. H. (2016). Event-related potentials reflecting smoking cue reactivity and cognitive control as predictors of smoking relapse and resumption. *Psychopharmacology* 233, 2857–2868. doi: 10.1007/s00213-016-4332-8

Malinowski, P. (2013). Neural mechanisms of attentional control in mindfulness meditation. *Front. Neurosci.* 7:8. doi: 10.3389/fnins.2013.00008

Miyake, A., Friedman, N. P., Emerson, M. J., Witzki, A. H., Howerter, A., and Wager, T. D. (2000). The unity and diversity of executive functions and their contributions to complex "Frontal Lobe" tasks: a latent variable analysis. *Cogn. Psychol.* 41, 49–100. doi: 10.1006/cogp.1999.0734

Ng, M., Fleming, T., Robinson, M., Thomson, B., Graetz, N., Margono, C., et al. (2014). Global, regional, and national prevalence of overweight and obesity in children and adults during 1980–2013: a systematic analysis for the Global Burden of Disease Study 2013. *Lancet* 384, 766–781.

O'Donovan, G., Owen, A., Bird, S. R., Kearney, E. M., Nevill, A. M., Jones, D. W., et al. (2005). Changes in cardiorespiratory fitness and coronary heart disease risk factors following 24 wk of moderate-or high-intensity exercise of equal energy cost. *J. Appl. Physiol.* 98, 1619–1625. doi: 10.1152/japplphysiol.01310.2004

Pontifex, M. B., Mcgowan, A. L., Chandler, M. C., Gwizdala, K. L., Parks, A. C., Fenn, K., et al. (2019). A primer on investigating the after effects of acute bouts of physical activity on cognition. *Psychol. Sport Exerc.* 40, 1–22. doi: 10.1016/j.psychsport.2018.08.015

Prickett, C., Brennan, L., and Stolwyk, R. (2015). Examining the relationship between obesity and cognitive function: a systematic literature review. *Obes. Res. Clin. Pract.* 9, 93–113. doi: 10.1016/j.orcp.2014.05.001

Quintero, A. P., Bonilla-Vargas, K. J., Correa-Bautista, J. E., Dominguez-Sanchez, M. A., Triana-Reina, H. R., Velasco-Orjuela, G. P., et al. (2018). Acute effect of three different exercise training modalities on executive function in overweight inactive men: a secondary analysis of the BrainFit study. *Physiol. Behav.* 197, 22–28. doi: 10.1016/j.physbeh.2018.09.010

Rognmo, Ø, Hetland, E., Helgerud, J., Hoff, J., and Slørdahl, S. A. (2004). High intensity aerobic interval exercise is superior to moderate intensity exercise for increasing aerobic capacity in patients with coronary artery disease. *Eur. J. Cardiovasc. Prev. Rehabil.* 11, 216–222. doi: 10.1097/01.hjr.0000131677.96762.0c

Russo, A., Buratta, L., Pippi, R., Aiello, C., Ranucci, C., Reginato, E., et al. (2017). Effect of training exercise on urinary brain-derived neurotrophic factor levels and cognitive performances in overweight and obese subjects. *Psychol. Rep.* 120, 70–87. doi: 10.1177/0033294116679122

Salih, S., and Sutton, P. (2013). Obesity, knee osteoarthritis and knee arthroplasty: a review. *Sports Med. Arthrosc. Rehabil. Ther. Technol.* 5:25.

Schupp, H. T., Junghöfer, M., Weike, A. I., and Hamm, A. O. (2003). Emotional facilitation of sensory processing in the visual cortex. *Psychol. Sci.* 14, 7–13. doi: 10.1111/1467-9280.01411

Smith, E., Hay, P., Campbell, L., and Trollor, J. N. (2011). A review of the association between obesity and cognitive function across the lifespan: implications for novel approaches to prevention and treatment. *Obes. Rev.* 12, 740–755. doi: 10.1111/j.1467-789x.2011.00920.x

Spencer, K. M., and Coles, M. G. H. (1999). The lateralized readiness potential: relationship between human data and response activation in a connectionist model. *Psychophysiology* 36, 364–370. doi: 10.1017/s0048577299970749

Themanson, J. R., and Hillman, C. H. (2006). Cardiorespiratory fitness and acute aerobic exercise effects on neuroelectric and behavioral measures of action monitoring. *Neurosciience* 141, 757–767. doi: 10.1016/j.neuroscience.2006.04.004

Thomas, S., Reading, J., and Shephard, R. J. (1992). Revision of the physical activity readiness questionnaire (PAR-Q). *Can. J. Sport Sci.* 17, 338–345.

Tsukamoto, H., Suga, T., Takenaka, S., Tanaka, D., Takeuchi, T., Hamaoka, T., et al. (2016). Greater impact of acute high-intensity interval exercise on post-exercise executive function compared to moderate-intensity continuous exercise. *Physiol. Behav.* 155, 224–230. doi: 10.1016/j.physbeh.2015.12.021

Van Strien, T., Frijters, J. E. R., Bergers, G. P. A., and Defares, P. B. (1986). The Dutch Eating Behavior Questionnaire (DEBQ) for assessment of restrained, emotional, and external eating behavior. *Int. J. Eat Disord.* 5, 295–315. doi: 10.1002/1098-108x(198602)5:2<295::aid-eat2260050209>3.0.co;2-t

Voss, M. W., Chaddock, L., Kim, J. S., Vanpatter, M., and Kramer, A. F. (2011). Aerobic fitness is associated with greater efficiency of the network underlying cognitive control in preadolescent children. *Neuroscience* 199, 166–176. doi: 10.1016/j.neuroscience.2011.10.009

Wang, D. S., Zhou, C. L., and Chang, Y. K. (2015). Acute exercise ameliorates craving and inhibitory deficits in methamphetamine: an ERP study. *Physiol. Behav.* 147, 38–46. doi: 10.1016/j.physbeh.2015.04.008

Wardle, J. (1987). Eating style: a validation study of the Dutch Eating Behaviour Questionnaire in normal subjects and women with eating disorders. *J. Psychosom. Res.* 31, 161–169. doi: 10.1016/0022-3999(87)90072-9

Watson, T. D., and Garvey, K. T. (2013). Neurocognitive correlates of processing food-related stimuli in a Go/No-go paradigm. *Appetite* 71, 40–47. doi: 10.1016/j.appet.2013.07.007

Wechsler, D. (1997). *WAIS-III: Adminiastration and Scoring Manual: Wechsler Adult Intelligence Scale: Psychological Corporation.* San Antonio, TX: Psychological Corporation.

Weston, K. S., Wisloff, U., and Coombes, J. S. (2014). High-intensity interval training in patients with lifestyle-induced cardiometabolic disease: a systematic review and meta-analysis. *Br. J. Sports Med.* 48, 1227–1234. doi: 10.1136/bjsports-2013-092576

Wewege, M., Van Den Berg, R., Ward, R. E., and Keech, A. (2017). The effects of high-intensity interval training vs. moderate-intensity continuous training on body composition in overweight and obese adults: a systematic review and meta-analysis. *Obes. Rev.* 18, 635–646. doi: 10.1111/obr.12532

Wilke, J., Giesche, F., Klier, K., Vogt, L., Herrmann, E., and Banzer, W. (2019). Acute effects of resistance exercise on cognitive function in healthy adults: a systematic review with multilevel meta-analysis. *Sports Med.* 49, 905–916. doi: 10.1007/s40279-019-01085-x

Yang, Y., Shields, G. S., Guo, C., and Liu, Y. (2018). Executive function performance in obesity and overweight individuals: a meta-analysis and review. *Neurosci. Biobehav. Rev.* 84, 225–244. doi: 10.1016/j.neubiorev.2017.11.020

12

Use of the Pittsburgh Sleep Quality Index in People with Schizophrenia Spectrum Disorders

Sophie Faulkner[1,2]* *and Chris Sidey-Gibbons*[3,4]

[1] School of Health Sciences, University of Manchester, Manchester, United Kingdom, [2] Greater Manchester Mental Health NHS Foundation Trust, Manchester, United Kingdom, [3] Patient Reported Outcomes, Value & Experience Center (PROVE), Brigham and Women's Hospital, Boston, MA, United States, [4] Faculty of Surgery, Harvard Medical School, Boston, MA, United States

Correspondence:
Sophie Faulkner
sophie.faulkner@manchester.ac.uk

The Pittsburgh Sleep Quality Index (PSQI) is a measure of self-reported sleep quality and sleep disturbance. Though the PSQI is widely used, it is unclear if it adequately assesses self-reported sleep disturbance in people with schizophrenia spectrum disorders. We used mixed methods to examine the relationship between scores on the PSQI and qualitative self-report during in-depth interview in a group of participants diagnosed with schizophrenia spectrum disorders (N = 15). Although the PSQI appears to accurately capture issues related to sleep initiation, average duration, and interruption by physical complaints, it did not adequately assess other salient issues including irregularity in sleep duration and timing, shallow unrefreshing sleep, prolonged sleep inertia, hypersomnia, and sleep interrupted by mental or psychological complaints. In interview by contrast these types of problems were readily reported and described as important by participants. Our findings suggest that using the PSQI summary score as a measurement of general sleep disturbance in this population may be misleading, as this failed to capture some of the types of sleep problems that are particularly common in this group.

Keywords: screening, outcome measure, psychometric, interview, qualitative, psychosis, circadian rhythm disorder, insomnia

INTRODUCTION

The Pittsburgh Sleep Quality Index (PSQI) is a widely used self-reported questionnaire measure of sleep (1). The PSQI is practical and brief, returning a single score representing overall sleep quality, which incorporates qualitative and quantitative aspects of sleep; scores above 5 are suggested as indicative of a potential sleep problem. The PSQI includes open-ended questions that can be used to identify the nature and possible causes of sleep problems to help direct treatment (2), and gives subscale scores that can indicate the type of sleep problems (sleep duration, latency, disturbances, quality, efficiency, daytime dysfunction, and use of sleep medication), as well as some questions on indicators of sleep apnea.

The PSQI was initially developed with a sample of people with depression, healthy sleepers, and people with sleep disorders (2). Many authors, including those who developed the PSQI, have subsequently developed new measures; some of which utilize more modern standards for patient involvement and psychometric analysis (1, 3). The widespread adoption of the PSQI has led to a large literature that appears to facilitate comparison between samples, and now acts as a motivating factor for researchers and clinicians to continue to use the PSQI in preference of other measures. This includes some populations for which it has not been validated (4).

The PSQI is often used as a global measure of self-reported sleep disturbance in people with schizophrenia spectrum disorders, but the validity of the PSQI (English version) as a global measure of sleep disturbance in this population has, to our knowledge, not been evaluated. We explored the content validity of the PSQI for assessing patient-reported sleep quality and sleep disturbance in people with schizophrenia spectrum disorders.

METHODS

We recruited 15 adults with schizophrenia spectrum disorders, who were in contact with specialist mental health services in the United Kingdom, and had a self-reported problem with sleep initiation, maintenance, quality, timing, or refreshingness. People whose predominant complaint was of parasomnia or sleep apnea were not included, in order to focus on insomnia and circadian rhythm problems. All participants' data are included in the current analysis. Written informed consent was obtained after participants reviewed the participant information sheet and had sufficient opportunity for further explanation or questions. Ethical approval was obtained through the NHS Research Ethics Committee Proportionate Review Service (14/NS/1085).

Demographic data were collected, and symptoms and functioning were rated using the Global Assessment of Functioning (GAF) split version (GAF-F and GAF-S). Participants completed the PSQI and were invited to report their experience as they went through the questionnaire; this was followed by an in-depth interview that further explored their sleep experiences and complaints (see **Supplementary File S1**). In addition to the planned questions, the interviewer used continuers and active listening techniques; interview questions later went on to cover other research aims including exploring acceptability of potential treatments, and barriers to improving sleep; these results are reported elsewhere (5). The use of in-depth interview is an additional complementary approach to quantitative psychometrics in evaluating the validity of standardized self-report questionnaires, and it has been used informatively to examine interpretation of other self-reported health measures (6).

Transcription noted long pauses and we made field notes on nonverbal expressions (e.g., frowning, and nonlexical utterances such as "Errrr..."). Analysis was facilitated by Nvivo (qualitative analysis software), creating an audit trail, and ensuring themes were linked back to the data. Transcript content was coded in relation to the PSQI question each section related to, and in relation to emergent themes and subthemes from in-depth analysis of participant interviews. The qualitative analysis used a framework approach, and samples of the data were independently analyzed by a second researcher to enhance reliability. The mixing of methods was approached through qualitization of individual PSQI component scores, and summarizing and classification of the sleep problems described in interviews, to facilitate comparison of component and total PSQI scores, with the clinical presentation as described in each participant's qualitative account (7).

RESULTS

Fifteen participants were recruited, including acute inpatients (n = 2), outpatients receiving intensive (daily) support (n = 3), those under Community Mental Health Teams (n = 8), and under outpatient clinic only (n = 2); none were currently in paid employment. There were 10 males and 5 females, with a mean age of 45.9 (SD = 10.55), diagnosed with schizophrenia (n = 8), schizoaffective disorder (n = 6), and delusional disorder (n = 1). All were prescribed either one (n = 8) or two antipsychotics (n = 7); dosages as a fraction of defined daily doses (8) ranged from 0.36 to 5.5 (mean 2.19, SD 1.28). GAF-F and GAF-S scores ranged from 38 to 85, and from 21 to 80, respectively (mean 62.3, SD 12.16 and mean 47.7, SD 19.40, respectively). For itemized PSQI component scores and raw values, see **Table 1**. Overall, the areas in which these participants scored higher (indicating worse problems) were sleep latency, sleep quality, and daytime dysfunction, while sleep duration scored very low (which should suggest minimal problems). **Table 2** shows summary statements describing the nature of sleep complaints described in interview, and a breakdown of participants endorsing various types of problems.

Acceptability

Most participants reported no problem completing the measure and felt it asked relevant questions. Although some noted a preference for open questions, this is not an issue specific to the PSQI. A minority of participants suggested there should be more questions relating to psychological or mental health-related causes of sleep disruption.

Sleep Duration

Nine participants scored 0 for sleep duration; however, four of these participants were sleeping 11 to 14.5 h, and expressed concerns about this:

> "I've looked it up on Google and it says things like, a higher risk of heart attack, diabetes or early death [laughs]. [...] I do feel guilty, quite a lot, yeah. I would like to be able to ... I would love to be able to just be a morning person" (r05, reported sleep duration = 14.5 h, score on this item = 0)

Hypersomnia was seen as a potential health concern, and a cause for negative self-concept:

> "you're lazy ... you're wasting your life away" (r12).

Participants who described a large amount of nightly variation found average sleep duration difficult to calculate accurately:

TABLE 1 | Participant itemized PSQI scores, hours of sleep, and minutes sleep latency.

Respondent	Hours of actual sleep: h/score[1]	Sleep latency: min/score[1]	Sleep disturbances[1]	Daytime dysfunction[1]	Habitual sleep efficiency[1]	Self-reported quality[1]	Use of sleeping medication[1]	Total PSQI score[2]
r01	11/0	60/3	0	0	0	0	0	**3**
r02	4.5/3	3/0	1	2	1	2	3	**12**
r03	12/0	10/0	1	2	0	0	3	**6**
r04	6/1	60/1	0	0	0	0	0	**2**
r05	14.5/0	180/3	1	3	0	1	0	**8**
r06	6.5/1	60/3	1	3	1	1	0	**10**
r07	4/3	120/3	1	1	2	2	3	**15**
r08	8.5/0	20/1	1	1	0	1	3	**7**
r09	11/0	30/2	2	1	1	1	0	**7**
r10	4.5/3	30/2	1	3	3	3	3	**18**
r11	8/0	30/1	1	0	1	1	0	**4**
r12	3/3	180/3	1	2	3	1	0	**13**
r13	8/0	60/3	1	0	0	2	3	**9**
r14	9/0	10/2	1	0	0	0	0	**3**
r15	7/0	60/3	2	2	1	2	3	**13**
Averages	7.83/0.9	61/2.0	1.0	1.3	0.9	1.1	1.4	**8.7**
Number of participants PSQI indicates have poor sleep quality = 11								

[1]Minimum score = 0 (better), maximum score = 3 (worse). [2]Minimum score = 0 (better), maximum score = 21 (worse), Total >5 associated with poor sleep quality. PSQI, Pittsburgh Sleep Quality Index.

TABLE 2 | Qualitative summaries of participant's description of their sleep problems.

Self-report regarding sleep	r01	r02	r03	r04	r05	r06	r07	r08	r09	r10	r11	r12	r13	r14	r15
Frequent problem with long sleep latency[1]				x			x					x	x		x
Occasional severe problem with long sleep latency[1]	x	x									x				
Problem maintaining sleep or excessively early rising[1]		x			x	x	x			x		x	x		
Problem with difficulty rising or waking[1]	x			x	x				x					x	x
Problem with too long sleep duration[1]			x		x					x				x	
Unusually long sleep, not a problem at present[2]	x								x						
Usually regularly naps[2]	x				x	x			x	x	x	x			x
Problem with prolonged sleep inertia[1]		x	x	x	x	x			x					x	
Significantly troubled by bad dreams[1]		x						x		x		x	x		x

[1]Items are selected where this was a major and consistent aspect of the participant's self-reported complaint; items are only selected where the participant subjectively perceived this as a problem.
[2]Items are selected where this was a frequent occurrence, may not subjectively be a problem.

> "sometimes [waking up] will be 6 o'clock for like three weeks, but very rarely it's 11 o'clock […] if I'm feeling too enthusiastic I'll be awake all night because of the excitement from the day […] yeah so it asks for a fixed time, but it's quite hard to estimate, it varies a lot" (r02, reported average sleep duration = 4.5 h, score on this item = 3)

Seven of the 15 participants tried to give ranges, which were sometimes several hours apart; three participants described nights of getting almost no sleep at all, followed by very long sleep when they did eventually sleep. These participants' mean total sleep time did not capture this issue as the very long and very short sleep times were averaged to a normal duration. Some distinguished "actual sleep" from light sleep/partial sleep, so were unsure how best to respond. Some answers weren't internally consistent (e.g., time to bed till time to wake, minus sleep latency and sleep interruptions, was inconsistent with reported total sleep time). It should be acknowledged that the latter of these issues could affect many retrospective self-report measures.

It is important also to note that daytime naps are not included within the sleep duration total, and for over half in this sample (eight participants), naps were a significant source of sleep:

> "Respondent: [...] I always go to sleep in the afternoon
>
> Interviewer: Most days?
>
> Respondent: Yeah I'd say every day.
>
> Interviewer: How long for?
>
> Respondent: One and a half to two hours" (r10, reported sleep duration = 4.5 h, score on this item = 3)

Other participants described 3- or 4-h naps; hence, the PSQI total sleep time question missed roughly half of their actual total sleep for that day.

Sleep Timing

Average sleep timings are measured by the PSQI, but do not contribute directly to the score. The times recorded give useful information for clinicians on circadian preference or social commitments when sleep timing is regular; in this group, however, times varied and averages may be less meaningful. This variability may have been missed altogether if times were averaged by participants without comment. Dissatisfaction with sleep timing, and unpredictability of sleep timing, were significant sources of dysfunction and distress in participant accounts; participants described the impact on their ability to take on work, education, or social commitments. Satisfaction with or regularity of sleep timing is not part of the PSQI scoring so a problem with sleep timing does not directly impact the score.

Sleep Latency

Sleep latencies reported in answering the PSQI and in interview were similar. While it is interesting that some participants had long sleep latency (60 min, score 3 = worst) and were untroubled by this, this constitutes a quantitative aspect of their sleep disturbance, which is accurately summarized by the PSQI.

Sleep Disturbance

It is not clear how decisions were made regarding what are considered normal frequencies for some of the listed types of sleep disturbance, resulting in floor and ceiling effects. Participants who described "problems" with going to the bathroom at night went several times per night, the highest option to select being ×3 per week. Someone who woke to use the toilet twice a week explained that they felt this was probably less than most people. With regards to the impact of bad dreams, it seemed that frequency of bad dreams bore limited relation to the distress caused; in this sample, no one endorsed 3× per week, but some described less frequent but intense bad dreams causing significant distress, which was not well captured:

> "Oh jeeze I'm always having bad dreams ... I'd say maybe twice a week." (r12)

Significantly, in interview the vast majority of the sample complained of problems with poor sleep maintenance and depth, in terms of "broken" sleep, sleep that was "not deep," or was not "proper sleep"; however, the average score for sleep disturbance was 1.0 (0 = best, 3 = worse). This can largely be attributed to the aggregation of scores from physical and psychological causes of sleep disturbance where there are more physical causes listed. It was noted that sleep, which was disturbed by a wide range of causes, scored higher than sleep very often disturbed, but generally by the same cause. Comparison of individual accounts and sleep disturbance scores showed that sleep that felt broken, but without a complete awakening, did not readily translate to a high score for "sleep disturbance."

"Another Reason..."

Although perhaps a trivial matter, the phrasing of this question proved problematic for well over half of participants, causing a pause in completion and questions regarding either the first part or both parts of this question:

> "...but what does that mean, how often during the past month have you had trouble sleeping because of this, because of what?" (r10)

It was also noted that this question rarely elicited information, as participants brought up many "other reasons" in interview (e.g., hypnopompic hallucinations), but wrote "N/A" on the PSQI. This may contribute to the unusually low scores for sleep disturbance, as these "other reasons" were not scored.

Daytime Dysfunction

The PSQI asks about trouble staying awake "while driving, eating meals, or engaging in social activity"; this question appeared not to be sensitive to sleepiness in those who did not drive and socialized infrequently:

> "My sleep's a bit spontaneous, my body don't plan it [...] I'm always falling asleep watching films [...] but no, I'm trying to think now how often I do a social activity, it's less than once a week isn't it. So it's less than once a week isn't it falling asleep." (r15, score on this item = 0)

Many asked if falling asleep in front of the television counted, and some then answered yes for this question.

The other question concerns "enthusiasm to get things done"; some noted they had difficulty with enthusiasm due to mood or psychotic symptoms, rather than their sleep. Daytime dysfunction questions did not pick up on the impact on daytime functioning, where participants were napping or sleeping for excessive periods to counter tiredness:

> "I'm really fed up because I'd like to get out and do things instead of sleeping the days away" (r01, daytime dysfunction score = 0)

> "It can be as short as half an hour or as long as two hours [...] I go to sleep because I'm tired in the day time, not because I'm bored." (r14, daytime dysfunction score = 0)

Sleep inertia and difficulty waking were also major complaints discussed by participants within the current study (n = 6 of 15). These should be detected as a form of daytime dysfunction; however, half of those expressing this complaint scored 0 for daytime dysfunction (see **Tables 1** and **2**).

Sleep Efficiency

Sleep efficiency has been found to be lower on average in groups with schizophrenia (9); in this sample, average sleep efficiency score does not suggest that this was a particular difficulty (average = 0.9). Interview accounts described difficulties initiating sleep, or maintaining sleep, suggesting poor sleep efficiency. Of those who reported one or more of these difficulties (n = 11), the average sleep efficiency score was 1.09; only four reporting such complaints scored 0. This suggests that the sleep efficiency score detected relevant problems to some extent in most cases.

Quality

Interestingly, over half of participants rated quality as very good (0) or fairly good (1), but went on to state significant concerns with their sleep and its impact on their life, including that their sleep was not restorative, that their poor sleep pattern was a barrier to getting a job, or that their sleep was "medicated sleep" and therefore substandard:

> "[If I wasn't on medication] That I'd actually sleep, yeah. And I think I'd be able to do more things as well, you know, in the day, if I wasn't on the medication, sometimes, if I managed to get natural sleep." (r03, sleep quality rated "very good" = 0)

For some, there seemed to be a direct contradiction between self-reported "sleep quality" on the PSQI and their view of their sleep during interview:

> "Interviewer: ...how would you describe your sleep, if you were sort of telling someone about it?
>
> Respondent: Umm, not very good.
>
> Interviewer: No?
>
> Respondent: No. Not like other people ... go on like sleep's supposed to be, you know?
>
> Interviewer: What?
>
> Respondent: Like, when they say have a nice sleep and you'll feel refreshed and all this nonsense.
>
> Interviewer: They say that.
>
> Respondent: Yes, and I don't feel like that.
>
> Interviewer: No.
>
> Respondent: I feel like, jeez, what's happened?" (r12, sleep quality rated "fairly good" = 1)

In the context of the rest of the analysis (5), this can be attributed to lowered expectations, so "fairly good" could mean good—when all is considered, good—compared to others with the same condition. It is also possible that participants responded regarding sleep quality by evaluating individual periods of sleep obtained, in contrast to the adequateness of their day-to-day sleep as a whole. Potentially also more rapport was built during the in-depth interview and participants felt more open and prepared to describe problems.

Sleeping Medication

The present sample's highest scoring domain was use of sleeping medication. This did not, however, represent high levels of hypnotic use in this sample; in six out of seven of those scoring 3 (highest), their answer related to their oral antipsychotic being "sleeping medication" (although some felt this was an ineffective sleeping medication). Some described in interview using their antipsychotic to control their sleep onset, but answered "never" to this question on the PSQI, and some raised the dilemma of whether their antipsychotic counted or not. Answers were therefore dictated by semantic interpretation rather than any meaningful differences between perceptions or behaviors.

Sleep Disordered Breathing

The PSQI includes questions regarding snoring or breathing among its sleep disturbance questions, and also a section for completion by the person's bed partner/roommate to screen for sleep disordered breathing, in acknowledgement of people's reduced awareness of their own breathing during sleep. Participants in this study did endorse snoring, but rarely endorsed "cannot breathe comfortably," rather clarifying that they breathed heavily, not had *difficulty* breathing:

> "...cause I'm a big lad as well so when I'm lying down ... I'd say not it's hard to breathe but I breathe heavily." (r15, cannot breathe comfortably = 1, cough or snore loudly = 3, circled 'loudly' for emphasis).

It was never designed as such, and it is important that the PSQI is not considered to be an effective screening for sleep disordered breathing, particularly without the bed partner/roommate questions being completed.

Total Scores

The total PSQI scores indicated that seven participants were either good sleepers or had only mild sleep problems (n = 4 score <5, n = 3, score 6–7). Of these seven, four described significant and severe concerns during interview, while the other three described milder but definite problems. Of those whose PSQI scores suggested moderate or severe problems (score 8–18), the global impression from the interview was also of moderate or severe problems.

DISCUSSION

The sample reported multiple and complex problems with sleep initiation, continuity, quality, and timing, with attendant daytime dysfunction; the PSQI was capable to assess some, but not all, of these issues. The PSQI appeared to be suitable for identifying self-reported short sleep, long sleep latency, or complete awakenings during the night, but poorly represented some other problems such as variable and inconsistent sleep length, poor sleep depth or quality, increased sleep inertia, hypersomnia, and inappropriate or inconsistent sleep timing. While issues with sleep timing are beyond the intended scope of the PSQI, sleep duration, quality, and daytime dysfunction are within its scope and were poorly captured. Furthermore, it is common for total PSQI scores to be treated as a global measure of sleep disturbance, which these findings suggest is not valid. Reliance on total PSQI score as a measure of sleep dysfunction is particularly inappropriate for those with schizophrenia spectrum disorders whose sleep problems include more circadian dysregulation than other groups (10), and who as a result experience more inconsistent and variable sleep, and more difficulties timing sleep patterns to fit with life expectations (5, 11, 12). Some of the measurement issues highlighted also have potential implications for interpretation of PSQI scores in other populations.

Measuring Sleep Duration, Variability, and Depth

As some participants feared, both excessively short and excessively long sleep are indeed associated with increased mortality (13), and it has previously been recommended that the relationship of sleep duration to assumed sleep quality on the PSQI should be U-shaped and not linear (14). Our findings support this suggestion, concurring that unusually long sleep, as well as too short sleep, caused concerns for participants. It is also important to note that in people taking significant naps, as was common in this sample, the PSQI can mischaracterize (underestimate) a person's total sleep time, as might also occur in regional populations in whom biphasic sleep is common. These issues with calculation and scoring of sleep duration of course affect the use of the PSQI in many other clinical and nonclinical samples, not just in those with schizophrenia spectrum disorders.

Participant PSQI scores were similar to those from research with the Japanese version of this instrument in a similar sample (14), where sleep latency, sleep quality, and daytime dysfunction received higher scores on the PSQI, while sleep duration scored very low [which should suggest minimal problems; Doi et al. (14) also noted hypersomnia was not captured]. In contrast to our study, the subgroup of the Japanese sample with schizophrenia (n = 24) scored low regarding sleeping medication, perhaps owing to different phrasing in the translation (14).

Insufficient detection of problems with sleep depth is significant particularly for this population, for whom levels of shallow sleep (stage 1) are often elevated, and deeper sleep (Stage 2 and Stage 3 non-REM sleep) is often reduced (9). Although objective assessment of sleep depth requires polysomnography or spectral analysis, the experience of deep sleep was important to participants. Even apart from importance to individuals, subjective evaluations of sleep have often been found to be equally if not more predictive of health and functioning outcomes than some more objective measures (15, 16), suggesting even "inaccurate" experiences may be equally important to capture.

Our findings are consistent with those of Waters et al. (12) who found only small and statistically nonsignificant differences in PSQI scores between people with schizophrenia and healthy controls, but found increased variability in sleep latency, efficiency, and duration in schizophrenia when using actigraphy. Actigraphy or sleep diaries can be recommended to assess variability. However, retrospective self-report is less burdensome and has the potential to offer some insight; a future measure might include questions that assess how frequently various sleep values deviate from the average, by more than a certain amount (e.g., "How many times in the last month? was it 2 h more or less than this?"). Appropriate phrasing, format, and content would require development and testing.

Clinical Assessment of Sleep

For current clinical practice, supplementary questions or additional measures should be used when using the PSQI as a screening for sleep problems. For instance, the PSQI should not be relied upon to screen for sleep disordered breathing; a ready alternative is the STOP-Bang questionnaire, which has been found to be reasonably accurate in detection (17) and is freely available and brief (18). Measures of circadian preference might be added (19, 20); however, these do not measure regularity of rhythm. It is possible to measure and quantify regularity of rest-activity rhythms through actigraphy, describing both amplitude (relative amplitude) and regularity of rhythm (interday stability) (21), as has been more extensively utilized in samples with dementia (22) who also experience circadian dysregulation. At least one retrospective self-report measure of regularity is available [e.g., (23)], although none has yet been tested in schizophrenia spectrum disorders. During clinical interview, therefore, additional questions are recommended regarding regularity of sleep timing, and the match between sleep timing and individual lifestyle choices and requirements.

Outcome Measurement

Whether for research or clinical outcome measurement for quality improvement, the findings of the present study caution against relying on the PSQI total score alone, as improvements in sleep timing or regularity (often accompanied by improved quality of life and functioning) may go undetected. There are more recently developed tools, including the PROMIS sleep dysfunction item bank (1), and the Glasgow Sleep Impact Scale (3), which have been specifically designed to act as a barometer of the patient's perceived standard of sleep. Both tools were developed with patient involvement and have undergone validation in healthy controls and those with sleep disorders, or in insomnia, respectively. These measures are very promising and may offer a useful adjunct to clinical assessments of sleep issues for people with schizophrenia spectrum disorders, and, by virtue of their use of modern psychometric methods, may also offer a reliable means of comparison across diagnostic groups.

These tools, however, are designed to measure change for research or clinical outcome measurement; they do not simultaneously help to characterize the sleep problem—as might be desired by a clinician. And in this respect, they do not replace the PSQI. Asking the patient to specify sleep latency, sleep times, and causes of sleep disturbance, as the PSQI does, can help identify the problem and therefore direct treatment. Unfortunately, the PSQI alone is likely to give an incomplete and sometimes misleading picture, in the case of people with schizophrenia spectrum disorders, and possibly many other groups.

Limitations and Future Directions

The generalizability of the findings from a small sample might be questioned, although as the types of problems described are similar to those found in larger samples studied using quantitative methodologies, we believe these findings are transferable. Although the diversity in the type and extent of problems is potentially representative of the diverse problems experienced in this group, it also limits the number of cases with each particular type of problem (e.g., with short sleep, or with hypersomnia). Furthermore, diversity in the environmental context of the participants, particularly the inclusion of both inpatients and outpatients, complicates interpretation. It would also have been useful to find out the approximate length of time since diagnosis, and length of time on antipsychotic medication, to better describe the sample and facilitate comparison with other studies. In hindsight, it would also have been useful if participants had been asked to comment on the recommended interpretation of their component or total PSQI scores (for instance, "This score suggests overall you have good/slightly disturbed/severely disturbed sleep. Do you agree?"), which might have provided a further point of reference.

This study did not set out to make statistical analysis of sensitivity or specificity, but these findings suggest a hypothesis of too low sensitivity, and missed cases, but no issues with overdetection. Future studies comparing PSQI to other measures such as actigraphy or polysomnography might confirm or quantify this, and could further examine which types of problem are underdetected in a larger sample. More detailed description of the weaknesses this study has highlighted would support improved interpretation of the considerable body of important work, which has used the PSQI to describe their sample or to measure change.

Our analysis demonstrates that the PSQI is insensitive to some sleep issues, which are described as important to people with schizophrenia spectrum disorders. This disparity between the range of issues highlighted in our interviews and those covered by the PSQI may suggest a need for a disease-specific measure to achieve high sensitivity to the particular problems of this group. Another possibility is the development of a measure of sleep disturbance, which can equally measure sleep problems of circadian, insomniac, or combined cause and nature, which could be used trans-diagnostically. A future measure could attempt also to take into account different environmental contexts; for instance, in many institutional settings, patients may more commonly go "to bed" far in advance of intending to sleep, as their bedroom may be the only private space in which to wind down for sleep. This can lead to underestimation of sleep efficiency, as has previously been noted in relation to sleep diaries (24); and alternative phrasing around "into bed" has been recommended. There may also be utility in a measure that examines or considers the impact of a mismatch between environment, occupational routine, and the individual, upon sleep, as well as factors that are more inherent to the person.

Self-Report Items versus Self-Evaluated Items

The PSQI is of course not unique among self-report measures in being affected by participants calibrating some of their responses in relation to their own context and peer group, as we found here regarding rating of sleep quality. Similar findings of peer group-dependent evaluations were presented by Adamson et al. (6) regarding the evaluation of general health:

> "Mrs K: Oh, I suppose for my age my health is excellent., I mean to say, it wasn't until I went up for the assessment I knew there was anything wrong with my heart" [(6), p142]

This context-dependent evaluation may equally measure a difference in a person's perceived peer group, as much as based on a change in self-perceived sleep, and makes it difficult to use exclusively self-evaluated items to compare between populations. It may therefore be desirable to include some quantitative self-report elements, which are more influenced by the individual's perception of their sleep than contextual factors.

CONCLUSION

Future research should develop a valid and reliable tool, with a similar shared utility for both clinicians and researchers as the PSQI has uniquely offered; this shared utility no doubt facilitates understanding between clinicians and researchers, and accounts for its enduring popularity. The authors suggest the development of a new measure that can act as a clinical screening and initial interview, and as an outcome measure in research.

ETHICS STATEMENT

Ethical approval was obtained through the NHS Research Ethics Committee Proportionate Review Service (14/NS/1085), North of Scotland Research Ethics Committee 1. Written informed consent was obtained after participants reviewed the participant information sheet and had sufficient opportunity for further explanation or questions. A disclosure or risk protocol and a distress protocol were followed during data collection, and information sharing with care providers was discussed with participants in advance (information was shared on participant's request, or if any immediate risks necessitated information sharing).

AUTHOR CONTRIBUTIONS

SF designed and conducted the study, collected and analyzed the data, and wrote the first draft of the manuscript. SF and CS-G were involved in editing, conceptual formulation, and discussion of the findings and implications of the study.

ACKNOWLEDGMENTS

Professor Penny Bee (School of Health Sciences, University of Manchester) is acknowledged for academic supervision and support of SF during study design, data collection, and analysis. Mr. Vik Veer [ENT Consultant, at Royal National Throat Nose & Ear Hospital, University College London Hospitals NHS Foundation Trust (UCLH), Sleep Surgery Department] is acknowledged for input regarding discussion of screening and assessment of sleep disordered breathing. The participants are thanked for their efforts in describing their experiences.

REFERENCES

Buysse DJ, Yu L, Moul DE, Germain A, Stover A, Dodds NE, et al. Development and validation of patient-reported outcome measures for sleep disturbance and sleep-related impairments. *Sleep* (2010) 33(6):781–92. [online]. Available from: https://www.ncbi.nlm.nih.gov/pmc/articles/ PMC2880437 doi: 10.1093/sleep/33.6.781

Buysse DJ, Reynolds CF 3rd, Monk TH, Berman SR, Kupfer DJ. The Pittsburgh Sleep Quality Index: a new instrument for psychiatric practice and research. *Psychiatry Res* (1989) 28(2):193–213. [online]. Available from: http://www. ncbi.nlm.nih.gov/pubmed/2748771 doi: 10.1016/0165-1781(89)90047-4

Kyle SD, Crawford MR, Morgan K, Spiegelhalder K, Clark AA, Espie CA. The Glasgow Sleep Impact Index (GSII): a novel patient-centred measure for assessing sleep-related quality of life impairment in insomnia disorder. *Sleep Med* (2013) 14(6):493–501. doi: 10.1016/j.sleep.2012.10.023

Garrow AP, Yorke J, Khan N, Vestbo J, Singh D, Tyson S. Systematic literature review of patient-reported outcome measures used in assessment and measurement of sleep disorders in chronic obstructive pulmonary disease. *Int J Chron Obstruct Pulmon Dis* (2015) 10:293–307. [online]. Available from: http://www.scopus.com/inward/record.url?eid=2-s2.0-84922743032&partnerID=tZOtx3y1

Faulkner S, Bee P. Experiences, perspectives and priorities of people with schizophrenia spectrum disorders regarding sleep disturbance and its treatment: a qualitative study. *BMC Psychiatry* (2017) 17(1):158. [online]. Available from: DOI 10.1186/s12888-017-1329-8 doi: 10.1186/ s12888-017-1329-8

Adamson J, Gooberman-Hill R, Woolhead G, Donovan J. 'Questerviews': using questionnaires in qualitative interviews as a method of integrating qualitative and quantitative health services research. *J Health Serv Res Policy* (2004) 9(3):139–45. [online]. Available from: http://www.ncbi.nlm.nih.gov/pubmed/15272971 [Accessed November 4, 2014]. doi: 10.1258/1355819041403268

Migiro SO, Magangi BA. Mixed methods: a review of literature and the future of the new research paradigm. *Afr J Bus Manage* (2011) 5(10):3757–64. [online]. Available from: http://www.academicjournals.org/AJBM

WHO. WHO Collaborating Centre for Drug Statistics Methodology., p. ATC/DDD Index. [online]. Available from: https://www.whocc.no/atc_ ddd_index/ [Accessed March 12, 2017].

Chan MS, Chung KF, Yung KP, Yeung WF. Sleep in schizophrenia: a systematic review and meta-analysis of polysomnographic findings in case- control studies. *Sleep Med Rev* (2017) 32:69–84. [online]. Available from: doi. org/10.1016/j.smrv.2016.03.001 doi: 10.1016/j.smrv.2016.03.001

Pritchett D, Wulff K, Oliver PL, Bannerman DM, Davies KE, Harrison PJ, et al. Evaluating the links between schizophrenia and sleep and circadian rhythm disruption. *J Neural Transm* (2012) 119(10):1061–75. doi: 10.1007/ s00702-012-0817-8

Waite F, Evans N, Myers E, Startup H, Lister R, Harvey AG, et al. The patient experience of sleep problems and their treatment in the context of current delusions and hallucinations. *Psychol Psychother: Theory Res Pract* (2015) 89:181–93. [online]. Available from: http://doi.wiley.com/10.1111/ papt.12073 doi: 10.1111/papt.12073

Waters F, Sinclair C, Rock D, Jablensky A, Foster RG, Wulff K. Daily variations in sleep-wake patterns and severity of psychopathology: a pilot study in community-dwelling individuals with chronic schizophrenia. *Psychiatry Res* (2011) 187(1–2):304–6. [online]. Available from: http://www. ncbi.nlm.nih.gov/pubmed/21272939 [Accessed October 28, 2014]. doi: 10.1016/j.psychres.2011.01.006

Cappuccio FP, D'Elia L, Strazzullo P, Miller MA. Sleep duration and all-cause mortality: a systematic review and meta-analysis of prospective studies. *Sleep* (2010) 33(5):585–92. [online]. Available from: http://www.pubmedcentral. nih.gov/articlerender.fcgi?artid=2864873&tool=pmcentrez&rendertype=ab stract doi: 10.1093/sleep/33.5.585

Doi Y, Minowa M, Uchiyama M, Okawa M, Kim K, Shibui K, et al. Psychometric assessment of subjective sleep quality using the Japanese version of the Pittsburgh Sleep Quality Index (PSQI-J) in psychiatric disordered and control subjects. *Psychiatry Res* (2000) 97:165–72. doi: 10.1016/S0165-1781(00)00232-8

Harvey AG, Tang NKY. (Mis)perception of sleep in insomnia: a puzzle and a resolution. *Psychol Bull* (2012) 138(1):77–101. [online]. Available from: http://www.pubmedcentral.nih.gov/articlerender.fcgi?artid=3277880&tool=pmcentrez&rendertype=abstract [Accessed October 22, 2014]. doi: 10.1037/a0025730

Pilcher JJ, Ginter DR, Sadowsky B. Sleep quality versus sleep quantity: relationships between sleep and measures of health, well-being and sleepiness in college students. *J Psychosom Res* (1997) 42(6):583–96. doi: 10.1016/S0022-3999(97)00004-4

Abrishami A, Khajehdehi A, Chung F. A systematic review of screening questionnaires for obstructive sleep apnea. *Can J Anaesth* (2010) 57(5):423– 38. doi: 10.1007/s12630-010-9280-x

Chung F, Subramanyam R, Liao P, Sasaki E, Shapiro C, Sun Y. *STOP-Bang Questionnaire.* Toronto: Toronto Western Hospital (2018). [online]. Available from: http://www.stopbang.ca/osa/screening.php [Accessed August 1, 2018].

Roenneberg T, Wirz-Justice A, Merrow M. Life between clocks: daily temporal patterns of human chronotypes. *J Biol Rhythms* (2003) 18(1):80– 90. doi: 10.1177/0748730402239679

Randler C, Díaz-Morales JF, Rahafar A, Vollmer C. Morningness–eveningness and amplitude—development and validation of an improved composite scale to measure circadian preference and stability (MESSi). *Chronobiol Int* (2016) 33(7):832–48. [online]. Available from: http://dx.doi.org/10.3109/07420528.2016.1171233 doi: 10.3109/07420528.2016.1171233

Van Someren EJW, Swaab DF, Colenda CC, Cohen W, McCall WV, Rosenquist PB. Bright light therapy: improved sensitivity to its effects on rest-activity rhythms in Alzheimer patients by application of nonparametric methods. *Chronobiol Int* (1999) 16(4):505–18. doi: 10.3109/07420529908998724

Gonçalves BSB, Adamowicz T, Louzada FM, Moreno CR, Araujo JF. A fresh look at the use of nonparametric analysis in actimetry. *Sleep Med Rev* (2015) 20:84–91. [online]. Available from: http://dx.doi.org/10.1016/j. smrv.2014.06.002 doi: 10.1016/j.smrv.2014.06.002

Monk TH, Buysse DJ, Kennedy KS, Pods JM, DeGrazia JM, Miewald JM. Measuring sleep habits without using a diary: the sleep timing questionnaire. *Sleep* (2003) 26(2):208–12. doi: 10.1093/sleep/26.2.208

Carney CE, Buysse DJ, Ancoli-israel S, Edinger JD, Krystal AD, Lichstein KL, et al. The Consensus Sleep Diary: standardizing prospective sleep self-monitoring. *Sleep* (2012) 35(2):287–302. doi: 10.5665/sleep.1642.

13

Correlation between Cognition and Balance among Middle-Aged and Older Adults Observed through a Tai Chi Intervention Program

Tao Xiao[1], *Lin Yang*[2,3], *Lee Smith*[4], *Paul D. Loprinzi*[5], *Nicola Veronese*[6], *Jie Yao*[7], *Zonghao Zhang*[8]* *and Jane Jie Yu*[9]*

[1] College of Mathematics and Statistics, Shenzhen University, Shenzhen, China, [2] Cancer Epidemiology and Prevention Research, Alberta Health Services, Calgary, AB, Canada, [3] Departments of Oncology and Community Health Sciences, Cumming School of Medicine, University of Calgary, Calgary, AB, Canada, [4] Cambridge Centre for Sport and Exercise Sciences, Anglia Ruskin University, Cambridge, United Kingdom, [5] Department of Health, Exercise Science and Recreation Management School of Applied Sciences, The University of Mississippi, Oxford, MS, United States, [6] Geriatrics Division, Department of Medicine–DIMED, University of Padova, Padua, Italy, [7] School of Humanities and Social Sciences, Harbin Institute of Technology (Shenzhen), Shenzhen, China, [8] College of Physical Education, Soochow University, Suzhou, China, [9] Department of Sports Science and Physical Education, The Chinese University of Hong Kong, Hong Kong, China

Correspondence:
Zonghao Zhang
zonghaozhang@163.com
Jane Jie Yu
jieyu0203@gmail.com

Background: Age-associated decline in cognition and balance may cause severe ability loss for daily living activities among middle-aged and older adults. The relationship between cognition and balance in this aging population remains to be explored.

Objective: The present study Is exploratory in nature and aimed to examine the relationship between balance (both static and dynamic components) and global cognitive function among middle-aged and older adults through Tai Chi (TC) practice as a research avenue.

Methods: A short-term (12 weeks) intervention of TC was conducted among middle-aged and older adults in the community setting. Global cognitive function (using the Chinese version of the Montreal Cognitive Assessment score (MoCA) and balance (i.e., one leg standing test score; Timed Up and Go Test score, TUGT) of all participants were assessed before and after the intervention. Age, body mass index (BMI), sex, and physical fitness variables (Chair Stand Test, CST; the 6-Meter Walk Test, 6MWT) were also collected as confounding factors.

Results: Significant moderator effects of baseline CST on the association between the dichotomized baseline MoCA score and the baseline left leg balance score ($p = 0.0247$), the baseline right leg balance score ($p = 0.0140$) and the baseline TUGT score ($p = 0.0346$) were found. Change score of left score balance ($p = 0.0192$) and change score of TUGT ($p = 0.0162$) were found to be significantly associated with change score of cognitive function.

Conclusion: Cognitive function and balance are interrelated in middle-aged and older adults. The association between global cognitive function and balance Is moderated by strength of lower limbs. The change scores of cognitive function and balance introduced by TC training were found to be positively correlated. Future research Is warranted to further confirm the cause-effect relationship of cognitive function and balance and its influencing factors among middle-aged and older adults utilizing intervention studies with larger sample sizes.

Keywords: cognition, alternative exercise, postural control, equilibrium, Tai Chi

INTRODUCTION

A large proportion of older adults live alone or are without children of any age at home. For example, in China, half (49.7%) of those 60 years and older live with no children, and this proportion increases to 56.1% in large and medium-sized cities (China Population Press, 2015). An increasing number of older adults living alone or without children exerts financial pressure on families and society as a whole (Asian Development Bank, 2014; Whetten-Goldstein et al., 2015). Moreover, greater financial pressures are more likely when older adults lose independence in activities of daily living such as walking, feeding, dressing and grooming, toileting, bathing, transferring, cooking, transportation, and shopping, etc. (Mlinac and Feng, 2016). Fall injuries and dementia are the most frequent and costly age-induced factors that may cause complete loss of independence in activities of daily living. According to the Centers for Disease Control and Prevention, falling Is the leading cause of fatal and non-fatal injuries among older adults, and more than one fourth of adults aged 65 years or above will fall each year (CDC Newsroom, 2016). For instance, among older Americans, around 29 million falls occur each year, resulting in 3 million emergency department visits, 800,000 hospitalizations, and 28,000 deaths. The average hospital cost of a fall encounter Is over US$30,000 and the annual Medicare costs for falls for individuals residing in the US aged 65 years and above was ~US$31 billion in the year 2015 (Laurence and Michel, 2017). According to the World Health Organization, around 50 million individuals, globally, are currently living with dementia and nearly 10 million new cases occur each year (World Health Organization [WHO], 2017). The consequences incurred by decline in cognition are as serious as those by falls among older people. Thus far, there has not been a curative treatment for dementia (Koller et al., 2016). Hence, it Is important to maintain or slow down the degrading processes of both balance and cognitive function among older adults and even at an earlier age stage (i.e., middle-aged adults) to reduce the risks of falling (Iwasaki and Yamasoba, 2015; Zou et al., 2017b, 2018a) and dementia (Morris, 2012; Petersen, 2016). A large 10-years study of middle-aged to older adults (45–70) found that cognitive decline begins in the 45–55 decade (Singh-Manoux et al., 2012). The central ability to inhibit balance destabilizing vision-related postural control processes was found among middle-aged and older adults to depend at least partially on striatal dopaminergic pathways (Cham et al., 2007). The relationship between cognitive function and balance among middle-aged and older adults calls for potentially effective interventions that might improve both cognition and balance for this population.

Physical activity or exercise (one domain of physical activity) intervention programs have been shown to delay age-related balance or cognitive decline (Chase et al., 2016; Zou et al., 2017a; Gheysen et al., 2018; Zhang et al., 2018). Tai Chi (TC) has been recognized to promote both fall-related balance ability and cognitive function in the aging population (Wayne et al., 2014; Huang et al., 2017). TC Is a mind-body exercise with special features that have shown to be effective for improving balance and cognition together. Transitions between double- and single-leg stance commonly occur throughout entire TC routines (Wayne et al., 2016) which can potentially strengthen lower-limb muscle and flexibility, improving postural control. Additionally, TC consists of relatively complex movement sequences, which may benefit practitioners with memory training opportunities. To perform such sequences smoothly and connectedly, higher-order cognition (e.g., visuospatial ability, orientation, attentional resource allocation, and executive function) Is needed. Thus, TC may help facilitate greater conscious control over the entire body. Such practice may lead to a combined promotion in cognitive function and balance over time (Liu et al., 2018, 2019; Zou et al., 2018b,c,d, 2019a; Kong et al., 2019). Therefore, TC training may be a potential research avenue for investigating the relationship of cognitive function and balance. However, previous studies that investigated the intervention effects of TC on age-related decline in cognition and balance, and that evaluated both outcomes simultaneously are limited. Recently, several large-scale epidemiological studies showed that balance and cognition are highly interdependent (Clouston et al., 2013; Smith-Ray et al., 2015; Demnitz et al., 2016). Synergistic effects on improvements in both balance control and cognitive functioning were found by exercises combining cognitive and balance training, including multimodal exercise (Marmeleira et al., 2018), unicycling training (Weber et al., 2019), and mind-body exercise like yoga (Subramaniam and Bhatt, 2017). In addition, cognitive functions were also reported to be highly associated with mobility among middle-aged and older adults (Buchman et al., 2011; Demnitz et al., 2016, 2018; Li et al., 2018). The authors of the present study conducted a randomized trial, with modified Chen-style TC as case and 24-style active TC as control, to verify the effectiveness of TC training on improving cognitive function and balance (Zou et al., 2019b). By re-exploring and pooling the data from this randomized trial, the main purpose of this study was to examine the relationship between balance (both static and dynamic components) and global cognitive function under a condition of TC training among middle-aged and older adults controlling for key covariates (e.g., age, sex, mobility level). It Is hypothesized that there would be a positive and interdependent relationship between global cognitive function and balance among middle-aged and older adults.

METHODS

Experimental Design

A 12-week intervention of TC was conducted among middle-aged and older adults. Baseline and posttest data on balance and cognitive function were collected; baseline and posttest data on confounding factors of fitness of lower limbs and aerobic exercise capacity were also collected; data on other confounding factors (i.e., age, gender, height, weight, and heart rate) were collected at baseline. Ethical approval was obtained from the research ethics committee before the commencement of this study.

Study Participants

Participants included 78 Chinese middle-aged and older adults (mean age: 58.92 ± 8.03 years) and consisted of 37 male individuals and 41 female individuals. Participants were recruited from Yongzhou city of Hunan province in China between December 2017 and March 2018. Individuals who had no physical limitations in participating in TC practice and had not received any exercise training programs or practiced TC regularly over the past 3 months were included. Those individuals who reported serious diseases (e.g., cardiovascular disease, clinical depression) or a history of alcohol abuse, and who were not able to understand and follow the instructions in the pilot training session were excluded. All participants voluntarily participated in this study and provided written informed consent.

Tai Chi Intervention Program

The intervention was a 12-week TC program consisting of two phases. All participants attended training for 1 h per session (including 10 min of warm-up, 40 min of TC practice, and 10 min of cool-down), 3 sessions per week for the first 6 weeks in a public park in the community of the city. The purpose of the first 6-week of the intervention was to guarantee that all participants understood the instructions and mastered the essentials of TC movements. The duration and frequency of practice were progressively increased during the last 6 weeks. During the latter half of the intervention, participants trained for one, and a half hours (including 10 min of warm-up, 70 min TC practice, and 10 min cool-down) in each session, five sessions per week for 6 weeks. In total, all participants practiced TC for 2,820 min over 12 weeks in a group format (~40 participants per class). The postures involved in TC practice were from two different TC styles (modified Chen-style and 24-style) with different difficulty levels. The intervention was led by one experienced TC instructor with more than 15 years of TC experience. The comparisons of the intervention effects between these two TC styles have been reported elsewhere (Zou et al., 2019b). The present study focuses on investigating correlations between improvements of cognition and balance through the TC intervention program and therefore the two TC groups were pooled together.

Outcome Measures

Global Cognitive Function

Global cognitive function was assessed using the Bejing version Montreal Cognitive Assessment (MoCA)[1] that has been used in Chinese in previous research (Lu et al., 2011). The MoCA Is a validated brief paper-and-pencil screening test for cognitive function and detecting cognitive impairments. It consists of 12 elements to assess a variety of cognitive domains, including visuospatial ability, attention, executive function, language, orientation, memory, and abstraction. The total score of MoCA ranges from 0 to 30, with high scores representing high global cognitive ability and a score of <26 considered as experiencing symptoms of cognitive impairments.

Balance

The one leg standing test was used to evaluate static balance in unilateral stance. With their eyes closed, the participants were instructed to stand on the leg they selected, lift the knee of the other leg to ~90°, keep their arms by their sides, and maintain balance without any assistive device. Both legs were tested successively with three attempts for each leg. To prevent falls or injuries, the tester stood close to the participants throughout the trials. The test was over when either the stance foot shifted or when the lifted foot was placed on the ground. The stance duration (in seconds) for each leg in each attempt was recorded using a stopwatch and the best (longest) score was chosen and included for data analyses (Michikawa et al., 2009).

The Timed Up and Go Test (TUGT), which Is widely used in elderly populations, was used to measure dynamic balance. The TUGT measures the time taken by an individual to rise from a standard chair (with the height of ~45 cm), walk three meters, turn around, walk back to the chair, and sit down without any assistive device throughout. The participants were asked to be seated on the chair with their arms resting on the chair's arms, and then stand up on the word "go" command. The recording time started on the "go" command and stopped as the participant sat down (Chan et al., 2017). Each participant had three attempts with the best (fastest) attempt used in the analysis.

Confounding Variables

Each participant provided demographic information in a survey, including age and sex. Participants' heart rate (HR), body height and weight (Healthometer 402 KL Beam Scale weight/Height Rod, PELSTAR, McCook, IL, United States) were assessed at baseline. Body mass index (BMI; kg/m^2) was calculated. The performance of balance has been widely reported as closely related to individuals' physical mobility and fitness level (Nakano et al., 2014). Chair Stand Test (CST) and the 6-Meter Walk Test (6MWT) were used to assess the strength of lower limbs

[1] www.mocatest.org

and aerobic endurance, respectively, at baseline and immediately after the intervention (12 weeks), and therefore considered as confounding factors in this study regarding the relation between cognition and balance. These two tests have been used in the elderly population, with further details discussed elsewhere (Zhou et al., 2019).

Statistical Analysis

All statistical analyses were carried out using R (version 3.6.1) (R Core Team, 2019). First, associations between the baseline score of the cognitive parameter MoCA and the baseline score of each of the three balance parameters, namely, left leg balance, right leg balance, and TUGT were assessed using regression analysis to control for potential confounders, with interaction effects between balance parameters and confounding variables considered. As the baseline MoCA scores in the present data were not normally distributed (Shapiro–Wilk Normality Test statistic $W = 0.94$, $p = 0.0007$), they were dichotomized at a recommended clinical cutoff of 26 (coded as 1 or normal: MoCA score $\geq$26; coded as 0 or cognitive impairment: MoCA score < 26) (Hu et al., 2013). The varImp (abbreviation for "variance importance") function of the caret package (version 6.0–84) in R was used to report the relative raw importance of all the available factors in the data that are potentially correlated to the dichotomized baseline MoCA, based on main-effect-only logistic regression model (Gevrey et al., 2003). Then three logistic regression analyses were used, with the dependent variable being the dichotomized baseline MoCA score, and independent variables being each of the three baseline balance parameters (i.e., Left Leg Balance score, Right Leg Balance score, or TUGT score) respectively, plus all of the six confounding variables (i.e., Gender, Age, HR, BMI, CST, and 6MWT), as well as their interaction terms with the corresponding baseline balance parameter. Second, four paired-sample t-tests were carried out to assess the change score volume of MoCA, left leg balance, right leg balance, and TUGT across time. Third, associations between the change score of MoCA and the change score of each of the three balance parameters were assessed by three linear regression models, controlling for change score of CST, change score of 6MWT, Gender, Age, HR, and BMI.

RESULTS

Seventeen out of the total 78 participants in this study were classified as having cognitive impairment (i.e., with MoCA score <26). The characteristics of all participants and descriptive information of confounding variables are presented in **Table 1**. Mean and standard deviation (M ± SD) of the raw data on all outcome measures at baseline and post-intervention, as well as the corresponding paired t-test results for these pre and post intervention data are presented in **Table 2**. All parameters were improved after the TC intervention. No participant had MoCA score less than 26 after the TC intervention. As noted earlier, these paired *t*-test results of significant improvements of cognitive function and balance introduced by TC intervention listed in **Table 2** have already been confirmed with a different statistical method (i.e., the generalized estimation equations) for randomized trials on these data in a previously published paper (Zou et al., 2019b). Therefore, these significant results are not new but consistent findings with different type of test statistic.

TABLE 1 | Confounder information of study participants at baseline and posttest ($N = 78$).

Variable	Distribution	
Gender	**Baseline**	**Posttest**
Male (*n*)	37	
Female (*n*)	41	
Age (years)	58.92 ± 8.03	
Heart Rate (HR)	74.51 ± 7.13	
Body mass index (BMI) (kg/m^2)	24.61 ± 2.42	
Chair stand test (CST)	9.36 ± 2.14	8.39 ± 1.61
6-meter walk test (6MWT)	5.12 ± 0.99	4.93 ± 0.83

Sample frequencies are displayed for each level of categorical variable; sample mean and standard deviation are displayed for each continuous variable as the form of "M ± SD".

TABLE 2 | Cognitive function and balance data at baseline and posttest, and their paired *t*-test results.

Variable	Baseline	Posttest	Paired *t*-test statistic	*p*
Global cognitive function (MoCA)	26.41 ± 1.40	29.86 ± 0.45	22.81	< 2.2e–16 ***
Static balance (left leg balance)	3.72 ± 2.54	5.63 ± 3.14	11.81	< 2.2e–16 ***
Static balance (right leg balance)	3.61 ± 2.82	5.46 ± 2.92	9.86	2.62e–15***
Dynamic balance (TUGT)	10.10 ± 2.47	8.95 ± 1.81	–9.01	1.16e–13***

*Sample mean and standard deviation are displayed for the data as the form of "M ± SD"; Significance code: '***'p < 0.001.*

Raw Relationships Between Cognitive Function *and* Balance Parameters *at* Baseline

Estimated logistic regression coefficients corresponding to the associations between the dichotomized baseline MoCA score and the baseline balance parameter scores controlling for other covariates with interaction terms are presented in **Table 3**. Similar significant tendencies were found for the correlations between the cognitive function and each of the three balance scores. A significant and positive (0.235) interaction effect between left leg balance and CST was found (95% CI 0.030–0.441, $p = 0.0247$) combined with the positively (3.287) estimated coefficient of the main effect of left leg balance score, this finding implies that high physical fitness Is associated with high positive correlation between the global cognitive function and the left leg balance. A significant and positive (11.922) coefficient estimate of the

TABLE 3 | Results of association analysis between the baseline MoCA and baseline balance scores.

Dependent variable	Dichotomized MoCA					
Independent variable	**Left leg balance**		**Right leg balance**		**TUGT**	
	Coef.	***p***	**Coef.**	***p***	**Coef.**	***p***
Balance	3.287	0.3639	11.922	0.0261*	−4.806	0.1914
Balance*HR	0.001	0.9756	−0.062	0.1821	0.031	0.3857
Balance*Gender	0.528	0.2097	−0.250	0.5874	−0.635	0.1613
Balance*Age	0.002	0.9468	−0.078	0.1166	0.057	0.1769
Balance*BMI	−0.189	0.0686	−0.187	0.1484	0.017	0.8864
Balance*CST	0.235	0.0247*	0.242	0.0140*	−0.274	0.0346*
Balance*6MWT	−0.252	0.1944	−0.130	0.6209	0.355	0.1213

MoCA; The Chinese version of the Montreal Cognitive Assessment; BMI, body mass index; CST, Chair Stand Test; TUGT, Timed Up and Go Test; Significance code: ''p < 0.05.*

TABLE 4 | Results of the association between the change scores of MoCA and those of the balance parameters.

Dependent Variable	MoCAΔ					
Independent Variable	**Left leg balanceΔ**		**Right leg balanceΔ**		**TUGTΔ**	
	Coef.	***p***	**Coef.**	***p***	**Coef.**	***p***
BalanceΔ	0.251	0.0192*	−0.025	0.7985	0.349	0.0162*
6MWTΔ	0.106	0.5693	0.069	0.7229	−0.050	0.7937
CSTΔ	−0.120	0.3866	−0.105	0.4812	−0.208	0.1507

Δ: change score; Significance code: ''p < 0.05.*

main effect of right leg balance score was found (95% CI 1.418–22.425, p = 0.00261), implying a significantly positive correlation between the global cognitive function and the right leg balance; a significant and positive (0.242) interaction effect between right leg balance and CST was also found (95% CI 0.049–0.435, p = 0.0140), implying that high physical fitness Is associated with high positive correlation between the global cognitive function and the left leg balance. A significant and negative (−0.274) interaction effect between TUGT and CST was found (95% CI −0.528 to −0.020, p = 0.0346) combined with the negatively (−4.806) estimated coefficient of the main effect of CST score, this finding implies that high physical fitness Is associated with high positive correlation between the global cognitive function and the dynamic balance (note that low TUGT score stands for high balance ability). These results indicate that the association between the baseline global cognitive function and the baseline static and dynamic balance abilities both increase with increased strength of lower limbs among middle-aged and older adults.

Relationship Between Improvements *in* Cognitive Function *and* Balance After TC Intervention

The associations between the change score of MoCA and the change score of each of the balance parameters are presented in **Table 4**. These associations are represented by regression coefficients and their p-values. As comparisons, we also provide association results between the change score of MoCA and the change scores of physical fitness parameters (CSTΔ and 6MWTΔ). The association between the change score of MoCA and the change score of left leg balance Is significantly positive with the corresponding regression coefficient estimated as 0.251 (95% CI 0.046–0.457, p = 0.0192). The association between the change score of MoCA and the change score of TUGT Is significantly positive with the corresponding regression coefficient estimated as 0.349 (95% CI 0.071–0.626, p = 0.0162). The change score of right leg balance, as well as the change scores of physical fitness parameters (CSTΔ and 6MWTΔ) do not present significant associations with change score of MoCA. These results indicate that the improvement of cognitive function introduced by TC training among middle-aged and older adults Is associated with change of left leg static balance and dynamic balance, but not with change of right leg static balance and physical fitness.

DISCUSSION

The primary purpose of this study was to investigate the dynamic relationship between cognitive function and balance among middle-aged and older adults through TC practice while considering influencing factors such as physical fitness (i.e., strength of lower limbs and aerobic endurance). Major findings of this study include: (1) cognitive function was related to static and dynamic balance, and such correlation increases with increased strength of lower limbs; (2) Improvements in cognitive function Is also potentially associated with improvements in left leg (usually non-dominant leg) static balance and dynamic balance, but not associated with improvements in right leg (usually dominant leg) balance and physical fitness introduced by TC training.

Cognitive function and balance remarkably decline with advancing age, which often restricts participation in activities of daily living and may contribute to secondary health risks (e.g., falls) in the elderly. In line with previous studies (Pichierri et al., 2011; Alonso et al., 2016), we found that cognitive function and balance are interrelated among middle-aged and older adults. This relationship can be explained by the competition of limited central attentional resources in maintaining posture and performing cognitive tasks during activities of daily living. Moreover, when compared to young individuals, middle-aged, and older adults usually experience more cognitive distractions and spend more attentional resources in generating complex movements due to the natural ageing process (Pichierri et al., 2011). Additionally, the results in this study demonstrated the importance of muscle strength as a moderator for the relationship between improvement of cognition and that of balance among middle-aged and older adults, which Is consistent with previous literature that muscle strength serves as an important role in performing activities requiring balance and cognitive functioning (Alonso et al., 2016), and that low levels of muscle training or physical activity are a risk factor for cognitive functioning or balance in middle-aged and older adults (Holviala et al., 2006; de Souto Barreto et al., 2016).

There Is a growing interest in merging physical and cognitive stimulation (mind-body exercise), such as TC and Yoga, in health promotion in aging individuals (Ni et al., 2014; Gothe et al., 2016; Marmeleira et al., 2018). Furthermore, a recent systematic review suggested that interventions incorporating both physical and cognitive components not only benefit cognitive function, but also physical functions, including balance (Booth et al., 2016). In the present study the association of cognitive function with balance through a TC intervention program Is comparable to a cross-sectional study (Leandri et al., 2015) that evaluated cognitive function using MoCA and static balance with participants eyes closed (similar to the present study). The study found a significant association between static and dynamic balance and cognitive function in middle-aged and older adults. These findings suggest that this relationship may due to the link between the vestibular system and the hippocampus in memory performance. Future research, using neuroimaging techniques, should investigate this in future.

The major strengths of this study include the assessment of both cognitive function and balance with the consideration of other key confounding factors and the advanced statistical analyses. Although this study was exploratory in nature, these findings will add to the current literature by improving our understanding of the relationship between cognitive function and balance and the mechanism behind the beneficial effects of TC on cognition. Such research will be valuable to professionals and practitioners who have concerns with the prevention and treatment of age-related deterioration in cognitive and physical functioning in the elderly.

Despite the above advantages, findings from this study must be interpreted in light of its limitations. First, MoCA evaluates global cognitive function as a diagnostic measurement, which may lack some degree of sensitivity to TC training. In addition, the dichotomization of the MoCA variable in the study may also limit its sensitivity to TC training, or perhaps over-emphasizes its effect. Future studies should focus on the specific components of cognitive function, such as executive function and memory. Second, all participants were Chinese, which limits the generalizability of our findings to other non-Chinese populations.

CONCLUSION

Cognitive function and balance are interrelated in middle-aged and older adults when using TC practice as a new research avenue for this investigation. The global cognitive function Is associated with balance, and such association Is moderated by strength of lower limbs. Trainings or exercise forms designed for improving balance may be also likely facilitate cognitive function among middle-aged and older adults. Future research Is warranted to further confirm the cause-effect relationship of cognitive function and balance among middle-aged and older adults and its influencing factors in intervention studies with larger sample size.

ETHICS STATEMENT

The studies involving human participants were reviewed and approved by Hunan University of Science and Technology College of Sport Science Research Ethics Committee. The patients/participants provided their written informed consent to participate in this study.

AUTHOR CONTRIBUTIONS

JY, TX, and ZZ: conceptualization. TX, JY, and LY: methodology. TX: formal analysis. TX, LY, LS, JY, PL, NV, ZZ, and JY: writing – original draft preparation and writing – review and editing.

REFERENCES

Alonso, A. C., Peterson, M. D., Busse, A. L., Jacob, W., Borges, M. T. A., Serra, M. M., et al. (2016). Muscle strength, postural balance, and cognition are associated with braking time during driving in older adults. *Exp Gerontol.* 85, 13–17.

Asian Development Bank (2014). *Challenges and Opportunities of Population Aging in the People's Republic of China*. Mandaluyong: Asian Development Bank.

Booth, V., Hood, V., and Kearney, F. (2016). Interventions incorporating physical and cognitive elements to reduce falls risk in cognitively impaired older adults: a systematic review. *JBI Database Syst. Rev. Implement. Rep.* 14, 110–135.

Buchman, A. S., Boyle, P. A., Leurgans, S. E., Barnes, L. L., and Bennett, D. A. (2011). Cognitive function is associated with the development of mobility impairments in community-dwelling elders. *Am. J. Geriatric Psychiatry* 19, 571–580.

CDC Newsroom (2016). *CDC Newsroom. Centers for Disease Control and Prevention.* https://www.cdc.gov/media/releases/2016/p0922-older-adult-falls.html.

Cham, R., Perera, S., Studenski, S. A., and Bohnen, N. I. (2007). Striatal dopamine denervation and sensory integration for balance in middle-aged and older adults. *Gait Posture* 1, 516–525.

Chan, P. P., Tou, J. I. S., Tse, M. M., and Ng, S. S. (2017). Reliability and validity of the timed up and go test with a motor task in people with chronic stroke. *Arch. Phys. Med. Rehabil.* 98, 2213–2220.

Chase, J. D., Phillips, L. J., and Brown, M. (2016). Physical activity intervention effects on physical function among community-dwelling older adults: a systematic review and meta-analysis. *J. Aging Phys. Act.* 25, 149–170. doi: 10.1123/japa.2016-0040

China Population Press (2015). *Report on the Family Development in China* Beijing: China Population Press.

Clouston, S. A., Brewster, P., Kuh, D., Richards, M., Cooper, R., Hardy, R., et al. (2013). The dynamic relationship between physical function and cognition in longitudinal aging cohorts. *Epidemiol. Rev.* 35, 33–50.

de Souto Barreto, P., Delrieu, J., Andrieu, S., Vellas, B., and Rolland, Y. (2016). Physical activity and cognitive function in middle-aged and older adults: an analysis of 104,909 people from 20 countries. *InMayo Clin. Proc.* 91, 1515–1524.

Demnitz, N., Esser, P., Dawes, H., Valkanova, V., Johansen-Berg, H., Ebmeier, K. P., et al. (2016). A systematic review and meta-analysis of cross-sectional studies examining the relationship between mobility and cognition in healthy older adults. *Gait Posture* 50, 164–174.

Demnitz, N., Hogan, D. B., Dawes, H., Johansen-Berg, H., Ebmeier, K. P., Poulin, M. J., et al. (2018). Cognition and mobility show a global association in middle- and late-adulthood: analyses from the Canadian longitudinal study on aging. *Gait Posture* 64, 238–243. doi: 10.1016/j.gaitpost.2018.06.116

Gevrey, M., Dimopoulos, I., and Lek, S. (2003). Review and comparison of methods to study the contribution of variables in artificial neural network models. *Ecol. Modell.* 160, 249–264.

Gheysen, F., Poppe, L., DeSmet, A., Swinnen, S., Cardon, G., De Bourdeaudhuij, I., et al. (2018). Physical activity to improve cognition in older adults: can physical activity programs enriched with cognitive challenges enhance the effects? A systematic review and meta-analysis. *Int. J. Behav. Nutr. Phys. Act.* 15:63. doi: 10.1186/s12966-018-0697-x

Gothe, N. P., Keswani, R. K., and McAuley, E. (2016). Yoga practice improves executive function by attenuating stress levels. *Biol. Psychol.* 121, 109–116.

Holviala, J. H., Sallinen, J. M., Kraemer, W. J., Alen, M. J., and Häkkinen, K. K. (2006). Effects of strength training on muscle strength characteristics, functional capabilities, and balance in middle-aged and older women. *J. Strength Condition. Res.* 20:336.

Hu, J. B., Zhou, W. H., Hu, S. H., Jb, H., and Sh, H. (2013). Cross-cultural difference and validation of the Chinese version of montreal cognitive assessment in older adults residing in Eastern China: preliminary findings. *Arch. Gerontol. Geriatr.* 56, 38–43.

Huang, Z. G., Feng, Y. H., Li, Y. H., and Lv, C. S. (2017). Systematic review and meta-analysis: Tai Chi for preventing falls in older adults. *BMJ Open* 7:e013661. doi: 10.1136/bmjopen-2016-013661

Iwasaki, S., and Yamasoba, T. (2015). Dizziness and imbalance in the elderly: age-related decline in the vestibular system. *Aging Dis.* 6:38.

Koller, D., Hua, T., and Bynum, J. P. (2016). Treatment patterns with antidementia drugs in the United States: medicare cohort study. *J. Am. Geriatr. Soc.* 64, 1540–1548. doi: 10.1111/jgs.14226

Kong, Z., Sze, T. M., Yu, J. J., Loprinzi, P. D., Xiao, T., Yeung, A. S., et al. (2019). Tai Chi as an alternative exercise to improve physical fitness for children and adolescents with intellectual disability. *Int. J. Environ. Res. Public Health* 16:E1152. doi: 10.3390/ijerph16071152

Laurence, B. D., and Michel, L. (2017). The fall in older adults: physical and cognitive problems. *Curr. Aging Sci.* 10, 185–200.

Leandri, M., Campbell, J., Molfetta, L., Barbera, C., and Tabaton, M. (2015). Relationship between balance and cognitive performance in older people. *J. Alzheimers Dis.* 45, 705–707.

Li, K. Z. H., Bruce, H., and Downey, R. (2018). Cognition and mobility with aging. *Oxf. Res. Encycl. Psychol.* 6, 63–69. doi: 10.1093/acrefore/9780190236557.013.370

Liu, J., Xie, H., Liu, M., Wang, Z., Zou, L., Yeung, A. S., et al. (2018). The effects of Tai Chi on heart rate variability in older chinese individuals with depression. *Int. J. Environ. Res. Public Health* 15:2771. doi: 10.3390/ijerph15122771

Liu, J., Yeung, A., Xiao, T., Tian, X., Kong, Z., Zou, L., et al. (2019). Chen-style tai chi for individuals (Aged 50 Years Old or Above) with chronic non-specific low back pain: a randomized controlled trial. *Int. J. Environ. Res. Public Health* 16:517. doi: 10.3390/ijerph16030517

Lu, J., Li, D., Li, F., Zhou, A., Wang, F., Zuo, X., et al. (2011). Montreal cognitive assessment in detecting cognitive impairment in chinese elderly individuals: a population-based study. *J. Geriatr. Psychiatry Neurol.* 24, 184–190.

Marmeleira, J., Galhardas, L., and Raimundo, A. (2018). Exercise merging physical and cognitive stimulation improves physical fitness and cognitive functioning in older nursing home residents: a pilot study. *Geriatr. Nurs.* 39, 303–309.

Michikawa, T., Nishiwaki, Y., Takebayashi, T., and Toyama, Y. (2009). One-leg standing test for elderly populations. *J. Orthop. Sci.* 14, 675–685.

Mlinac, M. E., and Feng, M. C. (2016). Assessment of activities of daily living, self-care, and independence. *Arch. Clin. Neuropsychol.* 31, 506–516. doi: 10.1093/arclin/acw049

Morris, J. C. (2012). Revised criteria for mild cognitive impairment may compromise the diagnosis of Alzheimer disease dementia. *Arch. Neurol.* 69, 700–708. doi: 10.1001/archneurol.2011.3152

Nakano, M. M., Otonari, T. S., Takara, K. S., Carmo, C. M., and Tanaka, C. (2014). Physical performance, balance, mobility, and muscle strength decline at different rates in elderly people. *J. Phys. Ther. Sci.* 26, 583–586. doi: 10.1589/jpts.26.583

Ni, M., Mooney, K., Richards, L., Balachandran, A., Sun, M., Harriell, K., et al. (2014). Comparative impacts of Tai Chi, balance training, and aspecially-designed yoga program on balance in older fallers. *Arch. Phys. MedRehabil.* 95, 1620–1628.

Petersen, R. C. (2016). Mild cognitive impairment. *Continuum* 22, 404–418. doi: 10.1212/CON.0000000000000313

Pichierri, G., Wolf, P., Murer, K., and de Bruin. (2011). Cognitive and cognitive-motor interventions affecting physical functioning: a systematic review. *BMC Geriatr.* 11:29. doi: 10.1186/1471-2318-11-29

R Core Team (2019). *R: A Language and Environment for Statistical Computing.* Vienna: R foundation for statistical computing.

Singh-Manoux, A., Kivimaki, M., Glymour, M. M., Elbaz, A., Berr, C., Ebmeier, K. P., et al. (2012). Timing of onset of cognitive decline: results from Whitehall II prospective cohort study. *BMJ* 5:d7622.

Smith-Ray, R. L., Hughes, S. L., Prohaska, T. R., Little, D. M., Jurivich, D. A., Hedeker, D., et al. (2015). Impact of cognitive training on balance and gait in older adults. *J. Gerontol. B Psychol. Sci. Soc. Sci.* 70, 357–366.

Subramaniam, S., and Bhatt, T. (2017). Effect of Yoga practice on reducing cognitive-motor interference for improving dynamic balance control in healthy adults. *Complement. Ther. Med.* 30, 30–35.

Wayne, P. M., Walsh, J. N., Taylor-Piliae, R. E., Wells, R. E., Papp, K. V., Donovan, N. J., et al. (2014). Effect of tai chi on cognitive performance in older adults: systematic review and meta-analysis. *J. Am. Geriatr. Soc.* 62, 25–39. doi: 10.1111/jgs.12611

Wayne, P. M., Yeh, G., and Mehta, D. (2016). Minding the mind-body literature. *J. Altern. Complement. Med.* 22, 849–852.

Weber, B., Koschutnig, K., Schwerdtfeger, A., Rominger, C., Papousek, I., Weiss, E. M., et al. (2019). Learning unicycling evokes manifold changes in gray and white matter networks related to motor and cognitive functions. *Sci. Rep.* 9:4324.

Whetten-Goldstein, K., Sloan, F., Kulas, E., Cutson, T., and Schenkman, M. (2015). The burden of Parkinson's disease on society, family, and the individual. *J. Am. Geriatr. Soc.* 45:7.

World Health Organization [WHO] (2017). *World Health Organization Fact sheets: Dementia*. Available from: https://www.who.int/news-room/fact-sheets/detail/dementia.

Zhang, Y., Li, C., Zou, L., Liu, X., and Song, W. (2018). The effects of mind-body exercise on cognitive performance in elderly: a systematic review and meta-analysis. *Int. J. Environ. Res. Public Health* 15:2791.

Zhou, S., Zhang, Y., Kong, Z., Loprinzi, P. D., Hu, Y., Ye, J., et al. (2019). The effects of tai chi on markers of atherosclerosis, lower-limb physical function, and cognitive ability in adults aged over 60: a randomized controlled trial. *Int. J. Environ. Res. Public Health* 16:753.

Zou, L., Han, J., Li, C., Yeung, A. S., Hui, S. S., Tsang, W. W. N., et al. (2018a). Effects of tai chi on lower limb proprioception in adults aged over 55: a systematic review and meta-analysis. *Arch. Phys. Med. Rehabil.*. 100, 1102–1113. doi: 10.1016/j.apmr.2018.07.425

Zou, L., Loprinzi, P. D., Yeung, A. S., Zeng, N., and Huang, T. (2019a). The beneficial effects of mind-body exercises for people with mild cognitive impairment: a systematic review with meta-analysis. *Arch. Phys. Med. Rehabil.* 100, 1556–1573. doi: 10.1016/j.apmr.2019.03.009

Zou, L., Loprinzi, P. D., Yu, J. J., Yang, L., Li, C., Yeung, A. S., et al. (2019b). Superior effects of modified chen-style tai chi versus 24-style tai chi on cognitive function, fitness, and balance performance in adults over 55. *Brain Sci.* 9:102.

Zou, L., Sasaki, J. E., Wei, G. X., Huang, T., Yeung, A. S., Neto, O. B., et al. (2018b). Effects of mind-body exercises (Tai Chi/Yoga) on heart rate variability parameters and perceived stress: a systematic review with meta-analysis of randomized controlled trials. *J. Clin. Med.* 7:404. doi: 10.3390/jcm7110404

Zou, L., Yeung, A., Li, C., Chiou, S. Y., Zeng, N., Tzeng, H. M., et al. (2018c). Effects of mind-body movements on balance function in stroke survivors: a meta-analysis of randomized controlled trials. *Int. J. Environ. Res. Public Health* 15:1292.

Zou, L., Yeung, A., Li, C., Wei, G. X., Chen, K. W., Kinser, P. A., et al. (2018d). Effects of meditative movements on major depressive disorder: a systematic review and meta-analysis of randomized controlled trials. *J. Clin. Med.* 7:195. doi: 10.3390/jcm7080195

Zou, L., Wang, C., Chen, K., Shu, Y., Chen, X., Luo, L., et al. (2017a). The effect of Taichi practice on attenuating bone mineral density loss: a systematic review and meta-analysis of randomized controlled trials. *Int. J. Environ. Res. Public Health* 14:1000.

Zou, L., Wang, C., Tian, Z., Wang, H., and Shu, Y. (2017b). Effect of yang-style tai chi on gait parameters and musculoskeletal flexibility in healthy chinese older women. *Sports* 5:52.

14

Effects of Probiotics on Cognitive Reactivity, Mood and Sleep Quality

Angela Marotta [1,2]*, *Eleonora Sarno* [3†], *Antonio Del Casale* [4†], *Marco Pane* [5], *Luca Mogna* [5], *Angela Amoruso* [5], *Giovanna E. Felis* [3] *and Mirta Fiorio* [1]*

[1] *Department of Neurosciences, Biomedicine and Movement Sciences, University of Verona, Verona, Italy,* [2] *Neurology Unit, Neuroscience Department, Azienda Ospedaliera Universitaria Integrata, Verona, Italy,* [3] *Department of Biotechnology, University of Verona, Verona, Italy,* [4] *Open Innovation Department, Microbion SRL, Verona, Italy,* [5] *BIOLAB RESEARCH SRL, Novara, Italy*

***Correspondence:**
Angela Marotta
angela.marotta@univr.it
Mirta Fiorio
mirta.fiorio@univr.it

† *These authors have contributed equally to this work*

Recent demonstration that probiotics administration has positive effects on mood state in healthy populations suggests its possible role as an adjunctive therapy for depression in clinical populations and as a non-invasive strategy to prevent depressive mood state in healthy individuals. The present study extends current knowledge on the beneficial effects of probiotics on psychological well-being, as measured by changes in mood (e.g., cognitive reactivity to sad mood, depression, and anxiety), personality dimensions, and quality of sleep, which have been considered as related to mood. For this double-blind, placebo-controlled study 38 healthy volunteers assigned to an experimental or control group assumed a daily dose of a probiotic mixture (containing *Lactobacillus fermentum* LF16, *L. rhamnosus* LR06, *L. plantarum* LP01, and *Bifidobacterium longum* BL04) or placebo, respectively, for 6 weeks. Mood, personality dimensions, and sleep quality were assessed four times (before the beginning of the study, at 3 and 6 weeks, and at 3 weeks of washout). A significant improvement in mood was observed in the experimental group, with a reduction in depressive mood state, anger, and fatigue, and an improvement in sleep quality. No between-groups differences were found. These findings corroborate the positive effect of probiotics on mood state and suggest that probiotics administration may improve psychological well-being by ameliorating aspects of mood and sleep quality.

Keywords: psychological well-being, probiotics, mood, sleep quality, personality traits

INTRODUCTION

Gut and brain communicate with each other via the gut-brain axis, a specific pathway that involves the neural, endocrine, and immune systems (1–4). The intestinal microbiota plays a crucial role in this bidirectional communication, since it can influence mood and cognitive functions by producing neurotransmitter precursors that reach the brain through the endocrine and the autonomic nervous systems where they regulate the level of specific neurotransmitters (5, 6).

It has been hypothesized that modifying the microbial environment by means of probiotics, for instance, may help to improve mood and cognitive functions. This hypothesis is supported by studies using animal models. Li et al. (7) found an improvement in spatial memory and problem solving in rats after probiotics supplementation. Other studies using rodent models showed beneficial effects of probiotics on anxiety and depression (8, 9). Research involving human participants is still scant. Among the existing literature on this topic, some studies showed no effects of probiotics on mood (10), but other found promising data. For instance, a recent fMRI study demonstrated that 4 weeks of probiotic intake reduced the activity of brain regions involved in emotional processing (11). Moreover, a recent triple blind, randomized, placebo-controlled study showed reduced cognitive reactivity to sad mood after a 4-week intervention with multispecies probiotics (12). Sleep quality also seems to benefit from probiotic supplementation. Takada et al. (13) reported an improvement in sleep quality in academic students during a period of increasing stress after 11 weeks of probiotics consumption. Beneficial effects of probiotics were also reported in studies involving clinical populations. For instance, Rao et al. (14) found that anxiety in patients with chronic fatigue syndrome was reduced after 2 months of probiotics intake. Overall, these studies suggest that probiotics administration might be used to improve mood and cognitive functions (e.g., emotional processing).

The aim of the present explorative study was to extend our current knowledge about the beneficial effects of probiotics on psychological well-being by investigating different aspects of mood (e.g., cognitive reactivity to sad mood, depression, and anxiety) and various dimensions of personality related to mood, including optimism, pessimism, and motivational drive. Also, we investigated the potential effects of probiotics on sleep quality, which is also known to affect mood (15). In line with previous findings, we expected an improvement in mood only in the group that received the probiotics. Additionally, we hypothesized an improvement in perceived sleep quality and personality dimensions known to be related to anxiety and depression.

Examining the ways in which probiotics influence mood, personality traits, and sleep may help to gain a better understanding of the relationship between the gut and the brain and to develop new applications for psychological well-being.

MATERIALS AND METHODS

Participants were recruited from students of the University of Verona (Italy) where the investigation took place and where data were collected. Computation of the sample size was performed with G-Power 3.1 (16), considering F-test within-between interaction with two groups (experimental and control) and four evaluation sessions (T0, T1, T2, T3) (see the procedure for details). Assuming a priori medium effect size of 0.25 (17), an α error probability of 0.05, and a power (1-β error probability) of 0.90, the resulting total sample size is 30. We recruited more participants to prevent reduction in statistical power due to potential drop-outs.

Thirty-eight male and female adults volunteered for the study (13 women, mean age $\pm$ SD, 22.00 $\pm$ 3.02, age range, 19–33 years). Inclusion criterion was an age between 18 and 35 years. Exclusion criteria were: psychiatric or neurological disorders, celiac disease, lactose intolerance, or allergies or other ongoing illnesses (i.e., irritable bowel syndrome, diabetes, ulcerative colitis, etc.) or recent antibiotic treatment (i.e., <3 months before the beginning of the study). Participants who smoked more than 10 cigarettes per day were excluded.

Participants were screened via structured interviews by three experimenters (MF, AM, ES) who collected data on demographics and physical activity. In order to account for potential bias due to premenstrual syndrome, the women were also asked about their monthly physical and emotional changes.

Participants were assigned to receive probiotics or placebo by means of stratified randomization method. Since the amount of physical activity can influence cognitive functions, mood and sleep quality (18, 19), we took this covariate into account in the randomization process. More precisely, we applied the stratified randomization method to address the need of balancing the groups for the amount of physical activity (20, 21). Following this method, participants were stratified into two blocks (Highs and Lows) of 19 participants each depending on the amount of physical activity. More precisely, according to the mean value of physical activity per week of the whole sample (2.87 $\pm$ 0.99 h), the block of Highs was made of participants with more than 2.87 h per week and the block of Lows was made of participants with <2.87 h per week). Then, participants were allocated to the experimental or control group by means of simple randomization through a computer generated list that guarantees the same number of subjects and equivalent physical activity by type of intervention. In this way, sample size and amount of physical activity were balanced in the experimental and control group. After randomization, we confirmed that the level of physical activity was balanced between the two groups [$t_{(34)} = 1.031$, $p = 0.310$]. Two experimenters (MA and ES) enrolled participants, generated the random allocation sequence, and assigned participants to interventions. The experimenters and the participants were blinded for group allocation.

The study was conducted according to the principles expressed in the Declaration of Helsinki and was approved by the Ethical committee of Verona Hospital (Azienda Ospedaliera Universitaria Intregrata, AOUI Verona, 766CESC). Written informed consent was obtained before the start of the study. The protocol is registered in ClinicalTrials.gov with the number ID: NCT03539263. The full trial protocol can be accessed upon request at Probiotical S.p.A. and to the principal investigator MF.

Procedure

The probiotic product or placebo was administered for 6 weeks followed by a 3-week washout period for a total duration of 9 weeks. The experimental group received 42 sachets of the product (one for each day), each containing 4×10^9 colony forming unit/active fluorescent unit (CFU/AFU) 2.5 g freeze-dried powder of the probiotic mixture containing *Lactobacillus fermentum* LF16 (DSM 26956), *L. rhamnosus* LR06 (DSM 21981), *L. plantarum* LP01 (LMG P-21021), and *Bifidobacterium longum* BL04 (DSM 23233) (Probiotical S.p.A., Novara, Italy).

The mixture was composed with commercially available probiotic strains extensively used for food supplement formulations.

The study materials were analyzed by Biolab Research S.r.l., Novara, Italy, via flow cytometry (ISO 19344:2015 IDF 232:2015, $> 4 \times 10^9$ AFU) and plate count method (Biolab Research Method 014-06, $>4 \times 10^9$ CFU) to confirm target cell count. The control group received 42 sachets of placebo, each containing 2.5 g of maltodextrin in powder form. The placebo powder was indistinguishable from the probiotics powder in color, taste, and smell, but contained no probiotic bacteria. Participants were instructed to dissolve the powder in water or milk and drink it in the morning with breakfast.

A mobile application developed *ad hoc* (AgendaQR, Bussola Labs, Verona, Italy) was installed on the participants' phones at the beginning of the study; adherence to the study protocol was facilitated by means of a daily reminder to take the probiotics product or placebo and to scan the QR code attached to the sachet. If a participant failed to scan the code, the application kept a record of the missed daily intake.

All participants completed an extensive battery of psychological questionnaires (see next paragraph for a details) at four time points: before intake of the probiotics product or placebo (baseline) (T0), at 3 (T1), and 6 (T2) weeks after the first intake, and then at 3 weeks of washout (T3). E-Prime 2.0 software (Psychology Software Tools Inc., Sharpsburg, PA, USA) was used to present the questionnaires and record the responses. Each session lasted about 45 min.

Questionnaires Measuring Mood-Related Aspects

Leiden Index of Depression Sensitivity-Revised Test

The primary outcome of our study was the difference in the scores at the Leiden Index of Depression Sensitivity-Revised test (LEIDS-R) (22) between the experimental and control groups. The LEIDS-R is a self-report questionnaire that tests cognitive reactivity to sad mood, which is an index of cognitive vulnerability to depression. It consists of 34 items describing different situations. Before answering the items, participants are asked to take a few minutes to imagine their feelings and thoughts when they experience a sad mood. They then rate how much each item applies to themselves on a 5-point scale ranging from 0 (*not at all*) to 4 (*very strongly*). Of note, the experimenter emphasizes that each item describes a situation happening on *a day that is not good, but you don't feel depressed.* The LEIDS-R consists of 6 subscales: Hopelessness/Suicidality (5 items), Acceptance/Coping (6 items), Aggression (5 items), Control/Perfectionism (6 items), Risk aversion (6 items), and Rumination (6 items). The total score for each subscale is obtained by adding the scores from the corresponding item. The range of the total score for the Aggression and Hopelessness/Suicidality subscales is from 0 to 20. The range of the total score for the other three scales is from 0 to 24. The higher the total subscale score, the higher the vulnerability to the assessed dimension.

State Trait Anxiety Inventory

The State Trait Anxiety Inventory, STAI, (23) is a self-report questionnaire that measures the presence and severity of current symptoms of anxiety and the propensity to be anxious (24). There are separate subscales for two anxiety components: state anxiety (STAI—form Y1) and trait anxiety (STAI—form Y2). Each subscale contains 20 items. The STAI—Y1 measures the current anxiety state by asking participants to rate how they actually feel (e.g., calm, tense, worried) on an intensity scale from 1 (*not at all*) to 4 (*very much so*). The STAI—Y2 measures the propensity to anxiety by asking participants to rate how they generally feel in their life (e.g., confident) on a frequency scale from 1 (*almost never*) to 4 (*almost always*). The total score for each subscale is obtained by adding the scores of all items. The score for the anxiety-absent items are reversed. The range of the total score for each subscale is 20–80, wherein the higher the score, the higher the degree of state or trait anxiety. Scores of 39–40 have been defined as a cut-off for clinically relevant symptoms of state anxiety (24).

Beck Depression Inventory

The Beck Depression Inventory, BDI-2 (25), is a self-report questionnaire that measures the occurrence and severity of current depressive symptoms. It consists of 21 groups of sentences describing different depression-related feelings and thoughts (e.g., self-dislike, loss of interest, irritability, changes in sleep pattern). Participants are asked to choose the statement from a group of sentences that best describes how they have been feeling in the past 2 weeks including the current day. Each statement corresponds to a specific severity score (range, 0–3). The total score is obtained by adding the statement scores (range, 0–63), wherein the higher the total score, the higher the severity of depressive state (minimal depression, 0–13; mild depression, 14–19; moderate depression, 20–28; severe depression, 29–63).

Profile of Mood State

The Profile of Mood State, POMS, (26) is a self-report questionnaire that assesses mood. It consists of 58 items (words or sentences) that describe feelings that people usually have. For each item, participants rate on a 5-point scale from 0 (*not at all*) to 4 (*extremely*) how they have been feeling the past week including the current day. The items are grouped in 6 subscales: Tension (9 items), Depression (15 items), Anger (12 items), Fatigue (7 items), Confusion (7 items), and Vigor (8 items). The Vigor scale is in inverted relationship with the other scales since it assesses positive feelings (e.g., to be lively, active, energetic). The total score for each scale is obtained by adding the related item, wherein the higher the total score of the scale, the higher the level of the related mood.

Sleep Quality Questionnaire

Pittsburgh Sleep Quality Index

The Pittsburgh Sleep Quality Index, PSQI, (27, 28) is a self-report questionnaire that assesses sleep quality for the majority of days and nights in the past months. It consists of 19 questions. The first four investigate usual bedtime, the number of minutes needed to fall asleep, the usual getting up time, and the hours of sleep per night. The other questions are related to other aspects of sleep quality rated on scales appropriate for the specific question. The items are weighted on a 0–3 interval scale and grouped in seven component scores (i.e., subjective sleep quality, sleep latency, sleep duration, use of sleeping medication, daytime dysfunction, sleep duration, habitual sleep efficiency). A global PSQI score (range, 0–21) is obtained by adding up the component scores, wherein the lower the PSQI global score, the better the sleep quality.

Questionnaires Measuring Personality-Related Aspects

Temperament and Character Inventory

The Temperament and Character Inventory, TCI, (29) is a self-report, true-false questionnaire that measures two components of personality: temperament and character. Temperament refers to automatic responses to perceptual stimuli likely reflecting hereditable biases in information processing (29). It consists of four dimensions: novelty seeking (system of behavioral activation), harm avoidance (system of behavioral inhibition), reward dependence (system for maintenance of ongoing behavior), and persistence (system of partial reinforcement and active behavior despite fatigue and frustration). Based on the psychobiological model of personality (29), each dimension is related to specific neurotransmitters: dopamine for novelty seeking; GABA and serotonin for harm avoidance; noradrenaline and serotonin for reward dependence, and glutamate and serotonin for persistence. Character refers to dimensions determined by the environment rather than by inheritance. These dimensions regulate the cognitive processes of perception and emotion defined by the person's temperament (30). The character dimensions are: self-directedness (identification with autonomous self and ability to solve situations); cooperativeness (extent to which other people are viewed as part of the self); and self-transcendence (identification with a unity of all things). Based on this model of personality, the TCI consists of 240 items grouped on four temperament scales (40 items for novelty seeking; 35 for harm avoidance; 24 for reward dependence; 8 for persistence) and three character scales (44 items for self-directedness; 42 for cooperativeness; 33 for self-transcendence). The total score for each scale is obtained by adding the related items (range of total scores: novelty seeking, 0–40; harm avoidance, 0–35; reward dependence, 0–24; persistence, 0–8; self-directedness, 0–44; cooperativeness, 0–42; self-transcendence 0–33). The higher the total score, the higher the level of the personality dimension described by the scale.

Cope Orientation to the Problems Experienced—New Italian Version

The Cope Orientation to Problem Experienced—New Italian Version, COPE-NIV, (31) is a self-report questionnaire that measures coping strategies: the cognitive and behavioral strategies people use to manage stressful situations (32). The COPE-NIV consists of 60 items that describe different coping strategies. Participants are asked to rate each item on a frequency scale from 1 (*I usually don't do this*) to 4 (*I usually do this*). The items are grouped in five essentially independent components: social support (12 items), avoidance strategies (16 items), positive attitude (12 items), problem solving (12 items), and turning to religion (8 items). The total score for the subscales is obtained by adding the corresponding item scores. The higher the total subscale score, the higher the frequency in adopting the coping strategy described by that subscale.

Behavioral Inhibition System and Behavioral Activation System Scale

The Behavioral Inhibition and Behavioral Activation Scale, BIS/BAS, (33) is a self-report questionnaire that measures an individual's sensitivity to behavioral inhibition and behavioral activation systems. The behavioral inhibition system (BIS) mediates responses to potential punishment and suppresses behavior that is expected to lead to threat, punishment or non-reward (34). Conversely, the behavioral activation or approach system mediates responses to rewards expectancy (34) and facilitates behavior that brings the person closer to expected rewards. The BIS/BAS scale consists of 24 items grouped in four subscales: BIS (7 items), BAS Drive (4 items), BAS Fun seeking (4 items), and BAS Reward responsiveness (5 items). Four items serve as control. Participants rate how much each statement describes themselves from 0 (*It does not describe me at all*) to 5 (*It completely describes me*). The total score for each scale is obtained by adding the items of the respective scale; the total BIS score ranges from 1 to 35 and the total BAS score ranges from 1 to 65. The higher the total score, the higher the sensitivity of behavioral inhibition and behavioral activation systems.

Life-Orientation Test-Revisited

The Life Orientation Test-revisited, LOT-R, (35) is a self-report measure of dispositional optimism and pessimism. It consists of 10 items: 3 are worded positively; 3 are worded negatively; and 4 are control items. Participants rate their agreement with each item on a 5-point scale from 0 (*strongly disagree*) to 4 (*strongly agree*). The LOT-R total score is obtained by adding all items except the 4 control items. The three negatively worded items are related to pessimism and are reverse scored. The LOT-R total score ranges from 0 to 24. The higher the total score, the higher the degree of optimism (high optimism, 19–24; moderate optimism, 14–18; low optimism, 0–13).

Data Analyses

Distribution of age and gender was analyzed with an independent sample t-test and a chi-square test, respectively. Questionnaire data were first checked for normality by means of the Shapiro–Wilk test ($p > 0.05$). Since the data were not normally distributed, non-parametric tests were used. The Friedman test was used to compare questionnaire scores across time points (T0, T1, T2, T3) separately for each group (experimental and control). *Post-hoc* comparisons were performed using the Wilcoxon signed-rank test. Bonferroni correction was applied and the adjusted critical level of significance for multiple comparisons was set at $p < 0.017$. The Mann–Whitney U-test was used to compare questionnaire scores between-groups. $P < 0.05$ were considered statistically significant. Spearman correlations were used to explore the relationship between mood and sleep quality, separately for each group. Mean and standard deviation of questionnaire data are reported in **Tables S1, S2**.

RESULTS

Nineteen participants assumed probiotics and made up the experimental group (7 women, mean age ± SD, 21.47 ± 2.22 years); 19 participants received placebo and made up the control group (6 women, mean age, 22.53 ± 3.64 years). One subject from the experimental group and four subjects from the control group did not complete the study because they underwent therapeutic interventions with antibiotics. The final study sample was 33 subjects: 18 in the experimental group (7 women, mean age, 21.61 ± 2.2 years) and 15 in the control group (5 women, mean age, 21.67 ± 2.19 years). The two groups did not differ by age [$t_{(31)} = -0.115$, $p = 0.909$] or gender distribution [$\chi^2_{(1)} = 0.109$, $p = 0.741$].

Recruitment started 28 November 2016 and follow-up finished 15 June 2017.

Mood-Related Aspects

Leiden Index of Depression Sensitivity-Revised Test

No significant time effect on the total score and subscale scores of the LEIDS-R was noted for the experimental and the control group. There was a significant between-group difference in the *acceptance* subscale scores at 6 weeks (T2). This difference was due to the higher scores recorded in the experimental group (mean ± SD, 5.33 ± 5.11) as compared to the control group (mean ± SD, 2.93 ± 3.51) ($Z = -2.162$, $p = 0.031$, effect size $= -0.376$) (**Figure 1**).

State Trait Anxiety Inventory

No significant time effect on STAI scores in the experimental and the control group was found: STAI-Y1 (state anxiety) (experimental group, $p = 0.612$; control group, $p = 0.412$) and STAI-Y2 (trait anxiety) (experimental group, $p = 0.161$; control group, $p = 0.085$). Moreover, there were no between-group differences in STAI-Y1 (all time points, $p > 0.218$) and STAI-Y2 (all time points, $p > 0.436$). The state and trait dimensions of anxiety remained constant in both groups at all four time points, discarding a potential effect of probiotics intake on both anxiety components.

Beck Depression Inventory

No significant time effect on BDI-2 scores in the experimental ($p = 0.137$) and the control group ($p = 0.409$) was found; there were no between-group differences at any of the four time points (all time points, $p > 0.383$). Probiotics intake had no effect on depressive symptoms as assessed by the BDI-2.

Profile of Mood State

A significant time effect on the *depression* subscale scores for the experimental group [$\chi^2_{(3)} = 12.43$, $p = 0.006$] was found. *Post-hoc* comparisons with Wilcoxon signed rank test (after Bonferroni correction, $p < 0.017$) showed that this result was due to lower scores after 6 weeks of treatment (T2) (mean ± SD, 6.22 ± 7.26) compared to baseline (T0) (mean ± SD, 11.00 ± 9.45) ($Z = -2.596$, $p = 0.009$, effect size $= -0.433$). Moreover, the effect was maintained after 3 weeks of washout, as revealed by a significant difference between T3 (mean ± SD, 5.67 ± 7.15) and T0 ($Z = -2.452$, $p = 0.014$, effect size $= -0.409$). These results suggest that the experimental group experienced a reduction in depressive mood state and that this effect remained nearly stable after 3 weeks of washout (**Figure 2A**).

A significant time effect [$\chi^2_{(3)} = 17.52$, $p = 0.001$] was also found on the *anger-hostility* scale scores for the experimental group. *Post-hoc* comparisons showed that this effect was due to lower scores after 3 weeks of probiotics intake (T1) (mean ± SD, 6.56 ± 4.87) compared to baseline (T0) (mean ± SD, 10.39 ± 6.79) ($Z = -2.695$, $p = 0.007$, effect size $= -0.449$), and after 6 weeks of probiotics intake (T2) (mean ± SD, 6.78 ± 5.11) compared to baseline ($Z = -2.411$, $p = 0.016$, effect size $= -0.402$), as well as after 3 weeks of washout (T3) (mean ± SD, 5.28 ± 4.66) compared to baseline ($Z = -2.921$, $p = 0.003$, effect size $= -0.487$) (**Figure 2B**).

A significant time effect was noted for the *fatigue* subscale scores [$\chi^2_{(3)} = 11.75$, $p = 0.008$]. This effect was due to a lower score at T2 (mean ± SD, 7.06 ± 4.24) compared to T0 (mean ± SD, 8.89 ± 4.30) ($Z = -2.802$, $p = 0.005$, effect size $= -0.467$) and at T3 (mean ± SD, 5.33 ± 4.12) compared to T0 ($Z = -2.556$, $p = 0.011$, effect size $= -0.426$) (**Figure 2C**). A significant time effect was also observed for the subscale *confusion* [$\chi^2_{(3)} = 14.45$, $p = 0.003$]. This effect was not further confirmed at *post-hoc* analysis, however ($p > 0.022$ for all comparisons). No significant time effect on any of the subscales for the control group. Finally, no between-group differences were found ($p > 0.079$ all-time points and subscales).

Sleep Quality

Pittsburgh Sleep Quality Index

A significant time effect in the experimental group [$\chi^2_{(3)} = 12.16$, $p = 0.007$] was found. *Post-hoc* comparisons showed that this effect was due to lower scores after 6 weeks of probiotics intake (T2) (mean ± SD, 4.00 ± 1.64) compared to baseline (T0) (mean ± SD, 5.61 ± 2.17) ($Z = -2.820$, $p = 0.005$, effect size $= -0.470$) (**Figure 3**). No significant time effect was noted for the control group nor were between-group differences found.

Correlations Between Mood and Sleep Quality

In the experimental group significant positive correlations were found between PSQI scores and STAI Y2 (T0, $r = 0.716$, $p = 0.001$; T1, $r = 0.623$ $p = 0.006$) and BDI2 (T2, $r = 0.634$, $p = 0.005$). PSQI positively correlated also with several scales of LEIDS-r: Hopelessness (T3, $r = 0.502$, $p = 0.034$); Acceptance (T3, $r = 0.834$, $p < 0.001$); Aggression (T0, $r = 0.544$, $p = 0.020$); Risk aversion (T0, $r = 0.472$, $p = 0.048$). Significant correlations were also found with different scales of POMS as well. Precisely, PSQI positively correlated with Tension (T0, $r = 0.628$, $p = 0.005$; T2, $r = 0.643$, $p = 0.004$), Depression (T0, $r = 0.709$, $p = 0.001$; T2, $r = 0.549$, $p = 0.018$), Anger (T0, $r = 0.829$, $p < 0.001$; T2, $r = 0.679$, $p = 0.002$), Fatigue (T0, $r = 0.595$, $p = 0.009$; T2, $r = 0.560$, $p = 0.016$), and Confusion (T0, $r = 0.595$, $p = 0.009$) subscales. Negative correlations, instead, were found with the Vigor subscale (T0, $r = -0.545$, $p = 0.019$; T3, $r = -0.507$, $p = 0.032$). As stated before, the higher the scores at PSQI, the lower the sleep quality. Thus, positive correlations with measures of anxiety (i.e., STAI Y2) and depression (i.e., BDI2) suggest that the lower the sleep quality, the higher the anxiety and depression. Similarly, poor sleep quality is related to higher hopelessness, acceptance, aggression, risk aversion as measured by the LEIDS-r subscales, and tension, depressive mood state, anger, fatigue, and confusions as measured by the POMS subscales. Conversely, the negative correlation with the Vigor subscale suggests that the better the sleep quality, the higher the level of vigor experimented by participants. In the control group PSQI positively correlated

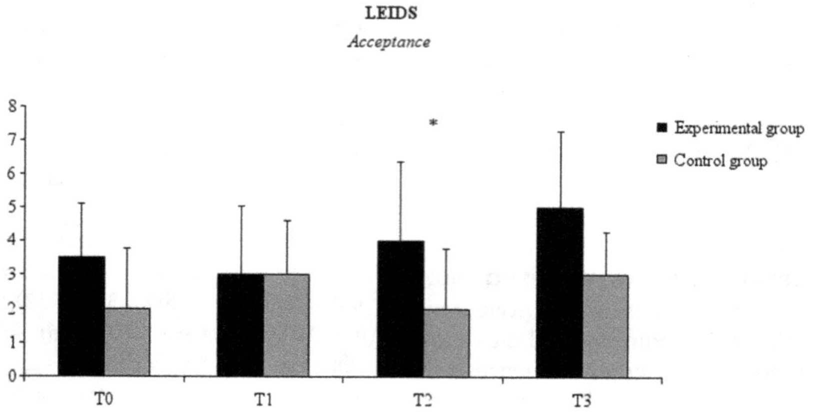

FIGURE 1 | Median LEIDS—R score, Acceptance subscale for the experimental (black columns) and the control (gray columns) groups at all-time points. Error bars represent 95% Confidence Interval. Asterisks indicate between-groups significant differences ($p < 0.05$).

with STAI-Y1 (T1, $r = 0.550, p = 0.034$; T2, $r = 0.638, p = 0.010$), STAI-Y2 (T1, $r = 0.707, p = 0.003$; T2, $r = 0.738, p = 0.002$) and BDI2 (T1, $r = 0.710, p = 0.003$). Significant correlations were also observed for several subscales of POMS. More precisely, sleep quality positively correlated with Tension (T0, $r = 0.537$, $p = 0.039$; T1, $r = 0.601, p = 0.018$; T2, $r = 0.595, p = 0.019$), Anger (T1, $r = 0.615, p = 0.015$), Fatigue (T2, $r = 0.677, p = 0.006$), and Confusion (T1, $r = 0.694$, $p = 0.004$) subscales, while negatively correlated with the Vigor subscale (T1, $r = -0.771$, $p = 0.001$; T2, $r = -0.537$, $p = 0.039$). These results suggest that a poor sleep quality relates to higher anxiety, depression, tension, anger, fatigue, and confusion. Conversely, a good sleep quality relates to higher vigor.

Personality-Related Aspects

Temperament and Character Inventory

No significant time effect on any of the TCI subscale scores in either the experimental or the control group was found. Significant between-group differences were found for four subscale scores at different time points. There was a significant group effect for the *novelty seeking* subscale score only at T3 ($Z = -2.209$, $p = 0.027$, effect size $= -0.385$), where the scores were higher for the experimental group. This finding might suggest that at the last assessment the participants who had taken probiotics for 6 weeks were more prone to look for new experiences; in other words, they may have been more activated by novel stimuli as compared to the controls. In addition, the *persistence* subscale scores differed between the groups; the difference was due to lower scores for the experimental group at all-time points (T0, $Z = -3.127, p = 0.002$, effect size $= -0.544$; T1, $Z = -2.906, p = 0.004$, effect size $= -0.506$; T2, $Z = -2.948$, $p = 0.003$, effect size $= -0.513$; T3, $Z = -2.820$, $p = 0.005$, effect size $= -0.491$). This means that starting from baseline, the experimental group was less persistent and that these differences remained constant independent of probiotics intake.

A significant group effect was found for the *self-directedness* subscale scores at T3 ($Z = -2.497$, $p = 0.013$, effect size $= -0.435$). This difference was due to the lower scores for the experimental group, suggesting that at 3 weeks since their last intake of the probiotic the experimental group was less self-directed than the controls.

Finally, there was a significant between-group difference in *cooperativeness* subscales scores at T2 ($Z = -2.233$, $p = 0.026$, effect size $= -0.389$), with lower scores noted for the experimental group. This finding might suggest that after 6 weeks of probiotics intake, the participants who had taken the probiotics were more self-focused than those who did not.

Coping Orientation to Problem Experienced

No significant time effect on any of the COPE subscale scores in either the experimental or the control group was noted. Significant between-group differences were found for the *Avoidance Strategies* subscale scores at T2 ($Z = -2.590, p = 0.010$, effect size $= -0.451$) and T3 ($Z = -2.728$, $p = 0.006$, effect size $= -0.475$), where the scores were higher for the experimental group, suggesting that they were more apt than the control group to use avoidance strategies after 6 weeks of probiotics intake and after 3 weeks of washout.

Moreover, there was a significant between-group difference in the *Positive Attitude* subscale scores at T1 ($Z = 2.412, p = 0.016$, effect size $= -0.420$) due to lower scores for the experimental group, suggesting that after 3 weeks of probiotics intake, the experimental group had a lower positive attitude toward problem solving than the controls. This difference was not observed at the other time points, however.

Behavioral Inhibition System and Behavioral Activation System Scale

No differences between time points for either group nor between-group differences were found. These results suggest that probiotics intake did not affect the inhibition or the activation system.

Life Orientation Test-Revisited Test (LOT-R)

No significant time effect on either group was found. Moreover, no differences between-groups were found. These results suggest

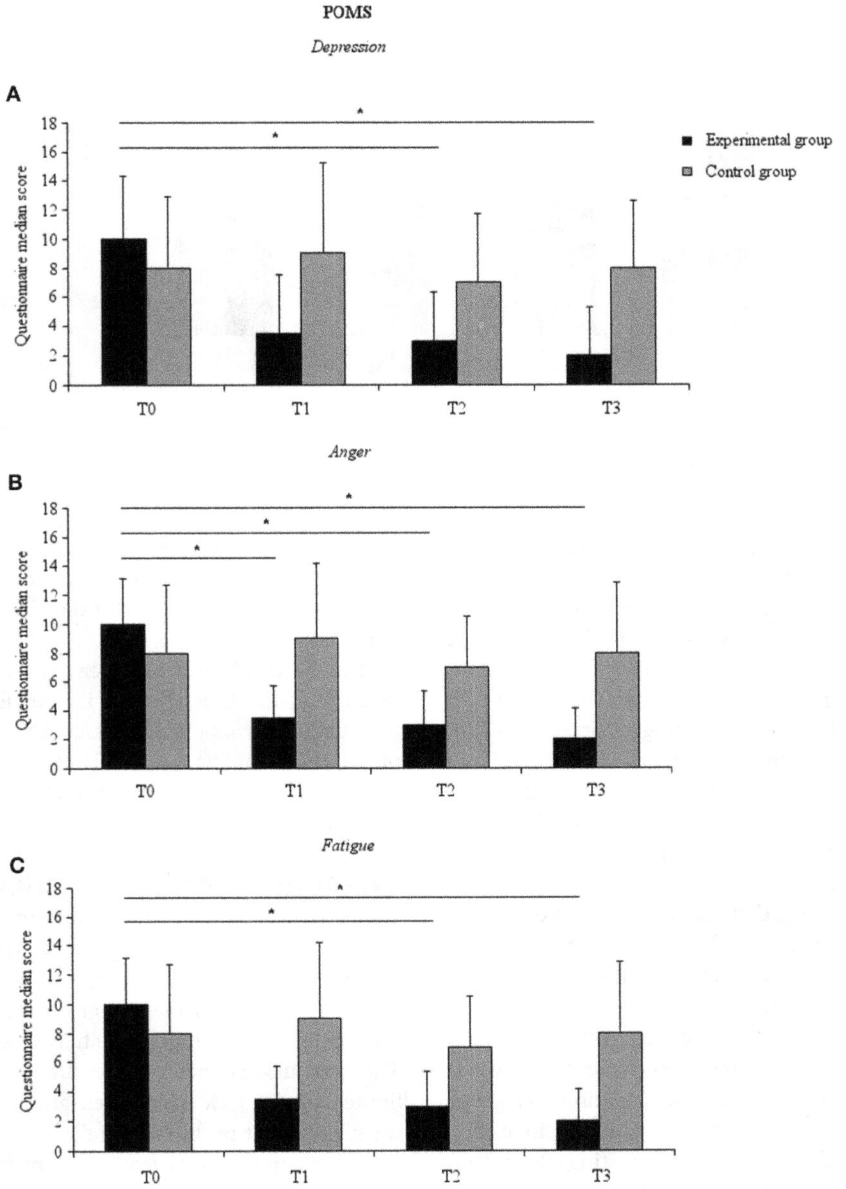

FIGURE 2 | Median POMS subscale score for the experimental (black columns) and the control (gray columns) groups at all-time points. **(A)** Depression subscale; **(B)** Anger subscale; **(C)** Fatigue subscale. Error bars represent 95% confidence interval. Asterisks indicate within-groups significant differences (Bonferroni corrected $p < 0.017$).

that probiotics intake did not influence the level of optimism in the experimental group.

DISCUSSION

With this exploratory study we investigated the effect of probiotics intake on different aspects of mood and dimensions of personality in healthy individuals. Overall, probiotics intake was noted to exert a positive effect on depressive mood state and sleep quality. This effect was specific for the experimental group, thus ruling out confounding factors like learning, expectations or maturation. We suggest, with caution, that these findings provide new support to the notion that probiotics may exert a beneficial psychological influence.

Effect of Probiotics on Mood-Related Aspects

Previous studies in non-clinical samples have demonstrated that multispecies probiotics have positive effects on mood (12, 36, 37). These studies focused mainly on depression and anxiety, whereas we extend previous findings with a more comprehensive assessment of these functions during and after 6 weeks of probiotics intake.

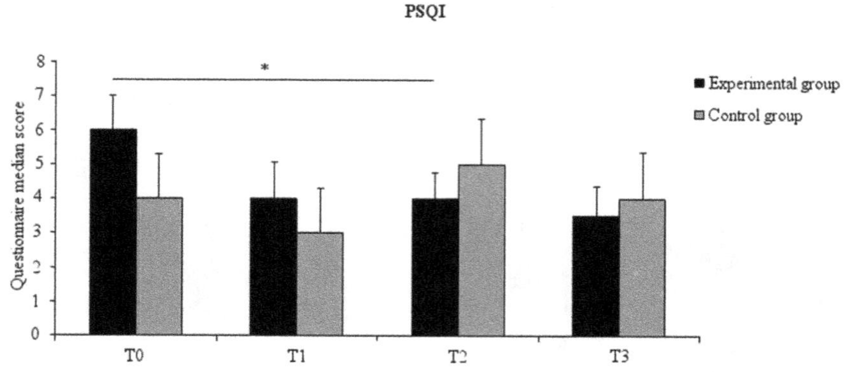

FIGURE 3 | Median PSQI score for the experimental (black columns) and the control (gray columns) groups at all time points. Error bars represent 95% confidence interval. Asterisks indicate within-groups significant differences (Bonferroni corrected $p < 0.017$).

Among the different indexes of cognitive reactivity to sad mood assessed by means of the LEIDS-R, the scores for *acceptance* were found to be higher in the experimental group than the control group after 6 weeks of probiotics intake. Acceptance is an emotion regulation strategy that facilitates recovery from depression in clinical populations (38). We speculate that increasing acceptance might protect healthy individuals from developing depressive mood.

Like Steenbergen et al. (12), we found no significant differences between-groups or across time points for depression scores as assessed by the BDI. This was not surprising since our participants all demonstrated being below the clinically relevant score for depression, suggesting that they did not have depressive symptoms. Nonetheless, using the POMS we were able to detect specific changes in positive and negative mood in healthy individuals. In line with previous studies (12, 36, 37), we found a reduction in depressive mood state in the group that received the probiotics. The *depression* subscale score was lower after 6 weeks of probiotics intake, suggesting that the experimental group benefited from probiotics intake. Interestingly, this positive effect was maintained after 3 weeks of washout, suggesting a long-term effect. Moreover, we found a reduction in anger as measured by the *anger* subscale of the POMS. This reduction appeared at the 3-week assessment and was consistent across other time points. Hence, the scores for anger were lower in the experimental group not only during the 6-week period of probiotics intake but also after 3 weeks of washout. The sense of *fatigue* was also lower in the experimental group at 6 weeks of probiotics intake and continued after the 3 weeks of washout. Since no between-group differences were detected, caution is needed in interpreting these findings. Nonetheless, we suggest that, overall, these findings hint at a beneficial effect of probiotics intake in the experimental group.

No significant differences were found for STAI scores, thus suggesting no changes in state and trait anxiety as assessed by STAI-Y1 and STAI-Y2. Of note, the STAY-Y1 measures the perceived anxiety level at a precise time point. In our study, this time point corresponded to the assessment sessions. The lack of differences between-groups and across time points may indicate that the study participants were relaxed and did not feel they were under pressure while completing the questionnaires, thus excluding potential biases due to anxiety.

The STAI-Y2, instead, measures a more stable dimension of anxiety, the trait anxiety, i.e., an individual's propensity to habitually give anxious responses. The lack of effect of probiotics on this trait could be explained by the fact that healthy individuals already have low anxiety scores that cannot be further lowered by probiotics intake.

Effect of Probiotics on Sleep Quality

Although we did not find significant differences between the experimental and control group at the PSQI, the former but not the latter reported an improvement in sleep quality. More precisely, the experimental group participants reported that their sleep quality improved after 6 weeks of probiotics intake. The conclusions that can be drawn from these findings are limited by the lack of between-group differences. At any rate, we suggest that probiotics intake had beneficial effects on sleep quality in experimental group. Recent studies have demonstrated that probiotics ameliorate sleep in patients with chronic fatigue syndrome (39), chronic pain (40), and in stressed medical students (41). Our finding extends previous observations, suggesting that the probiotics mixture we used was effective in improving sleep quality also in a healthy population. Moreover, the improvement in sleep quality fits well with the reduction in depressive mood state, anger, and fatigue we observed in the experimental group. Previous studies demonstrated a strong relationship between sleep quality and mood (15). This was also the case of our study. Correlation analysis indeed, showed that sleep quality correlated with different aspects of mood, like anxiety, depressive symptoms, fatigue, anger, confusion and vigor, and additionally, in the experimental group, with some aspects of cognitive reactivity to sad mood (e.g., aggression, risk aversion, acceptance and hopelessness). Probiotics might have positively influenced mood not only by influencing emotional processes, but also other related aspects such as sleep quality as well.

Effect of Probiotics on Aspects Related to Personality and its Relationship With Mood

We found no differences in personality traits across time points, suggesting that the two groups remained stable throughout the study. This suggests that personality dimensions are complex and consolidated features that cannot be easily modified over time. Whether the lack of effect was due to the duration of the study (too short) or to the dose of the probiotics (too small) will need to be investigated in a future study.

At certain time points and for specific TCI subscales, however, we found significant between-group differences. For instance, *novelty seeking* scores (i.e., exhilaration in response to novel stimuli) were higher for the experimental than the control group at T3, i.e., after 3 weeks of washout. Caution is warranted when interpreting these findings, however, since the between-group difference in novelty seeking was not consistent across time points. Nonetheless, we suggest that the improvement in mood induced by the probiotics could have facilitated novelty seeking in the experimental group. Support for this hypothesis derives from the evidence that positive emotions trigger exploratory behavior [for a review, see (42)]. Similarly, *self-directedness* and *cooperativeness* subscale scores were significantly different between the two groups only at T3 and at T2, respectively. Once again, because these differences were present only at single time points, it is difficult to draw strong associations with probiotics intake.

Two subscales in the COPE inventory, the *avoidance strategies* and *the positive attitude* subscales, revealed differences between the two groups at more than one time point. We found higher scores on the *avoidance strategies* subscale for the experimental group compared to the control group at T2 (after 6 weeks of probiotics intake) and at T3 (after 3 weeks of washout). This means that the experimental group participants were more likely to adopt strategies based on avoidance (e.g., through denial of stressful situations) when they experienced problems. Taking into account the findings on mood, we speculate that because the experimental group participants felt better, as shown by the reduced depressive mood state, anger and fatigue, they were also more likely to avoid negative thoughts or situations, which induced a positive bias in their responses. In this regard, it has been demonstrated that people who feel in a positive mood are motivated to maintain their positive state (43). For instance, studies on risk-taking behavior demonstrated that positive feelings can accentuate an aversion toward risky options related to a higher probability of loss (43). Of note, avoidance strategies allow to deny problems and related emotions that alter positive mood. In this sense, they might represent the "less risky option" to temporarily prevent loss of a positive state. Following this line of reasoning, we believe that the experimental group participants probably had a higher propensity to adopt avoidance strategies in order to preserve their acquired positive state. This is only speculative and cannot be completely supported by our data; nonetheless, it deserves further investigation.

Also, the *positive attitude* subscale scores were lower for the experimental compared to the control group at T1 (at 3 weeks into the study). Positive attitude is an adaptive coping strategy that allows individuals to positively reinterpret negative situations (44). Hence, a lower score for this subscale suggests that the experimental group participants were temporarily less prone than the controls to positively reinterpret a negative situation. How does this result fit with the amelioration of mood observed in the experimental group? It has been widely demonstrated that positive feelings can bias attention toward mood-congruent stimuli (45, 46). In virtue of this congruency effect, people who feel in a positive mood are apt to attend to positive rather than negative events (46). We speculate that, in virtue of a general positive mood, the experimental group participants subjects did not need to reinterpret negative situations probably because they tended to focus on positive events congruent with their mood rather than on negative events.

Limitations of the Study

Some limitations of this study should be acknowledged. For instance, the small sample size and the potential pre-existing group differences with regard to some personality traits (e.g., *persistence* subscale of the TCI) may limit generalizability of the findings. Future studies with larger sample will allow to apply a randomization method that allows to take into account more than one covariate (21). Moreover, due to time constraints, we used only dimensional questionnaires to assess personality, thus limiting our findings. Future investigations with categorical diagnostic tools (e.g., Structured Clinical Interview for DSM-IV, SCID-II) will allow to achieve a more comprehensive view by assessing personality disorders. Despite these limitations, we think that our study indicates that probiotics might help to promote psychological well-being. As one of the possible underlying mechanisms, we speculate that probiotics, by interacting with intestinal microbiota, facilitated the production of precursors of neuroactive substances involved in modulating emotional processing, sleep, and other brain functions (5, 6). Since the current study did not focus on changes in intestinal microbiota following probiotic intake, this is only a speculation based on previous findings (5, 6). Future studies on larger samples are needed to verify this hypothesis and to uncover the biological mechanisms at the basis of these effects by investigating the changes in the intestinal microbiota related to probiotics intake. Moreover, it would be interesting to extend these investigations to clinical populations and verify whether the positive effects of probiotics intake can be observed in such patients. If so, this would suggest the use of probiotics as adjunctive therapy for conditions characterized by altered mood and/or sleep disturbances.

CONCLUDING REMARKS

We did not find significant differences between the experimental and control group neither at mood-related questionnaires, nor at the questionnaire assessing the quality of sleep. Nonetheless, we found changes in mood state and sleep quality across sessions in the experimental and not in the control group. More precisely, our exploratory study shows an improvement across time in different aspects of the profile of mood state, like sad mood, anger, and fatigue only in healthy individuals which took probiotics. Sleep quality also reportedly improved after probiotics intake. Of note, sleep quality strongly relates to mood. More precisely, as suggested by the significant correlations between sleep quality and mood-related questionnaires, the higher the quality of sleep, the better the mood state in the experimental and in the control group. Finally, significant differences between-groups have been observed for some personality-related questionnaires. In this regard, our findings suggest that improving mood by means of probiotics intake might additionally determine changes in cognitive strategies to deal with problems by reducing sensitivity to negative situations, as well as the need to deal with them. Moreover, we speculate that ameliorating mood can differentially affect an individual's predisposition, for instance, by facilitating novelty seeking.

AUTHOR CONTRIBUTIONS

MF, GF, and AD conception and design of the research project. MF, GF, AD, and AM organization of the research project. AM and ES data acquisition. AM and MF data analysis. AM, MF, GF, and AD interpretation of the data. AM writing the first draft. MF, GF, ES, MP, AA, and AD revision and comments on the first draft. AM, ES, AD, MP, AA, LM, GF, and MF final approval of the manuscript.

ACKNOWLEDGMENTS

We wish to thank Alessio Papazzoni for mobile application development (AgendaQR, Bussola Labs, Verona, Italy), Kenneth Adolf Britsch for his assistance in proofreading the manuscript, and Alessia Masè and Cinzia Magotti for their support with data collection. This paper is dedicated to Dr. Giovanni Mogna, who strongly supported the research.

REFERENCES

Correll CU, Robinson DG, Schooler NR, Brunette MF, Mueser KT, Rosenheck RA, et al. Cardiometabolic risk in patients with first-episode schizophrenia spectrum disorders: baseline results from the RAISE-ETP study. *JAMA Psychiatry* (2014) 71:1350–63. doi: 10.1001/jamapsychiatry.20 14.1314

Curtis J, Henry C, Watkins A, Newall H, Samaras K, Ward PB. Metabolic abnormalities in an early psychosis service: a retrospective, naturalistic cross-sectional study. *Earl Interv Psychiatry* (2011) 5:108–14. doi: 10.1111/j.1751-7893.2011.00262.x

Zhang Q, Deng C, Huang X-F. The role of ghrelin signalling in second- generation antipsychotic-induced weight gain. *Psychoneuroendocrinology* (2013) 38:2423–38. doi: 10.1016/j.psyneuen.2013.07.010

Álvarez-Jiménez M, González-Blanch C, Crespo-Facorro B, Hetrick S, Rodriguez-Sánchez JM, Pérez-Iglesias R, et al. Antipsychotic-induced weight gain in chronic and first-episode psychotic disorders. *CNS Drugs* (2008) 22:547–62. doi: 10.2165/00023210-200822070-00002

Vancampfort D, Wampers M, Mitchell AJ, Correll CU, Herdt A, Probst M, et al. A meta-analysis of cardio-metabolic abnormalities in drug naïve, first-episode and multi-episode patients with schizophrenia versus general population controls. *World Psychiatry* (2013) 12:240–50. doi: 10.1002/wps.20069

Brown S, Kim M, Mitchell C, Inskip H. Twenty-five year mortality of a community cohort with schizophrenia. *Br J Psychiatry* (2010) 196:116–21. doi: 10.1192/bjp.bp.109.067512

Newcomer JW. Antipsychotic medications: metabolic and cardiovascular risk. *J Clin Psychiatry* (2007) 68:8–13.

Strassnig M, Kotov R, Cornaccio D, Fochtmann L, Harvey PD, Bromet EJ. 20- year progression of BMI in a county-wide cohort of people with schizophrenia and bipolar disorder identified at their first episode of psychosis. *Bipolar Disord.* (2017) 19:336–43. doi: 10.1111/bdi.12505

Fountaine RJ, Taylor AE, Mancuso JP, Greenway FL, Byerley LO, Smith SR, et al. Increased food intake and energy expenditure following administration of olanzapine to healthy men. *Obesity* (2010) 18:1646–51. doi: 10.1038/oby.2010.6

Dipasquale S, Pariante CM, Dazzan P, Aguglia E, McGuire P, Mondelli V. The dietary pattern of patients with schizophrenia: a systematic review. *J Psychiatr Res.* (2013) 47:197–207. doi: 10.1016/j.jpsychires.2012.10.005

Kluge M, Schuld A, Himmerich H, Dalal M, Schacht A, Wehmeier PM, et al. Clozapine and olanzapine are associated with food craving and binge eating: Results from a randomized double-blind study. *J Clin Psychopharmacol.* (2007) 27:662–6. doi: 10.1097/jcp.0b013e31815a8872

Stubbs B, Williams J, Gaughran F, Craig T. How sedentary are people with psychosis? a systematic review and meta-analysis. *Schizophr Res.* (2016) 171:103–9. doi: 10.1016/j.schres.2016.01.034

Lett TAP, Wallace TJM, Chowdhury NI, Tiwari AK, Kennedy JL, Müller DJ. Pharmacogenetics of antipsychotic-induced weight gain: review and clinical implications. *Mol Psychiatry* (2012) 17:242–66. doi: 10.1038/mp.2011.109

Minichino A, Francesconi M, Salatino A, Delle Chiaie R, Cadenhead K. Investigating the link between drug-naive first episode psychoses (FEPs), weight gain abnormalities and brain structural damages: relevance and implications for therapy. *Prog Neuropsychopharmacol Biol Psychiatry* (2017) 77:9–22. doi: 10.1016/j.pnpbp.2017.03.020

Knolle-Veentjer S, Huth V, Ferstl R, Aldenhoff JB, Hinze-Selch D. Delay of gratification and executive performance in individuals with schizophrenia: Putative role for eating behavior and body weight regulation. *J Psychiatric Res.* (2008) 42:98–105. doi: 10.1016/j.jpsychires.2006.10.003

Bauer UE, Briss PA, Goodman RA, Bowman BA. Prevention of chronic disease in the 21st century: elimination of the leading preventable causes of premature death and disability in the USA. *Lancet* (2014) 384:45–52. doi: 10.1016/S0140-6736(14)60648-6

American Psychiatric Association. *Diagnostic and Statistical Manual of Mental Disorders (DSM-5QR).* Washington DC: American Psychiatric Pub (2013).

Lachat C, Hawwash D, Ocké MC, Berg C, Forsum E, Hörnell A, et al. Strengthening the reporting of observational studies in epidemiology- nutritional epidemiology (STROBE-nut): An extension of the STROBE statement. *Nutr Bull.* (2016) 41:240–51. doi: 10.1371/journal.pmed.1002036

Burrows TL, Martin RJ, Collins CE. A systematic review of the validity of dietary assessment methods in children when compared with the method of doubly labeled water. *J Am Diet Assoc.* (2010) 110:1501–10. doi: 10.1016/j.jada.2010.07.008

Thompson FE, Subar AF. Dietary assessment methodology. In: Coulston ACB, editors. *Nutrition in the Prevention and Treatment of Disease.* 2nd edn. London: Elsevier (2008).

Curtis J, Newall HD, Samaras K. The heart of the matter: cardiometabolic care in youth with psychosis. *Earl Interv Psychiatry* (2012) 6:347–53. doi: 10.1111/j.1751-7893.2011.00315.x

Curtis J, Watkins A, Rosenbaum S, Teasdale S, Kalucy M, Samaras K, et al. Evaluating an individualized lifestyle and life skills intervention to prevent antipsychotic-induced weight gain in first-episode psychosis. *Earl Interv Psychiatry* (2016) 10:267–76. doi: 10.1111/eip.12230

National Health and Medical Research Council. *A ustralian D ietary Gui delines* Canberra: NHMRC (2013). Available online from: http://www.eatforhealth.gov.au.

Schofield WN. Predicting basal metabolic rate, new standards and review of previous work. *Hum Nutr Clin Nutr.* (1984) 39:5–41.

Black AE .Critical evaluation of energy intake using the Goldberg cut-off for energy intake: basal metabolic rate. A practical guide to its calculation, use and limitations. *Int J Obesity* (2000) 24:1119. doi: 10.1038/sj.ijo.0801376

Krenitsky J. Adjusted body weight, pro: evidence to support the use of adjusted body weight in calculating calorie requirements. *Nutr Clin Pract.* (2005) 20:468–73. doi: 10.1177/0115426505020004468

Goldberg G, Black A, Jebb S, Cole T, Murgatroyd P, Coward W, et al. Critical evaluation of energy intake data using fundamental principles of energy physiology: 1. Derivation of cut-off limits to identify under-recording. *Eur J Clin Nutr* (1991) 45:569–81.

World Health Organisation. *Global Database on Body Mass Index.* Geneva: WHO (2018) Available online at: https://www.who.int/gho/ncd/risk_factors/ bmi_text/ en/

Alberti KGMM, Zimmet P, Shaw J. Metabolic syndrome - a new world-wide definition. A consensus statement from the international diabetes federation. *Diabet Med.* (2006) 23:469–80. doi: 10.1111/j.1464-5491.2006.01858.x

Hall KD, Sacks G, Chandramohan D, Chow CC, Wang YC, Gortmaker SL, et al. Quantification of the effect of energy imbalance on bodyweight. *Lancet* (2011) 378:826–37. doi: 10.1016/S0140-6736(11)60812-X

Rosenbaum S, Tiedemann A, Sherrington C, Curtis J, Ward PB. Physical activity interventions for people with mental illness: a systematic review and meta-analysis. *J Clin Psychiatry* (2014) 75:964–74. doi: 10.4088/JCP.13r08765

Firth J, Carney R, Elliott R, French P, Parker S, McIntyre R, et al. Exercise as an intervention for first-episode psychosis: a feasibility study. *Earl Interv Psychiatry* (2016) 12:307–15. doi: 10.1111/eip.12329

McArdle WD, Katch FI, Katch VL. Energy expenditure at rest and during physical activity. In: McArdle WD, Katch FI, Katch VL, editors. *Essentials of Exercise Physiology.* 5th edn. Philidelphia, PA: Wolters Kluwer (2016).

Rummel-Kluge C, Komossa K, Schwarz S, Hunger H, Schmid F, Lobos CA, et al. Head-to-head comparisons of metabolic side effects of second generation antipsychotics in the treatment of schizophrenia: a systematic review and meta-analysis. *Schizophr Res.* (2010) 123:225–33. doi: 10.1016/j.schres.2010.07.012

Maayan L, Correll CU. Weight gain and metabolic risks associated with antipsychotic medications in children and adolescents. *J Child Adolesc Psychopharmacol.* (2011) 21:517–35. doi: 10.1089/cap.2011.0015

Australian Bureua of Statistics (ABS). *Australian Health Survey: Nutrition First Results - Foods and Nutrients 2011-12.* Canberra: ABS (2014). Available online at: http://www.abs.gov.au/ausstats/abs@.nsf/lookup/4364.0.55.007main$+$features12011-12

Teasdale SB, Ward PB, Rosenbaum S, Samaras K, Stubbs B. Solving a weighty problem: systematic review and meta-analysis of nutrition interventions in severe mental illness. *Br J Psychiatry* (2017) 210:110–8. doi: 10.1192/bjp.bp.115.177139

Shiers D, Curtis J. Cardiometabolic health in young people with psychosis. *Lancet Psychiatry* (2014) 1:492–4. doi: 10.1016/S2215-0366(14) 00072-8

Firth J, Rosenbaum S, Ward PB, Curtis J, Teasdale SB, Yung AR, et al. Adjunctive nutrients in first episode psychosis: a systematic review of efficacy, tolerability and neurobiological mechanisms. *Early Interv Psychiatry* (2018) 12:774–83. doi: 10.1111/eip.12544

Cadenhead KS, Minichino A, Kelsven S, Addington J, Bearden C, Cannon TD, et al. Metabolic abnormalities and low dietary Omega 3 are associated with symptom severity and worse functioning prior to the onset of psychosis:i findings from the North American Prodrome Longitudinal Studies Consortium. *Schizophr Res.* (2018) doi: 10.1016/j.schres.2018.09.022. [Epub ahead of print].

15

Combined Factors for Predicting Cognitive Impairment in Elderly Population Aged 75 Years and Older: From a Behavioral Perspective

Zhixiong Yan[1], Xia Zou[2,3] and Xiaohui Hou[1]*

[1] Psychology Department, Nanning Normal University, Nanning, China, [2] Guangxi College for Preschool Education, Nanning, China, [3] Faculty of Industrial Education and Technology, King Mongkut's Institute of Technology Ladkrabang, Bangkok, Thailand

***Correspondence:**
Zhixiong Yan
yanzx@nnnu.edu.cn

To unravel the combined effect of risk and protective factors that may contribute to preserve or impair cognitive status, this prospective cohort study systematically investigated a cluster of factors in elders aged 75 years and older from Guangxi Longitudinal Cohort (GLC) dataset. GLC has tracked 630 oldest-elders for two times within 2 years and will continue to follow two times in the next 4 years. At baseline geriatric assessment, sociodemographic information (e.g., education, Mandarin, marriage, and income), physical status [body mass index (BMI), chronic disease/medicine], lifestyle factors (smoking, alcohol, and exercise), and self-rated mental health (self-care, well-being, anxiety) were recorded by online interview. With 2 years' follow-up, Mini-Mental State Examination (MMSE) and memory test were performed through person-to-person interview. The performance of MMSE was applied to represent the responder's cognitive status which classified into cognitive impairment and normal group based on a cutoff point of 20. An age-related cognitive declining trend of 15 stratified factors was observed, though with a small effect size (R-square: 0.001–0.15). The odds of exposure or non-exposure on factors (memory, self-care, exercise, income, education, and literacy) had a significantly different effect on cognitive impairment through multivariate analysis after adjusting other confounding variables. Through stepwise multiple logistic regression analysis, the following 12 factors/index would be integrated to predict cognitive impairment: gender, physical health factors (BMI, chronic disease), socioeconomic and lifestyle factors (education, literacy, Mandarin, marriage, income, and exercise), and psychological health factors (memory, self-care cognition, and anxiety). Related clinical and nursing applications were also discussed.

Keywords: cognitive impairment, protective/risk factors, elderly population, lifestyle, logistic regression

INTRODUCTION

Cognitive impairment, such as deterioration in memory, attention, and language, was considered as an inevitable trend of aging experienced by majority of elderly people (Folstein et al., 1985), the extent of which is strongly affected by individual variables (e.g., lifestyle, socioeconomic status) and their interactions. For someone, even the detail of experienced things could clearly be recalled, while some peers could not remember their own name. In current decades, the prevalence of cognitive impairment (e.g., mild cognitive impairment and dementia) has increased dramatically (Boyle et al., 2006) and considerable interest was attached in science research community (Deary et al., 2009). Taking China as an example, the estimated annual expenditures for cognitive impairment in the elderly population are predicted to be US$69 billion in 2020, which stressed a detrimental effect on family and other carers (Xu et al., 2017). As chronic and complicated characteristics, the effect of medical intervention to modify the course of cognitive impairment has not been effective and even hard to clearly attenuate impairment progression (Rocca et al., 2011). For cognitive impairment may be an agent of lifestyle-based causes, potentially modifiable behavioral factors are alternative to delay the onset of cognitive impairment (Friedman et al., 2015).

Accumulating epidemiological evidence indicates that psychological, environmental, and social factors can help to alleviate cognitive impairment and improve cognitive preservation (Wang et al., 2006; Rocca et al., 2011; Roberts et al., 2015; Arnau et al., 2016; Clare et al., 2017; Klimova et al., 2017; Lamblin et al., 2017; Zhang et al., 2017). A healthy lifestyle (refraining from smoking, moderate alcohol consumption, more physical activity/cardiorespiratory fitness, a Mediterranean-style diet, and more social and mentally stimulating activity) was associated with better cognitive performance and resilience (Hughes and Ganguli, 2009; Fung et al., 2011; Bielak et al., 2014; Dardiotis et al., 2014; Satizabal et al., 2016; Bubbico et al., 2019). Socioeconomic adversities (e.g., illiteracy, poor occupational achievement, and low income) could be potentially attributed to dementia (Scazufca et al., 2010). However, the measurements of these studies were heterogeneous with cross-sectional design and partial epidemiological factors. Comprehensive factors assessment and prediction were still lacking. Few studies have systematically examined the odds of the exposure and non-exposure of lifestyle factors. Moreover, exploring factors in a comprehensive and aggregated way would be a promising direction for preserving cognitive capacity. Thus, a systematic exploration of these factors is needed, and aggregately considering them was emphasized in current research. To collect factors in multiple level and as rich as possible, we classified the factors in lifestyle, socioeconomic, psychological, and physical aspect. Several pivotal modifiable factors associated with cognitive impairment will be refined after exploring the effect of each factor. The application for elder people and clinicians was suggested.

Besides, the diagnostic methods such as mild cognitive impairment (MCI) measurement were time-consuming and impractical for aging community survey (Rohrer et al., 2005). As a valid and brief tool of mental state assessment, Mini-Mental State Examination (MMSE, 30 items as well as 5–10 min testing time) covered a variety of cognitive competencies including orientation, memory, attention, reading, and writing with good identification property (Folstein et al., 1975). Here, the current study applied MMSE as a primary tool to measure cognitive impairment of elder individuals aged 75 years above. The aim of this study is to conduct a systematic analysis of factors and explore which is the best combination of protective and risk factors of cognitive impairment.

MATERIALS AND METHODS

Subjects

A total of 788 subjects with normal cognitive function aged 75 years and above were randomly collected at baseline based on census track in 13 communities according to Guangxi Longevity Cohort Project (GLCP). After 2 years' interval, the final sample consisted of 630 subjects (259 males, 371 females, mean age: 84.23) through interview in person (**Figure 1**). Subjects who died (81), not reached (30), and disconnected (47) were excluded from the following data analysis. The following participation rate was 80%.

Factors and Stratified Criteria

At baseline, multidimensional factors were collected in sociodemographic characteristics (gender, the number of children, marriage, income, education, and Mandarin), lifestyle factors (smoking, alcohol, and exercise), physical status [body mass index (BMI), eyesight, chronic disease/medicine], and self-rated mental health factors (self-care, well-being, and anxiety) through telephone interview. Subjects were asked questions such as: How do you think your well-being? Are you a smoker? How many cigarettes do you smoke per day? The interviewer recorded the answer in specific points based on the subject's response. All variables were stratified into two or four levels.

Sociodemographic Characteristics

Sociodemographic information was available regarding gender, age, up-bring children, education, Mandarin, and income. The number of children was divided as three children or more and less than three children. Marriage was classified as married and unmarried (including single, divorced, or widowed). Income grouped by more than 500 RMB and less than 500 RMB. Education was grouped as uneducated (never received education), less than 5 years, and more than 5 years. Mandarin was classified as capable (understanding and speaking Mandarin) and unable (cannot understand and speak Mandarin) groups.

Physical Health Factors

A brief measure of physical functioning was based on three separate tests of physical ability, regarding BMI (subject's weight in kilograms divided by the square of height in meters), eyesight, and chronic disease/medicine condition. Subjects whose BMI < 18.5 were taken as underweight, > 24 as overweight and range between 18.5 and 24 as normal. Eyesight was divided by normal (eyesight test < 1.0) and abnormal (eyesight test > 1.0) groups. Chronic disease/Medicine had two levels (taking, none) according to having chronic disease

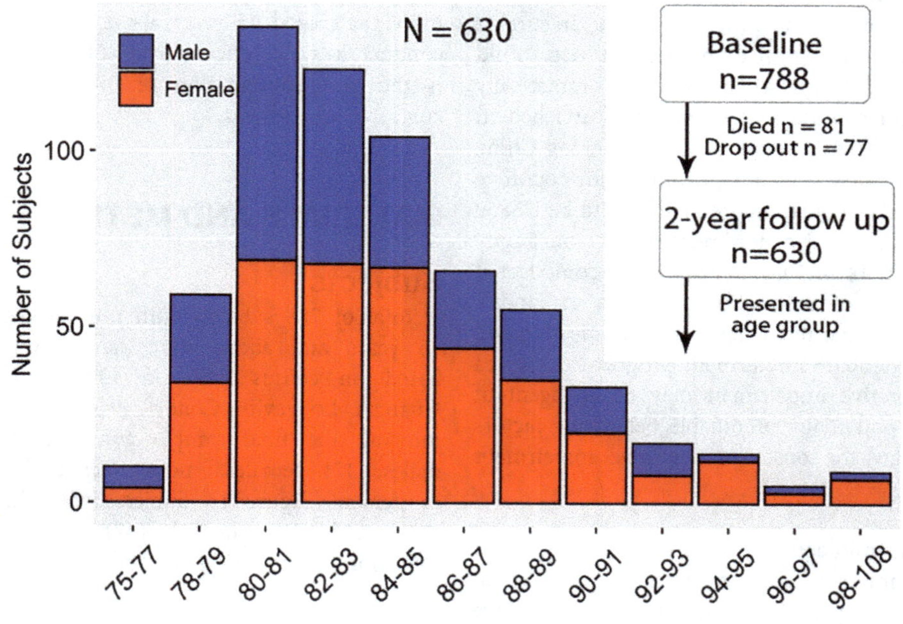

FIGURE 1 | Subjects age-group distribution and collection flowchart.

(like cardiovascular disease, respiratory disease) and taking medicines or not.

Lifestyle Factors

Smoking was classified as no smoking and smoking, whereas alcohol consumption was grouped into alcohol consumption and no alcohol consumption. Exercise was classified as > 50 min per day and < 50 min per day.

Self-Rated Mental Health

Self-rated mental health factors (anxiety, well-being, and self-care) were recorded by a single-item question with five alternative choices regarding excellent (receiving 5 points), very good (receiving 4 points), good (receiving 3 points), fair (receiving 2 points), and poor (receiving 1 point). Each specific component (like anxiety) was then divided into three stratified levels as low level (1–2 points), moderate level (3 points), and high level (4–5 points).

Follow-Up Assessment

With 2-year follow-up, the evaluation including two tests was conducted by coordinator interviewer in person. One test was MMSE (Molloy, 2014) as an index of cognitive status in which subjects are assigned into two groups, the cutoff point for the MMSE performance was 20. MMSE was commonly used to distinguish subjects into with and without cognitive impairment (Uffelen et al., 2008). MMSE score above 20 grouped into normal group, whereas score below 20 was treated as cognitive impairment group.

To validate the cognitive measurement, digit span test was utilized as supplemental cognitive measurement in addition to protective risk in which included 17 items (sequential memory: nine items; reversed order memory: eight items). Each item had 1 point if a subject gave a correct answer. According to the performance of the digit span task, memory was classified as four groups according to the sum of points: excellent (> 11.5), good (> 7.86), medial (≥ 4.2), weak (< 4.2).

In the spirit of collaboration and open science, the data are available for application and can be freely accessed at data sharing part in our lab web page: http://yanlab.club/index.php/info/128.html.

Statistical Analyses

All statistical analyses were performed in *Epicalc* (Chongsuvivatwong, 2007), an epidemiological data analysis tool in R. The data with missing records were omitted before statistical analyses. The function *lm* based on the least squares method was used to perform age-related linear modeling for each factor. The attributes of β (coefficients of the independent variables) and R-square (effect size) were calculated (**Figure 2**). Multivariate analyses using logistic regression models (*glm*) were conducted to identify the effect of exposure and non-exposure in specific factors on cognitive impairment in which crude odds ratio (OR) and adjusted OR (adjusted for other variables) were conducted (**Table 1**). Stepwise logistic regression (*step*) was followed for removing non-significant independent variables according to Akaike's Information Criterion (AIC) in which the optimal model with the lowest AIC value showed high likelihood or best fit. Specifically, the step removes each independent variable and compares the degrees of freedom reduced, the new deviance, and the

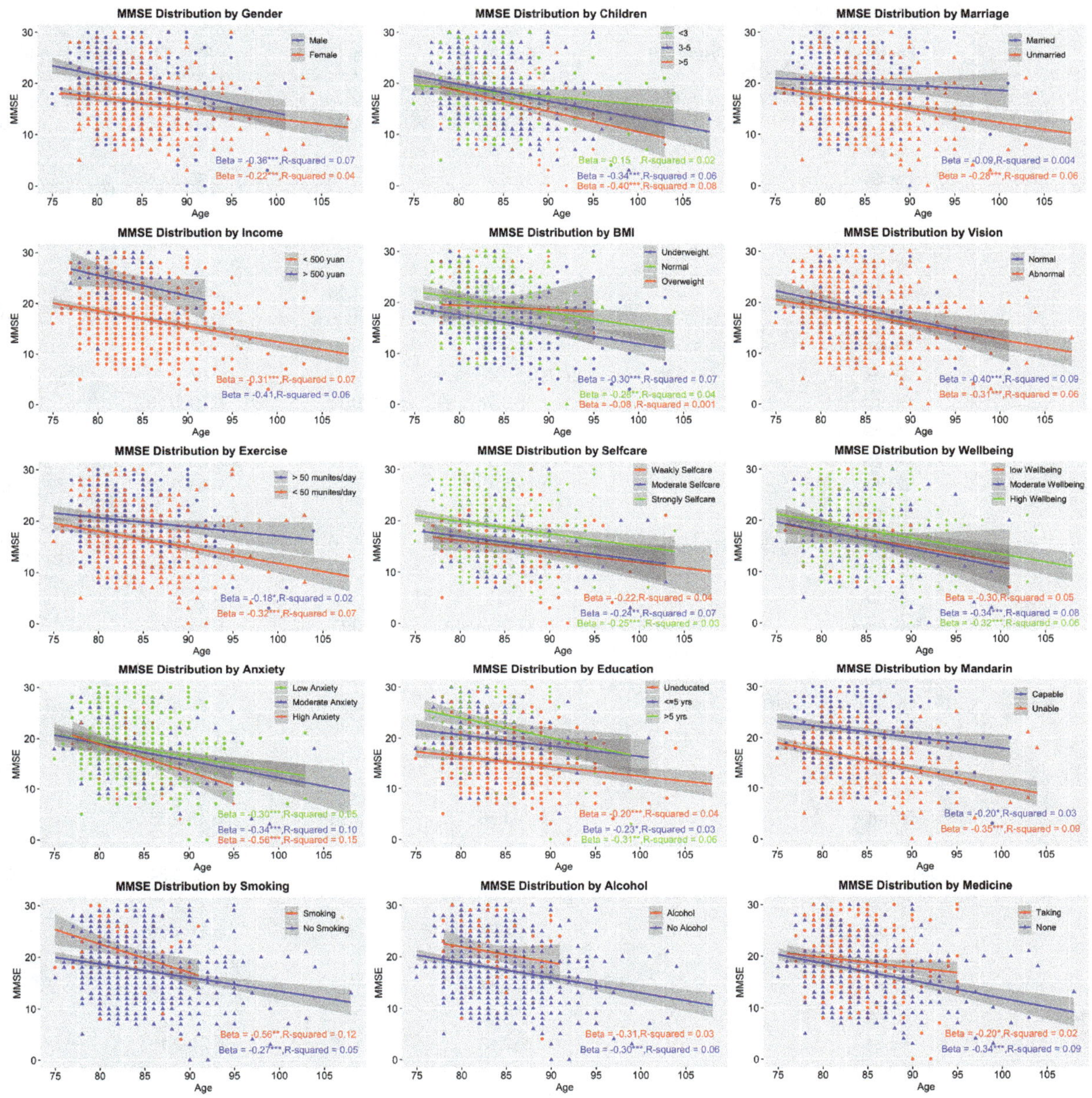

FIGURE 2 | Age-related trends of cognitive changes by stratified factors. The vertical axis presents Mini-Mental State Examination (MMSE) score symbolizing cognitive statue; the horizontal axis presents age. Beta (the strength of association) and R-square (effect size) of each stratified factor were also calculated. *$p < 0.05$; **$p < 0.01$; ***$p < 0.001$.

new AIC. The results are increasingly sorted by AIC. The top one having the lowest AIC is the best one (Step 6 in **Table 2**).

RESULTS

Age-Related Trajectories of Cognitive Changes via Stratified Factors

A linear declining trend was found in all factors stratified in two to four levels (**Figure 2**). Several factors showed stronger decreasing tendency such as high anxiety (β = -0.56) and smoking (β = -0.56), while others like married condition (β = -0.09) and overweight (β = -0.08) showed weaker associations. Unfortunately, all associations only reached small effect sizes (R^2 from 0.001 to 0.15).

The Effects of Exposure and Non-exposure in Specific Stratified Factors

In multivariate regression analysis on which the effects of exposure and non-exposure were checked (**Table 1**), the most significant factor that contributed to cognitive impairment was

TABLE 1 | The exposure and non-exposure effects of risk factors on cognitive impairment.

	Factors	Crude OR	95% CI	Adj. OR	95% CI	*p* (Wald's test)
Age	75	1.00				
	75 + 1	1.09	1.05–1.14	1.01	0.95–1.07	0.78
Gender	Male	1.00				
	Female	3.74	2.58–5.41	1.58	0.85–2.94	0.15
Children	0–2	1.00				
	> 3	1.01	0.66–1.55	1.11	0.58–2.10	0.75
BMI	Normal	1.00				
	Low-weight (< 18.5)	3.07	2.08–4.53	1.56	0.91–2.68	0.11
	Over-weight (> 24)	1.20	0.66–2.21	1.05	0.40–2.74	0.92
Self-care	Medial	1.00				
	Weak	0.63	0.28–1.44	0.22	0.07–0.70	0.01*
	Strong	0.23	0.11–0.43	0.21	0.09–0.50	<0.001***
Well-being	Medial	1.00				
	Weak	1.42	0.58–3.51	1.79	0.52–6.15	0.35
	Strong	0.74	0.46–1.18	1.26	0.63–2.52	0.52
Anxiety	Medial	1.00				
	Weak	1.02	0.64–1.65	1.76	0.89–3.49	0.10
	Strong	1.35	0.63–2.88	1.64	0.58–4.64	0.35
Education	None	1.00				
	1–5 years	0.21	0.13–0.32	0.77	0.38–1.55	0.46
	> 5 years	0.08	0.05–0.13	0.34	0.14–0.83	0.02*
Literacy	Literate	1.00				
	Illiterate	9.59	6.33–14.52	2.92	1.41–6.05	0.004**
Mandarin	Able	1.00				
	Unable	5.17	3.49–7.54	1.45	0.79–2.68	0.23
Marriage	Married	1.00				
	Unmarried	3.02	2.10–4.36	1.35	0.77–2.35	0.30
Income	Low (< 500 yuan)	1.00				
	High (> 500 yuan)	0.10	0.05–0.20	0.32	0.12–0.84	0.02*
Smoking	Smoking	1.00				
	Non-smoking	2.54	1.52–4.26	0.90	0.41–1.96	0.79
Alcohol	Drinking	1.00				
	Non-drinking	2.58	1.51–4.41	1.19	0.55–2.56	0.65
Chronic disease/	Taking	1.00				
Medicine	Never	1.51	1.06–2.15	1.26	0.74–2.13	0.39
Exercise	High (> 50)	1.00				
	Low (< 50)	2.50	1.74–3.58	3.10	1.80–5.31	<0.001***
Memory	Excellent	1.00				
	Good	6.14	3.27–11.56	4.84	2.25–10.39	<0.001***
	Medial	24.98	11.90–52.46	12.21	4.90–30.42	<0.001***
	Weak	55.05	21.00–144.30	36.78	11.62–136.44	<0.001***

*BMI, body mass index; CI, confidence interval. *p < 0.05, **p < 0.01, ***p < 0.001.*

memory. Compared to excellent memory subjects, five times increase in the odds of cognitive impairment, 12.21 times and 36.78 times for medial and weak memory subjects, respectively. Another significant mental health factor was self-care. Compared to medial level, weak level and strong level had only 0.22 and 0.21 times to developing cognitive impairment. Similarly, there are three sociodemographic factors that played as protective factors. As to non-education, subjects who received 1–5 years of education had only 0.77 times possibility resulting in cognitive impairment. If receiving education > 5 years, the odds decreased to 0.34 times. Similar to education, illiterate subjects had 2.92 times suffering cognitive impairment compared to literate subjects. Income is a representative index for subject's economic status, by which high-income subjects (> 500 yuan per month) had just 0.32 times led to cognitive abnormal referenced to low-income ones (< 500 yuan per month). Among lifestyle factors, the influence of physical exercise < 50 min/day had 3.1 times odds to lead to cognitive impairment compared to exercise > 50 min/day. Other factors did not show pronounced difference between exposure and non-exposure.

TABLE 2 | Crucial factors predicting cognitive impairment by stepwise regression.

	Step 1	Step 2	Step 3	Step 4	Step 5	Step 6
Age	+	+				
Gender	+	+	+	+	+	+
Children	+	+	+	+	+	
BMI	+	+	+	+	+	+
Self-care	+	+	+	+	+	+
Well-being	+					
Anxiety	+	+	+	+	+	+
Edu	+	+	+	+	+	+
Literacy	+	+	+	+	+	+
Mandarin	+	+	+	+	+	+
Marriage	+	+	+	+	+	+
Income	+	+	+	+	+	+
Smoke	+	+	+			
Alcohol	+	+	+	+		
Chronic disease/Medicine	+	+	+	+	+	+
Exercise	+	+	+	+	+	+
Memory	+	+	+	+	+	+
AIC	457.08	454.04	452.12	450.22	448.36	446.58

BMI, body mass index; Edu, received education years; AIC, Akaike's Information Criterion, in which a low value shows a high likelihood or a good fit. Each column shows an alternative model, the model of Step 6 was found as the optimal model with the lowest AIC.

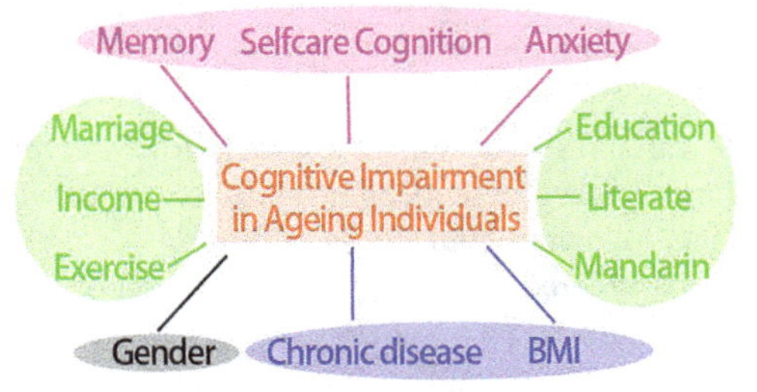

FIGURE 3 | Key potential modifiable factors that contribute to cognitive impairment in aging individuals. Blue ellipse: physical health factors, pink ellipse: psychological factors, green ellipse: socioeconomic and lifestyle factors, blank ellipse: generally unmodifiable factor.

The Aggregated Factors That Best Predict Cognitive Impairment

To check whether some crucial factors could combine to predict cognitive impairment as the optimal model, stepwise regression analysis was conducted (**Figure 3** and **Table 2**). The Step 6 was taken as the optimal model for which its lowest AIC value showed the best fitting results (466.58). The model encompassed Gender, BMI, Self-care cognition, Anxiety, Education, Literacy, Mandarin, Marriage, Income, Chronic disease/Medicine, Exercise, and Memory. Those factors may be more effective when they are combined to predict and intervene cognitive impairment for elderly populations aged 75 and older.

DISCUSSION

As lifestyle and other factors played an enduring and interacted way in the cognitive aging process, uncovering the protective or risk effect on cognitive impairment was a great challenge. Though numerous findings indicated that lifestyle and other sociodemographic factors impacted on cognitive performance (Mensink et al., 1997; Walsh, 2011; Roberts et al., 2015; Zhang et al., 2017; Clare et al., 2017), it is hard to explore the precise mechanism of each factor on cognitive change. Taking the determinants together would be a promising alternative to comprehensively consider protective or risk factors.

In the present study, a similar age-related decreasing trend of cognitive status was found in each stratified factor. Each factor independently contributed to cognitive impairment but with a limited effect size (Deary et al., 2009). Besides, a pronounced exposure effect was found in the following risks *via* multivariate regression analysis: lifestyle factor (physical activity/exercise), socioeconomic factors (education, literacy, income), psychological health factor (self-care cognition), and memory. Exposure in these factors made dramatically different chances to be onset of cognitive impairment. Taking memory as an illustration, the risks of cognitive impairment increased more than 36 times among weak memory individuals compared to that of excellent memory ones. It would be reasonable to infer that working memory stimulation tasks may be one of the most beneficial approaches for preserving and improving cognitive capacity in elder adults. A working memory intervention study also suggested that memory training was an effective way for maintaining normal cognitive function (Heinzel et al., 2014). As for other factors in the current study, low-level exercise (<50 min/day) responders had 3.1 times odds to suffer from cognitive impairment in comparison with high-level exercisers. It means that the value of physical activity was not limited in improving cardiovascular function but also can benefit psychological processes or brain health (e.g., delay cognitive decline) (Gregory et al., 2001). Regular fitness made great contribution to decreased mortality and morbidity rates (Gregory et al., 2001; Salmon, 2001; Uffelen et al., 2008). Other evidence also suggested that increased aerobic exercise was associated with structural and functional changes in elders' brain (Colcombe et al., 2006; Wei et al., 2014). Besides, other crucial sociodemographic factors such as education, literacy, and income also played a vital role in reserving cognitive status. Further evidence about their beneficial impact can be found in numerous aging studies (Perna et al., 2012; Calasanti, 2016; Livingston et al., 2017; Scarmeas et al., 2018).

Above all, as various causes led to cognitive decline in later life, exploring factors in an isolated approach was insufficient to explain cognitive impairment systematically. Instead, it would be appropriate to aggregate multifaceted factors into a unified profile. Only by doing so could clinical guidelines or healthy recommendation be efficient and appropriate, which was also suggested by review work (Plassman et al., 2010) from which a comprehensive consideration of risk and protective factors was necessary when drawing firm conclusions about associations with cognitive decline. The findings in the present study suggested that protective and risk factors were influenced by a number of potentially modifiable variables that could be targets for interventions to promote and reserve better cognitive function. Based on our analysis, the following four types including 12 factors/index would be considered to integrate for predicting cognitive impairment: gender, physical health factors (BMI, chronic disease), socioeconomic and lifestyle factors (education, literacy, Mandarin, marriage, income, and exercise), and psychological health factors (memory, self-care cognition, and anxiety). These potentially modifiable factors (gender excepted) showed promise in preserving cognitive capacity. Targeting these vital factors could help to reduce the incidence of cognitive impairment or substantially delay its onset (Colcombe et al., 2006). It would be constructive to encourage elder people using cognitive stimulation games/activities, like video games, playing cards, language learning, and so on, in which could enormously remedy deficiencies in education or literacy and improve well-being (Charness and Boot, 2009). Meanwhile, physical activity and psychological well-being are also recommended in nursing or clinical practice (McAuley and Rudolph, 1995; Ruuskanen and Ruoppila, 1995; McAuley et al., 2006). Taken together, each factor alone might manifest a spurious and faint association. A comprehensive considering those factors could be valid for predicting cognitive change and preserving cognitive capacity.

Besides, we did not observe significant associations between age and functional impairment. Previous study suggested that age was a major risk factor for cognitive decline (Deary et al., 2009). The reason may be the range of time in the current study was based on only 2 years, not a decade as a previous study (Guralnik et al., 1993). Therefore, the limited segment in our study would be insufficient to reflect the accumulated aging effect. Besides, the effects of smoking and alcohol drinking on cognitive decline were not found to be statistically significant, which was debated in previous evidence (Clare et al., 2017). Evidence was growing that moderate levels of alcohol intake may have a protective effect against dementia and cognitive decline compared with either abstinence or heavy drinking (Ganguli et al., 2005). Moreover, the crude dichotomous classification in our study might conceal the cognitive associations. More precise measurement according to actual consumption was necessary in future studies.

Several other limitations are also needed to be concerned carefully. Firstly, the subjects who participated in the present study came from a remote rural area of China. The external validity of cognitive status reduced and limited its generality. Also, an underestimated cognitive performance may occur for subjects who had relatively lower education and economic status than other older population living in an urban area. Thus, replicating investigation with larger samples and participants living in the city is necessary in future study. Secondly, we did not record information on genetic contribution, brain imaging evidence, healthy dietary habits, and emotional and social support factors, which have previously demonstrated associations with cognitive impairment (Dardiotis et al., 2014). Especially the related social factors, for social organizations are organism-like systems, such as in-group entitativity, which may play as a crucial protective factor for cognitive impairment and improve their life quality in terms of group support and well-being (Campbell, 1958; Pagliaro et al., 2013; Bubbico et al., 2019). Last but not least, we only utilized MMSE and digit span memory test as the measurement of cognitive function which limited the validation and generality of the results we found, though MMSE and digit memory test strongly associated and mutually confirmed the trends of cognitive aging process. Other objective measures, such as electrophysiological and brain imaging technologies, needed to address in future studies. More refined experimental design was also needed to make the protective and risk factors more valid and propel clinical application in cognitive aging field.

CONCLUSION

The comprehensive risk and protective effects of sociodemographic, lifestyle, and mental health on cognitive impairment were observed in subjects aged 75 years and older. We found an age-related declining trend of cognitive capacity in each stratified factor with slight diversity associations. The small effect size (R-square: 0.001–0.15) of individual factor suggests that a combined consideration of factors would be appropriate for clinical application and intervention.

ETHICS STATEMENT

The studies involving human participants were reviewed and approved by the Institutional Review Boards of Nanning Normal University. The patients/participants provided their written informed consent to participate in this study.

AUTHOR CONTRIBUTIONS

ZY conceived the idea, designed the study, analyzed and interpreted the data, and drafted part of the manuscript. XZ and XH assisted with the analysis and interpretation of data. XZ conducted the experiment. All authors contributed to the article and approved the submitted version.

REFERENCES

Arnau, A., Espaulella, J., Serrarols, M., Canudas, J., Formiga, F., and Ferrer, M. (2016). Risk factors for functional decline in a population aged 75 years and older without total dependence: a one-year follow-up. *Arch. Gerontol. Geriatr.* 65, 239–247. doi: 10.1016/j.archger.2016.04.002

Bielak, A. A. M., Cherbuin, N., Bunce, D., and Anstey, K. J. (2014). Preserved differentiation between physical activity and cognitive performance across young, middle, and older adulthood over 8 years. *J. Gerontol. Ser. B* 69, 523–532. doi: 10.1093/geronb/gbu016

Boyle, P., Wilson, R., Aggarwal, N., Tang, Y., and Bennett, D. (2006). Mild cognitive impairment: risk of Alzheimer disease and rate of cognitive decline. *Neurology* 67, 441–445. doi: 10.1212/01.wnl.0000228244.10416.20

Bubbico, G., Chiacchiaretta, P., Parenti, M., Di Marco, M., Panara, V., Sepede, G., et al. (2019). Effects of second language learning on the plastic aging brain: functional connectivity, cognitive decline, and reorganization. *Front. Neurosci.* 13:423. doi: 10.3389/fnins.2019.00423

Calasanti, T. (2016). Combating ageism: how successful is successful aging? *Gerontol.* 56, 1093–1101. doi: 10.1093/geront/gnv076

Campbell, D. T. (1958). Common fate, similarity, and other indices of the status of aggregates of persons as social entities. *Behav. Sci.* 3, 14–25. doi: 10.1002/bs.3830030103

Charness, N., and Boot, W. R. (2009). Aging and information technology use: potential and barriers. *Curr. Direct. Psychol. Sci.* 18, 253–258. doi: 10.1111/j.1467-8721.2009.01647.x

Chongsuvivatwong, V. (2007). *Analysis of Epidemiological Data Using R and Epicalc.* Thailand: Epidemiology Unit Prince of Songkla University. (pp. 1-314)

Clare, L., Wu, Y.-T., Teale, J. C., MacLeod, C., Matthews, F., and Brayne, C. (2017). Potentially modifiable lifestyle factors, cognitive reserve, and cognitive function in later life: a cross-sectional study. *PLoS Med.* 14:e1002259. doi: 10.1371/journal.pmed.1002259

Colcombe, S. J., Erickson, K. I, Scalf, P. E., Kim, J. S., Prakash, R., McAuley, E., et al. (2006). Aerobic exercise training increases brain volume in aging humans. *J. Gerontol. Ser. A* 61, 1166–1170. doi: 10.1093/gerona/61.11.1166

Dardiotis, E., Kosmidis, M. H., Yannakoulia, M., Hadjigeorgiou, G. M., and Scarmeas, N. (2014). The Hellenic Longitudinal Investigation of Aging and Diet (HELIAD): rationale, study design, and cohort description. *Neuroepidemiology* 43, 9–14. doi: 10.1159/000362723

Deary, I. J., Corley, J., Gow, A. J., Harris, S. E., Houlihan, L. M., Marioni, R. E., et al. (2009). Age-associated cognitive decline. *Br. Med. Bull.* 92, 135–152.

Folstein, M., Anthony, J. C., Parhad, I., Duffy, B., and Gruenberg, E. M. (1985). The meaning of cognitive impairment in the elderly. *J. Am. Geriatr. Soc.* 33, 228–235. doi: 10.1111/j.1532-5415.1985.tb07109.x

Folstein, M. F., Folstein, S. E., and McHugh, P. R. (1975). "Mini-mental state": a practical method for grading the cognitive state of patients for the clinician. *J. Psychiatr. Res.* 12, 189–198.

Friedman, D. B., Becofsky, K., Anderson, L. A., Bryant, L. L., Hunter, R. H., Ivey, S. L., et al. (2015). Public perceptions about risk and protective factors for cognitive health and impairment: a review of the literature. *Int. Psychogeriatr.* 27, 1263–1275. doi: 10.1017/s1041610214002877

Fung, A. W.-T., Leung, G. T.-Y., and Lam, L. C.-W. (2011). Modulating factors that preserve cognitive function in healthy ageing. *East Asian Arch. Psychiatry* 21, 152–156.

Ganguli, M., Vander Bilt, J., Saxton, J., Shen, C., and Dodge, H. (2005). Alcohol consumption and cognitive function in late life: a longitudinal community study. *Neurology* 65, 1210–1217. doi: 10.1212/01.wnl.0000180520.35181.24

Gregory, M. A., Gill, D. P., and Petrella, R. J. (2001). Brain health and exercise in older adults. *Curr. Sports Med. Rep.* 12, 256–271.

Guralnik, J. M., LaCroix, A. Z., Abbott, R. D., Berkman, L. F., Satterfield, S., Evans, D. A., et al. (1993). Maintaining mobility in late life. i. demographic characteristics and chronic conditions. *Am. J. Epidemiol.* 137, 845–857. doi: 10.1093/oxfordjournals.aje.a116746

Heinzel, S., Schulte, S., Onken, J., Duong, Q.-L., Riemer, T. G., Heinz, A., et al. (2014). Working memory training improvements and gains in non-trained cognitive tasks in young and older adults. *Aging Neuropsychol. Cogn.* 21, 146–173. doi: 10.1080/13825585.2013.790338

Hughes, T. F., and Ganguli, M. (2009). Modifiable midlife risk factors for late-life cognitive impairment and dementia. *Curr. Psychiatry Rev.* 5, 73–92. doi: 10.2174/157340009788167347

Klimova, B., Valis, M., and Kuca, K. (2017). Cognitive decline in normal aging and its prevention: a review on non-pharmacological lifestyle strategies. *Clin. Int. Aging* 12, 903–910. doi: 10.2147/cia.s132963

Lamblin, M., Murawski, C., Whittle, S., and Fornito, A. (2017). Social connectedness, mental health and the adolescent brain. *Neurosci. Biobehav. Rev.* 80, 57–68. doi: 10.1016/j.neubiorev.2017.05.010

Livingston, G., Sommerlad, A., Orgeta, V., Costafreda, S. G., Huntley, J., Ames, D., et al. (2017). Dementia prevention, intervention, and care. *Lancet* 390, 2673–2734.

McAuley, E., Konopack, J. F., Motl, R. W., Morris, K. S., Doerksen, S. E., and Rosengren, K. R. (2006). Physical activity and quality of life in older adults: influence of health status and self-efficacy. *Ann. Behav. Med.* 31, 99–103. doi: 10.1207/s15324796abm3101_14

McAuley, E., and Rudolph, D. (1995). Physical activity, aging, and psychological well-being. *J. Aging Phys. Act.* 3, 67–96. doi: 10.1123/japa.3.1.67

Mensink, G. B., Loose, N., and Oomen, C. M. (1997). Physical activity and its association with other lifestyle factors. *Eur. J. Epidemiol.* 13, 771–778.

Molloy, D. W. (2014).[[Au Query:
Please provide Accessed date for the reference "Molloy, 2014."]] *Standardised Mini-Mental State Examination (SMMSE):Guidelines for administration and scoring instructions.* Available online at: https://www.ihpa.gov.au/what-we-do/standardised-mini-mental-state-examination-smmse

Pagliaro, S., Alparone, F. R., Picconi, L., Paolini, D., and Aquino, A. (2013). Group based resiliency: contrasting the negative effects of threat to the ingroup. *Curr. Res. Soc. Psychol.* 21, 35–41.

Perna, L., Mielck, A., Lacruz, M. E., Emeny, R. T., Holle, R., Breitfelder, A., et al. (2012). Socioeconomic position, resilience, and health behaviour among elderly people. *Int. J. Public Health* 57, 341–349. doi: 10.1007/s00038-011-0294-0

Plassman, B. L., Williams, J. W., Burke, J. R., Holsinger, T., and Benjamin, S. (2010). Systematic review: factors associated with risk for and possible prevention of cognitive decline in later life. *Ann. Int. Med.* 153, 182–193. doi: 10.7326/0003-4819-153-3-201008030-00258

Roberts, R. O., Cha, R. H., Mielke, M. M., Geda, Y. E., Boeve, B. F., Machulda, M. M., et al. (2015). Risk and protective factors for cognitive impairment in persons aged 85 years and older. *Neurology* 84, 1854–1861. doi: 10.1212/wnl.0000000000001537

Rocca, W. A., Petersen, R. C., Knopman, D. S., Hebert, L. E., Evans, D. A., Hall, K. S., et al. (2011). Trends in the incidence and prevalence of Alzheimer's disease, dementia, and cognitive impairment in the United States. *Alzheimers Dement* 7, 80–93. doi: 10.1016/j.jalz.2010.11.002

Rohrer, J. E., Pierce, J. R. Jr., and Blackburn, C. (2005). Lifestyle and mental health. *Prev. Med.* 40, 438–443.

Ruuskanen, J. M., and Ruoppila, I. (1995). Physical activity and psychological well-being among people aged 65 to 84 years. *Age Ageing* 24, 292–296. doi: 10.1093/ageing/24.4.292

Salmon, P. (2001). Effects of physical exercise on anxiety, depression, and sensitivity to stress: a unifying theory. *Clin. Psychol. Rev.* 21, 33–61. doi: 10.1016/s0272-7358(99)00032-x

Satizabal, C. L., Beiser, A. S., Chouraki, V., Chêne, G., Dufouil, C., and Seshadri, S. (2016). Incidence of dementia over three decades in the framingham heart study. *N. Engl. J. Med.* 374, 523–532. doi: 10.1056/nejmoa1504327

Scarmeas, N., Anastasiou, C. A., and Yannakoulia, M. (2018). Nutrition and prevention of cognitive impairment. *Lancet Neurol.* 17, 1006–1015. doi: 10.1016/s1474-4422(18)30338-7

Scazufca, M., Almeida, O. P., and Menezes, P. R. (2010). The role of literacy, occupation and income in dementia prevention: the São Paulo Ageing & Health Study (SPAH). *Int. Psychogeriatr.* 22, 1209–1215. doi: 10.1017/s1041610210001213

Uffelen, J. G. Z. V., Chin A Paw, M. J. M., Hopman-Rock, M., and Mechelen, W. V. (2008). The effects of exercise on cognition in older adults with and without cognitive decline: a systematic review. *Clin. J. Sport Med.* 18, 486–500. doi: 10.1097/jsm.0b013e3181845f0b

Walsh, R. (2011). Lifestyle and mental health. *Am. Psychol.* 66, 579–592.

Wang, J. Y. J., Zhou, D. H. D., Li, J., Zhang, M., Deng, J., Tang, M., et al. (2006). Leisure activity and risk of cognitive impairment: the chongqing aging study. *Neurology* 66, 911–913. doi: 10.1212/01.wnl.0000192165.99963.2a

Wei, G.-X., Dong, H.-M., Yang, Z., Luo, J., and Zuo, X.-N. (2014). Tai Chi Chuan optimizes the functional organization of the intrinsic human brain architecture in older adults. *Front. Aging Neurosci.* 6:74. doi: 10.3389/fnagi.2014.00074

Xu, J., Wang, J., Wimo, A., Fratiglioni, L., and Qiu, C. (2017). The economic burden of dementia in China, 1990–2030: implications for health policy. *Bull. World Health Organ.* 12, 256–271.

Zhang, M., Jing, D., Liu, Y., Ning, S., Li, G., Yang, F., et al. (2017). Prevalence, incidence, risk and protective factors of amnestic mild cognitive impairment in the elderly in shanghai. *Curr. Alzheimer Res.* 14, 460–466.

16

Does Fruit and Vegetable Consumption during Adolescence Predict Adult Depression? A Longitudinal Study of US Adolescents

Erin Hoare[1]*, *Meghan Hockey*[1], *Anu Ruusunen*[1,2,3] *and Felice N. Jacka*[1]

[1] Food & Mood Centre, IMPACT SRC, School of Medicine, Deakin University, Geelong, VIC, Australia, [2] Department of Psychiatry, Kuopio University Hospital, Kuopio, Finland, [3] Institute of Public Health and Clinical Nutrition, University of Eastern Finland, Kuopio, Finland

***Correspondence:**
Erin Hoare
erin.hoare1@deakin.edu.au

The relationship between better diet quality and decreased depression across the life span is consistent and compelling. Fruit and vegetable consumption has been of particular interest. The nutritional benefits from the consumption of fruits and vegetables may mitigate non-communicable diseases and promote brain and mental health. This study aimed to determine whether fruit and vegetable consumption during adolescence was associated with a reduced risk of developing depression in adulthood in a large, representative sample of US individuals. Data from the Add Health Study were analyzed, which included 3,696 participants who were aged approximately 17 years at baseline (1994–1995), and 29 years at follow-up (2007–2008). The Center for Epidemiologic Studies Depression Scale was used to assess depression and a self-report item asked how many times the participant consumed fruit/vegetables on the previous day. Individuals who were depressed at both times points had the highest proportion who failed to consume any fruit (31%) or vegetables (42%) on the previous day. Fruit and vegetable consumption did not predict of adult depression in fully adjusted models. Cross sectional associations existed for diet and adolescent depression only. Our initial findings supported fruit and vegetable consumption as being protective against adult depression, but this association was subsequently attenuated on adjustment for other relevant factors. Future research will benefit from more precise measures of dietary intakes.

Keywords: depression, adolescents, fruit, vegetables, adulthood

INTRODUCTION

Healthful diets for the prevention and treatment of depression is a current major focus in nutritional psychiatric research. In particular, the Mediterranean Style Diet, traditional wholefood diets, and anti-oxidant rich foods have been promoted as supportive of positive mental health (1–4). Depression is a highly complex mental disorder and is the leading contributor to the global burden of disease (5). The causes and risk factors of depression span individual, familial, environmental, societal and other domains, thus prevention strategies are needed that account for the complexity within which depression occurs (6). Individuals experiencing depression are at greater risk of experiencing comorbid lifestyle driven diseases such as overweight/obesity, cardiovascular disease and some cancers (7). These conditions are all associated with underlying poor diet and it is therefore highly plausible that prevention strategies that target healthier diet could hold dual physical and mental health benefits. It is recognized that experiencing depression and associated symptoms such as low motivation, can also lead to poor dietary choices and overall unhealthy eating habits particularly as a form of coping (8). Indeed the typical diet of individuals living with mental illness is poorer at the population level, compared to individuals without mental illness (9). The diet and depression relationship is therefore assumed to be bi-directional. Whilst the etiology of depression is highly complex, targeting diet for prevention holds great promise given the population reach and the known dual benefits for physical health and non-communicable disease prevention.

The underlying components of diets considered beneficial for mental health are all similar in that they all promote the regular consumption of fruits and vegetables (4). Fruits and vegetables are micronutrient and anti-oxidant rich, which is thought to be protective against oxidative stress in the body (10, 11). In addition, vitamins and minerals found in fruit and vegetables have been shown to support healthy emotional and cognitive functioning (12). Diets high in fruit and vegetables have also been shown to impact directly on brain health. A study published in 2015 found that healthier dietary patterns, high in fruit and vegetables, were associated with larger hippocampal volume over time, compared to Western-style, unhealthy diets, low in fruit, and vegetables (13).

Evidence suggests that both low rates of common mental disorders including depression, low mood, stress, and anxiety (14, 15), and higher rates of positive mental health including life satisfaction, positive mood, and perceived life flourishing (16), co-occur with fruit and vegetable intake. Furthermore, research suggests that a dose-response relationship exists, whereby each serve increase in fruit and vegetables is associated with an improvement in mental health (17, 18). Given the evidence to date, treatment trials have been conducted examining the impact of dietary changes, including increased fruit and vegetable consumption, on depressive symptoms with significant positive outcomes being reported (3, 19).

Despite evidence to date, there are some research gaps in terms of the relationship between fruit and vegetable intake for the prevention of depression at a population-level. In particular, while it is known that a life span approach should be adopted, it remains unknown what the unique preventive potential of fruit and vegetable consumption during adolescence might be for reducing the risk of depression later in adulthood. This may be particularly critical given that depression often first occurs during adolescence (20). In addition, dietary habits formed in adolescence often track into adulthood, which has important implications for physical health later in life (21). Investigating the predictive potential of fruit and vegetable consumption during adolescence and adult depression outcomes thus has important implications for population-level prevention initiatives.

The aim of this study is to determine whether adolescent fruit and vegetable consumption predicts adult depression, and whether this predictive potential is independent of other factors known to be related to both diet and mental health outcomes, such as overweight/obesity, socio-economic status, and physical activity.

METHODS

Study Design

Add Health is a longitudinal, US population-based study of adolescent health (22). During the 1994–1995 school year, 132 secondary schools participated in a questionnaire data collection, which reflected a nationally representative sample of students aged between 12 and 18 years (n = 20,745). Additionally, four waves of in-home interviews were conducted in 1994–1994 (Wave 1), 1996 (Wave 2), 2001–2002 (Wave 3), and 2007-2008 (Wave 4), spanning a total of 18 years. The sampling strategy was stratified random sample that represented the entire US in regards to region, urban/rurality, size, and ethnicity. Further detailed information has been published elsewhere (22).

Our study examined data from the original participating adolescents from Wave 1, who also completed follow-up data collection at Wave 4, and had complete, public accessible data available (n = 4,807). Sample weights were employed to account for the baseline probabilities and potential clustering effects of school to which participant attended. Ethics approval for the Add Health study was approved by the Institutional Review Board of the University of North Carolina, Chapel Hill. Public-use data are available for research purposes and were accessed from http://www.cpc.unc.edu/projects/addhealth

Depression

Depression was measured by the Center for Epidemiologic Studies Depression Scale (CES-D) (23) at baseline in Wave 1 (1994–1995, mean age 16 years) and at Wave 4 (2007–2008, mean age 29 years). The CES-D is often used in population level epidemiological studies to measure the presence of symptoms typically resembling depression. The questionnaire includes items relating to how often in the past week the individual experienced symptoms such as restless sleep, feelings of loneliness and trouble in concentrating. Responses range from 0 to 3, where 0 = rarely or never and 3 = most or all of the time. Higher scores reflect greater depressive symptoms. The CES-D shows good sensitivity, specificity and high internal consistency and has been previously used across a broad range of age groups including adolescents (24). Reliability and validity has been previously shown.

At Wave 1, the 20-item CES-D was administered, and at Wave 4, participants received the 10-item version. A score of 16 or higher on the CES-D-20 and 11 or higher on the CES-D-10 was used to define probable depression, as per recommendations (23, 25). Adult (Wave 4) depression was the main outcome of interest and adolescent depression was controlled for as a covariate in analyses. We also ran models to examine the cross-sectional relationship between adolescent depression and fruit and vegetable consumption.

Fruit and Vegetable Consumption

Fruit and vegetable consumption was the main predictor of interest in this study. During Wave 1, participants completed questionnaires on habitual dietary intake including items asking whether they had eaten fruit or vegetables on the previous day. Specifically, participants were asked "How often did you eat fruit or drink fruit juice yesterday?" with responses "didn't eat," "ate once" or "ate twice or more." The same item with response options was asked for vegetable consumption. Single-item dietary measures for fruit and vegetable consumption are widely used in population level epidemiological questionnaires and have been shown to be indicative of overall dietary quality (26).

Covariates

Demographic, health behavioral, and anthropometric variables were selected for inclusion, based on evidence demonstrating potential to confound the relationship between diet and depression. Wave 1 questionnaires asked information relating to participants age, sex, total household income during 1994 (reported by parents) and ethnicity. Health behaviors including smoking status and physical activity levels were assessed at Wave 1 asking participants to report the number of times during the past week they did exercise, such as jogging, walking, karate, jumping rope, gymnastics, or dancing. Smoking status was also self-reported. Height and weight were objectively measured at Wave 4 and converted into body mass index, which was further converted into healthy weight and overweight/obese weight status categories (27). Because objective measures were only taken at Wave 4 (and not Wave 1), these data were used to control for weight status in analyses.

TABLE 1 | Participant characteristics, expressed as n (%) unless otherwise specified.

	Not depressed in adulthood (n = 3,003)	Depressed in adulthood (n = 693)	Total (n = 3,696)
Age, mean (SD)			
Baseline	15.9 (1.7)	15.9 (1.8)	15.9 (1.7)
Follow-up	28.9 (1.7)	28.9 (1.8)	28.9 (1.7)
Ethnicity			
Caucasian	2189 (72.9)	436 (62.9)	2625 (71.0)
African American	591 (19.7)	193 (27.9)*	784 (21.2)
Native American	34 (1.1)	Supressed	Supressed
Asian/pacific islander	85 (2.8)	Supressed	Supressed
Other	104 (3.5)	38 (5.5)	142 (3.8)
Household income during adolescence m SD ('000s)	50.8 (57.0)	40.2 (45.6)*	48.8 (55.2)
Smokers	565 (18.7)	150 (21.7)	712 (19.3)
Physical activity[a]			
Not at all	508 (16.9)	108 (15.6)	616 (16.7)
1 or 2 times	942 (31.4)	212 (30.6)	1,154 (31.2)
3 or 4 times	761 (25.3)	177 (25.5)	938 (25.4)
5 or more times	792 (26.4)	196 (28.3)	988 (26.7)
Overweight/obese in adulthood	2,013 (67.0)	469 (67.7)	2,482 (67.2)
Depression during adolescence	491 (16.4)	289 (41.7)*	780 (21.1)

**Significant (p < 0.05) difference between groups not depressed in adulthood and depressed in adulthood.*

Abbreviations: Standard deviation, SD.

[a]Participants were asked the number of times during the past week they did exercise, such as jogging, walking, karate, jumping rope, gymnastics, or dancing.

Statistical Analyses

All analyses were conducted in Stata/SE 15.0 (Stata Corporation) and significance was assumed at $p < 0.05$. Total CES-D scores were calculated and dichotomised using the cut off ≥16 for Wave 1 (CES-D-20) and ≥11 for Wave 4 (CES-D-10) as recommended by previous research (28).

Logistic regression models were used to examine whether adult depression was significantly predicted by adolescent fruit and vegetable consumption. Odds ratios with 95% confidence intervals assessed these relationships, with outcomes being whether or not depression was present (0 = no depression, 1 = depression present). Models were sex-specific given the known unique experiences of depression specific to sex. Univariate relationships were examined (Model 1) and then baseline depressive status were added (Model 2). Covariates age, household income during adolescence, ethnicity, physical activity, smoking status, and weight status were adjusted for in Model 3.

RESULTS

Participants were approximately 16 years at adolescence (baseline) and 29 years at adulthood (follow-up) (**Table 1**). Most participants were of Caucasian decent and depression significantly varied by ethnicity. The mean household income during adolescence was significantly lower among those with adult depression compared to those without adult depression. Physical activity and smoking status during adolescence, and adult overweight/obesity did not differ between those depressed as adults and those not depressed.

Individuals who never experienced depression were the highest consumers of fruit and vegetables during adolescence (**Figure 1**; **Supplementary Table 1**). Most (80%) of the individuals who did not ever experience depression ate fruit on the previous day. The proportion not eating fruit on previous day was higher among those who had depression during adolescence, and among those who went on to experience depression in adulthood. One third of those depressed at both time points did not consume fruit and 42% did not consume any vegetables on the previous day. Vegetable consumption was highest among those who did not experience depression at either time point (**Figure 2**).

Fruit consumption among males and vegetable consumption among females was prospectively associated with a reduced risk of adult depression in unadjusted models (**Table 2**). The association between vegetable consumption among females and the risk of adult depression remained significant after controlling for adolescent depression; however, this relationship was attenuated after controlling for age, household income, ethnicity,

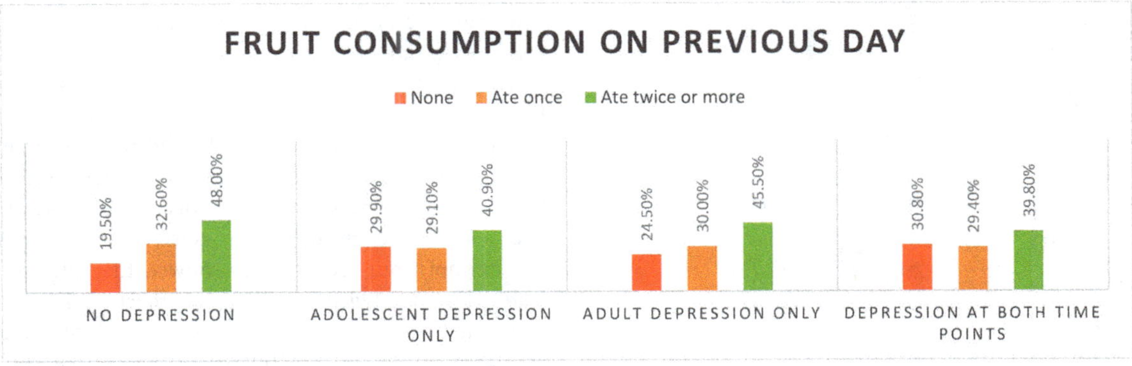

FIGURE 1 | Fruit consumption on previous day by depression status.

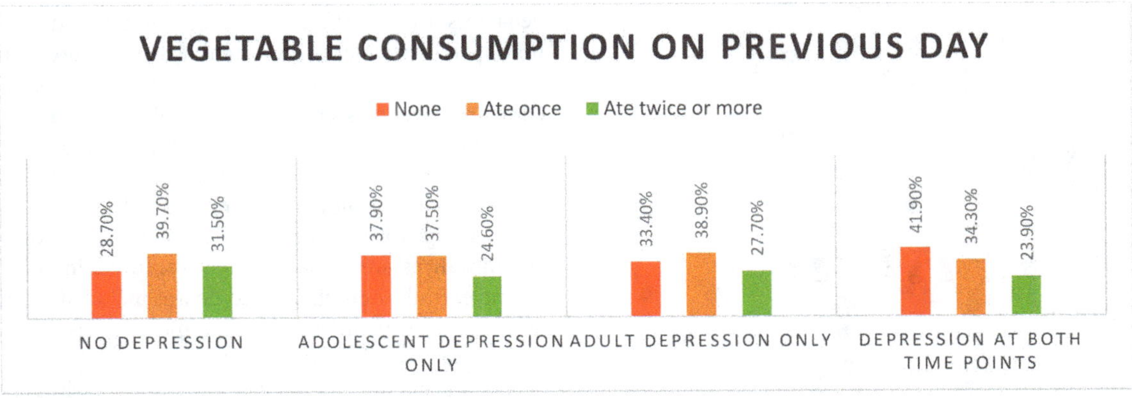

FIGURE 2 | Vegetables consumption on previous day by depression status.

physical activity and overweight/obesity. Fruit consumption was cross-sectionally related to reduced odds of depression in adolescence in both males and females, both before and after controlling for covariates (**Table 3**). Vegetable consumption among females was cross-sectionally associated with reduced odds of depression in adolescence.

DISCUSSION

Fruit and vegetable consumption during adolescence was predictive of adult depression in univariate models, however, this relationship was attenuated once adjusted for adolescent depression in males and by further adjustment for key confounding variables in females. In cross-sectional analyses, fruit (males and females) and vegetable (females only) consumption was related to adolescent depression, both before and after controlling for covariates. Consumption patterns by depressive status were as expected; fruit and vegetable consumption was highest among individuals who did not experience depression during adolescence or adulthood.

Our findings are somewhat inconsistent with previous literature that suggests that diet during adolescence is predictive of both concurrent and future mental health outcomes (26, 29). It has been suggested that it is fruit and vegetables, as a component of wider healthy diet, that promotes and supports mental and brain health (15, 26, 30). This was highlighted in research by (4) who proposed that it is the combination of foods and habitual dietary patterns over time, that hold implications for inflammation and oxidative stress which are contributing pathways to mood and emotional dysfunction that underpins depression (4). In light of the current results, it is possible that failing to incorporate the wider diet beyond fruit and vegetables, resulted in failure to capture potential predictive potential of future depression. In particular, given the established relationship between unhealthy diets and adolescent (31) and adult (1) depression, failure to assess and model the intake of other food groups, including processed and "junk" foods, may have limited our findings. This suggests that promoting fruit and vegetable consumption alone may not be enough to support prevention efforts. It is also known that mental health and diet relationship is considered bi-directional in that depressed states can impact upon appetite, hedonic capacity and food and dietary decisions (32). Recent evidence demonstrates poorer diet quality at a population level, among those living with mental illness, compared to those who do not experience mental illness (9). This relationship has been shown to be independent of relevant confounders

TABLE 2 | Prospective logistic regression models of adult depression (dependent variable) and associations with fruit and vegetable consumption during adolescence (independent variable).

Depress	*Model 1*						*Model 2*						*Model 3*					
	Males			Females			Males			Females			Males			Females		
Adult	**OR**	**95%CI**	***p***	**OR**	**95%CI**	***p***	**OR**	**95%CI**	***p***	**OR**	**95%CI**	***p***	**OR**	**95%CI**	***p***	**OR**	**95%CI**	***p***
Fruit																		
0	Ref.			Ref.			Ref.			Ref.			Ref.			Ref.		
Once	**0.62**	**0.41, 0.94**	**0.025**	0.81	0.57, 1.15	0.239	0.71	0.46, 1.10	0.123	0.93	0.65, 1.35	0.715	0.72	0.46, 1.11	0.139	0.92	0.63, 1.33	0.645
Twice +	**0.64**	**0.44, 0.94**	**0.021**	0.76	0.55, 1.05	0.098	0.73	0.49, 1.09	0.123	0.89	0.63, 1.26	0.526	0.71	0.47, 1.07	0.097	0.88	0.62, 1.26	0.478
Veg																		
0	Ref.			Ref.			Ref.			Ref.			Ref.					
Once	0.96	0.65, 1.40	0.815	**0.66**	**0.48, 0.89**	**0.007**	1.00	0.68, 1.48	0.986	**0.72**	**0.53, 1.00**	**0.047**	1.07	0.72, 1.57	0.752	0.74	0.54, 1.02	0.068
Twice +	0.97	0.64, 1.46	0.870	**0.68**	**0.49, 0.94**	**0.019**	1.01	0.66, 1.55	0.951	0.79	0.57, 1.10	0.168	1.02	0.66, 1.56	0.936	0.80	0.57, 1.12	0.201

Unadjusted (Model 1), adjusted for adolescent depression (Model 2) and further adjusted for age, household income, ethnicity, physical activity, and BMI (Model 3) models are presented.
BMI, body mass index; CI, confidence interval; OR, Odds ratio.
Bolding indicates significance at $p < 0.05$.

including age, gender, BMI, education, and social deprivation. The cross-sectional findings here during adolescence supports this bi-directionality.

Eating vegetables once a day during adolescence was predictive of reduced odds of depression as an adult among females, compared to females who did not consume vegetables on the previous day. Sex differences have been established both in experiences and trajectory of depressive disorders, and also in health behaviors across the life span (5, 33). For example, our recent study showed that adolescent females were close to twice as likely to meet fruit and vegetable consumption recommendations compared to males (33). In emerging adulthood (18–30 years), females were less likely to be habitual sugar sweetened beverage consumers and more likely to meet physical activity recommendations, compared to emerging adult males. It is possible that young females who are regular consumers of vegetables are also engaging in other protective behaviors that might in combination offset depression. This finding is particularly important with a disproportionate risk of depression increasing with age among adolescent females compared to adolescent males (5). Males and females experience similar level of risk of depression in early adolescence, and by early adulthood females are twice more likely to experience depression than males of the same age (34).

It is possible that the influence of socio-economic circumstances were inadequately captured in this study. For example, whilst household income was included in fully adjusted models, participants' socio-economic circumstances may have changed with their transition from adolescence to adulthood. It is possible that life experiences occurring in early adulthood such as leaving school, living independently, commencing studies or full-time employment, may have influenced adult mental health and the potential contribution of these factors was not adequately captured. Higher rates of depression are consistently seen in neighborhoods experiencing disproportionate socio-economic disadvantage (35). There are environmental challenges in such communities, such as greater density of fast food outlets in place of fresh wholefood stores (36). The influence of socio-economic circumstances on mental and physical health outcomes are well-established, and it is possible that the failure to identify significant relationships in this study was due to inadequate capturing of such circumstances.

The expectation for fruit and vegetable consumption to impact upon current and future mental health is supported by physiological mechanistic pathways. Several plausible mechanisms have been proposed as to why fruit and vegetable consumption may confer protective benefits. Fruits and vegetables are rich in essential micronutrients such as folate, magnesium and selenium. Deficiencies in nutrients, such as folate, have been implicated in the pathogenesis of depression (37). Folate is an essential co-factor in metabolic pathways required for the synthesis of neurotransmitters, such as noradrenaline and serotonin (38), and may further exert protective benefits by decreasing homocysteine levels (39). Further, adequate intake of magnesium may reduce inflammation (40), and protect against chronic, low-grade inflammation which is implicated in depression (11).

TABLE 3 | Cross-sectional logistic regression models of adolescent depression (dependent variable) and associations with fruit and vegetable consumption in adolescence (independent variable).

	Model 1						Model 2					
Depress	**Males**			**Females**			**Males**			**Females**		
Adoles	**OR**	**95%CI**	***p***	**OR**	**95%CI**	***p***	**OR**	**95%CI**	***p***	**OR**	**95%CI**	***p***
Fruit												
None	Ref.			Ref.			Ref.			Ref.		
Once	**0.48**	**0.33, 0.70**	**<0.001**	**0.59**	**0.43, 0.81**	**0.001**	**0.53**	**0.36, 0.77**	**0.001**	**0.68**	**0.49, 0.95**	**0.025**
Twice +	**0.50**	**0.35, 0.71**	**<0.001**	**0.54**	**0.40, 0.73**	**<0.001**	**0.55**	**0.38, 0.80**	**0.002**	**0.62**	**0.45, 0.85**	**0.003**
Veg												
None	Ref.			Ref.			Ref.			**Ref.**		
Once	0.79	0.56, 1.11	0.171	**0.65**	**0.49, 0.85**	**0.002**	0.80	0.56, 1.13	0.206	**0.69**	**0.52, 0.93**	**0.014**
Twice +	0.79	0.54, 1.16	0.232	**0.54**	**0.39, 0.73**	**<0.001**	0.87	0.59, 1.28	0.475	**0.64**	**0.46, 0.88**	**0.006**

Unadjusted (Model 1), and adjusted for age, household income, ethnicity, physical activity, and BMI (Model 2) models are presented. BMI, body mass index; CI, confidence interval; OR, Odds ratio.
Bolding indicates significance at $p < 0.05$.

Non-nutrient components of fruits and vegetables, such as polyphenols, also strengthen our rationale for fruit and vegetables to protect against depression. Polyphenols refers to a wide class of compounds that as antioxidants, may protect cells against oxidative damage (41) to positively influence brain health (42). Polyphenols may also act as prebiotics within the gut, and along with other dietary fibers, may contribute to the health of the commensal bacteria that reside within the gastrointestinal tract (i.e., the gut microbiota). Numerous studies suggest that the gut microbiota may play a key role in the pathophysiology of depression (43); thus, modulation of the microbiome by prebiotics and dietary fibers may have associated mental health benefits.

STRENGTHS AND LIMITATIONS

There were study design elements that limited this study. In particular, the measurement of fruit and vegetable consumption was self-reported, and this is likely to have introduced biases to the analysis such as social desirability bias. Moreover, there is large measurement error arising from dietary questionnaires and this would have attenuated the strength of the detected associations (44). On the other hand, single item fruit and vegetable consumption items have been shown to correlate with comprehensive dietary recall measures, and are widely used in population health research (44). In addition, our study examined fruit and vegetable consumption during adolescence only, and our findings could have been further explored with the inclusion of adult dietary behaviors. It is possible that dietary habits changed over time, but we did not have data to assess this. As identified, this study accounted for household income as a proxy for socio-economic status during adolescence. However, it is likely that social and economic changes were likely to have affected health behavioral and depressive outcomes in the transition from adolescence to adulthood. Our study failed to account for the impact of such changes. Our study was strengthened by the use of longitudinal cohort data, which were sampled to be representative of the US population. Despite this, the extent to which findings can translate to current adolescent health is limited. For example, the social environment and daily habitual lifestyle of adolescents is different to that experienced two decades ago and such experiences are likely to impact upon health outcomes adulthood. Lastly, the CES-D is a self-reported measurement of depression and our study was limited in that no clinical depression assessment was available. However, it has been commonly used in epidemiological studies and is widely accepted as an appropriate tool for the measurement of depression (23, 45).

CONCLUSION

The findings of this study offer further support for the role and importance of lifestyle behaviors, and in particular diet, for understanding experiences of mental health during adolescence. The wider evidence to date suggests that fruit and vegetable consumption could be an important predictor of future depression, and our null findings may be due to the limitations of our dietary assessment, which failed to capture overall dietary patterns and was likely affected by measurement error. Increasing consumption of fruit and vegetables is a highly valuable public health message in terms of preventing chronic and non-communicable diseases. The potential for prevention of depression to be included in this public health messaging is promising, given the current burden associated with depression and lifestyle-driven diseases. Given that diet and other lifestyle behaviors are largely shaped by social and economic circumstances, we propose that such factors, in addition to comprehensive dietary and other lifestyle behaviors, are incorporated into population-level mental health prevention research. Optimal prevention strategies are likely to be achieved through assuming complex interconnecting relationships between such drivers of health across the lifespan.

ETHICS STATEMENT

This study was carried out in accordance with the recommendations of University of North Carolina School of Public Health Institutional Review Board guidelines that are based on the Code of Federal Regulations on the Protection of Human Subjects 45CFR46: http://www.hhs.gov/ohrp/humansubjects/guidance/45cfr46.html Add Health participants provided written informed consent for participation in all aspects of Add Health.

AUTHOR CONTRIBUTIONS

EH developed the study design, conducted the analyses, and drafted the manuscript. MH contributed to the manuscript and revised for intellectual content. AR and FJ revised the manuscript for intellectual content. All authors read and approved the final draft for submission.

ACKNOWLEDGMENTS

This research uses data from Add Health, a program project directed by Kathleen Mullan Harris and designed by J. Richard Udry, Peter S. Bearman, and Kathleen Mullan Harris at the University of North Carolina at Chapel Hill, and funded by grant P01-HD31921 from the Eunice Kennedy Shriver National Institute of Child Health and Human Development, with cooperative funding from 23 other federal agencies and foundations. Special acknowledgment is due Ronald R. Rindfuss and Barbara Entwisle for assistance in the original design. Information on how to obtain the Add Health data files is available on the Add Health website (http://www.cpc.unc.edu/addhealth). No direct support was received from grant P01-HD31921 for this analysis. EH is supported by an Australian Rotary Health Postdoctoral Fellowship. MH is supported by a Deakin University Industry postgraduate scholarship. AR is supported by a Deakin University Postdoctoral Research Fellowship. FNJ is supported by an NHMRC Career Development Fellowship (2) (#1108125).

REFERENCES

Li Y, Lv MR, Wei YJ, Sun L, Zhang JX, Zhang HG, et al. Dietary patterns and depression risk: a meta-analysis. *Psychiatry Res.* (2017) 253:373–82. doi: 10.1016/j.psychres.2017.04.020

Psaltopoulou T, Sergentanis TN, Panagiotakos DB, Sergentanis IN, Kosti R, Scarmeas N. Mediterranean diet, stroke, cognitive impairment, and depression: a meta-analysis. *Ann Neurol.* (2013) 74:580–91. doi: 10.1002/ana.23944

Jacka FN, O'Neil A, Opie R, Itsiopoulos C, Cotton S, Mohebbi M, et al. A randomised controlled trial of dietary improvement for adults with major depression (the 'SMILES'trial). *BMC Med.* (2017) 15:23. doi: 10.1186/s12916-017-0791-y

Opie RS, Itsiopoulos C, Parletta N, Sanchez-Villegas A, Akbaraly TN, Ruusunen A, et al. Dietary recommendations for the prevention of depression. *Nutr Neurosci.* (2017) 20:161–71. doi: 10.1179/1476830515Y.0000000043

Ferrari AJ, Charlson FJ, Norman RE, Patten SB, Freedman G, Murray CJ, et al. Burden of depressive disorders by country, sex, age, and year: findings from the global burden of disease study (2010). *PLoS Med.* (2013) 10:e1001547. doi: 10.1371/journal.pmed.1001547

Schotte CK, Van Den Bossche B, De Doncker D, Claes S, Cosyns P. A biopsychosocial model as a guide for psychoeducation and treatment of depression. *Depression Anxiety* (2006) 23:312–24. doi: 10.1002/da.20177

Cohen BE, Edmondson D, Kronish IM. State of the art review: depression, stress, anxiety, and cardiovascular disease. *Am J Hypertens.* (2015) 28:1295– 1302. doi: 10.1093/ajh/hpv047

Hemmingsson E. A new model of the role of psychological and emotional distress in promoting obesity: conceptual review with implications for treatment and prevention. *Obes Rev.* (2014) 15:769–79. doi: 10.1111/obr.12197

Firth J, Stubbs B, Teasdale SB, Ward PB, Veronese N, Shivappa N, et al. Diet as a hot topic in psychiatry: a population-scale study of nutritional intake and inflammatory potential in severe mental illness. *World Psychiatry* (2018) 17:365–67. doi: 10.1002/wps.20571

Kaplan BJ, Crawford SG, Field CJ, Simpson JS. Vitamins, minerals, and mood. *Psychol Bull.* (2007) 133:747. doi: 10.1037/0033-2909.133.5.747

Berk M, Williams LJ, Jacka FN, O'Neil A, Pasco JA, Moylan S, et al. So depression is an inflammatory disease, but where does the inflammation come from? *BMC Med.* (2013) 11:200. doi: 10.1186/1741-7015- 11-200

Huskisson E, Maggini S, Ruf M. The role of vitamins and minerals in energy metabolism and well-being. *J Int Med Res.* (2007) 35:277–89. doi: 10.1177/147323000703500301

Jacka FN, Cherbuin N, Anstey KJ, Sachdev P, Butterworth P. Western diet is associated with a smaller hippocampus: a longitudinal investigation. *BMC Med.* (2015) 13:215. doi: 10.1186/s12916-015-0461-x

Jacka FN, Mykletun A, Berk M, Bjelland I, Tell GS. The association between habitual diet quality and the common mental disorders in community- dwelling adults: the Hordaland Health study. *Psychosomatic Med.* (2011) 73:483–90. doi: 10.1097/PSY.0b013e318222831a

Jacka FN, Berk M. Depression, diet and exercise. *Med J Aust.* (2013) 199:21– 23. doi: 10.5694/mja12.10508

Mujcic R, Oswald AJ. Evolution of well-being and happiness after increases in consumption of fruit and vegetables. *Am J Public Health* (2016) 106:1504–10. doi: 10.2105/AJPH.2016.303260

Liu X, et al. Fruit and vegetable consumption and the risk of depression: a meta-analysis. *Nutrition* (2016) 32:296–302. doi: 10.1016/j.nut.2015.09.009

Saghafian F, Malmir H, Saneei P, Milajerdi A, Larijani B, Esmaillzadeh A. Fruit and vegetable consumption and risk of depression: accumulative evidence from an updated systematic review and meta-analysis of epidemiological studies. *Br J Nutr.* (2018) 119:1087–1101. doi: 10.1017/S00071145180 00697

Parletta N, Zarnowiecki D, Cho J, Wilson A, Bogomolova S, Villani A, et al. A Mediterranean-style dietary intervention supplemented with fish oil improves diet quality and mental health in people with depression: a randomized controlled trial (HELFIMED). *Nutr Neurosci.* (2017) 1–14. doi: 10.1080/1028415X.2017.1411320

Schaakxs R, et al. Risk factors for depression: differential across age? *Am J Geriatr Psychiatry* (2017) 25:966–77. doi: 10.1016/j.jagp.2017.04.004

Pearson N, Biddle SJ. Sedentary behavior and dietary intake in children, adolescents, and adults: a systematic review. *Am J Prevent Med.* (2011) 41:178–88. doi: 10.1186/s12889-016-3708-3

Harris KM, Udry JR. *National Longitudinal Study of Adolescent Health (add health), 1994-2008:* Inter-university Consortium for Political and Social Research (2008).

Radloff LS. The CES-D scale: A self-report depression scale for research in the general population. *Appl Psychol Meas.* (1977) 1:385–401.

Lewinsohn PM, Seeley JR, Roberts RE, Allen NB. Center for epidemiologic studies depression Scale (CES-D) as a screening instrument for depression among community-residing older adults. *Psychol Aging* (1997) 12:277.

Andresen EM, Malmgren JA, Carter WB, Patrick DL. Screening for depression in well older adults: Evaluation of a short form of the CES-D . *Am J Prev Med.* (1994) 10:77–84.

Jacka FN, Kremer PJ, Berk M, de Silva-Sanigorski AM, Moodie M, Leslie ER, et al. A prospective study of diet quality and mental health in adolescents . *PLoS ONE* (2011) 6:e24805. doi: 10.1371/journal.pone.0024805

Entzel P, Whitsel E, Richardson AT, Joyce W, Hallquist S, Hussey J, et al. *Add Health Wave IV Documentation Report-Cardiovascular and Anthropometric*

Measures. Carolina Population Center (2013).

Sanders CE, Field TM, Diego M, Kaplan M. The relationship of Internet use to depression and social isolation among adolescents. *Adolescence* (2000) 35:237.

O'Neil A, Quirk SE, Housden S, Brennan SL, Williams LJ, Pasco JA, et al. Relationship between diet and mental health in children and adolescents: a systematic review. *Am J Public Health* (2014) 104:e31–42. doi: 10.2105/ AJPH.2014.302110

Jacka FN, Cherbuin N, Anstey KJ, Butterworth P. Dietary patterns and depressive symptoms over time: examining the relationships with socioeconomic position, health behaviours and cardiovascular risk. *PLoS ONE* (2014) 9:e87657. doi: 10.1371/journal.pone.0087657

Khalid S, Williams CM, Reynolds SA. Is there an association between diet and depression in children and adolescents? a Systematic review. *Br J Nutr.* (2016) 116:2097–108. doi: 10.1017/S0007114516004359

Kiecolt-Glaser JK. Stress, food, and inflammation: psychoneuroimmunology and nutrition at the cutting edge. *Psychosomat Med.* (2010) 72:365–9. doi: 10.1097/ PSY.0b013e3181dbf489

Hoare E, Dash SR, Jennings GL, Kingwell BA. Sex-specific associations in nutrition and activity-related risk factors for chronic disease: Australian evidence from childhood to emerging adulthood. *Int J Environ Res Public Health* (2018) 15:214. doi: 10.3390/ijerph15020214

Lawrence D, Johnson S, Hafekost J, Sawyer M, Ainley J, Zubrick SR, et al. *The Mental Health of Children and Adolescents: Report on the Second Australian Child and Adolescent Survey of Mental Health and Wellbeing.* Canberra, ACT: Department of Health (2015).

Miech RA, Shanahan MJ. Socioeconomic status and depression over the life course. *J Health Soc Behav.* (2000) 41:162–76. doi: 10.2307/2676303

Maguire ER, Burgoine T, Monsivais P. Area deprivation and the food environment over time: A repeated cross-sectional study on takeaway outlet density and supermarket presence in Norfolk, UK, 1990–2008. *Health Place* (2015) 33:142–7. doi: 10.1016/j.healthplace.2015.02.012

Gilbody ST, Lightfoot T, Sheldon T. Is low folate a risk factor for depression? a meta-analysis and exploration of heterogeneity. *J Epidemiol Community Health* (2007) 61:631–7. doi: 10.1136/jech.2006. 050385

Almeida OP, Ford AH, Flicker L. Systematic review and meta-analysis of randomized placebo-controlled trials of folate and vitamin B12 for depression. *Int Psychogeriatr.* (2015) 27:727–37. doi: 10.1017/S1041610215000046

Coppen A, Bolander-Gouaille C. Treatment of depression: time to consider folic acid and vitamin B12. *J Psychopharmacol.* (2005) 19:59–65. doi: 10.1177/0269881105048899

Dibaba DT, Xun P, He K. Dietary magnesium intake is inversely associated with serum C-reactive protein levels: meta-analysis and systematic review. *Eur J Clin Nutr.* (2014) 68:510–6. doi: 10.1038/ejcn.2014.7

Harasym J, Oledzki R. Effect of fruit and vegetable antioxidants on total antioxidant capacity of blood plasma. *Nutrition* (2014) 30:511–7. doi: 10.1016/j. nut.2013.08.019

McMartin SE, Jacka FN, Colman I. The association between fruit and vegetable consumption and mental health disorders: evidence from five waves of a national survey of Canadians. *Prev Med.* (2013) 56:225–30. doi: 10.1016/j. ypmed.2012.12.016

Cenit MC, Sanz Y, Codoñer-Franch P. Influence of gut microbiota on neuropsychiatric disorders. *World J Gastroenterol.* (2017) 23:5486–98. doi: 10.3748/wjg.v23.i30.5486

Subar AF, Freedman LS, Tooze JA, Kirkpatrick SI, Boushey C, Neuhouser ML, et al. Addressing Current Criticism Regarding the Value of Self-Report Dietary Data, 2. *J Nutr.* (2015) 145:2639–45. doi: 10.3945/jn.115.219634

Shafer AB. Meta-analysis of the factor structures of four depression questionnaires: beck, CES-D, Hamilton, and Zung. *J Clin Psychol.* (2006) 62:123–46. doi: 10.1002/jclp.20213

17

Acupuncture for Improving Cognitive Impairment after Stroke

Liang Zhou [1†], Yao Wang [2†], Jun Qiao [3], Qing Mei Wang [4] and Xun Luo [2,5]*

[1] Department of Reproductive Medicine, Peking University Shenzhen Hospital, Shenzhen, China, [2] Department of Rehabilitation Medicine, Dapeng New District Nan'ao People's Hospital, Shenzhen, China, [3] The Second Rehabilitation Hospital of Shanghai, Shanghai, China, [4] Stroke Biological Recovery Laboratory, Spaulding Rehabilitation Hospital, The Teaching Affiliate of Harvard Medical School, Boston, MA, United States, [5] Kerry Rehabilitation Medicine Research Institute, Shenzhen, China

***Correspondence:**
Xun Luo
larryluoxun@163.com

† These authors have contributed equally to this work

Objective: This meta-analysis evaluated the efficacy of acupuncture in improving cognitive impairment of post-stroke patients.

Design: Randomized controlled trials (RCTs) investigating the effects of acupuncture compared with no treatment or sham acupuncture on post-stroke cognitive impairment (PSCI) before December 2019 were identified from databases (PubMed, EMBASE, Ovid library, Cochrane Library, Chinese National Knowledge Infrastructure, VIP Chinese Periodical Database, Wanfang Database, and SinoMed). The literature searching and data extracting were independently performed by two investigators. Study quality was assessed using the Cochrane Handbook for Systematic Reviews of Interventions. Meta-analyses were performed for the eligible RCTs with Revman 5.3 software.

Results: Thirty-seven RCTs (2,869 patients) were included in this meta-analysis. Merged Random-effects estimates of the gain of MMSE (Mini-Mental State Examination) or MoCA (Montreal Cognitive Assessment) were calculated for the comparison of acupuncture with no acupuncture or sham acupuncture. Following 2–8 weeks of intervention with acupuncture, pooled results demonstrated significant effects of acupuncture in improving PSCI assessed by MMSE (MD [95% CI] = 2.88 [2.09, 3.66], $p < 0.00001$) or MoCA (MD [95% CI] = 2.66 [1.95, 3.37], $p < 0.00001$).

Conclusion: The results suggest that acupuncture was effective in improving PSCI and supported the needs of more rigorous design with large-scale randomized clinical trials to determine its therapeutic benefits.

Keywords: MMSE, cognitive impairment, electroacupuncture, acupuncture, post stroke

INTRODUCTION

Stroke is a disease that causes high rates of mortality and disability worldwide (Wu et al., 2010). Cognitive impairment is a frequent condition after stroke (Tatemichi et al., 1994; Patel et al., 2003), and its prevalence ranges from 17 to 92% (Pasi et al., 2012). Cognitive rehabilitation could enhance the quality of life for post-stroke patients, which included a comprehensive cognitive improvement program treating cognitive dysfunction involving disorientation, sensory disorders, attention disorders, executive function disorders, and memory disorders (Berrol, 1990; Choi and Twamley, 2013). The clinical depression is characterized by behavioral, cognitive, and emotional features (Merriman et al., 2019). Cognitive performance is associated with symptoms of depression (Nakling et al., 2017), and early cognitive impairment after stroke predicts long-term depressive symptoms in patients (Nys et al., 2006).

Acupuncture therapy has been used widely to promote motor recovery after stroke (Hu et al., 1993; Lee et al., 2003). Because of its low cost with low adverse events, acupuncture has also been used to improve the cognitive function of stroke patients, mostly in China, and it is receiving increasing attention among western countries (Johansson et al., 1993; NIH consensus conference, 1998). A considerable number of clinical trials showed the potential role of acupuncture as a promising treatment for post-stroke cognition impairment, but some trials suggest that acupuncture does not affect post-stroke cognitive impairment (PSCI) (Guo et al., 2007). The conflicting results may be caused by a small sample size of the trials and a flaw of study design.

Two systematic reviews (Liu et al., 2014; Wang, 2017) were performed; however, the studies were limited by small sample size. Liu et al. (2014) reported the meta-analysis results of 21 trials from 2006 to 2012; however, those trials had 12 different methods to evaluate cognitive function. Therefore, the largest dataset had only 116 patients from four studies [with Mini-Mental State Examination (MMSE) as the outcome measure]. In Wang's systematic review, only 15 studies with 1,085 subjects from 2008 to 2016 were included.

Since the last systematic review, many more clinical trials of acupuncture for post-stroke impairment were conducted; however, all of these clinical trials were limited by a small sample size or inconsistent selection criteria for the assessment of cognitive function. Therefore, with the further increased randomized controlled trials (RCT) evidence, there is a strong need to perform a systematic review to evaluate the therapeutic effect of acupuncture to treat PSCI.

In this study, we hypothesize that acupuncture is effective to improve cognitive function after stroke as compared to sham or no acupuncture. This systematic review and meta-analysis aimed to validate the efficacy of acupuncture in treatment for PSCI with MMSE or Montreal Cognitive Assessment (MoCA), which are the most generally used assessment tools for cognitive impairment (Foreman et al., 1996; Nasreddine et al., 2005).

MATERIALS AND METHODS

Inclusion Criteria and Exclusion Criteria

The inclusion criteria were the following: (1) type of studies: only randomized controlled trials (RCTs) of acupuncture for PSCI in English or Chinese language which were published before December 2019 were included; (2) type of participants: post-stroke patients (over 18 years old) with PSCI were included without restriction on gender, race, or nation; (3) type of interventions: the RCTs that used traditional acupuncture or electroacupuncture to treat PSCI were included; (4) outcome measurements: the outcome was assessed by MMSE or MoCA; and (5) type of comparators: the comparative interventions could be sham acupuncture or conventional treatment with rehabilitation. A RCT was included if acupuncture was used at acupoints as the sole treatment or as an adjunct to other treatments for cognition impairment after stroke. If studies included three or over three groups with only one group receiving acupuncture, and there is a control group without receiving acupuncture treated consistent with the acupuncture group, the data of acupuncture group, and control group were chosen for this study. If studies included three or over three groups with two or over two groups receiving acupuncture, a routine acupuncture group was chosen as the experiment group, and the group not receiving any acupuncture treated consistent with the acupuncture group was chosen as a control group.

The exclusion criteria were the following: (1) cognition impairment caused by other diseases except for stroke; (2) studies without a control group (control group treated consistent with the acupuncture group except receiving acupuncture); (3) studies compared different types of acupuncture; (4) studies compared the effect of acupuncture with a drug; (5) studies adopted complex treatment without specifying the sole effects of acupuncture; (6) cognition outcome measured by another assessing system except for MMSE or MoCA; (7) studies without standardized indices of curative effect or detailed results of treatment will be excluded; and (8) full texts cannot be obtained or the data cannot be extracted.

Identification of Eligible Trials

For search strategy, we searched articles published before December 2019 in the following databases: Chinese Science and Technology Periodical Database (VIP), China National Knowledge Infrastructure (CNKI), Wan Fang Database, PubMed, Embase, Web of Science, and the Ovid Library, and using the combining medical subject headings and keyword terms for stroke, acupuncture, and cognition. The search terms included "acupuncture/electroacupuncture" AND "stroke/stroke rehabilitation/cerebrovascular accident/brain ischemia/cerebral hemorrhage/CVA/cerebral embolism" AND "cognition/cognitive." At the same time, some studies were extracted from the references in the full-text articles. Articles were restricted to English and Chinese languages.

Assessment of Risk of Bias

The methodological quality and the risk of bias of the included studies were compiled using the risk of bias tool in the Cochrane Handbook for Systematic Reviews of Interventions (version 5.3) by two reviewers (L.Z. and Y.W.) independently. This instrument included seven specific domains: random sequence generation, allocation concealment, blinding of participants and personnel, blinding of outcome assessment, incomplete outcome data, selective reporting, and other bias.

Data Extraction

Studies were screened by two investigators independently. Disagreements were settled by consensus or a third investigator. The extracted data included general characteristics (author and year of publication), patient characteristics (sample size, mean age, and disease type), intervention characteristics (type and duration), and main outcomes and adverse events. When a given study reported the outcome with more than one cognitive function assessment, we gave preference primarily to MMSE or MoCA.

Statistical Analysis

All statistical analyses were performed with Revman 5.3 software (The Cochrane Collaboration software unpdate). Since the outcomes in studies were continuous variables, the mean differences (MDs) with 95% confidence intervals (CIs) were calculated. Heterogeneity was showed by I^2 index values with a p-value and percentage, respectively. A fixed-effects model would be used in a meta-analysis when heterogeneity was adopted ($I^2 <$ 25% or 50% $> I^2 \geq$ 25% with $p > 0.1$). Otherwise ($I^2 \geq$ 50% or 50% $> I^2 \geq$ 25% with $p \leq 0.1$) the random-effects model would be used.

The stability of the results was confirmed by sensitivity analysis. Publication bias was assessed by Begg's test with STATA software (version 12.0, Stata Corp). Quality of evidence was assessed with GRADEpro in website (www.gradepro.org).

RESULTS

Eligible Studies

The workflow of literature screening and inclusion is shown in **Figure 1**. The initial literature search yielded 977 studies. Out of 977 studies, 72 studies were duplicated. A total of 905 studies were assessed for eligibility by titles and abstracts screening. There were 69 papers that compared the effect of acupuncture in patients with PSCI. With full-text reading, 32 articles were excluded, and 37 studies were included in the synthesis. The 37 studies are 31 journal articles (Huang et al., 2008; Li and Zhang, 2008; Lin et al., 2010; Jia and Meng, 2011; Sun and Wu, 2011; Bai et al., 2012; Li et al., 2012, 2019; Liu and Feng, 2013; Song et al., 2013; Wang, 2014, 2019; Wang et al., 2014, 2019; Yang, 2014; Liu et al., 2015a,b; Zeng et al., 2015; Cai et al., 2016; Shao, 2016; Liu, 2017; Wang H. et al., 2017; Wang Z. et al., 2017; Zhang et al., 2017; Du et al., 2018; Jia and Lv, 2018; Ma et al., 2018; Wang and Li, 2018; Shi and Wei, 2019; Zhou H. et al., 2019; Zhou J. et al., 2019) and 6 dissertations (Jiang, 2011; Kang, 2011; Yang, 2011; Feng, 2013; Lu, 2014; Sun, 2017), which involved 2,869 patients (1,442 patients in the treatment group and 1,427 patients in the control group) in total. All those studies were conducted in China. Thirty-six papers were published in the Chinese language. **Table 1** shows the detailed information on the characteristics of the included studies. The ages of the patients range from 35 to 80 years. Seven trials did not describe the sex of the patients, while other trials included more male than female participants. The treatment period ranged from 2 to 12 weeks; the frequency of the sessions ranged from two sessions per day to five sessions per week. The chronicity of stroke ranged from 3 to 1,080 days, but most of those patients were treated within 6 months of onset. Twenty-three trials were conducted by manual acupuncture stimulation, and the other 14 trials used electroacupuncture only. The cognitive function assessment of all included studies was MMSE or MoCA.

Assessment of Risk of Bias

All RCTs had a low risk of bias (ROB) about adequate sequence generation. Eight RCTs had a low ROB with allocation concealment, while 9 RCTs had a high ROB, and 20 had an unclear ROB. Concerning participant blinding, one RCT had low ROB and the others had a high or unclear ROB. About assessor blinding, only three RCTs had a low ROB.

All 37 RCTs had a low ROB in incomplete outcome data addressed and selective outcome reporting. Thirty-four RCTs had an unclear ROB in other sources of bias. The results of the ROB assessment are shown in **Table 2, Figure 2**.

Meta-Analysis of the Results

The pooled meta-analysis of the data showed a weighted mean difference of 2.88 and 95% confidence intervals (CI) of 2.09–3.66 on the MMES ($p < 0.001$, $n = 2{,}349$; **Figure 3**).

Subgroup analyses showed weighted mean differences of 2.52 (95% CI: 1.86–3.18, n = 1,622) and 3.45 (95% CI: 2.09–3.66, n = 727) for acupuncture subgroup and electropuncture subgroup, respectively.

The pooled meta-analysis of the data showed a weighted mean difference of 2.66 and 95% confidence intervals of 1.95–3.37 on the MoCA ($p < 0.001$, $n = 1{,}129$; **Figure 4**).

Subgroup analyses showed weighted mean differences of 2.55 (95% CI: 1.71–3.39, n = 652) and 2.81 (95% CI: 1.42–4.02, n = 477) for acupuncture subgroup and electropuncture subgroup, respectively.

The results indicated that acupuncture had a significant effect on PSCI, and no adverse events were reported in those studies.

Sensitivity Analysis, Publication Bias, and Overall Quality of Evidence

High heterogeneity was shown in results (I^2 = 93 and 55 for MMSE and MoCA, respectively), so subgroup analyses were done based on different methods of acupuncture between manual acupuncture (acupuncture) and electropuncture. The results of subgroup analyses showed that intra-group heterogeneity remained high in subgroups ($I^2 > 50$), and the inter-group heterogeneity between subgroups was not too much ($I^2 <$ 50). Then sensitivity analysis was conducted by excluding the maximum weight studies in outcomes on subgroup analyses. The results showed that there was little influence on the pooled MD value. Then a study was removed at a time and the others analyzed to assess whether the results could have been influenced significantly by a single study. The results also showed no apparent fluctuation. These analyses confirmed the stability of the results of pooled MD value. Begg's tests showed no significant publication bias with symmetrical funnel plots. The overall quality of evidence was rated as moderate for MMSE and MoCA (**Figure 5**).

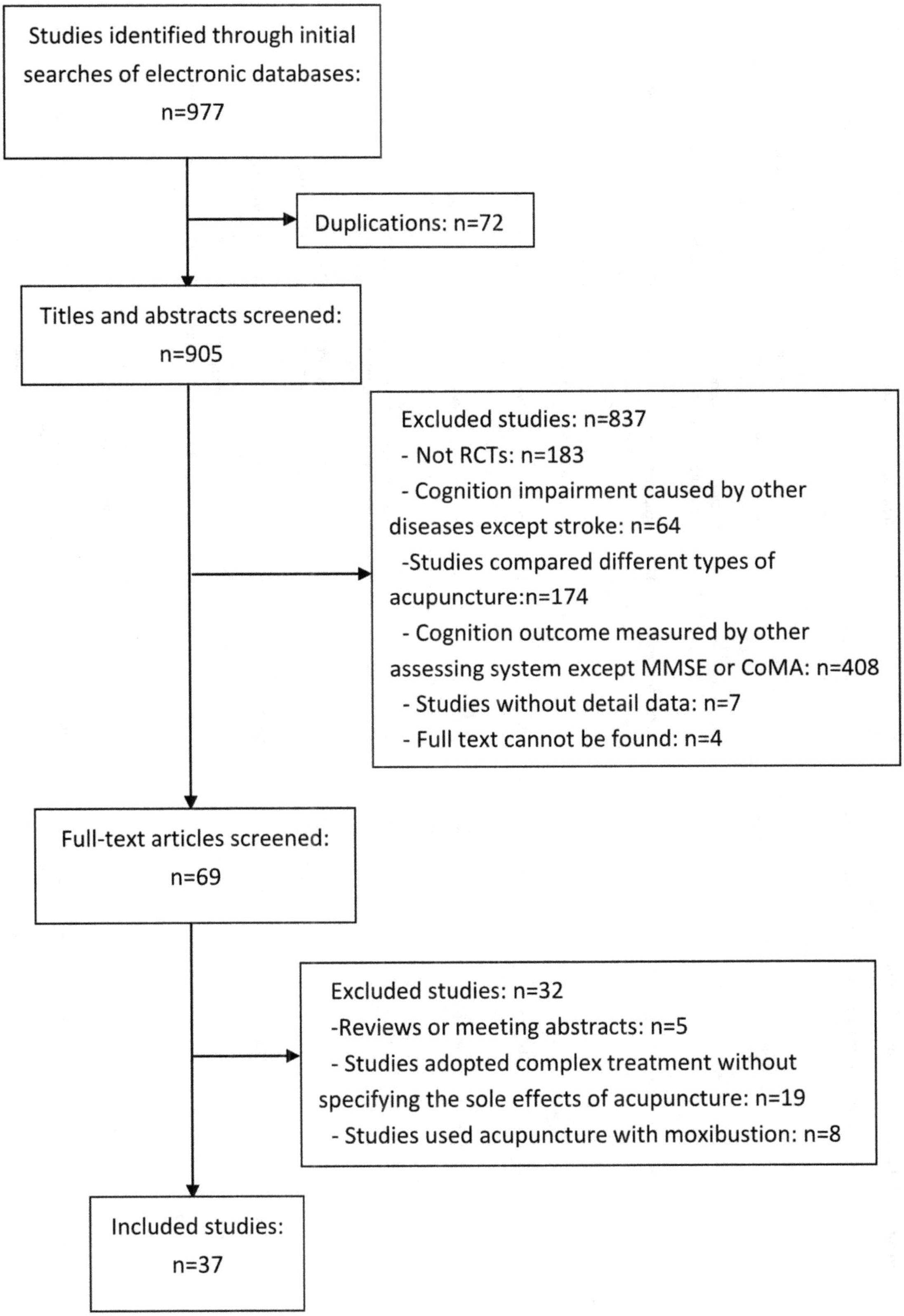

FIGURE 1 | Literature screening flow diagram.

TABLE 1 | Characteristics of included studies.

References	Patients no.		Ages (years)		Type of stroke	Outcome measures (MMSE/MoCA)	Therapy duration (wk)	Intervation		Source of diagnostic criteria for cerebral vascular diseases	Source of diagnostic criteria for PSCI
	Treatment	Control	Treatment	Control				Treatment	Control		
Sun (2017)	30	28	60.63 ± 8.273	61.29 ± 7.693	Ischemic stroke or hemorrhage	MMSE and MoCA	6	Acupuncture+ control treatment	Conventional treatment + rehabilitation	FNACCVD confirmed by head CT or MRI	DSM-IV
Shao (2016)	28	28	63 ± 5		Ischemic stroke or hemorrhage	MMSE	12	Acupuncture+ control treatment	Conventional treatment + rehabilitation	CECS, Chinese expert consensus standards	DSM-IV
Liu et al. (2015a)	32	30	51.97 ± 9.11	51.30 ± 10.57	Ischemic stroke or hemorrhage	MoCA	4	Electropuncture+ control treatment	Conventional treatment + rehabilitation	CECS, Chinese expert consensus standards	MoCA
Cai et al. (2016)	52	49	57.75 ± 13.74	56.18 ± 11.86	Ischemic stroke or hemorrhage	MMSE and MoCA	12	Acupuncture+ control treatment	Conventional treatment + rehabilitation	CECS, Chinese expert consensus standards	MMSE
Zeng et al. (2015)	50	50	66 ± 12	68 ± 10	Ischemic stroke or hemorrhage	MoCA	4/8	Electropuncture+ control treatment	Conventional treatment + rehabilitation	FNACCVD confirmed by head CT or MRI	MoCA
Wang (2014)	33	31	66.4 ± 3.0		Ischemic stroke or hemorrhage	MMSE	3	Acupuncture+ control treatment	Conventional treatment + xingnaojing	FNACCVD confirmed by head CT or MRI	Not shown
Lu (2014)	30	30	63.27 ± 11.88	63.90 ± 8.48	Ischemic stroke or hemorrhage	MoCA	4	Acupuncture+ control treatment	Conventional treatment + rehabilitation	CECS, Chinese expert consensus standards	MoCA
Zhai (2012)	55	55	59.2		Ischemic stroke	MMSE	12	Acupuncture+ control treatment	Conventional treatment + rehabilitation	FNACCVD confirmed by head CT or MRI	Not shown
Bai et al. (2012)	30	30	60 ± 6	60 ± 6	Ischemic stroke or hemorrhage	MMSE	4	Acupuncture+ control treatment	Conventional treatment + piracetam	FNACCVD confirmed by head CT or MRI	CCSE
Li et al. (2012)	48	46	68.29 ± 8.22	69.22 ± 7.88	Ischemic stroke or hemorrhage	MMSE	12	Acupuncture+ control treatment	Conventional treatment + nimodipine	FNACCVD confirmed by head CT or MRI	MMSE
Yang (2011)	20	20	59.00 ± 8.46	59.30 ± 8.42	Ischemic stroke or hemorrhage	MMSE	8	Acupuncture+ control treatment	Conventional treatment + rehabilitation	FNACCVD confirmed by head CT or MRI	MMSE
Sun and Wu (2011)	36	36	63.6 ± 5.8	64.1 ± 5.5	Ischemic stroke	MMSE	4	Acupuncture+ control treatment	Conventional treatment + aricept	FNACCVD confirmed by head CT or MRI	MMSE
Kang (2011)	24	24	60.67 ± 6.93	62.71 ± 5.34	Ischemic stroke or hemorrhage	MMSE	8	Electropuncture+ control treatment	Conventional treatment + rehabilitation	FNACCVD confirmed by head CT or MRI	MMSE
Jiang (2011)	20	20	62.85 ± 5.67	61.75 ± 6.35	Ischemic stroke or hemorrhage	MMSE	8	Electropuncture+ control treatment	Conventional treatment + rehabilitation	FNACCVD confirmed by head CT or MRI	CCSE

(Continued)

TABLE 1 | Continued

References	Patients no.		Ages (years)		Type of stroke	Outcome measures (MMSE/MoCA)	Therapy duration (wk)	Intervation		Source of diagnostic criteria for cerebral vascular diseases	Source of diagnostic criteria for PSCI
	Treatment	Control	Treatment	Control				Treatment	Control		
Jia and Meng (2011)	50	50	65 ± 2	58 ± 3	Ischemic stroke	MoCA	12	Acupuncture+ control treatment	Conventional treatment + rehabilitation + nimodipine	CECS, Chinese expert consensus standards	Diagnosis criteria shown in reference (Jia, 2004)
Lin et al. (2010)	30	30	63 ± 17	56 ± 13	Ischemic stroke	MMSE	3	Acupuncture+ control treatment	Conventional treatment + xingnaojing	FNACCVD confirmed by head CT or MRI	MMSE
Huang et al. (2008)	40	40	59.22 ± 10.6	61.05 ± 9.68	Ischemic stroke	MMSE	4	Acupuncture+ control treatment	Conventional treatment + xingnaojing	FNACCVD confirmed by head CT or MRI	CECVCI
Shi and Wei (2019)	55	55	60.31 ± 2.73	60.24 ± 2.65	Stroke	MMSE	4	Acupuncture+ control treatment	Conventional treatment + rehabilitation	Not shown	Not shown
Zhou J. et al. (2019)	60	60	61.44 ± 8.77	62.04 ± 8.69	Ischemic stroke or hemorrhage	MMSE and MoCA	4	Electropuncture+ control treatment	Conventional treatment + rehabilitation	CECS, Chinese expert consensus standards	DSM
Feng (2013)	40	40	51.65 ± 12.47	52.13 ± 12.77	Ischemic stroke or hemorrhage	MMSE and MoCA	4	Electropuncture+ control treatment	Conventional treatment + rehabilitation	FNACCVD confirmed by head CT or MRI	DSM-IV
Wang et al. (2019)	59	59	68.88 ± 3.64	67.71 ± 3.02	Ischemic stroke	MMSE	4	Acupuncture+ control treatment	Conventional treatment + Atorvastatin	FNACCVD confirmed by head CT or MRI	There are symptoms such as memory loss
Li et al. (2019)	40	40	66.9 ± 5.9	67.4 ± 6.1	Ischemic stroke or hemorrhage	MMSE and MoCA	6/12	Acupuncture+ control treatment	Conventional treatment+ Donepezil	FNACCVD confirmed by head CT or MRI	DSM-IV-R
Zhang et al. (2017)	42	42	62.28 ± 10.68	63.07 ± 10.59	Stroke	MMSE	4	Acupuncture+ control treatment	Conventional treatment + rehabilitation + Atorvastatin	FNACCVD confirmed by head CT or MRI	There are symptoms such as memory loss
Wang H. et al. (2017)	30	30	53.27 ± 11.62	56.73 ± 9.31	Ischemic stroke or hemorrhage	MMSE	8	Electropuncture+ control treatment	Conventional treatment + rehabilitation	FNACCVD confirmed by head CT or MRI	DSM-IV
Zhou H. et al. (2019)	40	40	61.5 ± 5.7	61.5 ± 4.4	Ischemic stroke	MMSE and MoCA	6	Electropuncture+ control treatment	Conventional treatment + rehabilitation + Perindopril	FNACCVD confirmed by head CT or MRI	Not shown
Wang Z. et al. (2017)	30	30	61.13 ± 11.42	60.06 ± 11.17	Ischemic stroke or hemorrhage	MMSE and MoCA	8	Acupuncture+ control treatment	Conventional treatment + rehabilitation	FNACCVD confirmed by head CT or MRI	DSM-IV-R

(Continued)

TABLE 1 | Continued

References	Patients no.		Ages (years)		Type of stroke	Outcome measures (MMSE/MoCA)	Therapy duration (wk)	Intervation		Source of diagnostic criteria for cerebral vascular diseases	Source of diagnostic criteria for PSCI
	Treatment	Control	Treatment	Control				Treatment	Control		
Wang et al. (2019)	78	78	69.04 ± 3.48	68.92 ± 3.65	stroke	MMSE	4	acupuncture+ control treatment	Conventional treatment + Tongluofuzheng decoction	Not shown	Not shown
Wang and Li (2018)	64	64	71.42 ± 8.67	69.33 ± 7.56	Ischemic stroke	MMSE and MoCA	6/10	Acupuncture+ control treatment	Conventional treatment + rehabilitation + nimodipine	CECS, Chinese expert consensus standards	Diagnosis criteria shown in reference (Zhang and Wang, 2004)
Yang (2014)	40	40	61.7 ± 4.8		Stroke	MMSE	3	Acupuncture+ control treatment	Conventional treatment + xingnaojing	FNACCVD confirmed by head CT or MRI	Not shown
Ma et al. (2018)	30	30	60.97 ± 7.15	60.17 ± 6.56	Ischemic stroke or hemorrhage	MMSE	2/4	Electropuncture+ control treatment	Conventional treatment + Oxiracetam + hyperbaric oxygen therapy	FNACCVD confirmed by head CT or MRI	MMSE
Jia and Lv (2018)	40	39	58.33 ± 11.13	57.45 ± 12.37	Ischemic stroke or hemorrhage	MMSE	4	Acupuncture+ control treatment	Conventional treatment + Huoxuetongluo decoction	FNACCVD confirmed by head CT or MRI	CCSE
Liu (2017)	32	32	56.9 ± 10.3	56.4 ± 10.1	Ischemic stroke or hemorrhage	MMSE	2	Electropuncture+ control treatment	Conventional treatment + rehabilitation	FNACCVD confirmed by head CT or MRI	Not shown
Liu et al. (2015b)	19	16	52.42 ± 7.62	51.06 ± 11.62	Ischemic stroke or hemorrhage	MMSE and MoCA	4	Electropuncture+ control treatment	Conventional treatment + rehabilitation	CECS, Chinese expert consensus standards	MMSE
Sun et al. (2013)	60	60	62.50 ± 4.52	63.01 ± 4.67	Ischemic stroke	MMSE	4	Electropuncture+ control treatment	Conventional treatment + rehabilitation + nimodipine	FNACCVD confirmed by head CT or MRI	MMSE
Liu and Feng (2013)	25	25	53.40 ± 8.48		Ischemic stroke or hemorrhage	MMSE	4	Electropuncture+ control treatment	Conventional treatment + rehabilitation	FNACCVD confirmed by head CT or MRI	DSM-IV-R
Wang et al. (2014)	30	30	45~80		Ischemic stroke	MoCA	12	Acupuncture+ control treatment	Conventional treatment + nimodipine	FNACCVD confirmed by head CT or MRI	Not shown
Li and Zhang (2008)	20	20	58~76		Ischemic stroke	MMSE	4	Electropuncture+ control treatment	Conventional treatment + rehabilitation	FNACCVD confirmed by head CT	Not shown

MMSE, Mini-Mental State Examination; MoCA, Montreal Cognitive Assessment; FNACCVD, Fourth National Academic Conference of Cerebral Vascular Diseases; CT, computed tomography; MRI, magnetic resonance imaging; DSM-IV,Diagnostic and Statistical Manual of Mental Disorders(the fourth edition); DSM-IV-R, DSM-IV-Revised edition; CECS, Chinese expert consensus standards, proposed in 2005 for the prevention and treatment of cognitive dysfunction; CCSE, Cognitive Capacity Screening Examination; CECVCI, Chinese Expert consensus on vascular cognitive impairment 2007.

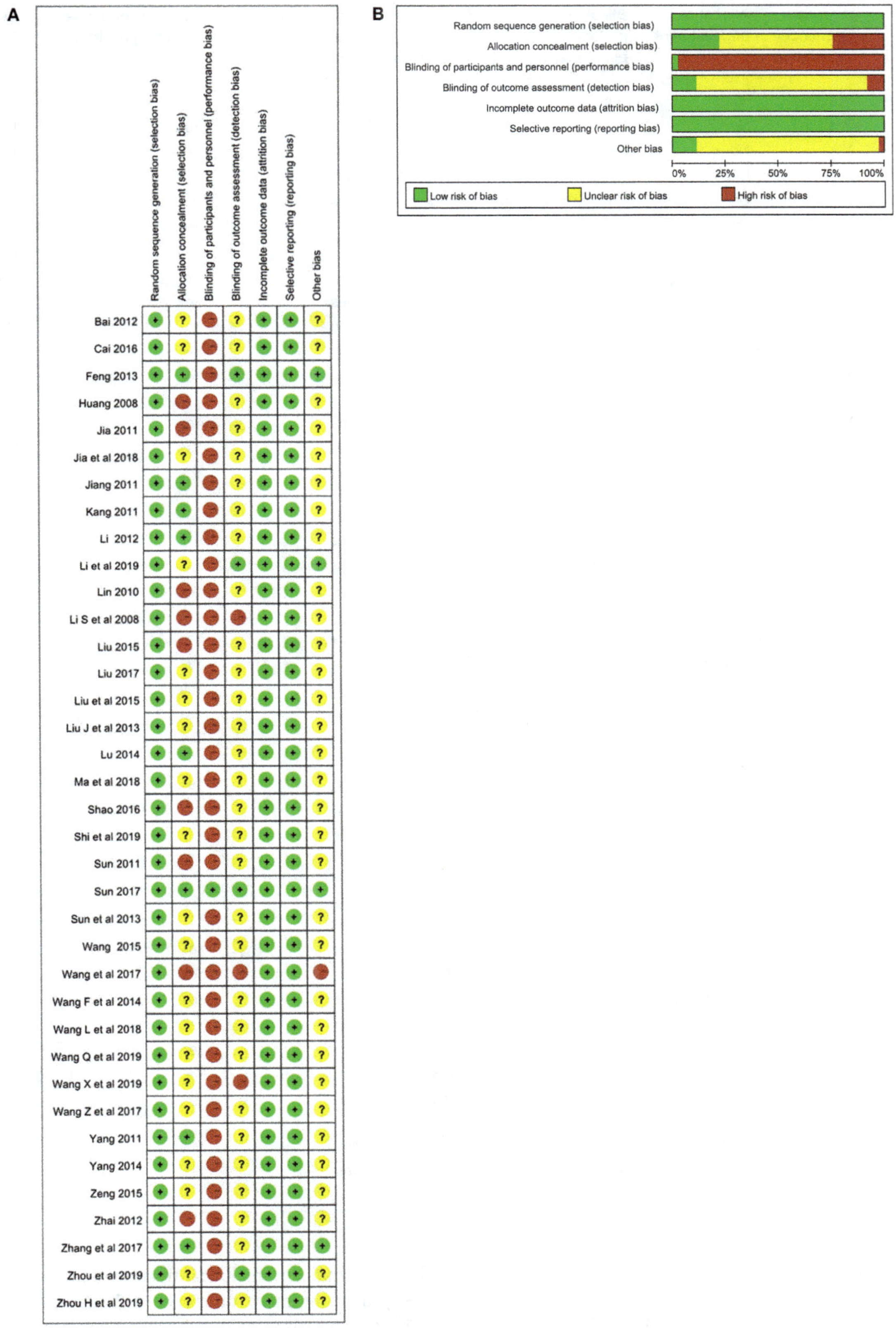

FIGURE 2 | **(A)** Assessment of risk of bias with selected studies. **(B)**. Risk of bias graph and summary.

TABLE 2 | Quality assessment of studies.

References	Adequate sequence generation	Allocation concealment	Blinding of participation and personnel	Blinding of outcome assessment	Incomplete outcome data addressed	Selective outcome reporting avoided	Other sources of bias
Sun (2017)	Yes	Yes	Yes	Yes	Yes	Yes	Unclear
Shao (2016)	Yes	No	No	Unclear	Yes	Yes	Unclear
Liu et al. (2015a)	Yes	No	No	Unclear	Yes	Yes	Unclear
Cai et al. (2016)	Yes	Unclear	No	Unclear	Yes	Yes	Unclear
Zeng et al. (2015)	Yes	Unclear	No	Unclear	Yes	Yes	Unclear
Wang (2014)	Yes	Unclear	No	Unclear	Yes	Yes	Unclear
Lu (2014)	Yes	Yes	No	Unclear	Yes	Yes	Unclear
Zhai (2012)	Yes	No	No	Unclear	Yes	Yes	Unclear
Bai et al. (2012)	Yes	Unclear	No	Unclear	Yes	Yes	Unclear
Li et al. (2012)	Yes	Yes	No	Unclear	Yes	Yes	Unclear
Yang (2011)	Yes	Yes	No	Unclear	Yes	Yes	Unclear
Sun and Wu (2011)	Yes	No	No	Unclear	Yes	Yes	Unclear
Kang (2011)	Yes	Yes	No	Unclear	Yes	Yes	Unclear
Jiang (2011)	Yes	Yes	No	Unclear	Yes	Yes	Unclear
Jia and Meng (2011)	Yes	No	No	Unclear	Yes	Yes	Unclear
Lin et al. (2010)	Yes	No	No	Unclear	Yes	Yes	Unclear
Huang et al. (2008)	Yes	No	No	Unclear	Yes	Yes	Unclear
Shi and Wei (2019)	Yes	Unclear	No	Unclear	Yes	Yes	Unclear
Zhou J. et al. (2019)	Yes	Unclear	No	Unclear	Yes	Yes	Unclear
Feng (2013)	Yes	Yes	No	Yes	Yes	Yes	No
Wang et al. (2019)	Yes	Unclear	No	Unclear	Yes	Yes	Unclear
Li et al. (2019)	Yes	Unclear	No	Yes	Yes	Yes	No
Zhang et al. (2017)	Yes	Yes	No	Unclear	Yes	Yes	No
Wang H. et al. (2017)	Yes	No	No	No	Yes	Yes	Unclear
Zhou H. et al. (2019)	Yes	Unclear	No	Unclear	Yes	Yes	Unclear
Wang Z. et al. (2017)	Yes	Unclear	No	Unclear	Yes	Yes	Unclear
Wang et al. (2019)	Yes	Unclear	No	Unclear	Yes	Yes	Unclear
Wang and Li (2018)	Yes	Unclear	No	Unclear	Yes	Yes	Unclear
Yang (2014)	Yes	Unclear	No	Unclear	Yes	Yes	Unclear
Ma et al. (2018)	Yes	Unclear	No	Unclear	Yes	Yes	Unclear
Jia and Lv (2018)	Yes	Unclear	No	Unclear	Yes	Yes	Unclear
Liu (2017)	Yes	Unclear	No	Unclear	Yes	Yes	Unclear
Liu et al. (2015b)	Yes	Unclear	No	Unclear	Yes	Yes	Unclear
Sun et al. (2013)	Yes	Unclear	No	Unclear	Yes	Yes	Unclear
Liu and Feng (2013)	Yes	Unclear	No	Unclear	Yes	Yes	Unclear
Wang et al. (2014)	Yes	Unclear	No	Unclear	Yes	Yes	Unclear
Li and Zhang (2008)	Yes	No	No	No	Yes	Yes	Unclear

DISCUSSION

Our findings showed that acupuncture or electroacupuncture therapy is effective in improving the cognitive impairment of post-stroke patients by assessing with MMSE and MoCA. The gain of the mean difference is 2.88 for MMSE (CI [2.09, 3.66]), which is significant in clinical treatment (Andrews et al., 2019). The gain of the mean difference is 2.66 for MoCA (CI [1.95, 3.37]), which is also significant in clinical treatment (Wong et al., 2017).

In this study, patients in the control group were treated with conventional treatment in all 37 trials, patients had

Study or Subgroup	Experimental Mean	Experimental SD	Experimental Total	Control Mean	Control SD	Control Total	Weight	Mean Difference IV, Random, 95% CI
1.3.1 acupuncture								
Bai 2012	4.72	5.16	30	1.75	3	30	2.9%	2.97 [0.83, 5.11]
Cai 2016	3.06	4.91	52	1.59	4.19	49	3.1%	1.47 [-0.31, 3.25]
Huang 2008	4.33	3.94	40	1.54	4.24	40	3.1%	2.79 [1.00, 4.58]
Jia et al 2018	6.08	2.31	40	3.22	2.22	39	3.5%	2.86 [1.86, 3.86]
Li 2012	3.25	2.55	48	2.09	2.13	46	3.5%	1.16 [0.21, 2.11]
Li et al 2019	3.14	2.34	40	1.58	2.12	40	3.5%	1.56 [0.58, 2.54]
Lin 2010	10.2	5.88	30	5.9	4.33	30	2.6%	4.30 [1.69, 6.91]
Shao 2016	3.53	5.41	28	1.66	6.41	28	2.4%	1.87 [-1.24, 4.98]
Shi et al 2019	8.88	2.19	55	4.66	2	55	3.6%	4.22 [3.44, 5.00]
Sun 2011	6.74	4.28	30	2.14	2.91	28	3.1%	4.60 [2.73, 6.47]
Sun 2017	3.59	3.65	36	1.72	3.56	36	3.2%	1.87 [0.20, 3.54]
Wang 2015	10.9	3.8	30	10.97	2.67	30	3.2%	-0.07 [-1.73, 1.59]
Wang L et al 2018	4.1	2.63	33	0.6	2.59	31	3.4%	3.50 [2.22, 4.78]
Wang Q et al 2019	4.22	1.9	59	2.75	1.5	59	3.7%	1.47 [0.85, 2.09]
Wang X et al 2019	8.93	3.74	78	4.75	3.96	78	3.4%	4.18 [2.97, 5.39]
Wang Z et al 2017	0.4	1.55	30	-0.04	1.5	30	3.6%	0.44 [-0.33, 1.21]
Yang 2011	3.75	2.91	20	1.15	3.02	20	3.1%	2.60 [0.76, 4.44]
Yang 2014	11.5	5.19	40	5.38	4.35	40	3.0%	6.12 [4.02, 8.22]
Zhai 2012	3.63	2.12	55	0.58	2.56	55	3.6%	3.05 [2.17, 3.93]
Zhang et al 2017	4.19	2.03	42	2.93	1.54	42	3.6%	1.26 [0.49, 2.03]
Subtotal (95% CI)			**816**			**806**	**65.3%**	**2.52 [1.86, 3.18]**
Heterogeneity: Tau² = 1.69; Chi² = 113.68, df = 19 (P < 0.00001); I² = 83%								
Test for overall effect: Z = 7.50 (P < 0.00001)								
1.3.2 electropuncture								
Jiang 2011	3.4	3.88	20	1.3	2.72	20	3.0%	2.10 [0.02, 4.18]
Kang 2011	2.37	2.37	24	0.96	2.28	24	3.4%	1.41 [0.09, 2.73]
Li S et al 2008	11.2	6.61	20	5.4	5.72	20	2.0%	5.80 [1.97, 9.63]
Liu 2015	15.08	1.14	25	8.8	0.96	25	3.7%	6.28 [5.70, 6.86]
Liu 2017	2.53	3.85	19	1.44	3.9	16	2.7%	1.09 [-1.49, 3.67]
Liu J et al 2013	15.14	1.04	32	9.21	0.89	32	3.7%	5.93 [5.46, 6.40]
Ma et al 2018	7.31	3.59	30	3.6	3.67	30	3.1%	3.71 [1.87, 5.55]
Sun et al 2013	4.08	2.31	60	2.01	2.45	60	3.6%	2.07 [1.22, 2.92]
Wang et al 2017	2.14	2.45	35	1.42	2.44	35	3.5%	0.72 [-0.43, 1.87]
Zhou et al 2019	8.1	3.92	60	3.25	3.86	60	3.3%	4.85 [3.46, 6.24]
Zhou H et al 2019	6.72	5.32	40	2.54	4.97	40	2.9%	4.18 [1.92, 6.44]
Subtotal (95% CI)			**365**			**362**	**34.7%**	**3.45 [2.04, 4.87]**
Heterogeneity: Tau² = 4.91; Chi² = 176.15, df = 10 (P < 0.00001); I² = 94%								
Test for overall effect: Z = 4.79 (P < 0.00001)								
Total (95% CI)			**1181**			**1168**	**100.0%**	**2.88 [2.09, 3.66]**
Heterogeneity: Tau² = 4.29; Chi² = 451.98, df = 30 (P < 0.00001); I² = 93%								
Test for overall effect: Z = 7.18 (P < 0.00001)								
Test for subgroup differences: Chi² = 1.38, df = 1 (P = 0.24), I² = 27.3%								

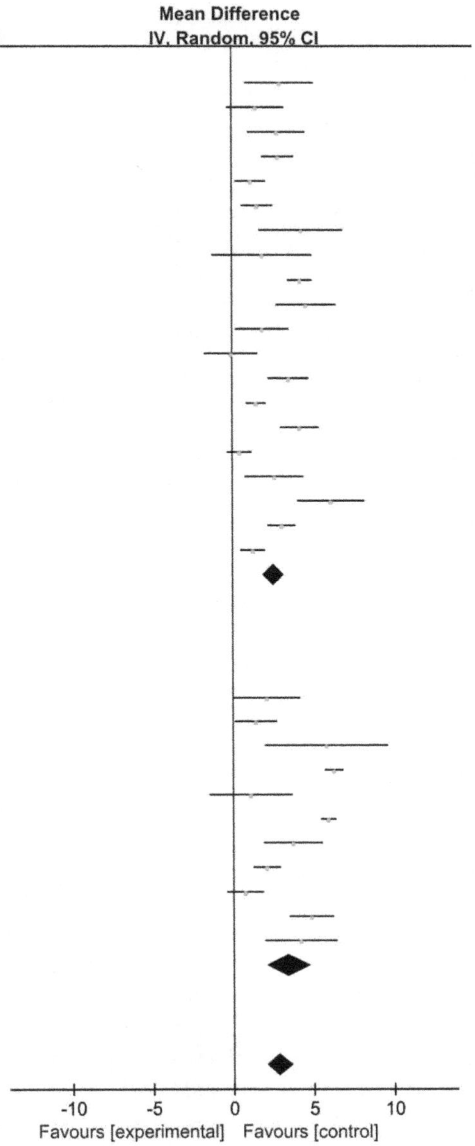

FIGURE 3 | Forest plot comparing the MMSE improved between acupuncture groups and control groups.

conventional rehabilitation done in the control groups in 23 trials, and patients had medicine in control groups in 17 trials. Patients in experiment groups combined the acupuncture or electroacupuncture and conventional rehabilitation or medicine used the same as in control groups in all trials. The merged results showed that synergistic effects of acupuncture or electroacupuncture therapy is clinically significant in improving PSCI, and there were no adverse events/incidents reported in those studies.

There was some inconsistent information in the included studies. The patients were all with ischemic stroke in 10 studies; the other 22 studies included patients with hemorrhage or ischemic stroke, and 4 studies only included post-stroke patients. In the 37 studies, 23 studies indicated that acupuncture treatment was within 6 months from stroke onset, 5 studies was under 1 year, 2 studies was under 14/36 months, and the other 7 studies did not report the accurate time. In this meta-analysis, 24 studies focused on the effects of acupuncture combined with conventional rehabilitation treatment, and the other 13 studies analyzed the effectiveness of acupuncture combined with medicine (Aricept, Xingnaojing, Nimodipine, Piracetam, etc.). Fourteen studies used electroacupuncture, and the other 23 studies used traditional manual acupuncture. The intervention period varied across studies from 2 to 12 weeks.

There were obvious heterogeneities of these articles, so the random effects model was used in this study. Subgroup analysis between acupuncture group and electropuncture did not significantly reduce heterogeneity in this study. This may

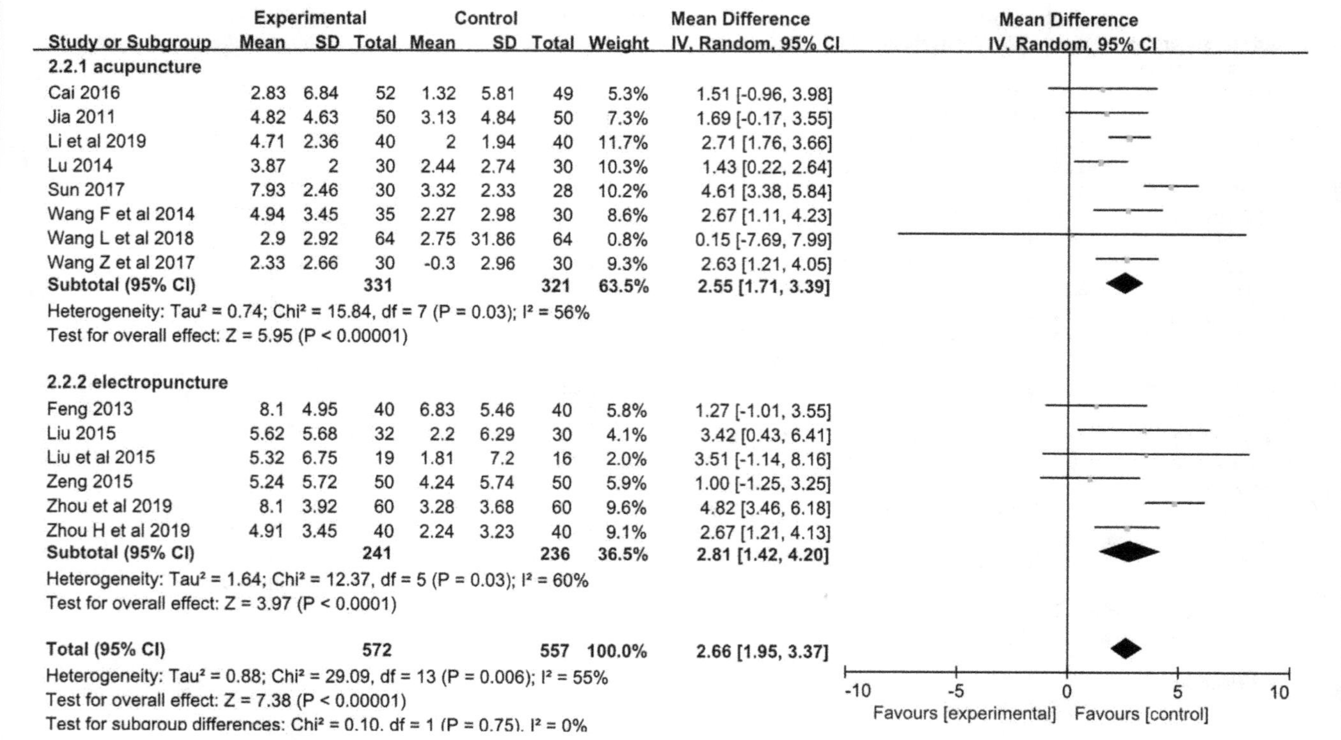

FIGURE 4 | Forest plot comparing the CoMA improved between acupuncture groups and control groups.

be caused by the unbalance of acupoints selection, the different treatment period, and the therapist's technical ability.

In the theoretical system of acupuncture, the Du Meridian is important for the cognitive brain function (Zhou et al., 2013; Liu et al., 2014), and acupoints "Baihui" and "Shenting" belong to the Du Meridian. Baihui and Shenting are both located in the head. To Chinese traditional medicine theoretical system, acupuncture Baihui and Shenting can lift the spirit, clear the mind, and promote resuscitation. In these 37 studies, 26 studies acupuncture the acupoints including "Baihui," and 19 studies involved the acupoint "Shenting" for the treatment of mental and emotional illness. Other acupoints, such as Feishu, Xinshu, Ganshu, Shenshu, and Pishu were shown involving the cognitive function in more than three studies. Other acupuncture points involved were Huiyin, Yintang, Neiguan, Yanglingquan, Taixi, Zulinqi, Sishencong, Fengchi, Fengfu, Gongxue, Yiming, Guanyuan, Taichong, Shenshu, Benshen, Hegu, Taichong, Fengshi, Quchi, Zusanli, Sanyingjiao, Xuehai, Renzhong, Shenmen, etc.

Acupuncture improves cognitive function and depressive disorder, because acupuncture on stroke patients can improve neurological function (Chen et al., 2018; Hung et al., 2019). Animal studies showed that acupuncture with Baihui may have a neuroprotective effect via decreasing MMP-9 expression or improving the endothelial nitric oxide synthase (eNOS)-mediated perfusion (Dong et al., 2009; Kim et al., 2013).

H Jiang et al.'s and J Liang et al.'s studies showed that acupuncture was associated with the potential of DNA methylation and histone modifications of brain-derived neurotropic factor in epigenetic mechanism, which can produce antidepressant effect in rats (Liang et al., 2012; Jiang et al., 2018). F Taya et al. showed that acupuncture may increase cerebral collateral circulation, promoting repair of the lesion (Taya et al., 2015). P.Y. Sun et al. showed that acupuncture repairs hippocampal neuronal damage, which is probably related to the contents of hippocampal monoamine neurotransmitters (NE, 5-HT and DA) (Sun et al., 2019). Other studies showed that electropuncture can improve cognitive function via synaptic plasticity by attenuating pathological lesions and increasing the density of dendritic spines and number of CA1 synapses in rats (Lin et al., 2016; Liu et al., 2017; Wen et al., 2018).

The selection criteria for the assessment of cognitive function were the Mini-Mental State Examination (MMSE) and the Montreal Cognitive Assessment (MoCA). MMSE is an effective tool that can be used to systematically and thoroughly assess mental status, which was validated and extensively used from 1975 (Foreman et al., 1996). MoCA is a widely used screening assessment for detecting cognitive impairment since 1996, which was validated in the setting of mild cognitive impairment (Nasreddine et al., 2005). There are other internationally recognized examinations of cognitive impairment including NCSE, NIHSS, LOTCA, HDS, and cognitive potential 300, but the most commonly used indicators are MMSE and MoCA. We restricted the inclusion criteria to a consistent standard of outcome assessing with MMSE or MoCA, so the number of RCTs included in this study was not so many

Acupuncture compared to conventional treatment for improving post strok cognitive impairment

Patient or population: Post strok patients
Setting: Peking University Shenzhen Hospital
Intervention: Acupuncture
Comparison: Conventional treatment

Outcomes	Anticipated absolute effects* (95% CI)		№ of participants (studies)	Certainty of the evidence (GRADE)
	Risk with conventional treatment	**Risk with acupuncture**		
Mental state improved (MMSE) assessed with: MMSE form follow up: 2-12 weeks	The mean mental state improved was **2.96** [a]	MD **2.88 higher** (2.09 higher to 3.66 higher)	3971 (31 RCTs)	⊕⊕⊕◯ MODERATE
Cognitive assessment improved (MoCA) assessed with: MoCA form follow up: 4-12 weeks	The mean cognitive assessment improved was **2.68** [b]	MD **2.66 higher** (1.95 higher to 3.77 higher)	1129 (14 RCTs)	⊕⊕⊕◯ MODERATE [c]

***The risk in the intervention group** (and its 95% confidence interval) is based on the assumed risk in the comparison group and the **relative effect** of the intervention (and its 95% CI).

CI: Confidence interval; **MD:** Mean difference

GRADE Working Group grades of evidence
High certainty: We are very confident that the true effect lies close to that of the estimate of the effect
Moderate certainty: We are moderately confident in the effect estimate: The true effect is likely to be close to the estimate of the effect, but there is a possibility that it is substantially different
Low certainty: Our confidence in the effect estimate is limited: The true effect may be substantially different from the estimate of the effect
Very low certainty: We have very little confidence in the effect estimate: The true effect is likely to be substantially different from the estimate of effect

Explanations

a. After conventional treatment, the MMSE score was improved by 2.97 than before.
b. After conventional treatment, the MoCA score was improved by 2.68 than before.
c. Many of the RCTs were low quality with an inadequate level of blinding because blindings in the acupuncture therapy were difficult for the therapists and patients.

FIGURE 5 | Evidence profile.

(only 37), but the results of meta-analyses were more clear and definite, and the quality of evidence was assessed to be moderate.

About the limitation, firstly, all studies were done in China, although the Cai et al. (2016) study was published in the English language. There might have been additional reports using non-Chinese or non-English languages that were not included which may limit the results of the study. Secondly, many of the trials were of low quality with an inadequate level of blinding; although blinding in the acupuncture therapy is difficult for the therapists and patients, blinding the assessor is necessary.

Despite these limitations, conclusions can be drawn from the results of our study.

CONCLUSIONS

Acupuncture therapy has positive synergistic effects in improving PSCI, but more rigorous design studies with large-scale sham are needed to determine the longevity of acupuncture effects.

AUTHOR CONTRIBUTIONS

LZ, QW, and XL: conceptualization and writing, review, and editing. LZ, YW, and JQ: data curation and methodology. LZ and XL: funding acquisition. QW and XL: supervision. LZ: writing the original draft. All authors contributed to the article and approved the submitted version.

REFERENCES

NIH consensus conference (1998). acupuncture. *JAMA* 280, 1518–1524. doi: 10.1001/jama.280.17.1518

Andrews, J., Desai, U., Kirson, N., Zichlin, M., Ball, D., and Matthews, B. (2019). Disease severity and minimal clinically important differences in clinical outcome assessments for Alzheimer's disease clinical trials. *Alzheimer's Dementia* 5, 354–363. doi: 10.1016/j.trci.2019.06.005

Bai, J., Li, B., and Wang, Q. (2012). Therapeutic observation on cluster needling at scalp acupoints plus cognitio training for post-stroke cognitive impairment. *Shanghai J. Acupunct. Moxibustion* 10, 711–713. doi: 10.3969/j.issn.1005-0957.2012.10.711

Berrol, S. (1990). Issues in cognitive rehabilitation. *Arch. Neurol.* 47, 219–220. doi: 10.1001/archneur.1990.00530020127025

Cai, J., Yang, S. L., Tao, J., Huang, J., Li, Y. Y., Ye, H. C., et al. (2016). Clinical efficacy of acupuncture treatment in combination with rehacom cognitive training for improving cognitive function in stroke: a 2 x 2 factorial design randomized controlled trial. *J. Am. Med. Dir. Assoc.* 17, 1114–1122. doi: 10.1016/j.jamda.2016.07.021

Chen, A., Gao, Y., Wang, G., Li, J., and Shen, W. (2018). Effect of early acupuncture intervention on post-stroke depression: a randomized controlled trial. *Zhongguo Zhen Jiu* 38, 1141–1144. doi: 10.13703/j.0255-2930.2018.11.001

Choi, J., and Twamley, E. W. (2013). Cognitive rehabilitation therapies for Alzheimer's disease: a review of methods to improve treatment engagement and self-efficacy. *Neuropsychol. Rev.* 23, 48–62. doi: 10.1007/s11065-013-9227-4

Dong, H., Fan, Y. H., Zhang, W., Wang, Q., Yang, Q. Z., and Xiong, L. Z. (2009). Repeated electroacupuncture preconditioning attenuates matrix metalloproteinase-9 expression and activity after focal cerebral ischemia in rats. *Neurol. Res.* 31, 853–858. doi: 10.1179/174313209X393960

Du, S. J., Su, X., Feng, W. F., Chen, X. J., Xu, C. Y., Feng, S. W., et al. (2018). Observation on the therapeutic effect of TiaoShenJiangPi acupuncture combined with tonepezil on cognitive impairment after stroke. *J. Pract. Tradit. Chinese Med.* 7, 810–811. doi: 10.3969/j.issn.1004-2814.2018.07.047

Feng, X. (2013). *The Studies of clinical Observation and Mechanism in Treating the Cognitive Impairment After Stroke by Electroacupuncture at Shenting and Baidui.* (M.D) Fujian University of Traditional Chinese Medicine, Fuzhou, China.

Foreman, M. D., Fletcher, K., Mion, L. C., and Simon, L. (1996). Assessing cognitive function. *Geriat. Nurs.* 17, 228–232. doi: 10.1016/S0197-4572(96)80210-2

Guo, R. Y., Liu, L. A., and Ma, X. W. (2007). Long-term effect of acupuncture on quality of life in patients with early stage of stroke. *Zhongguo Zhong Xi Yi Jie He Za Zhi* 7, 708–710. doi: 10.3321/j.issn:1003-5370.2007.08.012

Hu, H. H., Chung, C., Liu, T. J., Chen, R. C., Chen, C. H., Chou, P., et al. (1993). A randomized controlled trial on the treatment for acute partial ischemic stroke with acupuncture. *Neuroepidemiology* 12, 106–113. doi: 10.1159/000110308

Huang, F., Liu, Y., Zhou, F., Yao, G., and He, Q. (2008). Effect of acupuncture on vascular cognitive impairment after cerebral infarction. *Guangdong Med. J.* 11, 1918–1920. doi: 10.3969/j.issn.1001-9448.2008.11.071

Hung, C. Y., Wu, X. Y., Chung, V. C., Tang, E. C., Wu, J. C., and Lau, A. Y. (2019). Overview of systematic reviews with meta-analyses on acupuncture in post-stroke cognitive impairment and depression management. *Integrat. Med. Res.* 8, 145–159. doi: 10.1016/j.imr.2019.05.001

Jia, J. P. (2004). Attention should be paid to the establishment of diagnostic criteria and clinical research of vascular cognitive impairment. *Chinese J. Cerebrovas. Dis.* 1, 14–17. doi: 10.3969/j.issn.1672-5921.2004.01.004

Jia, X., and Meng, I. (2011). Observations on the efficacy of lower point selection for upper disease in treating cognitive impairment after acute cerebral infarction. *Shanghai J. Acupunct. Moxibustion* 30, 589–590. doi: 10.3969/j.issn.1005-0957.2011.09.589

Jia, Y., and Lv, X. (2018). Clinical study of acupuncture combined with Huoxue Tonglno Decoction in the treatment of post-stroke cognitive impairmen. *China Med. Herald* 4, 113–116.

Jiang, H., Zhang, X., Lu, J., Meng, H., Sun, Y., Yang, X., et al. (2018). Antidepressant-like effects of acupuncture insights from DNA methylation and histone modifications of brain-derived neurotrophic factor. *Front. Psychiatry* 9:102. doi: 10.3389/fpsyt.2018.00102

Jiang, Y. (2011). *Electroacupuncture DU20 and DU24 treatment on cognitive impairment.* (M.S) Fujian University of Traditional Chinese Medicine, Fuzhou, China.

Johansson, K., Lindgren, I., Widner, H., Wiklund, I., and Johansson, B. B. (1993). Can sensory stimulation improve the functional outcome in stroke patients? *Neurology* 43, 2189–2192. doi: 10.1212/WNL.43.11.2189

Kang, J. (2011). *Clinical study of effect of electroacupuncture on GV20 and EX-HN1 on stroke patients with cognitive impairment.* M.S. (Fujian University of Traditional Chinese Medicine).

Kim, J. H., Choi, K. H., Jang, Y. J., Bae, S. S., Shin, B. C., Choi, B. T., et al. (2013). Electroacupuncture acutely improves cerebral blood flow and attenuates moderate ischemic injury via an endothelial mechanism in mice. *PLoS ONE* 8:e56736. doi: 10.1371/journal.pone.0056736

Lee, J. D., Chon, J. S., Jeong, H. K., Kim, H., Yun, M., Kim, D. Y., Kim, D. I., et al. (2003). The cerebrovascular response to traditional acupuncture after stroke. *Neuroradiology* 45, 780–784. doi: 10.1007/s00234-003-1080-3

Li, L., Xiao, P., Chen, Q., and Tang, L. (2019). Effects of acupuncture combined with donepezil on cognitive impairment after stroke in elderly patients. *Chinese J. Prevent. Control Chronic Non-Commun Dis.* 27, 617–620. doi: 10.16386/j.cjpccd.issn.1004-6194.2019.08.015

Li, S. M., and Zhang, Z. X. (2008). The effect of acupuncture on the patients with cerebral infarction. *Zhejiang Chinese Med. Univ. xue bao* 24, 514–515. doi: 10.3969/j.issn.1005-5509.2008.04.051

Li, W., Cheng, Y. H., and Yu, X. G. (2012). Observation on therapeutic effect of acupuncture combined with medicine on mild cognition disorders in patients with post-stroke. *Chinese Acupunct. Moxibust.* 32, 3–7. doi: 10.13703/j.0255-2930.2012.01.005

Liang, J., Lu, J., Cui, S. F., Wang, J. R., and Tu, Y. (2012). Effect of acupuncture on expression ofbrain-derived neurotrophic factor gene and protein in frontal cortex and hip-pocampus of depress rats. *Zhen Ci Yan Jiu* 37, 20–24. doi: 10.13702/j.1000-0607.2012.01.009

Lin, H., Ding, X., and Fu, B. (2010). Effects of acupuncture combined with medicine on cognitive impairment of post-stroke patients. *Modern J. Integrat. Tradit. Chinese West. Med.* 1, 36–37. doi: 10.3969/j.issn.1008-8849.2010.01.017

Lin, R., Wu, Y., Tao, J., Chen, B., Chen, J., Zhao, C., et al. (2016). Electroacupuncture improves cognitive function through Rho GTPases and enhances dendriticspine plasticity in rats with cerebral ischemia-reperfusion. *Mol. Med. Rep.* 13, 2655–2660. doi: 10.3892/mmr.2016.4870

Liu, F., Li, Z. M., Jiang, Y. J., and Chen, L. D. (2014). A meta-analysis of acupuncture use in the treatment of cognitive impairment after stroke. *J. Alter. Complement. Med.* 20, 535–544. doi: 10.1089/acm.2013.0364

Liu, J., and Feng, X. (2013). Clinical observation of treating cognitive impairment after stroke by electroacupuncture at Baihui and Shenfing with cognitive rehabilitation training. *J. Chinese Med.* 4, 608–610. doi: 10.16368/j.issn.1674-8999.2013.04.020

Liu, L., Li, H., Chen, Z., Xu, J., and Lu, H. (2015b). Effects of electroacupuncture on head shen-acupoints on cognitive impairment after stroke. *Chinese J. Rehabil. Theory Pract.* 21, 575–578. doi: 10.3969/j.issn.1006-9771.2015.05.018

Liu, L., Li, H., and Xu, J. (2015a). Clinical study of electroacupuncture on memory dysfunction after stroke. *J. Emerg. Tradit. Chinese Med.* 5, 775–777. doi: 10.3969/j.issn.1004-745X.2015.05.008

Liu, R. (2017). Clinical study of electric acupuncture Shenting and Baihui point on mild cognitive impairment after stroke. *Clin. Res. Pract.* 29, 101–102. doi: 10.19347/j.cnki.2096-1413.201729049

Liu, W., Wu, J., Huang, J., Zhuo, P., Lin, Y., Wang, L., et al. (2017). Electroacupuncture regulateshippocampal synapitc plasticity via miR-134-mediated LIMK1 function in ratswith ischemic stroke. *Neural. Plast.* 2017:9545646. doi: 10.1155/2017/9545646

Lu, Z. (2014). *Clincal research of post-stroke vascular cognitive impairment treatent with needling back-shu point.* M.S. (Guangzhou University of Chinese Medicine).

Ma, Y., Han, Z., Wu, Y., Liu, P., and Peng, S. (2018). Effect of hyperharic oxygen combine with electroacupuncture at Siguan acupoint on early cognitive impairment in stroke patients. *Surg. Res. N. Techniq.* 1, 38–40. doi: 10.3969/j.issn.2095-378X.2018.01.011

Merriman, N. A., Sexton, E., McCabe, G., Walsh, M. E., Rohde, D., Gorman, A., et al. (2019). Addressing cognitive impairment following stroke: systematic review and meta-analysis of non-randomised controlled studies of psychological interventions. *BMJ Open* 9:e024429. doi: 10.1136/bmjopen-2018-024429

Nakling, A. E., Aarsland, D., Næss, H., Wollschlaeger, D., Fladby, T., Hofstad, H., et al. (2017). Cognitive deficits in chronic stroke patients: neuropsychological assessment. depression, and self-reports. *Dement. Geriatr. Cogn. Dis. Extra* 7, 283–296. doi: 10.1159/000478851

Nasreddine, Z. S., Phillips, N. A., Bédirian, V., Charbonneau, S., Whitehead, V., Collin, I., et al. (2005). The Montreal Cognitive Assessment, MoCA: a brief screening tool for mild cognitive impairment. *J. Am. Geriatr. Soc.* 53, 695–699. doi: 10.1111/j.1532-5415.2005.53221.x

Nys, G. M., van Zandvoot, M. J., van der Worp, H. B., de Kort, P. L., Jansen, B. P., Kappelle, L. J., et al. (2006). Early cognitive impairment predicts long-term depressive symptoms and qulity of life after stroke. *J. Neurol. Sci.* 247, 149–156. doi: 10.1016/j.jns.2006.04.005

Pasi, M., Poggesi, A., Salvadori, E., and Pantoni, L. (2012). Post-stroke dementia and cognitive impairment. *Front. Neurol. Neurosci.* 30, 65–69. doi: 10.1159/000333412

Patel, M., Coshall, C., Rudd, A. G., and Wolfe, C. D. (2003). Natural history of cognitive impairment after stroke and factors associated with its recovery. *Clin. Rehabil.* 17, 158–166. doi: 10.1191/0269215503cr596oa

Shao, D. (2016). The effect of scalp acupuncture and neck acupuncture and body acupuncture on the treatments of post-stroke cognitive impairment. *Chinese J. Geriatric Care* 3, 17–19. doi: 10.3969/j.issn.1672-4860.2016.03.007

Shi, C., and Wei, L. (2019). Effect of Xingnaokaiqiao acupuncture on hemiplegia after stroke. *Henan Med. Res.* 13, 2433–2434. doi: 10.3969/j.issn.1004-437X.2019.13.066

Song, S., Zhao, J., Tian, J., Wang, Z., Yang, L., and Xiu, X. (2013). The clinical curative efect of acupuncture combined with medicine on stroke patients with cognitive impairment. *J. Emerg. Tradit. Chinese Med.* 11, 1859–1860.

Sun, P. Y., Cai, R. L., Li, P. F., Zhu, Y., Wang, T., Wu, J., et al.

(2019). Protective effects on hippocampal neurons and the influence on hippocampal monoamine neurotransmitters with acupuncture for promoting the circulation of the governor vessel and regulating the mental state in rats with post-stroke depression. *Zhongguo Zhen Jiu* 39, 741–747. doi: 10.13703/j.0255-2930.2019.07.017

Sun, S. (2017). *The clinical study of the treatment in patients with moderate and severe post-stroke cognitive impairment by acupuncture at RN 1.* M.S. (Fujian University of Traditional Chinese Medicine).

Sun, S. C., Zhao, J. W., Tian, J. B., Wang, Z. Y., Yang, L. J., and Liu, X. F. (2013). The clinical curative effect of acupuncture combined with medicine on stroke patients with cognitive impairment. *J. Emerg. Tradit. Chinese Med.* 22, 1859–1860.

Sun, Y., and Wu, W. (2011). The effect of scalp acupuncture of 36 cases of cognitive dysfunction after ischemic stroke. (translation from Chinese by author). *J. Clin. Acupunct. Moxibust.* 9, 11–13. doi: 10.3969/j.issn.1005-0779.2011.09.004

Tatemichi, T. K., Desmond, D. W., Stern, Y., Paik, M., Sano, M., and Bagiella, E. (1994). Cognitive impairment after stroke: frequency, patterns, and relationship to functional abilities. *J. Neurol. Neurosurg. Psychiatr* 57, 202–207. doi: 10.1136/jnnp.57.2.202

Taya, F., Sun, Y., Babiloni, F., Thakor, N., and Bezerianos, A. (2015). Brain enhancement through cognitive training: a new insight from brain connectome. *Front. Syst. Neurosci.* 9:44. doi: 10.3389/fnsys.2015.00044

Wang, F., Liang, H., Chen, S., Huang, J., and Lin, Q. Y. (2014). Magnetic resonance spectroscopy of acupuncture regulating brain tissue metabolism in treatment of mild cognitive impairment after stroke. (translation from Chinese by author). *J. Emerg. Tradit. Chinese Med.* 10, 1928–1930. doi: 10.3969/j.issn.1004-745X.2014.10.072

Wang, H., Feng, X., and Chen, Z. (2017). Clinical efficacy of electro-acupuncturing on Baihui and Zusanli points plus rehabilitation training on post-stroke cognitive impairment. *Clin. J. Chinese Med.* 5, 67–70.

Wang, J. (2017). *The Literature Evaluation and Clinical Research of Treating PSCI With Acupuncture and Moxibustion.* (M.D.), Guangzhou University of Chinese Medicine, Guangzhou, China.

Wang, L., and Li, W. (2018). Effect of Xingnao Kaiqiao acupuncture on clinical efficacy of patients with mild cognitive impairment after stroke and its mechanism. *Chinese J. Integrat. Tradit. West. Med. Intens. Critical Care* 3, 260–263. doi: 10.3969/j.issn.1008-9691.2018.03.010

Wang, Q. (2014). Analysis of cognitive impairment after stroke treated by acupuncture combined with drugs. *Chinese J. Moderm Drug Appl.* 8:239. doi: 10.14164/j.cnki.cn11-5581/r.2014.14.199

Wang, Q., Dong, J., and Sun, L. (2019). Effect of acupuncture combined with atorvastatin on hemorheology and cognitive status in elderly patients with mild cognitive impairment after ischemic stroke(translation from Chinese by author). *Chinese J. Gerontol.* 21, 5180–5183. doi: 10.3969/j.issn.1005-9202.2019.21.012

Wang, X. (2019). Effects of tongluo fuzheng decoction combined with acupuncture on limb function and cognitive function in elderly patients with post-stroke hemiplegia. *Nei Mongol J. Tradit. Chinese Med.* 2, 30–31. doi: 10.3969/j.issn.1006-0979.2019.02.022

Wang, Z., Zhang, H., Zhang, Y., and Gu, Z. (2017). A clinical study on the treatment of vascular mild cognitive impairment with kidney-tonifying turbid acupuncture. *Chinese J. Woman Child Health Res.* 28:127. doi: 10.3969/j.issn.1674-7860.2017.05.035

Wen, T., Zhang, X., Liang, S., Li, Z., Xing, X., Liu, W., et al. (2018). Electroacupuncture amelio-rates cognitive impairment and spontaneous low-frequency brain activity inrats with ischemic stroke. *J. Stroke Cerebrovas. Dis.* 27, 2596–2605. doi: 10.1016/j.jstrokecerebrovasdis.2018.05.021

Wong, G. K. C., Mak, J. S. Y., Wong, A., Zheng, V. Z. Y., Poon, W. S., Abrigo, J., et al. (2017). Minimum clinically important difference of montreal cognitive assessment in aneurysmal subarachnoid hemorrhage patients. *J. Clin. Neurosci.* 46, 41–44. doi: 10.1016/j.jocn.2017.08.039

Wu, P., Mills, E., Moher, D., and Seely, D. (2010). Acupuncture in poststroke rehabilitation: a systematic review and meta-analysis of randomized trials. *Stroke* 41, e171–179. doi: 10.1161/STROKEAHA.109.573576

Yang, H. (2014). Observation on the effect of acupuncture combined with drugs on cognitive impairment after stroke(translation from Chinese by author). *Guangming J. Chinese Med.* 29, 1680–1681. doi: 10.3969/j.issn.1003-8914.2014.08.051

Yang, J. (2011). *The Clinical study on cognitive impairment after stroke by using the treatment of electroacupuncture given at DU20 and GB20.* M.S. (Fujian University of Traditional Chinese Medicine).

Zeng, Y., Bao, Y., Zhu, M., Chen, S., and Fang, J. (2015). Mild cognitive impairment of stroke at subacute stage treated with acupuncture: a randomized controlled trial. *Chinese Acupunct. Moxibust.* 35, 979–982. doi: 10.13703/j.0255-2930.2015.10.001

Zhai, W. Q. (2012). Effect of acupuncture combined with rehabilitation training on cognitive dysfunction after cerebral infarction. *Healthy People.* 6, 18–19.

Zhang, X., Y. Z., Guo, Z., Liu, J., and Jiao, X. (2017). Effect of acupuncture at cervical Jiaji point and Du Channel Point combined with atorvastatin on hemodynamics in patients with mild cognitive impairment after stroke. *J. Hunan Normal Univ.* 14, 131–134. doi: 10.3969/j.issn.1673-016X.2017.02.041

Zhang, Y. Y., and Wang, L. Y. (2004). Diagnosis and intervention of mild cognitive impairment. *Chinese J. Epidemiol.* 25, 905–907. doi: 10.3760/j.issn:0254-6450.2004.10.021

Zhou, H., Qing, S., Huang, D., and Huang, C. (2019). Effect of acupuncture combined with perindopril on cognitive function in ischemic stroke patients. (translation from Chinese by author). *Chinese Commun. Doct.* 4, 129–131. doi: 10.3969/j.issn.1007-614x.2019.04.085

Zhou, J., Zuo, J., Chen, B., and Lu, J. (2019). Effects of electroacupuncture at Baihui (GV20) and Shenting (GV24) on mild cognitive impairment after stroke. *World Chinese Med.* 2, 486–489. doi: 10.3969/j.issn.1673-7202.2019.02.050

Zhou, L., Zhang, Y. L., Cao, H. J., and Hu, H. (2013). Treating vascular mild cognitive impairment by acupuncture: a systematic review of randomized controlled trials. *Chinese J. Integrat. Tradit. West. Med.* 33, 1626–1630. doi: 10.7661/CJIM.2013.12.1626

18

Investigating the Agreement between Cardiovascular Disease Risk Calculators among People Diagnosed with Schizophrenia

Alexandra Berry [1], Richard J. Drake [1,2], Roger T. Webb [1], Darren M. Ashcroft [3], Matthew J. Carr [1] and Alison R. Yung [1,2,4]*

[1] Division of Psychology & Mental Health, School of Health Sciences, Faculty of Biology, Medicine and Health, Manchester Academic Health Sciences Centre (MAHSC), University of Manchester, Manchester, United Kingdom, [2] Greater Manchester Mental Health NHS Foundation Trust, Manchester, United Kingdom, [3] Division of Pharmacy & Optometry, School of Health Sciences, Faculty of Biology, Medicine and Health, Manchester Academic Health Sciences Centre (MAHSC), University of Manchester, Manchester, United Kingdom, [4] Orygen, The National Centre of Excellence in Youth Mental Health, The University of Melbourne, Parkville, VIC, Australia

***Correspondence:**
Alexandra Berry
alexandra.berry-2@postgrad.manchester.ac.uk

Background: People diagnosed with schizophrenia have a much reduced life expectancy compared to the general population, and a more than doubled risk of dying from cardiovascular disease (CVD). Existing CVD risk calculators can be used to detect people with an elevated predicted risk of CVD to inform interventions to reduce risk.

Aims: This study aimed to compare four different risk calculators for 10-year predicted CVD risk in a sample of people with schizophrenia.

Methods: Thirty participants with a diagnosis of schizophrenia spectrum disorders living within Greater Manchester, United Kingdom took part. Ten-year predicted cardiovascular risk scores were calculated using four different models: QRISK3, Framingham, PRIMROSE BMI, and PRIMROSE lipid. Risk estimates and classified risk categories were compared.

Results: QRISK3 identified 11 (39%) as having >10% risk of a CV event within 10 years, 4 (14%) of whom exceeded 20%. The Framingham model identified 4 (14%) as exceeding 10%, none of whom exceeded 20%. PRIMROSE risk calculators identified no participants as having >10% risk of a CV event within 10 years. Pairwise concordance correlation coefficients between types of model ranged 0.22–0.77. Mean (± SD) age was 40 (± 10) years but QRISK3's mean "Heart age" was 58 (± 14) years.

Conclusion: Risk calculators generate differing predicted CVD risk scores for patients with schizophrenia. Using one risk calculator might yield different recommended monitoring and treatment plans compared to another. Clinicians should therefore take into account other patient-related factors, such as patients' preferences and other underlying physical conditions when making treatment decisions.

Keywords: schizophrenia, cardiovascular risk, risk calculator, cardiovascular disease, risk score

INTRODUCTION

Globally, people diagnosed with schizophrenia have a mortality rate 2–3 times that of the general population (1) and their life expectancy is reduced by 10 to 30 years (1–3). As in the general population, cardiovascular disease (CVD) is the most common cause of death among these individuals (4–6). A meta-analysis of over 3 million patients with severe mental illness (SMI) and over 113 million controls from 92 studies with a cross-sectional or retrospective/prospective longitudinal design showed that people with schizophrenia are at more than double the risk of dying from CVD and are at 59% greater risk of developing coronary heart disease (CHD) compared to the remainder of the population (7).

CVD risk calculators are used to estimate an individual's absolute risk of having a heart attack or stroke within a specified amount of time, such as 5 or 10 years. These calculators have been developed in large population studies and their validity and reproducibility assessed using population-level statistics that measure calibration and discrimination (8–11). CVD risk prediction scores are used in clinical practice with the general population to guide whether early intervention could be beneficial, such as prescribing medication to lower blood pressure and cholesterol (12). Moreover, in the United Kingdom (UK), the National Institute for Health and Care Excellence (NICE), which issues national clinical guidelines in the UK to improve health and social care (13) recommend routine monitoring of cardiovascular risk in people with schizophrenia (14).

Risk prediction scores can also be used as surrogate endpoints for intervention studies; that is, an outcome in a clinical trial would be change in CVD risk score after a certain period of time (15). In the schizophrenia population, risk prediction scores have been used as surrogate endpoints in intervention studies, for example the Clinical Antipsychotic Trials of Intervention Effectiveness (CATIE) trial included 1,125 people with schizophrenia and compared change in predicted 10-year CHD risk using the Framingham risk score (16) during antipsychotic treatment.

There are currently more than 360 CVD risk calculators available (17). A previously published review reported that 25 different calculators allocated the same person to a different risk category 33% of the time (18). Given the differences between risk calculators when applied in the general population, it would be useful to know whether or not consistency is similarly poor when the calculators are applied specifically to people with schizophrenia. Therefore, the aim of this study was to compare the 10-year absolute CVD risk score in a sample of 30 people with schizophrenia using four different risk calculators: QRISK3 (9), Framingham (11), The PRedIction, and Management of cardiovascular Risk in peOple with SEvere mental illnesses (PRIMROSE) body mass index (BMI) and PRIMROSE lipid (10). Whilst there are a large number of calculators to select from, we decided to focus on risk calculators that include risk factors applicable to people with schizophrenia, such as an SMI diagnosis and antipsychotic use. Such risk factors may confer additional risk for CVD, independent of traditional predictors (19, 20). Furthermore, we chose to assess Framingham due to it being a calculator still commonly used worldwide, including in this patient group. **Table 1** shows a comparison of risk factors measured in each model that we have selected: QRISK3, Framingham, PRIMROSE BMI, and PRIMROSE Lipid.

TABLE 1 | Comparison of risk factors included in four cardiovascular risk calculators.

Variables	Cardiovascular risk calculators			
	Framingham	QRISK3	PRIMROSE Lipid	PRIMROSE BMI
Age	✓	✓	✓	✓
Gender	✓	✓	✓	✓
Ethnicity	✗	✓	✗	✗
HDL cholesterol	✓	✓	✓	✗
Total cholesterol	✓	✓	✓	✗
Systolic blood pressure	✓	✓	✓	✓
SD of two systolic blood pressure readings	✗	✓	✗	✗
Type 2 diabetes	✓	✓	✓	✓
Type 1 diabetes	✗	✓	✗	✗
Current smoker	✓	✓	✓	✓
Ex-smoker	✗	✓	✓	✓
Light/moderate/heavy smoker	✗	✓	✗	✗
Hypertension treatment	✓	✓	✓	✓
BMI	✗	✓	✗	✓
Townsend index of deprivation	✗	✓	✓	✓
Family history of CVD	✗	✓	✗	✗
Chronic kidney disease	✗	✓	✗	✗
Migraines	✗	✓	✗	✗
Lupus (SLE)	✗	✓	✗	✗
Rheumatoid arthritis	✗	✓	✗	✗
Erectile dysfunction	✗	✓	✗	✗
Atrial fibrillation	✗	✓	✗	✗
History of heavy drinking	✗	✗	✓	✓
SMI diagnosis	✗	✓	✓	✓
Prescription for atypical antipsychotics	✗	✓	✓	✓
Prescription for typical antipsychotics	✗	✗	✗	✓
Prescription for antidepressants	✗	✗	✓	✓
Oral steroids	✗	✓	✗	✗

METHODS

Sample

Individuals were eligible to take part if they were aged 18–65 and had a diagnosis of schizophrenia or related psychosis, according to the ICD-10 classification system (21). Individuals were excluded if they were non-English speaking, were unable to give their informed consent, or they had a history of CVD as specified by the CVD risk calculators used (9, 11), as well as NICE guidelines (22). These individuals are already considered at high-risk of CVD events, therefore generating a risk score does not add useful additional information (22). Participants were recruited from Greater Manchester Mental Health NHS Foundation Trust services in England. All were given an information sheet to read and provided their written informed consent. The study received ethical approval from the North West Research Ethics Committee (17/NW/0368). Thirty participants were included in the study. Seventeen participants resided in the community and 13 were inpatients on mental health or rehabilitation wards. Participants' histories of diagnosed CVD were established by reviewing their medical records for related diagnoses and for any prescribed medication associated with cardiometabolic conditions.

CVD Risk Calculators

Framingham

The Framingham risk scores (11) apply an algorithm that calculates the predicted CVD risk from risk factors such as diabetes, dyslipidemia, hypertension (23–25), smoking, and obesity (26, 27). This risk calculator is frequently used in the general population but has also been applied to population groups with SMI (28). The prevalence of these risk factors is considerably raised in people with schizophrenia (4, 29–31) and people with schizophrenia have been shown to have higher risk scores than the general population (32–34). However, people with SMI were excluded from the Framingham cohort. As such, risk factors of particular relevance to those with an SMI diagnosis, such as antipsychotic use are not included. Yet antipsychotic use can cause significant morbidity, including weight gain (35, 36) and diabetes (37), conditions that are associated with an increased risk of CVD.

When applying the Framingham risk calculator to patients in the United Kingdom (UK), NICE recommends using the modified version (38). The modified version entails multiplying the results of the US Framingham score by 1.4 for south Asian men in the UK. Patients are considered to be at high risk of a CVD event over the next 10 years if they score 20% or greater (11). Estimates of risk include several CVD outcomes, including coronary death, myocardial infarction, coronary insufficiency, angina pectoris, ischaemic stroke, haemorrhagic stroke, transient ischaemic attack, peripheral artery disease, and heart failure (39).

PRIMROSE

The PRIMROSE BMI and lipid models are 10-year predicted cardiovascular risk calculators specifically designed for people with SMI (10). They include risk factors relevant to people with SMI, such as prescription of antipsychotic medication, antidepressant medication, history of heavy alcohol consumption, area-level Townsend index of deprivation (in quintiles) (40) and diagnosis of an SMI. These models were validated using The Health Improvement Network (THIN) UK primary care database (10).

The PRIMROSE BMI risk calculator excludes lipid profile. Patients are considered to be at high risk of a CVD event over the next 10 years if they score 20% or greater (10). The PRIMROSE lipid model excludes BMI and, again, patients are considered to be at high risk of a CVD event over the next 10 years if they score 20% or greater (10). Outcomes for which risks are in predicted in both PRIMROSE risk calculators cover both fatal and non-fatal cardiovascular events including myocardial infarction, angina pectoris, coronary heart disease, major coronary surgery and revascularization, cerebrovascular accident, and transient ischaemic attack (10).

QRISK3

The QRISK2 risk calculator is recommended for use with the UK general population by NICE (41). NICE also recommends QRISK2 for use in those with medical conditions including SMI, whilst acknowledging it may underestimate risk in such groups (22). QRISK2 is about to be superseded by QRISK3, which includes both typical risk indicators and specific factors for SMI (i.e., an SMI diagnosis and antipsychotic use) in patients aged 25–84 years (9) and may enable more accurate assessment. The QRISK algorithms have been validated using UK primary care databases including the Clinical Practice Research Datalink (CPRD) (42) and THIN (43–45). As well as calculating the 10-year risk of CVD, QRISK3 also estimates a "heart age." This is calculated by comparing the ideal age of healthy individuals who receive the same predicted CVD risk score and have the same sex and ethnicity (46). A heart age older than the current age suggests increased risk that is modifiable (46). It is important to emphasize that this is a relative measure and heart age has been found on average to be older than chronological age in every age strata (47). It may be a useful tool to encourage lifestyle modification rather than to inform medication recommendations (48).

Using the QRISK3, patients are considered to be at high risk of a CVD event over the next 10 years if they score 10% or greater (9). This threshold was set following health economics modeling for when to offer medical intervention, such as with statins prescription (38). Risks are estimated for the following CVD outcomes: transient ischaemic attack and related syndromes, angina pectoris, myocardial infarction, subsequent myocardial infarction, complications after myocardial infarction, other acute ischaemic heart disease, chronic ischaemic heart disease, cerebral infarction, and stroke not specified as hemorrhage or infarction (9).

Anthropometric Measurements

BMI was calculated as weight/height^2 (kg/m^2). Participants were classified according to the World Health Organization (WHO) criteria as underweight (BMI $<$18.5), normal (BMI 18.5–24.99), overweight (BMI 25–29.99) obese (BMI 30–39.99), or severe obesity (BMI $\geq$40) (49). Medical records were reviewed for any diagnosed physical and mental health conditions, prescribed medication and to confirm self-reported demographic information.

Statistical Analyses

Data were analyzed using STATA (version 11; Statacorp, TX, USA). Descriptive statistics were reported as medians, means, standard deviations (SDs) and percentages. 10-year predicted cardiovascular risk scores were calculated using published algorithms (9–11). The relationship between each CVD risk calculator model was assessed using concordance correlation coefficients (P_c). This correlation measures how far the best-fit line differs from the line y = x, by adjusting the *r*-value using a bias correction factor. P_c therefore provides a measure of correlation and agreement. Bland-Altman plots were generated to plot the difference against mean between pairs of CVD risk calculators.

RESULTS

Sociodemographic and Summary Data

The study sample included 30 participants. Their mean age was 40.4 ± 10.2 years and 83% were male. Most of the participants were overweight, with 33% being either obese (BMI ≥30 kg/m²) or severely obese (BMI ≥40 kg/m²) and the mean BMI was in the overweight range (29.9 ± 7.9; **Table 2**). Atypical antipsychotics were prescribed to 83% of participants; typical antipsychotics were prescribed to 27% of participants. Both atypical and typical antipsychotics were prescribed to 10% of these participants.

TABLE 2 | Distribution of sociodemographic and clinical factors in the sample of patients diagnosed with schizophrenia.

	N	%	Mean ± SD	Median
GENDER				
Male	25	83		
Female	5	17		
Age			40.4 ± 10.2	40
18–34	9	30		
35–64	21	70		
ETHNICITY				
White British	19	63		
Black British/African	4	13		
Black British/Caribbean	2	7		
Other ethnic groups	5	17		
SMOKING				
Current smoker	22	73		
Ex-smoker	5	17		
Never smoked	3	10		
DIAGNOSIS OF TYPE 2 DIABETES				
Yes	4	13		
No	26	87		
PRESCRIBED ANTI-DEPRESSANT MEDICATION				
Yes	12	40		
No	18	60		
PRESCRIBED STATINS				
Yes	7	23		
No	23	77		
PRESCRIBED HYPERTENSIVE TREATMENT				
Yes	7	23		
No	23	77		
Systolic blood pressure			125.9 ± 16.7	125.5
<120 mmHg	11	37		
≥120–139 mmHg	12	40		
≥140 mmHg	7	23		
BMI			29.9 ± 7.9	27.5
Underweight (<18.5)	0	0		
Normal (18.5–24.99)	8	27		
Overweight (25–29.99)	12	40		
Obese (30–39.99)	7	23		
Severe obesity (≥40)	3	10		

Systolic Blood Pressure.

10-Year Predicted CVD Risk

Participants' absolute 10-year risk of CVD was calculated using four different risk calculators: QRISK3, Framingham, PRIMROSE BMI, and PRIMROSE lipid. Two participants were excluded from the QRISK3 analysis due to their age being below 25 years. One participant was excluded from the Framingham and PRIMROSE lipid analyses due to an inability to draw blood and obtain their lipid profile. QRISK3 identified 11 participants (39%) who were classified into the high-risk category of having a CVD event within 10 years (range 0.4–38.5%), based on a 10% threshold for high-risk. No participants were classified into the high risk category for the PRIMROSE lipid (range 0.1–8.5%), PRIMROSE BMI (range 0.2–7.4%), or Framingham (range 0.1–15.6%) risk calculators, based on a 20% threshold for high-risk. However, if a 10% threshold is imposed across all four calculators, 39% of patients are categorized as high-risk with QRISK3, 14% with Framingham and none with PRIMROSE risk calculators. If a 20% threshold is imposed across all four calculators, 14% are categorized as high risk by QRISK3 and none with other the other risk calculators (**Table 3**).

Heart Age

Frequency distributions of age and heart age calculated using QRISK3 can be seen in **Figures 1, 2**. The mean heart age was 58.4 ± 13.5. The mean difference between age and calculated heart age was found to be over 16 years with one individual scoring a heart age 40 years above their actual age (**Figure 3**).

Agreement Between 10-Year Predicted CVD Risk Models

Pairwise concordance correlation coefficients were highest between the two PRIMROSE measures but the QRISK3 and PRIMROSE metrics had notably poor correlations, not even reaching the acceptable range at their upper CIs and close to zero at the lower CIs (**Table 4**; **Figure 4**).

DISCUSSION

We applied four risk calculators to determine the predicted CVD risk for 30 patients with schizophrenia over the next 10 years. Mean QRISK3 calculated risk estimates were approximately 4 times higher than the PRIMROSE lipid calculated risk estimates, and roughly 3 times higher than PRIMROSE BMI. Moreover, agreement between calculators was poorest between QRISK3 and the PRIMROSE calculators, despite these calculators taking into account diagnosis of SMI and use of antipsychotic medication within their algorithms. These risk factors are known to have

TABLE 3 | Ten-year predicted CVD risk scores according to 4 different risk calculators.

	<10%		10–19%		20% or more		Mean* ± SD
	N	%	*N*	%	*N*	%	
QRISK3	17	61	7	25	4	14	9.3 ± 8.8
Framingham	25	86	4	14	0	0	4.1 ± 4.1
PRIMROSE Lipid	29	100	0	0	0	0	2.0 ± 2.0
PRIMROSE BMI	30	100	0	0	0	0	2.9 ± 2.1

**Mean % of 10-year predicted CVD risk.*

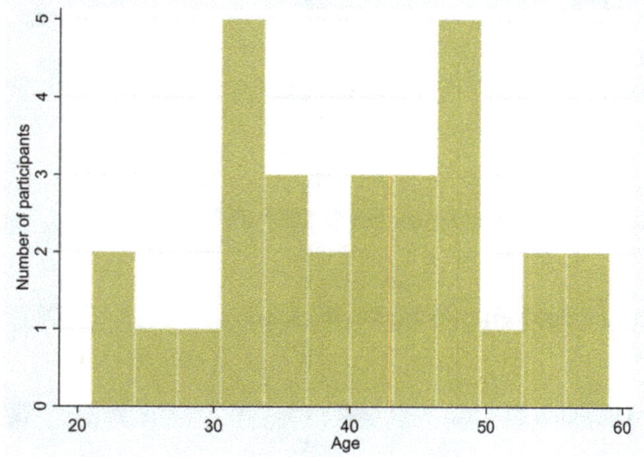

FIGURE 1 | Distribution of age.

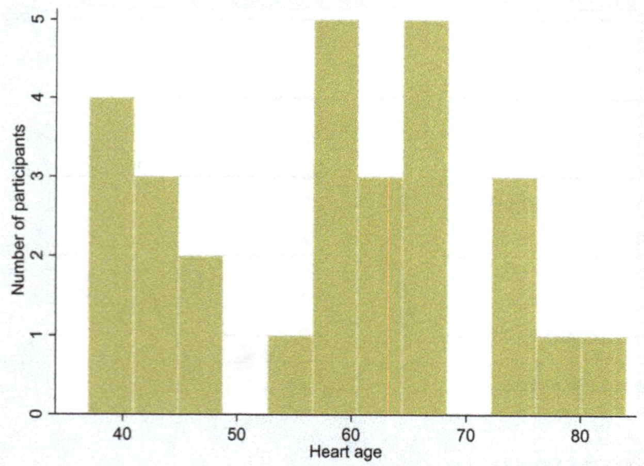

FIGURE 2 | Distribution of heart age.

a complex effect on cardiovascular risk (9) and the lack of agreement highlights the variability in the weighting of risk factors between these models, which impacts the relative risk. Agreement between Framingham and the three other risk calculators was more acceptable but not high. People with SMI were excluded from the Framingham heart study cohort and

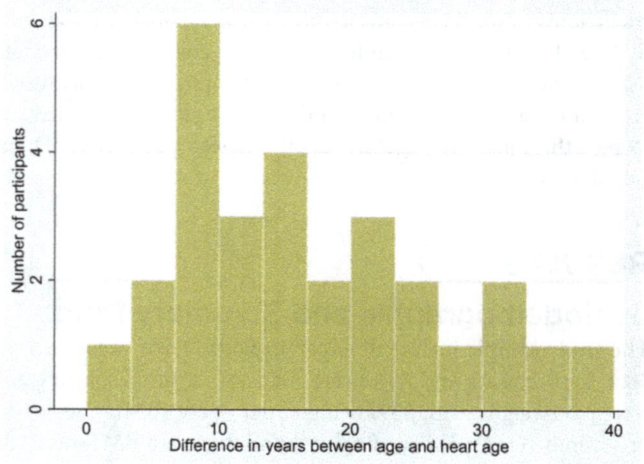

FIGURE 3 | Difference between age and heart age.

previous research comparing cardiovascular risk calculators in the general population has recommended selecting calculators that have been developed from a population similar to the patient (50).

People with schizophrenia and related conditions are recommended to attend for regular physical health assessments, including checking for cardiometabolic indicators specifically so that clinicians may offer any required interventions (51). For the purposes of CVD prevention, it is therefore important for clinicians to be able to identify individuals at highest risk of developing CVD. There is currently a lack of reliable evidence indicating the superiority of one CVD risk calculator over another, particularly in relation to persons with SMI. Our data suggest that there are important differences between calculators.

The threshold for classifying a patient as high-risk of having a CVD event over the next 10 years differed between the models. Thirty nine percent of participants were classified as high-risk using QRISK3, but all were classified as low-risk using the other calculators. Framingham and the PRIMROSE risk calculators both set the threshold as 20% or greater, while QRISK3 sets the threshold as 10% or greater. NICE guidelines recommend using a 10% threshold for initiating preventative therapy with statins (52). It is however not clear whether this is the optimal threshold for modifying risk in people with schizophrenia. For clinicians it is therefore not clear when to initiate preventative therapy or which risk calculator to use with patients with SMI. NICE emphasizes that faced with the challenge of applying population-based measures to individuals, clinicians should exercise their judgement and include patients' preferences when making clinical decisions in relation to CVD risk scores (53). There may also be other patient-related factors that should be considered, such as socioeconomic status or other underlying medical conditions (53).

The risk factors included in the algorithms for CVD risk calculators typically include age, gender, medical diagnoses, prescription to medications, BMI, blood pressure, and lipid profile. With the exception of smoking in all risk calculators,

TABLE 4 | Agreement among 10-year predicted CVD risk models (%).

	Difference		95% Limits of agreement	P_C (95% CI)
	Mean	**SD**		
QRISK3 vs. Framingham	5.0	5.4	−5.7 to 15.7	0.549 (0.41 to 0.69)
QRISK3 vs. PRIMROSE Lipid	7.2	7.3	−7.1 to 21.6	0.224 (0.12 to 0.32)
QRISK3 vs. PRIMROSE BMI	6.2	7.4	−8.2 to 20.6	0.226 (0.12 to 0.33)
Framingham vs. PRIMROSE Lipid	2.1	2.6	−3.0 to 7.3	0.543 (0.38 to 0.70)
Framingham vs. PRIMROSE BMI	1.2	2.8	−4.3 to 6.7	0.581 (0.41 to 0.75)
PRIMROSE Lipid vs. PRIMROSE BMI	−0.9	1.2	−3.2 to 1.4	0.767 (0.63 to 0.91)

P_C, Concordance correlation coefficient; CI, confidence intervals.

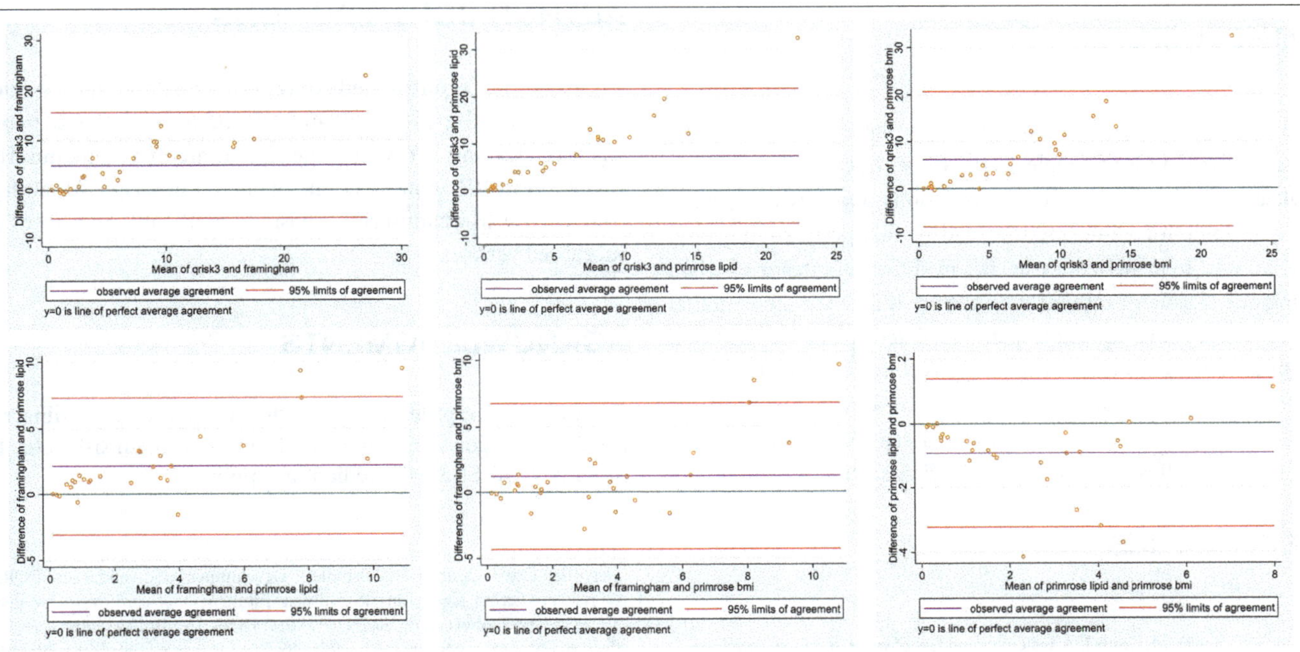

FIGURE 4 | Difference against mean between 10-year predicted CVD risk calculators.

and history of heavy drinking within PRIMROSE risk calculators (10), lifestyle screening is not included. Lifestyle screening contributes little to CVD risk calculator algorithms, partly because resource limitations mean lifestyle factors are not routinely recorded within primary care databases from which risk models derive. However, many lifestyle factors have been found to increase the risk of CVD both in the general population and SMI groups. Meta-analyses show that sedentary behavior in the general population is associated with increased risks of diabetes, CVD and cardiovascular and all-cause mortality (54); and that those with schizophrenia group engage in high levels of sedentary behavior (55). Furthermore, sleep disorders are reported in 30–80% of people with schizophrenia (56, 57). They take longer to fall asleep, sleep longer, take daytime naps and have severely fragmented sleep compared to healthy controls (58). There is emerging evidence that disrupting sleep can cause health problems, such as CVD (59). It may be that sleep quality needs to be routinely enquired about and its role in CVD risk calculators investigated

Comparing models, it is notable that the low PRIMROSE and Framingham risk scores seem at odds with clinical impressions of participants and with studies of life expectancy, CVD and CVD risk factor prevalence in people with schizophrenia. People with schizophrenia have 2.5 times the risk of dying compared to the general population (1), and a mean age of death from CVD in schizophrenia patients was found to be 51 years (60). Moreover, general population life expectancy in the UK is lowest in northern urban England, including Manchester (61), with healthy male life expectancy at birth in Greater Manchester in the 50s (54). This implies that a substantial proportion of this sample should be in a high-risk category. QRISK3 estimated our participant heart ages to be a mean of 16 years older than chronological age. Whilst "heart age" may not be an accurate enough tool to inform medical decision-making (48), an age adjustment of this size may be similar to the substantial reduction in life expectancy in this group.

Our study was limited by its small sample size, which makes it difficult to draw generalisable conclusions and we therefore recommend repeating this study on a considerably large scale. The sample was recruited from Greater Manchester in England by volunteers. This is an area where health and life expectancy is unusually poor in the general population (54), so this sample may well not be representative. However, this may have enabled us to detect higher rates of predicted CVD risk in this group. A longitudinal study of a representative cohort of sufficient size to accurately estimate agreement among CVD risk calculators is indicated. This study underlines the importance of such work in that, even in a small study, differences were observed between algorithms in their risk predictions.

CONCLUSIONS

Existing CVD risk calculators have low agreement with each other in our sample of people diagnosed with schizophrenia. This makes it challenging to draw conclusions about which tool is most suitable for clinicians to use with this population group, and how to treat patients who fall in different categories when using one calculator rather than another. It is recommended that clinicians consider multiple patient-related factors in addition to predicted CVD risk score when recommending treatment. Furthermore, participants in our study had a calculated heart age that was much older than their actual ages. Of interest would be whether adjusting the age of patients with schizophrenia more accurately predicts CVD events. Further research is needed with larger numbers and with longitudinal follow-up to assess actual CVD events to understand this further. Also of interest would be the use of large datasets to examine the question of CVD risk in schizophrenia. Such studies should also investigate if any of the factors known to increase risk of CVD in the general population that are also common in schizophrenia, such as physical inactivity (55–57), high rates of sedentary behavior (58), and sleep disturbance (59, 62) impact on CVD risk, independent of the risk factors already included in existing CVD risk calculators.

AUTHOR CONTRIBUTIONS

AB, AY, and RD contributed conception and design of the study. AB collected the data. AB and RD performed the statistical analysis. AB and AY wrote the first draft of the manuscript. AB, AY, and RD wrote sections of the manuscript. All authors contributed to manuscript revision, read and approved the submitted version.

ACKNOWLEDGMENTS

Dr. Stephen Hippisley-Cox is acknowledged for providing risk prediction algorithm support. Thanks to ClinRisk Ltd for providing QRISK3 risk prediction support.

REFERENCES

Saha S, Chant D, McGrath J. A systematic review of mortality in schizophrenia: is the differential mortality gap worsening over time? *Arch Gen Psychiatry* (2007) 64:1123–31. doi: 10.1001/archpsyc.64.10.1123

Wahlbeck K, Westman J, Nordentoft M, Gissler M, Laursen TM. Outcomes of nordic mental health systems: life expectancy of patients with mental disorders. *Br J Psychiatry* (2011) 199:453–8. doi: 10.1192/bjp.bp.110.085100

De Hert M, Cohen D, Bobes J, Cetkovich-Bakmas M, Leucht S, Ndetei DM, et al. Physical illness in patients with severe mental disorders. II. barriers to care, monitoring and treatment guidelines, plus recommendations at the system and individual level. *World Psychiatry* (2011) 10:138. doi: 10.1002/j.2051-5545.2011.tb00014.x

Hennekens CH, Hennekens AR, Hollar D, Casey DE. Schizophrenia and increased risks of cardiovascular disease. *Am Heart J.* (2005) 150:1115–21. doi: 10.1016/j.ahj.2005.02.007

Brown S. Excess mortality of schizophrenia. a meta-analysis. *Br J Psychiatry* (1997) 171:502–8. doi: 10.1192/bjp.171.6.502

Westman J, Eriksson SV, Gissler M, Hallgren J, Prieto ML, Bobo WV, et al. Increased cardiovascular mortality in people with schizophrenia: a 24-year national register study. *Epidemiol Psychiatr Sci.* (2017) 5:1–9. doi: 10.1017/S2045796017000166

Correll CU, Solmi M, Veronese N, Bortolato B, Rosson S, Santonastaso P, et al. Prevalence, incidence and mortality from cardiovascular disease in patients with pooled and specific severe mental illness: a large-scale meta- analysis of 3,211,768 patients and 113,383,368 controls. *World Psychiatry* (2017) 16:163–80. doi: 10.1002/wps.20420

Hippisley-Cox J, Coupland C, Vinogradova Y, Robson J, Minhas R, Sheikh A, et al. Predicting cardiovascular risk in England and Wales: prospective derivation and validation of QRISK2. *BMJ* (2008) 336:a332. doi: 10.1136/bmj.39609.449676.25

Hippisley-Cox J, Coupland C, Brindle P. Development and validation of QRISK3 risk prediction algorithms to estimate future risk of cardiovascular disease: prospective cohort study. *BMJ* (2017) 357: j2099. doi: 10.1136/bmj.j2099

Osborn DP, Hardoon S, Omar RZ, Holt RIG, King M, Larsen J, et al. The PRIMROSE cardiovascular risk prediction models for people with severe mental illness: results from the PRIMROSE Research Programme: prediction and management of cardiovascular risk in people with severe mental illnesses. *JAMA Psychiatry* (2015) 72:143–51. doi: 10.1001/jamapsychiatry. 2014.2133

D'Agostino RS, Vasan RS, Pencina MJ. General cardiovascular risk profile for use in primary care: the Framingham Heart Study. *Circulation* (2008) 117:743–53. doi: 10.1161/CIRCULATIONAHA.107. 699579

Jackson R, Lawes CMM, Bennett DA, Milne RJ, Rodgers A. Treatment with drugs to lower blood pressure and blood cholesterol based on an individual's absolute cardiovascular risk. *Lancet* (2005) 365:434–41. doi: 10.1016/S0140-6736(05)70240-3

National Institute for Health and Care Excellence (NICE). *About 2018.* Available online: https://www.nice.org.uk/about (Accessed October 2, 2018).

National Institute for Health and Care Excellence (NICE). *Psychosis and Schizophrenia in Adults: Prevention and Management* 2014 Available online at:https://www.nice.org.uk/guidance/cg178/chapter/1-Recommendations (Accessed November 5, 2018).

Maruthur NM, Wang NY, Appel LJ. Lifestyle interventions reduce coronary heart disease risk: results from the PREMIER trial. *Circulation* (2009) 119:2026–31. doi: 10.1161/CIRCULATIONAHA.108.809491

Daumit GL, Goff DC, Meyer JM, Davis VG, Nasrallah HA, McEvoy JP, et al. Antipsychotic effects on estimated 10-year coronary heart disease risk in the CATIE schizophrenia study. *Schizophr Res.* (2008) 105:175–87. doi: 10.1016/j.schres.2008.07.006

Damen JAAG, Hooft L, Schuit E, Debray TPA, Collins GS, Tzoulaki I, et al. Prediction models for cardiovascular disease risk in the general population: systematic review. *BMJ* (2016) 353:i2416. doi: 10.1136/bmj.i2416

Allan GM, Nouri F, Korownyk C, Kolber MR, Vandermeer B, McCormack J. Agreement among cardiovascular disease risk calculators. *Circulation* (2013) 127:1948-56. doi: 10.1161/CIRCULATIONAHA.112.000412

De Hert M, Detraux J, van Winkel R, Yu W, Correll CU. Metabolic and cardiovascular adverse effects associated with antipsychotic drugs. *Nat Rev Endocrinol.* (2011) 8:114. doi: 10.1038/nrendo.2011.156

Ösby U, Westman J, Hällgren J, Gissler M. Mortality trends in cardiovascular causes in schizophrenia, bipolar and unipolar mood disorder in Sweden 1987–2010. *Eur J Public Health* (2016) 26:867–71. doi: 10.1093/eurpub/ ckv245

World Health Organization. *The ICD-10 Classification of Mental and Behavioural Disorders. Diagnostic Criteria for Research.* Geneva: World Health Organization (1993).

National Institute for Health and Care Excellence (NICE). *Cardiovascular Risk Assessment and Lipid Modification* 2015. Available online at: https:// www. nice. org.uk/guidance/qs100/resources/cardiovascular-risk-assessment- and- lipid-modification-pdf-75545230925509 (Accessed October 30, 2018).

Kannel WB, Gordon T, Schwartz MJ. Systolic versus diastolic blood pressure and risk of coronary heart disease: the Framingham Study. *Am J Cardiol.* (1971) 27:335–46. doi: 10.1016/0002-9149(71)90428-0

Castelli WP, Garrison RJ, Wilson PWF, Abbott RD, Kalousdian S, Kannel WB. Incidence of coronary heart disease and lipoprotein cholesterol levels the Framingham Study. *JAMA* (1986) 256:2835–8. doi: 10.1001/ jama.1986.03380200073024

Kannel WB, McGee DL. Diabetes and cardiovascular disease. *JAMA* (1979) 241:2035–8. doi: 10.1001/jama.1979.03290450033020

Doyle JT, Dawber TR, Kannel WB, Heslin AS, Kahn HA. Cigarette smoking and coronary heart disease: combined experience of the Albany and Framingham studies. *N Eng J Med.* (1962) 26:796–801. doi: 10.1056/ NEJM196204192661602

Hubert HB, Feinleib M, McNamara PM, Castelli WP, Hubert MF, McNamara PM, et al. Obesity as an independent risk factor for cardiovascular disease: a 26-year follow-up of participants in the Framingham Heart Study. *Circulation* (1983) 67:968–77. doi: 10.1161/01.CIR.67.5.968

Foguet-Boreu Q, Fernandez-San-Martin MI, Flores-Mateo G, Zabaleta- del-Olmo E, Garcia-Morzon LA, Perez-Pinar Lopez M, et al. Cardiovascular risk assessment in patients with a severe mental illness: a systematic review and meta-analysis. *BMC Psychiatry* (2016) 16:141. doi: 10.1186/s12888-016- 0833-6

Kelly DL, McMahon HJ, Wehring HJ, Liu F, Mackowick KM, Boggs DL, et al. Cigarette smoking and mortality risk in people with schizophrenia. *Schizophr Bull.* (2011) 37:832–8. doi: 10.1093/schbul/sbp152

Chuang HT, Mansell C, Patten SB. Lifestyle characteristics of psychiatric outpatients. *Canad J Psychiatry* (2008) 53:260–6. doi: 10.1177/070674370805300407

Liao CH, Chang CS, Wei WC, Chang SN, Liao CC, Lane HY, et al. Schizophrenia patients at higher risk of diabetes, hypertension and hyperlipidemia: a population-based study. *Schizophr Res.* (2011) 126:110–6. doi: 10.1016/j. schres.2010.12.007

McCreadie RG. Diet, smoking and cardiovascular risk in people with schizophrenia. *Br J Psychiatry* (2003) 183:534–9. doi: 10.1192/bjp.183.6.534

Ratliff JC, Palmese LB, Reutenauer E, Srihari V, Tek C. Obese schizophrenia spectrum patients have significantly higher 10-year general cardiovascular risk and vascular ages than obese individuals without severe mental illness. *Psychosomatics* (2013) 54:67–73. doi: 10.1016/j.psym.2012.03.001

Tay Y, Nurjono M, Lee J. Increased Framingham 10-year CVD risk in Chinese patients with schizophrenia. *Schizophr Res.* (2013) 147:187–92. doi: 10.1016/j. schres.2013.03.023

Bak M, Fransen A, Janssen J, van Os J, Drukker M. Almost All Antipsychotics result in weight gain: a meta-analysis. *PLoS ONE* (2014) 9:e94112. doi: 10.1371/ journal.pone.0094112

Allison D, Mentore J, Heo M, Chandler L, Cappelleri J, Infante M, et al. Antipsychotic-induced weight gain: a comprehensive research synthesis. *Am J Psychiatry* (1999) 156:1686–96.

Vancampfort D, Correll CU, Galling B, Probst M, De Hert M, Ward PB, et al. Diabetes mellitus in people with schizophrenia, bipolar disorder and major depressive disorder: a systematic review and large scale meta-analysis. *World Psychiatry* (2016) 15:166–74. doi: 10.1002/wps.20309

National Collaborating Centre for Primary Care (UK). *Lipid Modifi ation: Cardiovascular Risk Assessment and the Modification of Blood Lipids for the Primary and Secondary Prevention of Cardiovascular Disease.* London: Royal College of General Practitioners (UK) (2008) Available online at: https://www. ncbi.nlm.nih.gov/books/NBK55501/?report=classic. [Accessed June 14th 2018].

Cupples LA, D'Agostino RB. Section 34: some risk factors related to the annual incidence of cardiovascular disease and death in pooled repeated biennial measurements. In: Kannel WB, Wolf PA, Garrison RJ, editors. *Framingham Heart Study: 30 Year Follow-Up.* Bethesda, MD: Department of Health and Human Services (1987).

Townsend P, Phillimore P, Beattie A. *Health and Deprivation: Inequality and the North.* London: Routledge (1988).

National Institute for Health and Care Excellence (NICE). *Surveillance Report 2018 - Cardiovascular Disease: Risk Assessment and Reduction, Including Lipid Modifi ation* (2014) *NICE guideline CG181*: NICE. (2018). Available onlione at: https://www.nice.org.uk/guidance/cg181/resources/ surveillance-report-2018-cardiovascular-disease-risk-assessment-and- reduction-including-lipid-modifi ation-2014-nice-guideline-cg181-pdf- 6123288665797 (Accessed 25th September 2018).

Hippisley-Cox J, Coupland C, Brindle P. The performance of seven QPrediction risk scores in an independent external sample of patients from general practice: a validation study. *BMJ Open.* (2014) 4:5809. doi: 10.1136/ bmjopen-2014-005809

Collins GS, Altman DG. Predicting the 10 year risk of cardiovascular disease in the United Kingdom: independent and external validation of an updated version of QRISK2. *BMJ* (2012) 2012:344. doi: 10.1136/bmj.e4181

Riley RD, Ensor J, Snell KIE, Debray TPA, Altman DG, Moons KGM, et al. External validation of clinical prediction models using big datasets from e-health records or IPD meta-analysis: opportunities and challenges. *BMJ* (2016) 2016:353. doi: 10.1136/bmj.i3140

Collins GS, Altman DG. An independent and external validation of QRISK2 cardiovascular disease risk score: a prospective open cohort study. *BMJ* (2010) 2010:340. doi: 10.1136/bmj.c2442

Wells S, Kerr A, Eadie S, Wiltshire C, Jackson R. 'Your Heart Forecast': a new approach for describing and communicating cardiovascular risk? *Heart* (2010) 96:708. doi: 10.1136/hrt.2009.191320

Yang Q, Zhong Y, Ritchey M, Cobain M, Gillespie C, Merritt R, et al. *Vital Signs: Predicted Heart Age and Racial Disparities in Heart Age Among U.S. Adults at the State Level.* MMWR Morb Mortal Wkly Rep [Internet]. (2015). Available online at: http://europepmc.org/abstract/MED/26335037

Bonner C, Bell K, Jansen J, Glasziou P, Irwig L, Doust J, et al. Should heart age calculators be used alongside absolute cardiovascular disease risk assessment? *BMC Cardiovasc Disord.* (2018) 18:19. doi: 10.1186/s12872-018-0760-1

World Health Organization. *Physical Status: The Use and Interpretation of Anthropometry. Report of a WHO Expert Committee. WHO Technical Report Series 854.* Geneva: World Health Organization (1995).

Allan GM, Garrison S, McCormack J. Comparison of cardiovascular disease risk calculators. *Curr Opin Lipidol.* (2014) 25:254–65. doi: 10.1097/ MOL.0000000000000095

National Institute for Health and Care Excellence (NICE). *NICE Impact Cardiovascular Disease Prevention.* London: National Insitute for Health and Care Excellence (2018). Available online at: https://www.nice.org.uk/media/ default/about/what-we-do/into-practice/measuring-uptake/nice-impact-cardiovascular-disease-prevention.pdf. (Accessed September 24th 2018).

Majeed A. Statins for primary prevention of cardiovascular disease. *BMJ* (2014) 2014:348. doi: 10.1136/bmj.g3491

National Institute for Health and Care Excellence (NICE). *Cardiovascular Disease: Risk Assessment and Reduction, Including Lipid Modification.* (2014). Available online at: https://www.nice.org.uk/guidance/cg181/resources/ cardiovascular-disease-risk-assessment-and-reduction-including-lipid- modification-pdf-35109807660997 (Accessed October 5th 2018).

Office for National Statistics (ONS). *Health State Life Expectancy by 2011 Census Wards, England and Wales: 2009 to 2013.* (2018). Available onlineat:https://www.ons.gov.uk/peoplepopulationandcommunity/ h e a l t h a n d s o c i a l c a r e/ h e a l t h a n d li f e e x p e c t a n ci e s/ a r t ic l e s / healthstatelifeexpectancyby2011censuswardsenglandandwales/2009to2013 (Accessed 5th October 2018).

Gardner-Sood P, Lally J, Smith S. Cardiovascular risk factors and metabolic syndrome in people with established psychotic illnesses: baseline data from the IMPaCT randomized controlled trial. *Psychol. Med.* (2015) 45:2619–29. doi: 10.1017/S0033291715000562

Snethen GA, McCormick BP, Lysaker PH. Physical activity and psychiatric symptoms in adults with schizophrenia spectrum disorders. *J Nerv Mental Dis.* (2014) 202. doi: 10.1097/NMD.0000000000000216

Vancampfort D, Probst M, Knapen J, Carraro A, De Hert M. Associations between sedentary behaviour and metabolic parameters in patients with schizophrenia.

Stubbs B, Williams J, Gaughran F, Craig T. How sedentary are people with psychosis? A systematic review and meta-analysis. *Schizophr Res.* (2016) 171:103–9. doi: 10.1016/j.schres.2016.01.034

Tandon R, Shipley JE, Taylor S. Electroencephalographic sleep abnormalities in schizophrenia. Relationship to positive/negative symptoms and prior neuroleptic treatment. *Arch General Psychiatry* (1992) 49:185–94. doi: 10.1001/archpsyc.1992.01820030017003

Sweeting J, Duflou J, Semsarian C. Postmortem analysis of cardiovascular deaths in schizophrenia: a 10-year review. *Schizophr Res.* (2013) 150:398–403. doi: 10.1016/j.schres.2013.08.029

Bennett JE, Li G, Foreman K, Best N, Kontis V, Pearson C, et al. The future of life expectancy and life expectancy inequalities in England and Wales: Bayesian spatiotemporal forecasting. *Lancet* (2015) 386:163–70. doi: 10.1016/S0140-6736(15)60296-3

Keshavan MS, Keshavan MS, Saisps PM. Sleep abnormalities in schizophrenia: pathophysiological significance. *Psychol Med.* (1993) 23:831–5. doi: 10.1017/S0033291700026313

19

Depression-, Anxiety-, and Anger and Cognitive Functions: Findings from a Longitudinal Prospective Study

Jutta Lindert[1,2*], *Kimberley C. Paul*[3], *Margie E. Lachman*[4], *Beate Ritz*[3] *and Teresa E. Seeman*[4,5]

[1] Department of Health and Social Work, University of Applied Sciences Emden/Leer, Emden, Germany, [2] Women's Research Center at Brandeis University, Waltham, MA, United States, [3] Department of Epidemiology, Jonathan and Karin Fielding School of Public Health, University of California, Los Angeles, Los Angeles, CA, United States, [4] The Heller School for Social Policy and Management, Brandeis University, Waltham, MA, United States, [5] Division of Geriatrics, David Geffen School of Medicine at UCLA, Los Angeles, CA, United States

Correspondence:
Jutta Lindert
jutta.lindert@hs-emden-leer.de

Background: Determinants of changes in cognitive function during aging are not well-understood. We aimed to estimate the effects of depression-, anxiety- and anger symptoms on cognition and on cognition changes, especially on changes in episodic memory (EM) and executive functioning (EF).

Methods: We analyze data from the Mid-Life in the Midlife in the United States Biomarker study at two time points including n = 710 women, and n = 542 men (1996/1997) at the first assessment and n = 669 women, and n = 514 men at the second assessment (2013/2014). To assess cognition we used the Brief Test of Adult Cognition (BTACT). To measure depression-, anxiety- and anger symptoms we used the Mood and Anxiety Symptom Questionnaire (MASQ), the Center for Epidemiologic Studies Depression Scale (CES-D) and the State-Trait Anger Expression Inventory (STAXI). We used repeated models analyses to explore changes in cognition, and repeated measures linear mixed-effects models to investigate depression, anxiety and anger effects on cognition. All analyses were adjusted for potential confounders (cognition at baseline, age, education, income).

Results: At the first assessment, women had significantly better episodic memory functioning than men; men in the oldest age group had significant better executive functioning. At the second assessment, more education, and white ethnicity were associated with less negative changes on episodic memory and executive functioning. Depression- and anger symptoms were associated with declines in episodic memory among women; anxiety symptoms were associated with declines in episodic memory and executive functioning in both gender in men (EF: β: −0.02, (95% CI: −0.03, −0.01; EM: β −0.02 (−0.02, 95% CI: −0.03, −0.01) and in women (EF: β −0.01, 95% CI: −0.02, −0.0004; EM: β −0.013, 95% CI: −0.03, −0.001).

Conclusions: Depression-, anxiety- and anger symptoms were associated with changes in episodic memory and executive functioning. Further longitudinal studies are critical in populations in more countries to better understand the impact of depression, anxiety and anger symptoms on cognition changes.

Keywords: depression, anxiety, cognitive function, longitudinal, anger

INTRODUCTION

Decline in cognitive function is a significant Public Health problem associated with disability, personal, and family suffering, institutionalization and increased risk for dementia. Cognitive function refers to the mental processes, which are critical for the conduct of everyday activities (1). Such mental processes include attention, short and long-term memory [episodic memory (EM)], reasoning and planning of tasks (executive function (EF) (2). Declines in cognitive function are possible with increasing age (3, 4). However, cognitive changes trajectories are heterogeneous and knowledge about modifiable risk factors is needed given the rising number of older people, worldwide (5) and the lack of effective treatments for cognitive function decline (6).

Studies suggest that a variety of socio-demographic and lifestyle factors are associated with cognitive function changes in the aging population such as gender and increasing age (7, 8), low childhood education (9, 10), smoking (11, 12), alcohol abuse (1) and social contact (13). The evidence for gender related cognitive function changes is mixed. In Northern Europe, women show higher EM levels than men, and in Southern Europe, women and men do not differ in cognitive function changes (14). Additionally to regional differences, gender differences in cognitive function tend to disappear among recently born cohorts (15, 16).

Additional to the socio-demographic and behavioral factors several aspects of emotions, especially depression and anxiety, have been implicated in risk of cognition decline (17–19). Studies suggest that ~20% of individuals aged 55+ experience depression- or anxiety symptoms (20, 21). Depression-, and anxiety symptoms are not only associated with physical health outcomes (22–24) such as cardiovascular diseases (25–27), and higher allostatic load (28) but with cognition decline (29–35).

Recent studies suggest that depression, anxiety and anger are associated with cognition decline and dementia risk. Depression has been recognized as potential risk factor for cognitive decline in a meta-analysis investigating risk and protective factors for cognition decline including 32 studies with 62 598 participants and a follow-up from 2 to 17 years, depression symptoms were a risk factor for dementia. However, studies showed substantial heterogeneity and main effects of depression on cognition decline was obvious in older cohorts of 80 years and older but less in younger individuals (36). Anxiety has been recognized as potential risk factor for cognitive in meta-analyses which found that people with anxiety disorders have a 29–45% greater risk of cognitive decline (37, 38). However, depression and anxiety are also part of the prodrome of dementia and associated with early stages of dementia. Therefore, reverse causation is possible whereby depression or anxiety symptoms result from changes in emotions long before cognition declines become recognizable (1). Additionally, there is some evidence, that more anger symptoms are associated with greater declines in cognitive function across long follow-ups (19, 39).

Finally, some studies suggest gender differences in cognitive function changes (40, 41). However, the gender differences in cognitive function vary across cohorts and regions (15, 16). To understand and support cognition changes in aging men and women a better understanding of the impact of depression-, anxiety- and anger symptoms on cognition changes is needed. This study aims to fill the gap in knowledge by investigating the association between depression-, anxiety- and anger symptoms and cognition changes. Specifically, our objective was to evaluate the association of depression-, anxiety- and anger symptoms on cognition changes, longitudinally.

METHODS

Design

The study design is a longitudinal prospective cohort study.

Participants

Participants were drawn from two waves of the Midlife in the US-Study (MIDUS-II (2004/2005) and MIDUS—III (2013/2014), i.e., the longitudinal follow-up of the original MIDUS-I cohort (1995/1996) (n = 7,108 participants, mean age 46 years, SD = 13). The original MIDUS-I cohort is a sample of non-institutionalized English speaking adults living in the 48 United States funded by the National Institute on Aging (42). The MIDUS participants were selected with a random digit dialing sampling procedure (43).

Our analytical sample consists of a subsample of MIDUS participants who provided information on anxiety-, depression-, and anger symptoms at MIDUS -II (the "Biomarker" subsample) and on cognition at MIDUS-II and MIDUS-III (44) (**Supplemental Material Table 1**: Flowchart of the analytical sample).

Cognitive Function

Cognitive function was assessed with the Brief Test of Adult Cognition by Telephone (BTACT) (45) administered by telephone (46, 47). EM was assessed by the ability to correctly recall as many words read aloud from a 15-word list (word list immediate) and at the end of each BTACT interview after 20 min (word list delayed). Scoring is the number of unique words produced in 60 s or the number of unique words at the end of the interview. For the assessment of EF the following tests were used: Verbal fluency was tested in a test which asks participants to generate as many animals within 60 s as possible (score: number of animals produced in the 60 s); inductive reasoning was tested with the Number Series Test, which requires responding with the correct number in a series of numbers by inferring a pattern; processing speed is assessed with the 30-s-and-Counting-Task, which requires counting backwards from 100 within 30 s (score: total number of correct numbers reported); Attention switching/reaction time was assessed with the "stop" and "go" task. Following Lachman (46, 48), each score on EF was standardized and averaged to obtain a global EF score. The subtests were standardized using means and standard deviations from MIDUS-II. All cognitive assessment were administered by telephone interview.

Depression-, Anxiety-, and Anger Symptoms

Participants reported on depression-, anxiety- or anger symptoms in the Mood and Anxiety Symptom Questionnaire (MASQ), the Center for Epidemiologic Studies Depression Scale (CES-D) and the State-Trait Anger Expression Inventory (STAXI) (**Supplementary Material Table 1**). The MASQ was designed to assess symptoms of distress, depression, and anxiety (49) on two subscales. The distress scale contains mixed anxiety and somatic symptoms (11 items) and the anxiety scale contains anxiety symptoms (17 items) (50). The Center for Epidemiological Studies Depression (CES-D) Scale is a self-report scale designed to measure depression symptoms in the (51) with 20-items on a four-point Likert scale. We measured furthermore anger using the STAXI. The STAXI assesses anger-in and anger out with each eight items on a four-point Likert scale; and anger control with four items on a seven-point scale (52, 53). For each scale, we calculated the mean score of all items allowing for up to one missing item per respondent.

Co-variates

Socio-demographic- and economic variables were measured at baseline with the MIDUS questionnaire. We assessed chronological age (in categories), gender (female, male), race/ethnicity (White, Latino, other), marital status (married, not married), educational level (high school or less, some college or more), working status (employed, unemployed, retired/other not working), and income. Income was measured adjusted for household size to generate a measure relative to the Federal Poverty Level (FPL); i.e., a measure of annual cash income issued every year by the Department of Health and Human Services in the US (for 2018: $12,140 for individuals). To categorize FPL for this study, we calculated FPL-tertiles for the respective study years (tertile 1: <305 FPL, tertile 2: 306–564 FPL, tertile 3: >565%).

Data Analyses

First, we calculated cross-sectional descriptive statistics by gender and age (including standardized means for EF and EM). Second, we assessed the correlations between emotional items with Pearson's R. Next, we assessed cross-sectional associations between depression, anxiety and anger and EM and EF age, gender, marital status, race/ethnicity, educational level, and income cross-sectionally using linear regression analyses. To investigate changes in EM and EF from time-point one to time-point two, we estimated linear mixed-effects repeated measures models. We conducted longitudinal hierarchical block-wise linear repeated measures regression analysis. In a block-wise manner, we adjusted for baseline cognition and performed blockwise regression analyses. First we regressed the EM and EF scores on sociodemographic variables (gender, marital status, race/ethnicity, and education), forming residuals. Then we regressed these residuals on working status and household income, forming a second set of residuals without the variance explained by block one and two. Third mental condition symptoms (distress, depression, and anger), were entered into the regression model. Missing data in the sample were handled based on a missing-at-random assumption. To investigate the robustness of our findings we conducted sensitivity analyses in which we excluded one of two siblings who were enrolled in the study or non-white participants. All analyses were conducted in SASv9.4 (SAS Institute Inc.).

RESULTS

We included $n = 1,252$ ($n = 542$ (43.3% male) at MIDUS II, and $n = 1,183$ [$n = 514$ male (43.5% male)] at MIDUS-III (**Supplementary Material Table 1**). The majority of participants were white ($N = 821$, 87%) with a mean age of 54.9 (S.D. = 11.8) at the first time point and 63.4 (S.D. = 11.1) at the second time point, and slightly more were women (56.5%). A majority of the male participants reported some college education or more (75.9%). Female participants were less often married than men

TABLE 1 | Means and standard deviations for EM and EF scores by gender at the two exams.

	First exam							Second exam						
	Men			Women				Men			Women			
Age group	n	Mean, SD	Range	n	Mean, SD	Range	p-value	n	Mean, SD	Range	n	Mean, SD	Range	p-value
All	493	−0.25, 0.89	−2.10–2.57	652	0.25, 0.89	−2.50–3.23	<0.0001	414	−0.34, 0.84	−2.10–2.63	552	0.26, 1.04	−2.50–3.64	<0.0001
40–49	132	−0.01, 0.72	−1.88–2.41	169	0.45, 0.79	−1.47–2.44	<0.0001	33	0.10, 0.89	−1.44–2.03	60	0.60, 1.09	−1.47–3.42	0.028
50–59	147	−0.19, 0.71	−1.88–1.56	205	0.32, 0.90	−1.66–3.23	<0.0001	105	0.05, 0.85	−1.88–2.63	132	0.55, 1.00	−1.44–3.64	<0.0001
60–69	105	−0.50, 0.74	−2.10–2.57	137	0.12, 0.74	−1.66–2.44	<0.0001	124	−0.32, 0.72	−2.10–2.60	145	0.40, 0.91	−1.88–2.79	<0.0001
≥70	73	−0.69, 0.73	−2.10–0.96	72	−0.33, 0.56	−1.66–2.82	0.006	119	−0.75, 0.69	−1.88–1.56	142	−0.13, 1.04	−2.50–2.65	<0.0001
All	495	0.13, 0.65	−2.58–2.01	654	−0.001, 0.65	−3.07–1.93	0.001	415	−0.01, 0.69	−2.22–1.97	553	−0.19, 0.74	−3.15–1.71	0.002
40–49	132	0.40, 0.64	−0.99–2.01	169	0.22, 0.62	−2.01–1.51	0.018	33	0.34, 0.66	−1.07–1.49	60	0.23, 0.63	−1.06–1.71	0.445
50–59	147	0.17, 0.58	−1.38–1.50	206	0.05, 0.61	−1.77–1.56	0.051	105	0.38, 0.67	−1.41–1.97	132	0.18, 0.59	−1.74–1.41	0.016
60–69	105	−0.06, 0.55	−1.16–1.33	138	−0.19, 0.63	−3.07–1.30	0.088	124	0.04, 0.55	−1.26–1.35	145	−0.05, 0.64	−1.66–1.58	0.194
≥70	73	−0.29, 0.63	−2.58–1.30	72	−0.50, 0.51	−2.02–0.64	0.025	120	−0.34, 0.55	−1.58–0.96	143	−0.57, 0.65	−3.15–1.36	0.002

TABLE 2 | Associations of socio-demographic, work related, and mental conditions (depressive-, anxiety-, and anger symptoms) and executive function and episodic memory by gender in cross-sectional analyses.

	Men				Women			
	Executive function (n = 558)		Episodic memory (n = 556)		Executive function (n = 558)		Episodic memory (n = 556)	
	β	95% CI	β	95% CI	β	95% CI	β	95% CI
Socio-Demographics								
Baseline age	−0.02	−0.02, −0.01*	−0.02	−0.02, −0.01*	−0.02	−0.02 −0.02*	−0.02	0.03, −0.02*
Ethnicity (Reference:White)								
Latino	−0.42	−0.73, −0.11*	0.02	−0.46, −0.01*	−0.25	−0.47, −0.03*	−0.06	−0.41, 0.28
Other	−0.09	−0.33, − 0.12*	−0.17	−0.69, −0.29*	−0.45	−0.65, −0.25*	−0.38	−0.70, −0.07*
Education (Reference: Less Than College Education)								
Some college	0.30	0.17, 0.43*	0.27	−0.18, 0.01	0.33	0.25, 0.43*	0.25	0.11, 0.39*
Marital status (reference: married)								
Not married	−0.12	−0.25, 0.01	0.02	−0.18, 0.01	−0.12	−0.21, −0.02	0.02	−0.13, 0.16
Economic Variables								
Working status (reference: working)								
Unemployed	−0.55	−0.92, −0.17*	−0.73	−0.22, 0.05	−0.14	−0.27, −0.01*	0.08	−0.13, 0.29
Retired/other	−0.09	−0.24, 0.07	−0.17	−0.30, −0.05*	−0.19	−0.31, −0.07*	−0.13	−0.32, 0.06
Household income (reference: tertile 3)								
Tertile 1	−0.12	−0.26, 0.02	−0.11	−0.35, −0.11*	−0.22	−0.34, −0.10*	−0.27	−0.46, 0.09
Tertile 2	−0.02	−0.14, 0.11	−0.17	−0.21, 0.02	0.08	−0.19, 0.04	−0.14	−0.31, 0.04
Mental Health								
Depression 1*	−0.004	−0.01, 0.004	−0.01	−0.02, −0.01*	−0.01	−0.02, −0.01*	−0.01	−0.02, 0.001
Distress	0.003	−0.01, 0.01	0.000	−0.02, −0.003*	−0.01	−0.02, −0.01*	−0.01	−0.02, −0.01*
Depression 2**	0.01	−0.01, 0.02	0.002	−0.02, −0.003*	−0.01	−0.02, −0.003*	−0.01	−0.02, −0.001*
Anxiety*	−0.01	−0.03, −0.001*	−0.02	−0.02, −0.003*	−0.02	−0.02, −0.006*	−0.01	−0.02, 0.003
Anger* **								
State anger (reference: no state anger)								
Anger—in	0.01	−0.003, 0.03	0.01	−0.02, 0.003	−0.01	−0.02, −0.01*	−0.01	−0.03, 0.01
Anger—out	0.004	−0.01, 0.02	0.01	−0.02, 0.02	−0.002	−0.02, 0.01	−0.01	−0.02, −0.001*
Trait Anger/Reference: No Trait Anger)								
Trait anger	0.006	−0.004, 0.02	0.01	−0.01, 0.01	−0.003	−0.01, 0.01	0.000	−0.01, 0.01

**Assessed with the MASQ; **Assessed with the CESD; ***Assessed with the STAXI.*

were. Mean levels of household income were higher in men than in women.

To describe cognition and depression-, anxiety-, and anger symptoms in the analytical sample, we analyzed means and standard deviations for EM and EF scores in men and women at the two exams (**Table 1**). Consistent with other findings on the MIDUS sample (48), in our analytical sample women had higher EM mean scores across all age groups at both exams compared to men, while men had higher EF scores across all age groups at both exams (**Table 1**). Among participants, mean EM and EF declined with increasing age. Women exhibited higher levels of anxiety and depression than men at the second exam (**Table 1**).

Correlations among the variables are shown in **Supplementary Material Table 2**. Measures for depression and anxiety symptoms correlated strongly.

An initial set of analyses examined within person changes in EM and EF. For EM, significant within-person changes between exams were not observed until participants reached 70 years of age (women) and 60 years of age (men) (**Supplementary Material Table 3**).

Depression-, Anxiety-, and Anger Symptoms and Cognition

We observed different associations between depression-, anxiety-, and anger symptoms with EM and EF (**Table 2**). At the first exam, higher age, being of race/ethnicity other than white, lower education, being unemployed and lower income was associated with worse EM and EF scores. More anxiety symptoms were associated with worse EM and EF, while less anger symptoms was associated with better EF. In women, higher age, being of race/ethnicity other than white and lower education was associated with worse EM and EF. However, not being married and low income were associated with worse EF only. Additionally, depression- and anxiety symptoms but not anger symptoms were associated with worse EM and EF.

In repeated measures analyses, we assessed the impact of a variety of socio-demographic,- and work related mental conditions related factors on EM and EF in block-wise analyses (**Table 3**). In men, lower levels in EF at follow-up were associated

TABLE 3 | Effects of socio-demographic and -economic variables on executive function (EF) and episodic memory (EM) 10 years after baseline, adjusted for baseline age, time, socio-demographic and—economic variables.

	Men				Women			
	Executive function		Episodic memory		Executive function		Episodic memory	
	β	95% CI	β	95% CI	β	95% CI	β	95% CI
	$N = 365$		$N = 364$		$N = 465$		$N = 463$	
Variable								
Follow-up time	−0.02	−0.03, −0.01	−0.02	−0.03, 0.004	−0.03	−0.03, −0.02	−0.004	−0.02, 0.01
Baseline age	−0.02	−0.03, −0.02	−0.03	−0.03, −0.02	−0.03	−0.03, −0.02	−0.02	−0.03, −0.02
Socio-Demographics								
Ethnicity (reference: white)								
Latino	−0.77	−0.63, −0.12	−0.04	−0.25, 0.28	−0.19	−0.37, −0.001	−0.09	−0.39, 0.20
Other	−0.23	−0.43, −0.04	−0.13	−0.36, 0.11	−0.47	−0.64, 0.29	−0.33	−0.60, −0.05
Education								
Some college	0.21	0.11, 0.31	0.20	0.06, 0.34	0.36	0.28, 0.43	0.27	0.15, 0.38
Marital status (reference: married)								
Not married	−0.09	−0.20, 0.03	0.07	−0.07, 0.20	−0.10	−0.18, −0.03	0.01	−0.11, 0.12
Economic Variables								
	$n = 357$	$n = 356$	$n = 459$	$n = 459$				
Working status (reference: employed)								
Unemployed	−0.54	−0.87, 0.20	−0.45	−0.86, −0.04	−0.09	−0.21, 0.02	0.11	−0.07, 0.28
Retired/other	−0.08	−0.20, 0.04	−0.08	−0.22, 0.66	−0.12	−0.20, −0.04	−0.01	−0.15, 0.12
Household income (reference: tertile 3)								
Tertile 1+	−0.08	−0.19, 0.04	−0.11	−0.25, 0.03	−0.16	−0.24, 0.08	−0.17	−0.30, −0.03
Tertile 2++	−0.002	−0.10, 0.10	−0.14	−0.25, −0.02	−0.07	−0.15, 0.01	−0.06	−0.20, 0.08

+Tertile 1<305%FPL, ++Tertile 2: 306–564%FPL.

with higher age, race/ethnicity other than white and being unemployed, and lower levels in EM were associated with being unemployed and lower household income. In women, lower levels in EF were associated with higher age, and race/ethnicity other than white, not being married, being retired and lower household income. A decline in EM was associated with race/ethnicity other than white and lower education.

Finally, we examined whether depression-, anxiety- or anger symptoms influence EM and EF change over a decade, accounting for s *socio-demographic,- and work related* covariates (**Table 4**). We found that in both, in men and women, more anxiety symptoms were statistically significantly associated with worse EM and EF. Additionally, in women higher depression symptoms were significantly associated with worse EM and EF. In men, more trait anger symptoms were associated with better EM. In contrast, in women, more sate anger symptoms contributed to worse EM.

Sensitivity Analyses

We conducted two sensitivity analyses. First, to investigate whether the twins which are included in the sample influenced results, we analyzed data excluding one twin from each pair from all analyses. Results were robust and any differences are likely related to the reduction of statistical power in the smaller sample. Second, to investigate whether race/ethnicity (white, Latino, and Latina) had an impact on the results, we analyzed participants of white race/ethnicity vs. race/ethnicity other than white and found no more than minor changes in effect estimates.

DISCUSSION

Using data of a large longitudinal sample of middle aged and older individuals, the present study examined the long-term associations between depression-, anxiety-, and anger symptoms and EM and EF. Consistently, our analyses suggest that depression-, anxiety-, and anger symptoms are related to cognition. In repeated measures analysis, higher anxiety was associated with lower levels of EM and EF. Analyzing the data by female and male gender, we found that in women, more depression symptoms were associated with worse EM; and that in men, more anger symptoms were associated with better EM.

Overall, we found age-related EM and EF changes which have been found previously in studies analyzing the MIDUS data (48). We observed decreases in cognition after age 70. Prior studies with other samples suggested age-related changes after age 60 (54). The difference of a decade might be related to worldwide increases in cognitive performances favoring later born cohorts in many population groups. Cognitive performance increases have been found in more recent birth cohorts and have been attributed to changes in living conditions, family size, health, and better education (15, 16).

TABLE 4 | Effects of mental health (depressive-, anxiety-, or anger symptoms) on executive function and episodic memory 10 years after baseline on men and women, adjusted for baseline age, time, socio-demographic and—economic variables United States, 2016.

	Men				Women			
	Executive function		Episodic memory		Executive function		Episodic memory	
Variable	β	95% CI	β	95% CI	β	95% CI	β	95% CI
	N = 365		N = 364		N = 465		N = 463	
Mental conditions								
Distress (reference: no distress)								
Distress*	0.001	−0.01, 0.01	−0.003	−0.01, 0.01	−0.008	−0.01, −0.002*	−0.012	−0.02, −0.003
Depression (referencce: no depression)								
Depression 1*	0.001	−0.01, 0.01	−0.003	−0.01, 0.01	−0.008	−0.01, −0.002	−0.012	−0.02, −0.002
Anxiety (reference: no anxiety)								
Anxiety*	−0.02	−0.03, −0.01	−0.02	−0.03, −0.01	−0.01	−0.02, −0.004	−0.013	−0.03, −0.001
Depression 2 (reference: no depression 2)								
Depression 2**	−0.002	−0.01, 0.01	−0.006	−0.01, 0.002	−0.008	−0.01, −0.004	−0.01	−0.02, 0.002
Anger								
State anger (Anger-in)***	0.007	−0.02, 0.001	0.002	−0.01, 0.02	0.007	−0.02, 0.001	−0.006	−0.02, −0.01
Trait anger***	0.004	−0.004, 0.01	0.01	0.002, 0.02	0.004	−0.002, 0.01	0.001	−0.01, 0.01

**Assessed with the MASQ; **Assessed with the CESD; ***Assessed with the STAXI.*

The pattern for cognition confirms the results of previous studies with data from respondents ages 50–93 years from other longitudinal surveys (14), suggesting that women outperform same age men on EM (55). Studies conducted in non-Western societies, such as China and India, however, have reported a disadvantage for older women compared with men in the same age group in measures of EM and word fluency.

Depression and Cognition

Adjusting for all covariates, more depression symptoms were associated with worse EM and EF in women. The findings are in line with previous research which suggested that individuals with mood disorders have worse cognition (56), and that positive emotions help maintain cognitive function (57, 58). Furthermore, in women, depression symptoms are associated with worse EM and EF. Depression symptoms may trigger hypercortisolemia (59, 60), increase autonomic responses associated with cardiovascular disease (61, 62), contribute to inflammation (63), and herewith to neurotoxicity. These processes may accelerate cognitive decline during aging (64).

Anxiety and Cognition

We show that higher levels of anxiety symptoms are associated with lower levels of EM and EF in men and women. An explanation for the adverse effects of increased anxiety on decreases in EF and EM is given by the attentional control theory (65, 66). Attentional control theory predicts that anxiety impairs various functions (66, 67), specifically, the inhibition, shifting and updating functions and herewith reduces resources for EM and EF (68, 69). A further explanation might be that anxiety is associated with anxiety induced hypothalamic-pituitary-adrenal (HPA) over-activation, and chronic changes in cortisol levels, which may lead to dysregulation of the immune system, damage of the hippocampus and subsequent changes in cognition.

Anger and Cognition

More anger symptoms are associated with better EM and worse EF. It has been suggested that anger symptoms are associated with reductions in cortisol (70, 71). The associations were small, however, they are important from a Public Health perspective as small changes in a huge population are of huge importance from a Public Health Point of view.

Strengths of our study include the longitudinal design, well-validated measures and the 10 years of follow-up. Additional strengths are that we were able to investigate these effects in a large population-based sample with information on multiple cognitive domains as well as detailed confounding variables. The study used measures that are useful in community-based studies of non-clinical populations. An additional strength of this study is that we analyzed data separately for men and women. Assessment of depression-, anxiety- and anger symptoms was based on self-report and therefore some misclassification is likely. Any such misclassification, however, is expected to bias our results toward the null. The findings concerning non-white populations are based on a small sample size. It might be that the results of the findings are limited due to this sample size. Additionally, this study is an observational study, which does not test mental health symptoms, EM, and EF under standardized conditions. However, sensitivity analyses analyzing a "white only" sample yielded the same results, suggesting an association of increased depression and anxiety symptoms with decreased EM and EF. Attrition is a concern when carrying out longitudinal research. It might be that individuals in poorer health tend not to participate in longitudinal cohort studies. We can report changes between two time points but not trajectories based on multiple assessments. The MIDUS sample underrepresents those with lower levels of education. A further limitation might be that the sample we used is based on the Biomarker study only, which is a subsample of the MIDUS II study. However, these respondents were quite similar to the sample, which they were recruited from (44). The differences between the baseline sample and the follow up sample might have introduced some selection bias if loss was differential according to exposure and outcome. Specifically, as individuals with more severe cognitive limitations tend to participate less in studies at follow-up and those with certain mood disorders specifically depression also are more likely lost, we may have underestimated the impact of such emotions on cognitive outcomes.

The findings of this study suggest a long-term association between depression-, anxiety- and anger symptoms in midlife and EM and EF in later life. EM and EF in aging populations can be improved by reducing depression-, anxiety- and anger symptoms. In the future differences between men in women in the effect of the different emotional factors on cognitive changes over time should be assessed. Our findings have important implications for preventive interventions. Although some aspects of early life cannot be modified such as early life education, later lie conditions such as depression-, anxiety-, or anger symptoms might be modifiable. Interventions to reduce depression-, anxiety-, and anger symptoms in midlife may benefit EM and EF in later life.

ETHICS STATEMENT

Data collection for all phases of the MIDUS studies was approved by Institutional Review Boards and all participants provided informed consent.

AUTHOR CONTRIBUTIONS

JL, BR, MEL, and TES designed this study. TES and MEL collected the data for the MIDUS studies. JL, BR, and KCP developed the analysis strategy. KCP analyzed the data. JL wrote the manuscript. All authors commented on the manuscript and approved the manuscript.

FUNDING

The MIDUS data collection was supported, in part, by Grant P01-AG020166 from the National Institute on Aging to conduct a longitudinal follow-up of the MIDUS (Midlife in the United States) investigation. MIDUS II data collection was further supported by the following Grants: M01-RR023942 (Georgetown University), M01-RR00865 (University of California, Los Angeles) from the General Clinical Research Centers Program, and UL1TR000427 (University of Wisconsin) and UL1TR001881 (University of California, Los Angeles) from the National Center for Advancing Translational Sciences, National Institutes of Health. Additional support was provided by the USC/UCLA Biodemography & Population Health Center (P30-AG017265) as well as from the original MIDUS study was supported by the John D. and Catherine T. MacArthur Foundation Research Network on Successful Midlife Development.

REFERENCES

Livingston G, Huntley J, Sommerlad A, Ames D, Ballard C, Banerjee S, et al. Dementia prevention, intervention, and care: 2020 report of the lancet commission. *Lancet.* (2020) 396:413–46. doi: 10.1016/S0140-6736(20) 30367-6

Gallagher D, Ni Mhaolain A, Crosby L, Ryan D, Lacey L, Coen RF, et al. Dependence and caregiver burden in alzheimer's disease and mild cognitive impairment. *Am J Alzheimers Dis Other Demen.* (2011) 26:110– 4. doi: 10.1177/1533317510394649

MacDonald SW, Hultsch DF, Dixon RA. Aging and the shape of cognitive change before death: terminal decline or terminal drop? *J Gerontol B Psychol Sci Soc Sci.* (2011) 66:292–301. doi: 10.1093/geronb/gbr001

Zahodne LB, Manly JJ, Smith J, Seeman T, Lachman ME. Socioeconomic, health, and psychosocial mediators of racial disparities in cognition in early, middle, late adulthood. *Psychol Aging.* (2017) 32:118–30. doi: 10.1037/pag0000154

Patterson C. (2018) *World Alzheimer report* Retrieved from London:

Dumas JA. Strategies for preventing cognitive decline in healthy older adults. *Can J Psychiatry.* (2017) 62:754–60. doi: 10.1177/0706743717720691

Mayeux R, Stern Y. Epidemiology of Alzheimer disease. *Cold Spring Harb Perspect Med.* (2012) 2:6239. doi: 10.1101/cshperspect.a006239

Meng X, D'Arcy C. Education and dementia in the context of the cognitive reserve hypothesis: a systematic review with meta-analyses and qualitative analyses. *PLoS ONE.* (2012) 7:e38268. doi: 10.1371/journal.pone.0038268

Albert MS, Jones K, Savage CR, Berkman L, Seeman T, Blazer D, et al. Predictors of cognitive change in older persons: macArthur studies of successful aging. *Psychol Aging.* (1995) 10:578–589.

Lyu J, Burr JA. Socioeconomic status across the life course and cognitive function among older adults: an examination of the latency, pathways, accumulation hypotheses. *J Aging Health.* (2016) 28:40–67. doi: 10.1177/0898264315585504

Berryman N, Bherer L, Nadeau S, Lauziere S, Lehr L, Bobeuf F, et al. Multiple roads lead to rome: combined high-intensity aerobic and strength training vs. gross motor activities leads to equivalent improvement in executive functions in a cohort of healthy older adults. *Age (Dordr).* (2014) 36:9710. doi: 10.1007/s11357-014-9710-8

Kramer AF, Erickson KI. Capitalizing on cortical plasticity: influence of physical activity on cognition and brain function. *Trends Cogn Sci.* (2007) 11:342–8. doi: 10.1016/j.tics.2007.06.009

Seeman TE, Lusignolo TM, Albert M, Berkman L. Social relationships, social support, and patterns of cognitive aging in healthy, high-functioning older adults: macarthur studies of successful aging. *Health Psychol.* (2001) 20:243–55. doi: 10.1037/0278-6133.20.4.243

Weber D, Skirbekk V, Freund I, Herlitz A. The changing face of cognitive gender differences in europe. *Proc Natl Acad Sci USA.* (2014) 111:11673– 8. doi: 10.1073/pnas.1319538111

Dodge HH, Zhu J, Hughes TF, Snitz BE, Chang CH, Jacobsen EP, et al. Cohort effects in verbal memory function and practice effects: a population- based study. *Int Psychogeriatr.* (2017) 29:137–48. doi: 10.1017/S104161021600 1551

Leggett A, Clarke P, Zivin K, McCammon RJ, Elliott MR, Langa KM. Recent improvements in cognitive functioning among older u.S. Adults: how much does increasing educational attainment explain? *J Gerontol B Psychol Sci Soc Sci.* (2017). doi: 10.1093/geronb/gbw210

Cherbuin N, Kim S, Anstey KJ. Dementia risk estimates associated with measures of depression: a systematic review and meta-analysis. *BMJ Open.* (2015) 5:e008853. doi: 10.1136/bmjopen-2015-008853

Low LF, Harrison F, Lackersteen SM. Does personality affect risk for dementia? A systematic review and meta-analysis. *Am J Geriatr Psychiatry.* (2013) 21:713–28. doi: 10.1016/j.jagp.2012.08.004

Terracciano A, Stephan Y, Luchetti M, Albanese E, Sutin AR. Personality traits and risk of cognitive impairment and dementia. *J Psychiatr Res.* (2017) 89:22–7. doi: 10.1016/j.jpsychires.2017.01.011

Baxter AJ, Scott KM, Vos T, Whiteford HA. Global prevalence of anxiety disorders: a systematic review and meta-regression. *Psychol Med.* (2013) 43:897–910. doi: 10.1017/S003329171200147X

Petkus AJ, Reynolds CA, Wetherell JL, Kremen WS, Gatz M. Temporal dynamics of cognitive performance and anxiety across older adulthood. *Psychol Aging.* (2017) 32:278–92. doi: 10.1037/pag0000164

Chirinos DA, Murdock KW, LeRoy AS, Fagundes C. Depressive symptom profiles, cardio-metabolic risk and inflammation: results from the mIDUS study. *Psychoneuroendocrinology.* (2017) 82:17–25. doi: 10.1016/j.psyneuen.2017.04.011

Eng PM, Fitzmaurice G, Kubzansky LD, Rimm EB, Kawachi I. Anger expression and risk of stroke and coronary heart disease among male health professionals. *Psychosom Med.* (2003) 65:100–10. doi: 10.1097/01.psy.0000040949.22044.c6

Pressman SD, Cohen S. Does positive affect influence health? *Psychol Bull.* (2005) 131:925–71. doi: 10.1037/0033-2909.131.6.925

Chida Y, Steptoe A. The association of anger and hostility with future coronary heart disease: a meta-analytic review of prospective evidence. *J Am Coll Cardiol.* (2009) 53:936–46. doi: 10.1016/j.jacc.2008. 11.044

Mostofsky E, Maclure M, Tofler GH, Muller JE, Mittleman MA. Relation of outbursts of anger and risk of acute myocardial infarction. *Am J Cardiol.* (2013) 112:343–8. doi: 10.1016/j.amjcard.2013.03.035

Pimple P, Shah A, Rooks C, Bremner JD, Nye J, Ibeanu I, et al. Association between anger and mental stress-induced myocardial ischemia. *Am Heart J.* (2015) 175:115–21.e112. doi: 10.1016/j.ahj.2014.07.031

Zilioli S, Imami L, Ong AD, Lumley MA, Gruenewald T. Discrimination and anger control as pathways linking socioeconomic disadvantage to allostatic load in midlife. *J Psychosom Res.* (2017) 103:83–90. doi: 10.1016/j.jpsychores.2017.10.002

Bierman EJ, Comijs HC, Rijmen F, Jonker C, Beekman AT. Anxiety symptoms and cognitive performance in later life: results from the longitudinal aging study amsterdam. *Aging Ment Health.* (2008) 12:517– 23. doi: 10.1080/13607860802224276

Brodaty H, Heffernan M, Draper B, Reppermund S, Kochan NA, Slavin MJ, et al. Neuropsychiatric symptoms in older people with and without cognitive impairment. *J Alzheimers Dis.* (2012) 31:411– 20. doi: 10.3233/JAD-2012-120169

Bunce D, Batterham PJ, Mackinnon AJ, Christensen H. Depression, anxiety and cognition in community-dwelling adults aged 70 years and over. *J Psychiatr Res.* (2012) 46:1662–6. doi: 10.1016/j.jpsychires.2012.08.023

Chapman B, Duberstein P, Tindle HA, Sink KM, Robbins J, Tancredi DJ, et al. Personality predicts cognitive function over 7 years in older persons. *Am J Geriatr Psychiatry.* (2012) 20:612–21. doi: 10.1097/JGP.0b013e31822cc9cb

Ganguli M, Du Y, Dodge HH, Ratcliff GG, Chang CC. Depressive symptoms and cognitive decline in late life: a prospective epidemiological study. *Arch Gen Psychiatry.* (2006) 63:153–60. doi: 10.1001/archpsyc.63.2.153

Okereke OI, Grodstein F. Phobic anxiety and cognitive performance over 4 years among community-dwelling older women in the nurses' health study. *Am J Geriatr Psychiatry.* (2013) 21:1125–34. doi: 10.1016/j.jagp.2013. 01.050

Pietrzak RH, Maruff P, Woodward M, Fredrickson J, Fredrickson A, Krystal JH, et al. Mild worry symptoms predict decline in learning and memory in healthy older adults: a 2-year prospective cohort study. *Am J Geriatr Psychiatry.* (2012) 20:266–75. doi: 10.1097/JGP.0b013e3182107e24

Gulpers B, Ramakers I, Hamel R, Kohler S, Oude Voshaar R, Verhey F. Anxiety as a predictor for cognitive decline and dementia: a Systematic review and meta-Analysis. *Am J Geriatr Psychiatry.* (2016) 24:823– 42. doi: 10.1016/j.jagp.2016.05.015

Lipnicki DM, Makkar SR, Crawford JD, Thalamuthu A, Kochan NA, Lima- Costa MF, et al. Determinants of cognitive performance and decline in 20 diverse ethno-regional groups: a COSMIC collaboration cohort study. *PLoS Med.* (2019) 16:e1002853. doi: 10.1371/journal.pmed.1002853

Santabarbara J, Lipnicki DM, Bueno-Notivol J, Olaya-Guzman B, Villagrasa B, Lopez-Anton R. Updating the evidence for an association between anxiety and risk of Alzheimer's disease: a meta-analysis of prospective cohort studies. *J Affect Disord.* (2020) 262:397–404. doi: 10.1016/j.jad.2019. 11.065

Sutin AR, Stephan Y, Terracciano A. Psychological distress, self-Beliefs, and risk of cognitive impairment and dementia. *J Alzheimers Dis.* (2018) 65:1041– 50. doi: 10.3233/JAD-180119

Herlitz A, Nilsson LG, Backman L. Gender differences in episodic memory. *Mem Cognit.* (1997) 25:801–11.

Jäncke L. Sex/gender differences in cognition, neurophysiology, and neuroanatomy. *F1000Res.* (2018) 7. doi: 10.12688/f1000research.13917.1

Brim OG, Baltes PB, Marmot MG, Ryff CD, Rossi AS, Bumpass LL, et al. *Midlife in the United States (MIDUS 1), 1995-1996. Interuniversity Consortium for Political and Social Research (distributor)*, 2020-09-28. (2017). p. 1995- 1996. doi: 10.3886/ICPSR02760.v19

Radler BT, Ryff CD. Who participates? Accounting for longitudinal retention in the MIDUS national study of health and well-being. *J Aging Health.* (2010) 22:307–31. doi: 10.1177/0898264309358617

Dienberg Love G, Seeman TE, Weinstein M, Ryff CD. Bioindicators in the mIDUS national study: protocol, measures, sample, comparative context. *J Aging Health.* (2010) 22:1059–80. doi: 10.1177/0898264310374355

Tun PA, Lachman ME. Telephone assessment of cognitive function in adulthood: the brief test of adult cognition by telephone. *Age Ageing.* (2006) 35:629–32. doi: 10.1093/ageing/afl095

Lachman ME, Agrigoroaei S, Tun PA, Weaver SL. Monitoring cognitive functioning: psychometric properties of the brief test of adult cognition by telephone. *Assessment.* (2014) 21:404–17. doi: 10.1177/10731911135 08807

Tun PA, Lachman ME. Age differences in reaction time and attention in a national telephone sample of adults: education, sex, and task complexity matter. *Dev Psychol.* (2008) 44:1421–9. doi: 10.1037/a0012845

Hughes ML, Agrigoroaei S, Jeon M, Bruzzese M, Lachman ME. Change in cognitive performance from midlife into old age: findings from the midlife in the united states (MIDUS) study. *J Int Neuropsychol Soc.* (2018) 24:1- 16. doi: 10.1017/S1355617718000425

Morozink JA, Friedman EM, Coe CL, Ryff CD. Socioeconomic and psychosocial predictors of interleukin-6 in the MIDUS national sample. *Health Psychol.* (2010) 29:626–35. doi: 10.1037/a0021360

Watson D, Weber K, Assenheimer JS, Clark LA, Strauss ME, McCormick RA. Testing a tripartite model: i. Evaluating the convergent and discriminant validity of anxiety and depression symptom scales. *J Abnorm Psychol.* (1995) 104:3–14.

Radloff LS. The use of the center for epidemiologic studies depression scale in adolescents and young adults. *J Youth Adolesc.* (1991) 20:149– 66. doi: 10.1007/BF01537606

Forgays DK, Spielberger CD, Ottaway SA, Forgays DG. Factor structure of the state-Trait anger expression inventory for middle-aged men and women. *Assessment.* (1998) 5:141–55. doi: 10.1177/107319119800500205

Goodstein LD, Spielberger CD, Williams JE, Dahlstrom WG. The effects of serial position and design difficulty on recall of the bender-Gestalt test designs. *J Consult Psychol.* (1955) 19:230–4.

Drewelies J, Agrigoroaei S, Lachman ME, Gerstorf D. Age variations in cohort differences in the united states: older adults report fewer constraints nowadays than those 18 years ago, but mastery beliefs are diminished among younger adults. *Dev Psychol.* (2018) 54:1408–25. doi: 10.1037/dev0000527

Bonsang E, Skirbekk V, Staudinger UM. As you sow, so shall you reap: gender-Role attitudes and late-Life cognition. *Psychol Sci.* (2017) 28:1201– 13. doi: 10.1177/0956797617708634

Beaudreau SA, O'Hara R. Late-life anxiety and cognitive impairment: a review. *Am J Geriatr Psychiatry.* (2008) 16:790– 803. doi: 10.1097/JGP.0b013e31817945c3

Lee PL. A joyful heart is good medicine: positive affect predicts memory complaints. *Am J Geriatr Psychiatry.* (2016) 24:662– 70. doi: 10.1016/j.jagp.2016.04.001

Yang H, Yang S, Isen AM. Positive affect improves working memory: implications for controlled cognitive processing. *Cogn Emot.* (2013) 27:474– 82. doi: 10.1080/02699931.2012.713325

Green KN, Billings LM, Roozendaal B, McGaugh JL, LaFerla FM. Glucocorticoids increase amyloid-beta and tau pathology in a mouse model of Alzheimer's disease. *J Neurosci.* (2006) 26:9047–56. doi: 10.1523/JNEUROSCI.2797-06.2006

Sapolsky RM. Glucocorticoids and hippocampal atrophy in neuropsychiatric disorders. *Arch Gen Psychiatry.* (2000) 57:925–35. doi: 10.1001/archpsyc.57.10.925

Batelaan NM, Seldenrijk A, Bot M, van Balkom AJ, Penninx BW. Anxiety and new onset of cardiovascular disease: critical review and meta-analysis. *Br J Psychiatry.* (2016) 208:223–31. doi: 10.1192/bjp.bp.114.156554

Lambiase MJ, Kubzansky LD, Thurston RC. Prospective study of anxiety and incident stroke. *Stroke.* (2014) 45:438– 43. doi: 10.1161/STROKEAHA.113.003741

Furtado M, Katzman MA. Neuroinflammatory pathways in anxiety, posttraumatic stress, and obsessive compulsive disorders. *Psychiatry Res.* (2015) 229:37–48. doi: 10.1016/j.psychres.2015.05.036

Fung AWT, Lee JSW, Lee ATC, Lam LCW. Anxiety symptoms predicted decline in episodic memory in cognitively healthy older adults: a 3- year prospective study. *Int J Geriatr Psychiatry*. (2018). doi: 10.1002/gps. 4850

Englert C, Bertrams A. Integrating attentional control theory and the strength model of self-control. *Front Psychol.* (2015) 6:824. doi: 10.3389/fpsyg.2015.00824

Eysenck MW, Derakshan N, Santos R, Calvo MG. Anxiety and cognitive performance: attentional control theory. *Emotion.* (2007) 7:336–53. doi: 10.1037/1528-3542.7.2.336

Derakshan N, Smyth S, Eysenck MW. Effects of state anxiety on performance using a task-switching paradigm: an investigation of attentional control theory. *Psychon Bull Rev.* (2009) 16:1112–7. doi: 10.3758/PBR.16.6.1112

Cocks AJ, Jackson RC, Bishop DT, Williams AM. Anxiety, anticipation and contextual information: a test of attentional control theory. *Cogn Emot.* (2016) 30:1037–48. doi: 10.1080/02699931.2015.1044424

Edwards EJ, Edwards MS, Lyvers M. Cognitive trait anxiety, situational stress, and mental effort predict shifting efficiency: implications for attentional control theory. *Emotion.* (2015) 15:350–9. doi: 10.1037/emo0000051

Owen JM. Transdiagnostic cognitive processes in high trait anger. *Clin Psychol Rev.* (2011) 31:193–202. doi: 10.1016/j.cpr.2010.10.003

Shields GS, Moons WG, Tewell CA, Yonelinas AP. The effect of negative affect on cognition: anxiety, not anger, impairs executive function. *Emotion.* (2016) 16:792–7. doi: 10.1037/emo0000151

20

Lifestyle Modifications to Help Prevent Headache at a Developmental Age

Umberto Raucci[1], *Alessandra Boni*[2], *Melania Evangelisti*[3], *Nicoletta Della Vecchia*[1], *Margherita Velardi*[3], *Fabiana Ursitti*[4], *Gianluca Terrin*[5], *Giovanni Di Nardo*[3], *Antonino Reale*[1], *Alberto Villani*[1] *and Pasquale Parisi*[3*]

[1] Pediatric Emergency Department, Bambino Gesù Children's Hospital, Institute for Research, Hospitalization and Health Care (IRCCS), Rome, Italy, [2] Department of Pediatrics, Sapienza University, Rome, Italy, [3] Department of Pediatrics, Department of Neuroscience, Mental Health & Sense Organs (NESMOS), Faculty of Medicine & Psychology, c/o Sant'Andrea Hospital, Sapienza University, Rome, Italy, [4] Division of Neurology, Bambino Gesù Children's Hospital, Institute for Research, Hospitalization and Health Care (IRCCS), Rome, Italy, [5] Department of Gynecological Obstetric and Urological Sciences, Faculty of Medicine and Dentistry, Sapienza University of Rome, Rome, Italy

***Correspondence:**
Pasquale Parisi
pasquale.parisi@uniroma1.it

Headache is the world's seventh most significant cause of disability-adjusted-life in people aged between 10 and 14 years. Therapeutic management is based on pharmacological approaches and lifestyle recommendations. Many studies show associations between each migraine-promoting lifestyle, behavioral triggers, frequency, and intensity of headaches. Nevertheless, the overall aspects of this topic lack any definitive evidence. Educational programs advise that pediatric patients who suffer from migraines follow a correct lifestyle and that this is of the utmost importance in childhood, as it will improve quality of life and assist adult patients in avoiding headache chronicity, increasing general well-being. These data are important due to the scarcity of scientific evidence on drug therapy for prophylaxis during the developmental age. The "lifestyle recommendations" described in the literature include a perfect balance between regular sleep and meal, adequate hydration, limited consumption of caffeine, tobacco, and alcohol, regular physical activity to avoid being overweight as well as any other elements causing stress. The ketogenic diet is a possible new therapeutic strategy for the control of headache in adults, however, the possible role of dietary factors requires more specific studies among children and adolescents. Educational programs advise that the improvement of lifestyle as a central element in the management of pediatric headache will be of particular importance in the future to improve the quality of life of these patients and reduce the severity of cephalalgic episodes and increase their well-being in adulthood. The present review highlights how changes in different aspects of daily life may determine significant improvements in the management of headaches in people of developmental age.

Keywords: headache, migraine, tension-type headache, lifestyle, risk factors, pediatric, quality of life

INTRODUCTION

Migraine and other headache syndromes represent an enormous source of morbidity, especially among the pediatric population. In a 2016 study, the Global Burden of Disease (GBD) indicated that migraine is the second leading cause of years lived with disability (1), up from the seventh cause in GBD 2010 (2). Particularly in adolescence, headache is a cause for common neurological conditions in Europe, especially in women, with an estimated average prevalence of 54.4% (3, 4). This represents the seventh most significant cause in the world for years of life adjusted for disabilities in subjects between 10 and 14 years (5).

Headache frequency is not better controlled with a pharmacological approach compared to placebo as demonstrated in The Childhood and Adolescent Migraine Prevention (CHAMP) study which matched the results of amitriptyline vs. topiramate vs. placebo for migraine prevention in 8 to 17-year-old patients and was stopped early for emptiness. This study hypothesized that active co-interventions, such as management of lifestyle, limiting the use of medications only to cases of acute attacks, may have contributed to the high placebo response rate. In the CHAMP study, the healthy habits prescribed to children and adolescents for the prevention of migraine attacks were: adequate hydration, regular exercise, avoidance of skipping meals, and maintaining regular sleep (6).

Education about lifestyle factors is an important part of any headache management plan. Since headache management is also based on non-pharmacologic complementary and integrative treatments, healthy lifestyle habits should be a focus in the treatment approach (**Figures 1**, **2**). Potentially modifiable lifestyle factors associated with headache are advocated. High consumption of caffeine, insufficient fluid intake, and irregular intake of meals were identified as contributing to trigger or prolong headache attacks or headache frequency; other lifestyle factors, such as physical inactivity, smoking, or excess of alcohol were also reported to be associated with headache in adults (7). Physical inactivity in pediatric age is known to be an important predictive factor for obesity in adulthood. In particular, recent data show an association between obesity and headache disorders also in children (8, 9); in fact, the same pathophysiological mechanisms appear to be implicated in obesity and migraine such as thalamic activation, and the release of serotonin as a neurotransmitter along with adiponectin as an immune modulator, suggesting that lifestyle and behavioral differences may contribute to the migraine-obesity connection (10).

In clinical practice, it may be observed the growing use of ketogenic diet (KD) on the hypothesis that KD should contribute to restore brain excitability and metabolism and counteract the neuroinflammation present in migraine, although its specific mechanism remains unclear (11). Meal skipping should also be linked to subjective somatic and psychological health complaints in a pediatric population, as shown in the CASPIAN-V study (12). Another lifestyle factor contributing as a "trigger" for headaches is stress. This is particularly true at adolescent age. Due

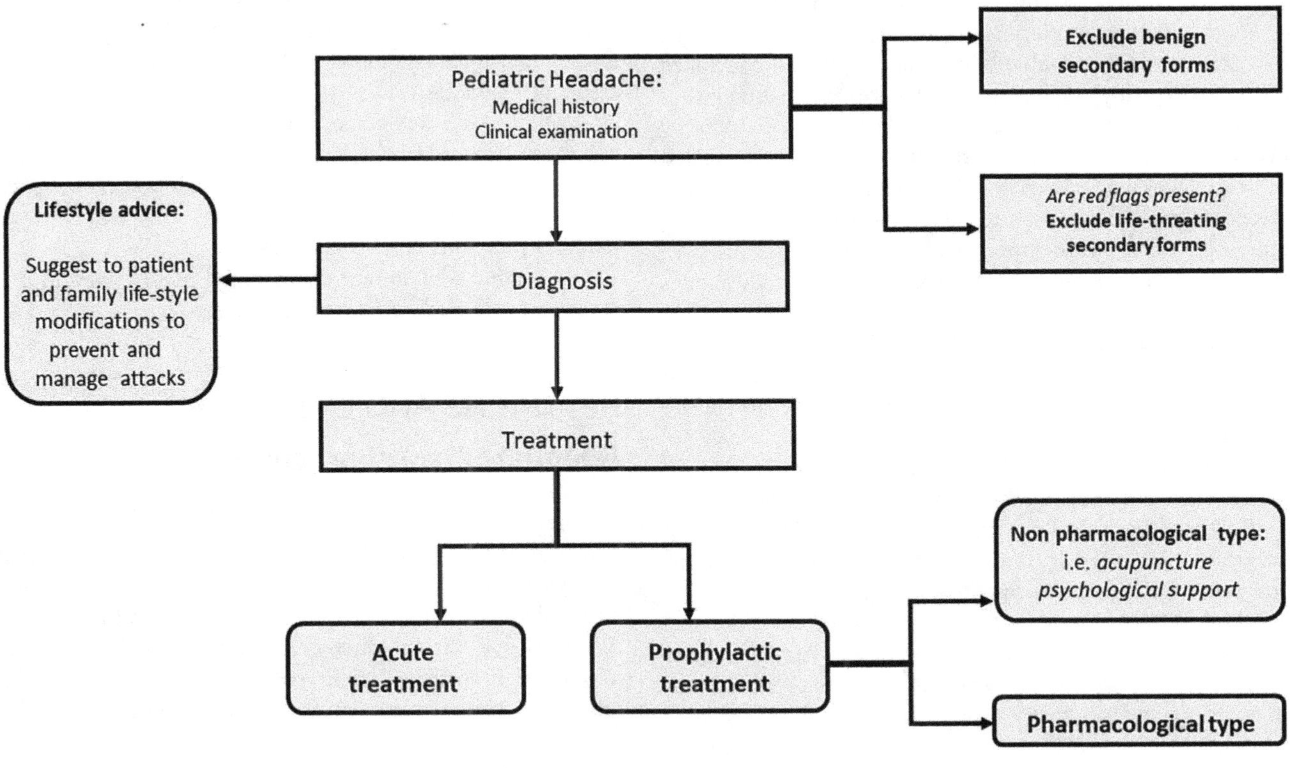

FIGURE 1 | Lifestyle advise in headache management plan.

Dietary triggers

- ✓ Do you skip breakfast or other meals during the day?
- ✓ How much water do you drink per day?
- ✓ How much coffee do you drink per day?
- ✓ How many carbohydrates do you eat during the day?

Cronobiology trigger

- ✓ How many hours of sleep do you get per day?
- ✓ Do you wake up tired in the morning?

Physical and psycological triggers

- ✓ How much physical activity do you do per week or per day? How much water do you drink per day?
- ✓ Check the patient's BMI
- ✓ Is this a stressful time in your life?
- ✓ Is your child having problems at school?

Voluptuous habits triggers

- ✓ How many hours do you spend a day using your mobile phone or playing video games?
- ✓ How many hours do you spend a day watching TV series?
- ✓ Do you smoke? How many cigarettes per day?
- ✓ Do you drink? How many spirits per week?
- ✓ Do you use drugs?

FIGURE 2 | Lifestyle habits to be investigate in pediatric headache management.

to its physical, psychological, and biological changes, it is indeed considered a transitional and critical period.

The use of "life-style rules" in the management of pediatric headache is of vital importance as these strategies may also improve the quality of life in future adulthood, provided that educational promotion starts during the pediatric age. Many randomized, double-blind, and placebo-controlled trials have recently suggested that there is no significant decrease in headache frequency or headache-related disability in childhood and adolescent migraine when it is treated with the available drugs. In particular, no significant differences have been reported in pediatric studies when comparing pharmacotherapy with placebo (6, 12–14). Moreover, the active drugs are associated with higher rates of adverse events.

In pediatric age, these aspects should be taken into account more carefully than in adults, as the placebo response, in children, may have a more significant impact on the sample size under investigation.

Based on these pieces of evidence, pediatricians should help migraine-children in limiting the impact of lifestyle triggers, thereby mitigating the severity and frequency of their attacks by offering lifestyle programs. Sleep, exercise, eat/obesity, cognitive impairment, bullying, and other family and school-related stressors as well as other comorbidities may play a crucial role in this respect. This review highlights how at the developmental age, modifications of various aspects of daily life may lead to improving changes in headache. The search for the best pieces of evidence associated with each one of these factors may produce best-practice recommendations.

METHODS

Papers published up to August 2020 were selected through a computerized literature search using PubMed, ISI Web of Science databases. The following terms were entered, individually or in combinations: lifestyle, sleep, skipping meals, diet, breakfast, caffeine, hydration, overweight, obesity, smoking, alcohol, stress, physical activity, inactivity, technology, electronic device, ketogenic diet, children, pediatric, headache, and migraine/headache.

No restrictions were made on the publication date, study design, and language. A cross-reference search was carried out to identify any further relevant data.

We conducted a literature search and papers relevant to this review are included in the list of references.

HEADACHE AND LIFESTYLE

Adequate Hydration and Headache

According to reports and literature, the clinical practice lifestyle recommendations for migraine management include consistent intake of non-caffeinated fluid (on average 8–10 cups per day, adolescent population) (15). Nevertheless, to the best of our knowledge, no data are reported in the literature regarding the likelihood that an increased intake of water in children may help to decrease the frequency of headache in pediatric migraine. On the other hand, there is evidence, from studies on adults affected by migraine, that an increased water intake might decrease headache severity, frequency, and duration. A randomized clinical trial, conducted in a primary care setting

TABLE 1 | Adequate hydratation.

		Institute of medicine recommendations		European food safety authority	
		Total water intake (fluids + foods)	**Total water intake (only fluids)**	**Total water intake (fluids + foods)**	**Total water intake (only fluids)**
Gender	Boys	2.4 l/day	1.9 l/day	2.1 l/day	1.7 l/day
	Girls	2.1 l/day	1.7 l/day	1.9 l/day	1.5 l/day

Modified by Suh and Kavouras (18).

among 102 adult patients evaluated through the Migraine-Specific Quality of Life (MSQOL) test, concluded that drinking more water determined a statistically significant improvement by 4.5 points on MSQOL. In addition, a 6 point improvement on a 10-point scale was demonstrated among patients who drank more water (in 47% of patients) compared with the control group.

According to these data, this non-invasive protocol for a short period of time could be a reasonable recommendation, at least to verify any improvements that result from an increase in water intake (16).

Kenney et al. (17) examined systematically the adherence to medication and lifestyle in adolescents with migraines and concluded that the population in the study did not drink enough non-caffeinated fluids each day. Indeed, most children and especially adolescents tend to be quite dehydrated. The study evaluated the hydration status of Unity States children and adolescents (4,134 participants, 6–19 years old) and calculated the mean urine osmolality and the relation to inadequate hydration (urine osmolality >800 mOsm/kg); the prevalence of inadequate hydration was 54.5% (17). A recent review of 32 studies also indicated that under-hydration was one of the main problems, suggesting that children are not drinking enough water to be adequately hydrated (18).

The observation that water deprivation can provoke migraine was recognized also by migraineurs; 34 of 95 (36%) adult subjects interviewed indicated that insufficient fluid intake is a factor that precipitates migraine (19).

Therefore, adequate hydration is important in the management of headache (**Table 1**). From the pathogenetic point of view, fluids can help increase blood volume, resulting in better oxygen delivery to the brain (20), and maintain the balance of cellular ion concentrations to ensure a correct plasma osmolality and sodium concentration (21, 22).

TABLE 2 | Headache attributed to a substance or its withdrawal.

Headache attributed to use of or exposure to a substance
Nitric oxide (NO) donor-induced headache
Phosphodiesterase (PDE) inhibitor-induced headache
Carbon monoxide (CO)-induced headache
Alcohol-induced headache
Cocaine-induced headache
Histamine-induced headache
Calcitonin gene-related peptide (CGRP)-induced headache
Headache attributed to exogenous acute pressor agent
Headache attributed to occasional use of non-headache medication
Headache attributed to long-term use of non-headache medication
Headache attributed to use of or exposure to other substance
Medication-overuse headache (MOH)
Ergotamine-overuse headache
Triptan-overuse headache
Non-opioid analgesic-overuse headache
Opioid-overuse headache
Combination-analgesic-overuse headache
Medication-overuse headache attributed to multiple drug classes not individually overused
Medication-overuse headache attributed to unspecified or unverified overuse of multiple drug classes
Medication-overuse headache attributed to other medication
Headache attributed to substance withdrawal
Caffeine-withdrawal headache
Opioid-withdrawal headache
Oestrozen-withdrawal headache
Headache attributed to withdrawal from chronic use of other substance

Modified by Headache Classification Committee of the International Headache Society (IHS) (25).

Overuse of Caffeine and Headache

Caffeine abuse among teens is an increasing practice in age-related behaviors and can lead to triggering or exacerbating headaches. Children (but especially adolescents) also drink large volumes of caffeine-containing carbonated drinks daily. Adolescent girls frequently utilize diet colas as substitutes for food, unaware of the risk of caffeine dependency (23). Approximately 55% of caffeine is consumed as a soft drink by young American schoolchildren (24).

Caffeine withdrawal has also been identified as a cause of headache by the International Headache Society (**Table 2**). However, excessive caffeine consumption, particularly in the form of coffee and tea, seems to be an as yet unrecognized cause of headache and migraine (25). Caffeine-withdrawal headache has been reported in the case of the customary daily consumption of as much caffeine as for about 1 cup of coffee per day (26).

Hering-Hanit and Gadot (27), described a correlation between the reduction in headache recurrence and the use of caffeine-drinks in a pediatric population. The study cohort was composed of 36 children and adolescents (17 girls and 9 boys), enrolled for 5 years, with daily or near-daily headaches related to excessive caffeine intake in the form of cola drinks. All enrolled subjects were heavy cola drinkers; at least 1.5 L of cola drinks per day (192.88 mg of caffeine per day) and an average of 11 (range 10.5–21) L of cola drinks per week, which equals 1414.5 mg of caffeine (range 1350.1–2700.3). The gradual withdrawal of cola drinks resulted in the complete cessation of all headaches in 33 subjects over a 24-week follow-up. In addition, the importance of creating lifestyle guidelines between parents and headache patients was advocated, showing that gradual withdrawal could have been achieved without withdrawal headache (27).

In the TEENs study, a cross-sectional observational study conducted in Spain on students (12–18 years old) from six different schools, headaches were significantly more frequent in people who overused caffeine (30.9 vs. 24.7%, $p = 0.009$). Moreover, caffeine consumption was particularly decisive in older adolescents (14–18 years old) (28).

In a large cross-sectional study among high-school students, elevated consumption of coffee was significantly associated with migraine and tension-type headache, with an about twice relative risk (OR = 2.4; 95% confidence interval 1.3–4.7). Markedly, migraine demonstrated a 3 times higher relative risk (OR = 3.4; 95% confidence interval 1.6–7.0) (7).

As reported in a population-based case/control study on an adult population (26), case-patients manifesting chronic daily headache (CDH) (by convention occurring ≥15 days/month), were more likely to have been high caffeine consumers before the onset of CDH (OR = 1.50, $p = 0.05$), compared with control-patients affected by episodic headache.

Physical Activity and Headache

Physical activity, especially aerobics, may represent a non-pharmacologic option in headache management and can play a role in modulating pain processing: opioid, serotonin, and NMDA mechanisms acting in the rostral ventromedial medulla, promoting analgesia when associated with exercise (29). Exercise does not only reduce pain perception but also has a positive influence on conditions such as stress, depression, anxiety, and mental health, which are often associated with chronic pain.

Large population-based studies indicate that a reduction in physical activity and fitness level, as well as becoming overweight, are lifestyle-related risk factors for migraine and are associated with a higher prevalence and frequency of migraine (30–33). In school-aged children, subjects with migraine mostly prefer sedentary activities and less exercise in their leisure time, compared to the general population (34). A cross-sectional study demonstrated that adolescents with headaches have a sedentary life and exercise less frequently than teenagers who do not suffer from migraines (28).

Furthermore, some evidence states that, in patients with migraine, aerobic physical therapy reduces the number of migraine episodes, with an associated tendency to decrease pain intensity and the duration of migraine attacks (35–38).

Evers S. demonstrated in 2008 that Topiramate is both effective and well-tolerated in preventing migraine, and was elected as a first choice in adult prophylactic treatment (39). Varkey et al. (40) proposed a randomized controlled trial to study in migraine adult patients, the effect of prophylactic use of topiramate compared with non-pharmacological prophylactic treatments, such as relaxation and aerobic physical exercise. The absence of a significant difference in the number of episodes between the two groups highlights the efficacy of non-pharmacological prophylactic treatments and supported the opinion that exercise may be an option in preventing migraine attacks in patients who do not benefit from (or do not want to take) daily medication.

Although, in the long run, physical activity can help prevent migraines, acute phase biological effects can be triggered by physical exercise, some of which could have a role in the pathogenesis of migraine. Koppen et al. (41) interviewed a group of people who suffer from regular migraines and concluded that 38% of them reported exercise-triggered attacks, so much to, that more than half of them had to quit the sports activity as a result. Varkey et al. (42) showed that maximal aerobic exercise might trigger a migraine, but it does not always provoke an attack, even in the migraineur population who suffer from exercise-related migraines. The individuals who consistently experience physical activity-related pain worsening may require tailored interventions to gradually increase exercise to reach a chronic adaptation and benefit from the other long-term advantages of a more active lifestyle.

Hanssen et al. (43) compared a mild continuous training program with an elevated intensity interval training program in a group of migraineurs. After a 12-week intervention period, both exercises appeared to be effective in reducing migraine days, although an intensive interval training program seemed more effective than continuous training.

In light of the aforementioned evidence, to obtain the most advantageous result, migraine patients should be encouraged to use physical activity with cautiously increased modalities (in terms of intensity, frequency, and duration), adapting the training pattern to the individual patient.

Ketogenic Diet and Headache

The ketogenic diet consists of a dietary regimen that induces and maintains a basal state of ketosis. In this metabolic condition ketone bodies are used as an energy source for the body. Ketone bodies include three compounds, such as acetone, acetoacetic acid, and beta-hydroxybutyric acid, and are present in the blood in small quantities.

Fasting is the first condition in which the production of ketone bodies is activated. Low-calorie or particularly high-fat diets have the same result of activating the production of ketone bodies.

The ketogenic diet has been used for years to treat various clinical conditions in both the adult and pediatric population, including pharmaco-resistant epilepsy. Recent studies, including randomized trials, are applying this dietary regimen in adult patients with chronic migraine.

The underlying mechanisms of action of the ketogenic diet in these neurological conditions are currently being investigated. The hypothesized and supported mechanisms were recently described as follows: (1) Reduction of glycolysis and increase of lipid oxidation with the supply of substrates for energy production in the Krebs cycle; (2) Mitochondrial biogenesis and increase in brain energy reserves; (3) Alteration of brain neurotransmitters with increased levels of gamma-aminobutyric acid (GABA) and inhibition of glutamatergic synaptic transmission; (4) Activation of cytoplasmic or membrane ATP-dependent potassium channels; (5) Neuroprotective effects through an increase in energy reserves and a reduction in the production of free radicals; (6) Positive effects against cortical spreading depression; (7) Reduction of the inflammation generated by macrophages; (8) Alteration of the microbiome and its beneficial effects on intestinal permeability, the synthesis of metabolites and neuropeptides (44).

Few studies reported in the literature have demonstrated the efficacy of the ketogenic diet in adult patients with migraine, while rare cases have been reported in pediatric age.

Strahlman was one of the first authors to report on the efficacy of the ketogenic diet as a migraine prophylaxis approach. In 2006 he reported on a woman (his wife) who had been suffering for years from chronic migraine attacks treated with different prophylactic drugs, in which the ketogenic diet seemed to have resolved migraine (45).

Kossoff et al. (46) were among the first in 2010 to run a prospective, open-label study that included adolescents aged 12–19 years with chronic migraine treated with the modified Atkins diet (MAD). Eight patients were enrolled for 2 years (three males and five females, aged 13–16 years). Three patients completed the 3 months period of the study, while the remaining five completed the study before week 6 due to the absence of effects and poor adherence to the diet. The results of this study were not favorable for the use of the ketogenic diet in migraine. No patient showed a reduction in the frequency of migraine attacks. Only 2 patients, male and younger, reported an improvement in the intensity of the attacks. In any case, it is interesting to observe that this study represents the first published prospective study on dietary treatment for migraine in a pediatric population (46).

In another report in 2010, Urbizu et al. described the cases of two monochorionic twins who, between 5 and 10 years of age, developed a mixed neurological condition consisting of exercise-induced paroxysmal dyskinesia, migraine with and without aura, absence seizures, and cramping pains while writing. Genetic investigations documented a *de novo* heterozygous missense mutation in exon 4 of the SLC2A1 gene, associated with the GLUT1 deficiency syndrome. It is interesting to note that both twins responded positively to the ketogenic diet. Therefore, this study confirmed that in the intermediate form of the clinical spectrum of GLUT1 deficiency, the ketogenic diet remains a cornerstone from a therapeutic point of view, although not specific for migraine (47).

In 2013, Di Lorenzo et al. (48) reported cases of two 47 year old twin sisters suffering from high-frequency migraines, whose migraine attacks were reduced by a ketogenic weight loss diet. This accidental and retrospective observation led to the hypothesis that a ketogenic diet could be useful for patients with migraine (48).

In contrast, Bond et al. (49) proposed that weight loss could improve migraines in obese women. Despite several other factors, such as the reduction of analgesia, restraint from trigger foods, and nutrient intake could have contributed to the unexpected outcome observed in the twin sisters, and the authors concluded that KD improved migraine. The first observation documented that migraine had improved before the final weight loss. In addition, the withdrawal of KD has been linked with the recurrence of migraine, despite the persistence of body weight. The second observation demonstrated that nutraceuticals do not play a role in migraine improvement, since they must have been taken at higher concentrations and for a longer time to induce some effects. Finally, triggers for migraine, such as phenylethylamine, tyramine, aspartame, monosodium glutamate, nitrates, and nitrites were not avoided during KD. Consequently, the observed improvement was due more probably to ketogenesis. The authors hypothesized that the improvement of migraine may have been explained with the dampening of inflammation and modified neuro-inflammatory phenomena, the modulation of cortical excitability, the inhibition of oxidative stress in neurons, the depression of the phenomenon of cortical diffusion, together with the activation of cerebral mitochondrial metabolism. However, these cases provided only class IV evidence, as the authors' hypothesis that KD weight loss may lead to an improvement in migraine was based only on retrospective observation of a small number of cases (48).

Later in 2015, Di Lorenzo et al. (50) reported that the mechanisms underlying the effectiveness of KD could be related to its ability to improve mitochondrial energy metabolism and counteract neural inflammation. In this study, the authors included overweight female patients with migraine (96 patients in total) and examined whether the ketogenic diet could improve headache characteristics regardless of weight loss. Their most innovative result was that while on the ketogenic diet, patients experienced a significant reduction in the number of headache days, frequency of attacks, and medication intake for the attack per month, compared to the baseline period (50).

In 2016, Di Lorenzo et al. (51) showed that characteristics of migraine had improved during 1 month of the ketogenic diet, in terms of frequency and duration, confirming their previous clinical findings. The most surprising discovery of this study was that KD significantly normalized the addiction deficit on evoked potentials, provided that the clinical features of migraine improved. Various mechanisms, such as the induction of neural plasticity, changes in cortical excitability, and increased energy metabolism, could explain these results. The results of this study suggested that KD selectively affected delayed habituation by reducing cortical hyperreactivity in migraineurs. Both the increase in rapid GABAergic neurotransmission (GABAA) and decrease in the probability of release of excitatory neurotransmitters from presynaptic neurons have been implicated in the anticonvulsant actions of KD. Considering that the brain of migraineurs is in an imbalance between arousal and inhibition in sensory cortices, it is very interesting that KD, as reported, plays a role in increasing and maintaining synaptosomal GABA content at a higher value, in increasing intracellular concentration, and in causing a presynaptic reduction in glutamate input (51).

In a subsequent study in 2019, Di Lorenzo et al. (52) reported that the positive clinical effects observed in a population of migraineurs with 1-month of KD treatment coexisted with a normalization of the typical addictive inter-ictal deficit at the cortical level, although not in the brainstem. These results suggest that the cerebral cortex could have been the primary site of KD-related modulation (52).

Yet again, in 2019, Di Lorenzo et al. (53) confirmed, in a double-blind study, that VLCKD (Very Low Calorie Ketogenic Diet) was effective for a rapid and short-term improvement of migraine in overweight patients in contrast to VLCnKD (Very Low Calorie non-Ketogenic Diet). The duration of this dietary strategy and the selection of overweight patients with migraine should be determined in future studies (53).

Recently, Gross et al. launched a study on the efficacy and safety of the use of ketone bodies as a prophylactic treatment for adult migraine patients, which consists of a randomized, placebo-controlled, double-blind, crossover study (54).

Finally, in a recent study by Moavero et al. (55), the efficacy and safety of KD in pediatric patients with chronic migraine was evaluated. In this study, patients (10–18 years of age) with chronic migraine, who did not respond to previous prophylactic treatments or refused other therapies, were enrolled. As a first step, the patients underwent a biochemical screening to rule out inborn errors of metabolism. KD was started in a 1:1 ratio. Sixteen patients, 3 males, and 13 females were enrolled to initiate KD. Among them, 8 decided not to start KD, so reducing the number of patients enrolled in the KD group to 8 patients, 1 male, and 7 female, with ages ranging from 11 to 18 years. In this study, the difficulties found in enrolling patients for KD were primarily due to the palatability of the diet itself. In the enrolled patients, partial efficacy was observed in 50% of cases. However, the benefits were transient in 2 of them. These final results were not considered sufficiently encouraging to justify such a diet in these patients (55). Although expressing a potential efficacy in treating chronic migraine, KD involved significant stress for both patients and parents and appeared to be a difficult treatment option during childhood and adolescence. Whereas, KD is increasingly used in adults affected by migraines, to date, data on efficacy in childhood and adolescence are still lacking.

Overweight and Headache

In pediatric ages and adulthood, migraine and overweight/obesity are common conditions with negative impacts on the quality of life. Due to the increased prevalence of overweight and obesity in pediatric patients over the last decade, the occurrence of migraine in the pediatric population has increased as well. Between 1980 and 2013 the prevalence of overweight or obesity in pediatric age children was 23,8% in boys and 22.6% in girls in developed countries, while it settled at 8.1–12.9% among boys and 8.4–13.4% among girls in developing countries (56).

Most interestingly, in recent years many authors have analyzed the association between obesity and migraine in adulthood and pediatric age patients (8, 9). Robberstad et al. (30) conducted a cross-sectional lifestyle analysis of 5,847 Norwegian adolescents, in which students were interviewed about headaches. The results showed that the relative risk of migraine was two times higher in overweight or obese subjects (OR 1.6; 95% CI 1.4–2.2, $p < 0.0001$). Furthermore, the recurrence of headaches in adolescent age appeared to be linked to being overweight, smoking, and sedentary lifestyles, whether the items were analyzed as independent factors or in combination (30). Ravid, in a retrospective study on 181 children evaluated because of headache, concluded that a higher prevalence (39.8%) of obesity occurred in pediatric groups relative to the general population. Unlike the tension-type headache, the diagnosis of migraine was undoubtedly associated with an increased risk of being overweight (OR $= 2.37$, $p = 0.01$) or overweight (OR $= 2.29$, $p = 0.04$). A significant independent risk for being overweight was present in females with migraine (OR $= 4.93$, $p = 0.006$). Disregarding the type of headache, a high body mass index percentile was associated with increased headache frequency and disability, except for the duration of attacks (57).

Several studies have reported that being overweight has a specific role in headache severity and the conversion from episodic to chronic migraine (58–60). Lu et al. (60) reported a more than doubled risk for chronic migraine in obese patients. Comparable results were observed in the Kinik et al. study (61) on 77 females (10–16 years of age). It has been also reported that obese patients have higher rates of headache frequency (considering both migraine and tension-type headaches) and intensity with more nausea and more missed school days (62).

Once more, as described by different reports, there is clear evidence of a beneficial effect of weight loss on headache severity (49, 63–65).

Considering that some authors did not confirm the association between overweight and migraine (66, 67), it is nevertheless necessary to implement research data to achieve more conclusive results.

It seems to be likely that the association between obesity and migraine in pediatric age is a multifactorial event involving both central and peripheral pathways (9). Currently, the role played in migraine attacks by the hypothalamus and the bioactive neurotransmitters and neuropeptides modulating the energy homeostasis, namely serotonin, orexin, and adiponectins (68) are current subjects of focus.

No Breakfast and Headache

Diet plays an important role in headache: fasting meals, eating high-sugar foods, dieting too rigorously, and skipping meals could act as a trigger or make children and adults more likely to complain of headache (69–72). Headache brought on by skipping meals is often quite severe and accompanied by mild nausea. Premonitory signs of headache, such as yawning, pallor, sweating, a craving for sweet things, and mood changes are similar to the symptoms manifested when skipping meals.

Several dietary habits may be associated with headaches or chronicity.

Milde-Busch et al. studied the association between diet, lifestyle factors, and different types of headache among a total of 1,260 adolescents. They used questionnaires to evaluate the intake of meals, coffee, non-alcoholic, and alcoholic drinks, the event of smoking, and the quality of physical activity undertaken. They found no correlation between different types and skipping meals (7).

An Italian population-based study among pre-adolescent and adolescent students reported that 365 of over 800 subjects complained about headache episodes (45, 6%) associated with anorexia. In more than 50% of cases, the event caused the patients to miss school. A strict association between the headache, irregular intake of meals (especially irregular breakfast), and sleep disturbance were also documented (73).

The preliminary results of a population-based study on preadolescent/adolescent students (800, divided into two groups: with headache and without headache) showed that headache patients were mostly women ($P = 0.006$), and were irregular meal consumers ($P < 0.0001$), particularly breakfast ($P < 0.0001$). More frequent and painful attacks were reported among the population who skipped more often the meals (74).

On the basis of the results of a cross-sectional study (based on an anonymous questionnaire on demographic, lifestyle, medical data, presence of headaches and its features) and administered to 1,619 Spanish adolescents from six different schools, Torres-Ferrus et al. (28), reported that 30.5% of the subjects suffered recurrent headaches, of which 11.3% manifested migraine features. Univariate analysis of the results demonstrated, with a statistically significant difference, that headaches were more common in girls, teenagers, were significantly associated with a sedentary life, with the habit of skipping breakfast, smoking, and overusing caffeine.

The results reported are of clear importance to the design of educational programs and to improving the clinical practice for children and more specifically, adolescents.

Technology and Headache

The exposure of children to technological devices, in terms of time spent using smart-phones, watching television, or playing videogames, has increased enormously during the last few decades, concurrent with a shortened engagement in physical activities. A large epidemiological study (involving 1,501,914 subjects) showed that 63% of adolescents (11–15 years of age) use mobile phones and, among them, 23% suffered from migraine, and 5% suffer from insomnia (that is known as strictly connected to migraine) (75). In a single-center, cross-sectional study involving a total of 123 patients, Demir and Sumer observed that the use of smartphones increases headache duration and frequency of migraine among adult patients due to ensuing poor sleep quality and daytime sleepiness (76).

The prevalence of 15 predefined trigger factors was considered in a retrospective descriptive study among 102 children and adolescents. Videogame overuse was reported as the fourth most common trigger referred by children with migraine (77).

Xavier et al. (78) reported a prevalence of 80.6% headache episodes in adolescents and its association with excessive use of electronic devices and games (OR 1,21). In terms of classification, 17.9% of cases were tension-type headaches, 19.3% were migraines, and 43.4% other types of headaches. Adolescents between 14 and 16 years were less likely (OR ≤ 0.68) to report the tension-type headache and other types of headache. The excessive use of digital equipment, electronic games, or attending the third year of high school proved to be risk factors for the development of migraine-type (OR ≥ 1.84) (78).

An epidemiological study on 11-year-old children failed to demonstrate that watching television was a trigger to improve migraine or tension-type headache (79) while a positive link between television watching combined with obesity and depression was proven in children and adolescents (80).

More detailed and long-term studies need to be implemented to explore the harmful effects of smartphone and videogame overuse, as well as an excess of time spent watching television, and to prevent effects on health.

TABLE 3 | Relationship between sleep and headache in children and adolescents.

1. Sleep could be a trigger factor for headache (excessive, reduced, or disrupted)
2. Sleep is often used by the patient to relieve headache
3. Bad sleep hygiene can worsen a pre-existing headache
4. Headache can be related to specific sleep stages (REM or SWS)
5. Headache occurs mostly during sleep or just after sleep; the association between headache and sleep is mediated by the same neurotransmitters (serotonin/dopamine)
6. Sleep disorders are often present in headache patients (restless legs syndrome, periodic limb movements during sleep, parasomnias, sleep-disordered breathing, narcolepsy)

REM, Rapid Eye Movement; SWS, Slow Wave Sleep.

Regular Sleep and Headache

Sleep and headache are related by common neuroanatomical and neurophysiological substrates (81, 82). Studies necessarily rule out headache episodes that occur during sleep, those that are secondary to intracranial hypertension, or other life-threatening conditions.

"Sleep hygiene" refers to programs based on environmental conditions and practices, promoting continuous and restful sleep and including recommendations aimed at improving sleep habits. The programs advocate regularity of bedtime and waking time, encourage adequate time spent in bed for sustained and individually suitable sleep, endorse the restriction of beverages, foods, and the intake before bedtime of any substance able to disrupt sleep. Conversely, exercise, nutrition, and environmental factors enhancing sleep should be implemented to encourage "good sleep quality" (83), since sleep alterations (excessive, reduced or disrupted, deep sleep increase) may facilitate the onset of headache and migraine attack (84, 85).

To promote optimal health, the American Academy of Sleep Medicine recommends 9–12 h of sleep every 24 h for children aged 6–12 years of age, while teenagers 13–18 years of age should sleep 8–10 h per 24 h (86).

Due to the close relationship between regular sleep habits and headache in children and adolescents, several features of sleep are associated with episodes of headache (**Table 3**) Torres et al., in a survey dealing with adolescents, reported that 69.3% had regular sleeping habits (7.7 ± 1.1 mean sleep hours a day), while only 30.3% rated their sleep as restful (28). Specifically, students with headaches had shorter sleep time (7.6 ± 1.1 vs. 7.9 ± 1.1 h, $p < 0.01$) and reported non-regular sleeping habits, insomnia, daytime sleepiness, and unrestful sleep ($p < 0.001$), even when the data were adjusted by sleep time (28).

Teenagers manifest variable sleep timing, chronically insufficient sleep, excessive daytime sleepiness, deficits in mood stability, learning ability, and control of impulsiveness. All these phenomena could be referred to as a delayed sleep phase and resulting from the negative consequences of the adolescent lifestyles on sleep bio-regulatory changes (87, 88).

Insomnia and sleeping <8 h are significant predictors for headaches in children and adolescents (28, 89).

Sleep state has been related to the occurrence of headache syndromes, and headache patients are more prone to sleep disorders (81, 83).

Headaches may occur during sleep, after sleep, and in relation to different sleep stages. Lack of sleep and excessive sleep are both considered possible triggers for headaches in children and adults. Indeed, especially in children, sleep constitutes the decisive factor for the resolution of a migraine attack (84, 90).

Both sleep and headache disorders are frequent health problems during childhood: the weighted aggregate migraine headache rate in children is 10.1%, while about as much as 25% of children had at least one type of sleep problem (81, 91, 92). Literature reports that children with headache usually manifest a higher rate of sleep difficulties, including co-sleeping, insufficient sleep, anxiety related to sleep, difficulties falling asleep, restless sleep, night waking, nightmares, and fatigue during the day (81, 93, 94). Different surveys based on large pediatric populations include the symptoms associated with headaches, such as parasomnias, insomnia, sleep-breathing disorders, and daytime sleepiness (81, 95–97).

As demonstrated by Roth-Isigkeit in a large population study (based on 662 children and adolescents), pain is strictly associated with sleep disturbances (53.6%), an inability to pursue hobbies (53.3%), eating problems (51.1%), and skipping school (48.8%). It is interesting to note that 60% of the population suffered from headaches (98).

A preferential occurrence of headache during REM sleep has been demonstrated. This observation could be explained by the silencing of the anti-nociceptive network of the periaqueductal gray matter (PAG), locus ceruleus, and dorsal raphe nucleus during REM sleep. Headaches triggered by sleep disorders can be classified as:

1. Headaches associated with obstructive sleep apnea (OSA), which include cluster headache, hypnic headache, and headache related to OSA.
2. Headaches related to insomnia, medication overuse, and psychiatric co-morbidity, including chronic migraine and tension-type headaches (90, 99).

Armoni et al. observed that children who were referred to the Sleep Clinic because of migraine episodes reported various sleep problems: in 40% of cases obstructive sleep apnea (OSA); in 27% of cases, insomnia; in 15% of cases periodic limb movement disorder (PLMD). Finally, 6 % of cases complained of hypersomnia (a Central Nervous System disorder). As for sleep patterns, children with migraine had significantly higher NREM 2 phase ($p < 0.001$) and a lower percentage of NREM3 phase ($p < 0.001$) compared to controls (after adjustment for demographics and the presence of sleep-disordered breathing) (100).

A strong link between cluster headache and hypnic headache, with the involvement of the hypothalamus, emerges from other literature. During REM sleep, a preferential presence of cluster headache, hypnic headache, and paroxysmal migraine may be observed. These preferential patterns could be explained by the silencing of the anti-nociceptive network of periaqueductal gray matter (PAG), locus ceruleus, and dorsal raphe nucleus during REM sleep.

The idiopathic hypnic headache usually occurs in adult age. However, it can be observed even in pediatric age, thus amplifying the clinical spectrum of this disorder, and suggesting a possible revision of the diagnostic criteria, with particular regard to the developmental age (101).

Recent research has expanded the comorbidity to several sleep disorders, such as restless legs syndrome, periodic limb movements during sleep, parasomnias, sleep-disordered breathing, and narcolepsy (82).

A detailed sleep anamnesis, relating to sleep hygiene, lifestyle habits, and the presence of sleep disorders, is mandatory in patients with headaches since it could improve the welfare of migraineur patients by correcting inappropriate sleep behaviors.

Smoking and Headache

The correlation between smoking and headache has been hard to study in a systematic fashion (102) due to the difficulties of rigorously categorizing the type, amount, and frequency of the smoking habit. For this reason, the role of smoking in the pathogenesis or trigger role of headache is extremely controversial.

The pharmacological aspects of nicotine have been extensively studied, although they are not yet fully understood, while other toxic products of tobacco remain largely untested (103).

It is unclear whether tobacco addiction is a risk factor for headache, or headache sufferers use tobacco as an analgesic therapy for headache attacks or, at least, some kind of association between the two eventualities may be reported.

The nicotine contained in tobacco (in the form of the highly effective isomer S-nicotine) readily crosses the blood-brain barrier through passive diffusion and active transport from the choroid plexus (103). S-nicotine binds to the cortex, hippocampus, nigrostriatal, mesolimbic, thalamic, hypothalamic, midbrain, and brain stem receptors (104). Relating to some types of headache, it has been hypothesized that the Central Nervous System action of nicotine is directed in a cluster to the hypothalamus (105, 106).

Cluster Headache (CH) represents a unique feature among primary headache syndromes, due to its association with cigarette smoking or any kind of tobacco exposure (107).

Strong evidence, based on large population studies, is available to support the association between CH and smoking. In 2018 Rozen evaluated 1,134 subjects affected by cluster headache. This study observed that, in subjects who did not smoke cigarettes, the age for the onset of CH was lower and there was also a marked familiarity for CH, to suggest a greater genetic predisposition to CH. On the contrary, the later age for the CH onset in smokers could suggest the consequences of tobacco exposure and secondary toxicity from harmful metabolites (108).

Several studies have been devoted to the effect of smoking on headaches in adolescent patients.

All of them agree in defining cigarette smoking as an environmental risk factor for headache in adolescents.

In the Nord-Trøndelag Health Study, in which 8,040 adolescent students between 13 and 18 years of age underwent a self-administered questionnaire and an interview, an association between headache and smoking was reported (OR 1.5, 95% CI 1.3–1.7, $P < 0.0001$) (109).

A larger American study from the U.S. National Institute of Health, based on a group of 10.36 million students, showed that teenagers who smoked cigarettes every day exhibited symptoms such as headache, stomach ache, back pain, and morning fatigue 1.5 times more frequently than non-Smokers (110).

A more recent cross-sectional study on 5,741 students carried out in Croatia showed that teenage smokers have more frequent headaches than those who refrained from smoking (OR 1.94, CI 1.45–2.59) (111).

Alcohol and Headache

Epidemiological studies show that more than 90% of the population had at least one episode of headache and that many have had headaches triggered by alcohol. In particular, in the work by Dueland, 75% of patients with migraines indicated alcohol consumption among the other dietary triggers, as the most frequent cause for their migraine attacks (112).

The International Classification of Headache Disorders (ICHD-3 beta revised) is an essential standpoint to classify the types of headache associated with alcohol intake. It identifies headache episodes as "secondary" when they are part of the hangover syndrome and they are not associated with any known primary headaches; they are recognized as "immediate alcohol-induced" and "delayed alcohol-induced" headaches. The first form develops within 3 h of alcohol intake; while the second form occurs after 5–12 h after drinking alcohol. Both headache forms fade out within 72 h and in both cases, they manifest characteristics different from primary headache forms (ICHD-3 beta revision) (25).

In migraineurs, on the other hand, alcohol-related headache often manifests the same features and symptoms as regular migraines. In this case, the most correct diagnosis is probably migraine or cluster headache triggered by alcohol consumption (25).

Multiple observational studies (113–116) have shown that subjects with primary headaches have a lower alcohol intake than subjects who do not suffer from headaches. Onderwatera et al. carried out a study on 1,547 patients with headaches. Close to half of the subjects were completely abstemious (much less than the general population) and just less than half of the commonly identified alcohol intake as a certain or presumed trigger for headache. The study illustrated that alcoholic drinks are commonly identified as migraine trigger factors and have an important effect on alcohol consumption behavior (117).

According to the data just described, it does not seem that alcohol may be considered the triggering factor for headache as it seems to happen in subjects with migraine and cluster headache.

Although some chemical compounds such as histamine, sulfites, tyramine, and tannins are unable to cause headache alone, they can contribute to headaches. The possibility of an inflammatory response to alcohol, triggering migraines has also been suggested (118).

In contrast to what happens in adults, in the adolescent population, the ingestion of alcohol is a risk factor for headache. In the study by Milde-Busch et al., dealing with 1,260 students aged 13–19 years and run by self-administered questionnaire and interviews, there was three times relative risk of headache disclosed among high school students in case of cocktail drinking (OR 3.4) (7).

An interesting population-based study by Arruda et al. considered the possible effects of prenatal alcohol exposure and demonstrated its association with chronic daily headaches, notably in girls, showing the correlations between headache and alcohol intake (119).

Substances of Abuse and Headache

Substance abuse is associated with a variety of neurological complications, including headaches. Psychoactive substance abuse is growing up among adolescents in the last few decades. These substances can provoke headaches but the exact mechanisms are still unknown. In literature, there are not studies among pediatric age and what is known comes from a careful review of the literature relating to adulthood. In a large Turkish questionnaire study of 1,055 psychoactive abuse users were included and 18% of patients reported having headaches attributed to a substance or its withdrawal with a prevalence of around 30% (120). 94.5% of substance users described headaches after the onset of substance use suggesting a causal relationship. It is also reported that the substances more responsible for headache are methylamphetamine, cocaine, heroin, volatile solvent abusers (120). This large population study demonstrated that younger abusers were more inclined to primary headaches such as migraines and tension-type headaches than older users. The characteristics of headaches in abusers have reported a prevalence of bilateral location and particularly temporal ones with pulsatility (120–122).

Marinis et al. studied the relationship between headache and opiates comparing drug abusers with a control group with a higher ($p < 0.001$) incidence of headache among opiate abusers (60%), particularly those with a long history of addiction (121). The authors have reported 37.5% of patients who completed detoxification therapy configuring opiate withdrawal headache (121).

Another hypothesis was formulated by El-Mallakh et al. who analyzed self-reported questionnaires completed by 236 patients. The results showed that the onset of migraines occurred before the onset of substance use, while the onset of tension headaches occurred after the onset of substance use. Based on this data, the study proposed the probability that migraines may play a role in the genesis of substance use, while substance use may play a role in the genesis of tension headaches (123).

The pathophysiological mechanisms hypothesized underlying this type of headache may be related to chemical irritative effects on trigeminal afferents or to excitation of cortical neurons by the blockage of descending sensory inhibition, originating in the brainstem by these substances (124).

Although there are no pediatric studies in the literature, we recommend that headache patients do not take drugs because of the known complications but also because they are possible triggers of headache.

Stress and Headache

For a long time, research has speculated that stress responses to external or internal factors may influence headaches. The origin of this belief is rooted in the neurochemical links between stress and chronic pain: on the one hand, stress produces hyperalgesia, mediated by NMDA receptors and μ receptors (125). On the other hand, it leads to a reduction of the inhibiting pain pathways (126). One more factor contributing to a chronic headache is activation, in subjects prone to chronic stress of the inflammatory process at the neuronal level, which is mediated by cytokines (127).

Acute stress is frequently reported in the literature as one of the most powerful triggers of migraine attacks in the general population. According to different studies, 50–80% of migraine episodes are caused by a stressful event both in adults (128–132) and in the pediatric population (71, 133).

Apart from being a trigger, stress has been also correlated with the development of chronic headache disease (134). De Benedittis et al. (135) retrospectively demonstrated that, in the year preceding the onset of a migraine, patients had significantly more stressful events compared to the general population. More recently, in a prospective study, Scher et al. (136) highlighted that in the general population, stressful events were more frequent in the 2 years preceding the onset of a chronic headache than in previous years. These data suggest that chronic negative events on predisposed patients could lead to migraines.

In the pediatric population, school-related stress, defined as problems with peers, teachers, and school commitments, is considered one of the primary phenomena associated with headache, (137, 138). School-related stress can also be associated with family background and adolescents with demanding parents experience a higher amount of primary headache (139).

Family background is also an important impact stressor and is frequently reported as being associated with headaches and migraines. Family dysfunctions, punitive parenting, frequent quarrels in the domestic environment, and higher parental depressive symptomatology in early life are associated with a greater likelihood of migraine in children and adolescents (140–142). In most cases in which headache is linked to comorbid stress conditions such as a dysthymic disorder (i.e., depression and bipolar syndromes), the migraine type is rarely an exclusive clinical presentation. On the contrary, a "double pattern" or even a clear picture of "tension-type headache" is often observed. Aromaa et al. (143) reported that an unhappy family atmosphere, a poorer family environment, and a bad relationship between parents are more often associated with a tension-type headache than with migraine.

Awareness that stress may have a negative impact both on the acute episodes of headache and on the severity of chronic headache disease has led to suggestions that improving the management of stress could have short and long-term positive effects on those patients. In a meta-analysis, Campbell et al. (144) showed that relaxation therapy can reduce the cephalalgia index by 33%. These results were confirmed in a more recent randomized-controlled study (145, 146). Moreover, Nestoriuc and Martin (147) conducted a meta-analytic study on the effectiveness of biofeedback in reducing the recurrence of headache attacks. These results were confirmed by Kang et al. in a successive study (148). A more detailed meta-analytic study by Hermann et al. reported that in the pediatric population, non-pharmacological prophylactic treatments such as biofeedback and relaxation therapy manifested an even more positive impact compared to the adult population: in 70% of the pediatric population studied, Hermann et al. detailed a reduction by half of the cephalalgia index (149). Therefore, it might be useful to implement good practices (relaxation therapy and biofeedback) as a prophylactic treatment for migraine in the pediatric population. This may be specifically helpful for those patients who do not manage stressful events well. This kind of intervention could also be used in association with medical treatment or the event of bad compliance, inefficacy, or contraindications for pharmacological therapies.

TABLE 4 | Lifestyle recommendations.

1. Adequate hydration: ingest 1 ounce of fluid per kilogram of body weight (89)
Expected intake of fluids: 4–8 y (all) 1.2 L
9–13 y: 1.8 L (boys); 1.6 L (girls)
14–18 y: 2.6 L (boys); 1.8 L (girls)
2. Limit or avoid the use of caffeine-drinks and cup of coffee
3. Limit or avoid the use of smoking
4. Limit or avoid the use of alcohol
5. Limit or avoid the use of videogames, watching TV, and electronic devices
6. Regular exercise: start with a 5–10 min to walk for 3/5 days a week
7. Regular sleep: at least 8 h of sleep per night are recommended
8. No skipping meals
9. Avoid the use of substances of abuse

High consumption of cocktails (odds ratio = 3.4; 95% confidence interval 1.9–6.0) and coffee (2.4; 1.3–4.7), smoking (2.7; 1.4–5.1), and lack of physical activity (2.2; 1.3–3.7) were significantly associated with migraine plus TTH episodes, consumption of coffee, and physical inactivity particularly with migraine (3.4; 1.6–7.0; and 4.2; 2.2–7.9, respectively) and physical inactivity with TTH (1.7; 1.1–2.7). Couturier et al. (150), supposed that cerebral vasoconstriction during caffeine intake is followed by a rebound vasodillatation and increased arterial blood flow when caffeine is discontinued. Acute consumption of caffeine causes stimulation of the central nervous system, diuresis, gastric and muscle contraction, mucus secretions. It also decreased peripheral vascular resistance concomitant and increased cerebrovascular resistance and decreases smooth muscle tone, especially of the bronchial tree (27).

CONCLUSIONS

Homeostasis and regularity are important in the pediatric population that suffers from headaches, particularly during the challenging time of childhood and adolescent life. Lifestyle recommendations should play a crucial role in the management of headache (**Table 4**).

Although many studies deal with the correlation between pediatric headache and lifestyle advice, no comprehensive reviews consider all triggering factors as a whole, showing the current state of evidence. Drug treatment for acute migraine attacks is often unsatisfactory and the long-term pharmacological treatment for the prophylaxis of migraine attacks has been questioned, due to the lack of evidence on the efficacy and safety of these treatments at a developmental age. As a consequence, lifestyle recommendations play an important role in the management of this significant source of morbidity during childhood and, notably, adolescence.

Accordingly, children and teenagers with headaches should be advised to aim for a life-balance that includes regular sleep and meals, adequate hydration, adequate consumption of caffeine, reduced smoking and alcohol consumption, and regular physical activities should be promoted to prevent them from becoming overweight and to avoid stressors. An important dietary benefit for the management of migraine in adulthood may come from the ketogenic diet, which could be a new strategy in the treatment of patients of pediatric age, but further studies among the pediatric and adolescent population need to be conducted. This lifestyle advice should be considered as a first preventive treatment and be regarded as a central step in the management of programs aimed at controlling the recurrence of migraine attacks. Since headache attacks are recognized as one of the main factors influencing or even limiting the health and welfare of young people. We would expect that these educational practices be promoted with the encouragement of the International Headache Society. These lifestyle programs could promote a healthier adulthood, reducing the occasions for headache chronicity and intensifying general well-being.

AUTHOR CONTRIBUTIONS

UR and PP conceived and directed the review. This article's content was made by consensus of all the authors. All authors listed have made a substantial, direct and intellectual contribution to the work, and approved it for publication.

REFERENCES

GBD 2016 Disease and Injury Incidence and Prevalence Collaborators. Global, regional, and national incidence, prevalence, and years lived with disability for 328 diseases and injuries for 195 countries, 1990–2016: a systematic analysis for the Global Burden of Disease Study 2016. *Lancet.* (2017) 390:1211–59. doi: 10.1016/S0140-6736(17)32154-2

Vos T, Flaxman AD, Naghavi M, Lozano R, Michaud C, Ezzati M et al. Years lived with disability (YLDs) for 1160 sequelae of 289 diseases and injuries 1990–2010: a systematic analysis for the global burden of disease study 2010. *Lancet.* (2012) 380:2163–96. doi: 10.1016/S0140-6736(12)61729-2

Wittchen HU, Jacobi F, Rehm J, Gustavsson A, Svensson M, Jönsson B, et al. The size and burden of mental disorders and other disorders of the brain in Europe 2010. *Eur Neuropsychopharmacol.* (2011) 21:655–79. doi: 10.1016/j.euroneuro.2011.07.018

Wöber-Bingöl C. Epidemiology of migraine and headache in children and adolescents. *Curr Pain Headache Rep.* (2013) 17:341. doi: 10.1007/s11916-013-0341-z

Gore FM, Bloem PJN, Patton GC, Ferguson J, Joseph V, Coffey C, et al. Global burden of disease in young people aged 10–24 years? A systematic analysis. *Lancet.* (2011) 377:2093–102. doi: 10.1016/S0140-6736(11)60512-6

Powers SW, Coffey CS, Chamberlin LA, Ecklund DJ, Klingner EA, Yankey JW, et al. Trial of amitriptyline, topiramate, and placebo for pediatric migraine. *N Engl J Med.* (2017) 376:115–24. doi: 10.1056/NEJMoa1610384

Milde-Busch A, Blaschek A, Borggräfe I, Heinen F, Straube A, von Kries R. Associations of diet and lifestyle with headache in high-school students: results from a cross-sectional tudy. *Headache.* (2010) 50:1104–14. doi: 10.1111/j.1526-4610.2010.01706.x

Chai NC, Scher AI, Moghekar A, Bond DS, Peterlin BL. Obesity and headache: part I—a systematic review of the epidemiology of obesity and headache. *Headache.* (2014) 54:219–34. doi: 10.1111/head.12296

Chai NC, Bond DS, Moghekar A, Scher AI, Peterlin BL. Obesity and headache: part II—potential mechanism and treatment considerations. *Headache.* (2014) 54:459–71. doi: 10.1111/head.12297

Oakley CB, Scher AI, Recober A, Peterlin BL. Headache and obesity in the pediatric population. *Curr Pain Headache Rep.* (2014) 18:416. doi: 10.1007/s11916-014-0416-5

Barbanti P, Fofi L, Aurilia C, Egeo G, Caprio M. Ketogenic diet in migraine: rationale, findings and perspectives. *Neurol Sci.* (2017) 38:S111–5. doi: 10.1007/s10072-017-2889-6

Azemati B, Heshmat R, Qorbani M, Ahadi Z, Azemati A, Shafiee G, et al. Association of meal skipping with subjective health complaints in childre and adolescents: the CASPIAN-V study. *Eat Weight Disord.* (2020) 25:241–6. doi: 10.1007/s40519-018-0559-1

Papetti L, Ursitti F, Moavero R, Ferilli M, Sforza G, Tarantino S, et al. Prophylactic treatment of pediatric migraine: is there anything new in the last decade? *Front Neurol.* (2019) 10:771. doi: 10.3389/fneur.2019.00771

Oskoui M, Pringsheim T, Billinghurst L, Potrebic S, Gersz EM, Gloss D, et al. Practice guideline update summary: pharmacologic treatment for pediatric migraine prevention: report of the guideline development, dissemination, and implementation subcommittee of the American Academy of Neurology and the American Headache Society. *Neurology.* (2019) 93:500–9. doi: 10.1212/WNL.0000000000008105

Kroon Van Diest AM, Ramsey R, Aylward B, Kroner JW, Sullivan SM, Nause K, et al. Adherence to biobehavioral recommendations in pediatric migraine as measured by electronic monitoring: the Adherence in Migraine (AIM) study. *Headache.* (2016) 56:1137–46. doi: 10.1111/head.12836

Spigt M, Weerkamp N, Troost J, van Schayck CP, Knottnerus JA. A randomized trial on the effects of regular water intake in patients with recurrent headaches. *Fam Pract.* (2012) 29:370–5. doi: 10.1093/fampra/cmr112

Kenney EL, Long MW, Cradock AL, Gortmaker SL. Prevalence of inadequate hydration among US children and disparities by gender and race/ethnicity: national health and nutrition examination survey, 2009- 2012. *Am J Public Health.* (2015) 105:e113–8. doi: 10.2105/AJPH.2015. 302572

Suh H, Kavouras SA. Water intake and hydration state in children. *Eur J Nutr.* (2019) 58:475–96. doi: 10.1007/s00394-018-1869-9

Blau JN. Water deprivation: a new migraine precipitant. *Headache.* (2005) 45:757–9. doi: 10.1111/j.1526-4610.2005.05143_3.x

Langdon R, DiSabella MT. Pediatric headache: an overview. *Curr Probl Pediatr Adolesc Health Care.* (2017) 47:44–65. doi: 10.1016/j.cppeds.2017.01.002

Blau JN, Kell CA, Sperling JM. Water-deprivation headache. A new headache with two variants. *Headache.* (2004) 44:79–83. doi: 10.1111/j.1526-4610.2004.04014.x

Rolls BJ, Wood RJ, Rolls ET, Lind H, Lind W, Ledingham JG. Thirst following water deprivation in humans. *Am J Physiol.* (1980) 239:R476–82. doi: 10.1152/ajpregu.1980.239.5.R476

Millichap JG, Yee MM. The diet factor in pediatric and adolescent migraine. *Pediatr Neurol.* (2003) 28:9–15. doi: 10.1016/S0887-8994(02)00466-6

Ellison RC, Singer MR, Moore LL, Nguyen UDT, Garrahie EL, Marmor JK. Current caffeine intake of young children: amount and sources. *J Am Diet Assoc.* (1995) 95:802–4. doi: 10.1016/S0002-8223(95)00222-7

Headache Classification Committee of the International Headache Society (IHS). The international classification of headache disorders, 3rd edition. *Cephalalgia.* (2018) 38:1–211. doi: 10.1177/0333102417738202

Scher AI, Stewart WF, Lipton RB. Caffeine as a risk factor for chronic daily headache: a population-based study. *Neurology.* (2004) 63:2022–7. doi: 10.1212/01.WNL.0000145760.37852.ED

Hering-Hanit R, Gadoth N. Caffeine-induced headache in children and adolescents. *Cephalalgia.* (2003) 23:332–5. doi: 10.1046/j.1468-2982.2003.00576.x

Torres-Ferrus M, Vila-Sala C, Quintana M, Ajanovic S, Gallardo VJ, Gomez JB, et al. Headache, comorbidities and lifestyle in an adolescent population (the TEENs Study). *Cephalalgia.* (2019) 39:91–9. doi: 10.1177/0333102418777509

Lima LV, Abner TSS, Sluka KA. Does exercise increase or decrease pain? Central mechanisms underlying these two phenomena. *J Physiol.* (2017) 595:4141–50. doi: 10.1113/JP273355

Robberstad L, Dyb G, Hagen K, Stovner LJ, Holmen TL, Zwart JA. An unfavorable lifestyle and recurrent headaches among adolescents: the HUNT study. *Neurology.* (2010) 75:712–7. doi: 10.1212/WNL.0b013e3181eee244

Casucci G, Villani V, d'Onofrio F, Russo A. Migraine and lifestyle in childhood. Neurol Sci. (2015) 36(Suppl. 1):S97–100. doi: 10.1007/s10072-015-2168-3

Queiroz LP, Peres MF, Piovesan EJ, Kowacs F, Ciciarelli MC, Souza JA, et al. A nationwide population-based study of migraine in Brazil. *Cephalalgia.* (2009) 29:642–9. doi: 10.1111/j.1468-2982.2008.01782.x

Varkey E, Hagen K, Zwart JA, Linde M. Physical activity and headache: results from the Nord-Trøndelag Health Study (HUNT). *Cephalalgia.* (2008) 28:1292–7. doi: 10.1111/j.1468-2982.2008.01678.x

Bektaş Ö, Ugur C, Gençtürk ZB, Aysev A, Sireli Ö, Deda G. Relationship of childhood headaches with preferences in leisure time activities, depression, anxiety and eating habits: a population-based, cross-sectional study. *Cephalalgia.* (2015) 35:527–37. doi: 10.1177/0333102414547134

Darabaneanu S, Overath CH, Rubin D, Lüthje S, Sye W, Niederberger U, et al. Aerobic exercise as a therapy option for migraine: a pilot study. *Int J Sports Med.* (2011) 32:455–60. doi: 10.1055/s-0030-1269928

Krøll LS, Hammarlund CS, Linde M, Gard G, Jensen RH. The effects of aerobic exercise for persons with migraine and co-existing tension- type headache and neck pain. A randomized, controlled, clinical trial. *Cephalalgia.* (2018) 38:1805–16. doi: 10.1177/0333102417752119

Domingues RB, Teixeira AL, Domingues SA. Physical practice is associated with less functional disability in medical students with migraine. *Arq Neuropsiquiatr.* (2011) 69:39–43. doi: 10.1590/S0004-282X2011000100009

Narin SO, Pinar L, Erbas D, Oztürk V, Idiman F. The effects of exercise and exercise-related changes in blood nitric oxide level on migraine headache. *Clin Rehabil.* (2003) 17:624–30. doi: 10.1191/0269215503cr657oa

Evers S. Treatment of migraine with prophylactic drugs. *Expert Opin Pharmacother.* (2008) 9:2565–73. doi: 10.1517/14656566.9.15.2565

Varkey E, Cider A, Carlsson J, Linde M. Exercise as migraine prophylaxis: a randomized study using relaxation and topiramate as controls. *Cephalalgia.* (2011) 31:1428–38. doi: 10.1177/0333102411419681

Koppen H, van Veldhoven PL. Migraineurs with exercise-triggered attacks have a distinct migraine. *J Headache Pain.* (2013) 14:99. doi: 10.1186/1129-2377-14-99

Varkey E, Grüner Sveälv B, Edin F, Ravn-Fischer A, Cider Å. Provocation of migraine after maximal exercise: a test-retest study. *Eur Neurol.* (2017) 78:22–7. doi: 10.1159/000477166

Hanssen H, Minghetti A, Magon S, Rossmeissl A, Rasenack M, Papadopoulou A, et al. Effects of different endurance exercise modalities on migraine days and cerebrovascular health in episodic migraineurs: a randomized controlled trial. *Scand J Med Sci Sports.* (2018) 28:1103–12. doi: 10.1111/sms.13023

Gross E, Klement RJ, Schoenen J, D'Agostino DP, Fischer D. Potential protective mechanisms of ketone bodies in migraine prevention. *Nutrients.* (2019) 11:811. doi: 10.3390/nu11040811

Strahlman RS. Can ketosis help migraine sufferers? A case report. *Headache.* (2006) 46:182. doi: 10.1111/j.1526-4610.2006.00321_5.x

Kossoff EH, Huffman J, Turner Z, Gladstein J. Use of the modified Atkins diet for adolescents with chronic daily headache. *Cephalalgia.* (2010) 30:1014–6.

Urbizu A, Cuenca-León E, Raspall-Chaure M, Gratacòs M, Conill J, Redecillas S, et al. Paroxysmal exercise-induced dyskinesia, writer's cramp, migraine with aura and absence epilepsy in twin brothers with a novel SLC2A1 missense mutation. *J Neurol Sci.* (2010) 295:110–3. doi: 10.1016/j.jns.2010.05.017

Di Lorenzo C, Currà A, Sirianni G, Coppola G, Bracaglia M, Cardillo A, et al. Diet transiently improves migraine in two twin sisters: possible role of ketogenesis? *Funct Neurol.* (2013) 28:305–8. doi: 10.11138/FNeur/2013.28.4.305

Bond DS, O'Leary KC, Thomas JG, Lipton RB, Papandonatos GD, Roth J, et al. Can weight loss improve migraine headaches in obese women? Rationale and design of the Women's Health and Migraine (WHAM) randomized controlled trial. *Contemp Clin Trials.* (2013) 35:133–44. doi: 10.1016/j.cct.2013.03.004

Di Lorenzo C, Coppola G, Sirianni G, Di Lorenzo G, Bracaglia M, Di Lenola D, et al. Migraine improvement during short lasting ketogenesis: a proof-of- concept study. *Eur J Neurol.* (2015) 22:170–7. doi: 10.1111/ene.12550

Di Lorenzo C, Coppola G, Bracaglia M, Di Lenola D, Evangelista M, Sirianni G, et al. Cortical functional correlates of responsiveness to short-lasting preventive intervention with ketogenic diet in migraine: a multimodal evoked potentials study. *J Headache Pain.* (2016) 17:58. doi: 10.1186/s10194-016-0650-9

Di Lorenzo C, Coppola G, Bracaglia M, Di Lenola D, Sirianni G, Rossi P, et al. A ketogenic diet normalizes interictal cortical but not subcortical responsivity in migraineurs. *BMC Neurol.* (2019) 19:136. doi: 10.1186/s12883-019-1351-1

Di Lorenzo C, Pinto A, Ienca R, Coppola G, Sirianni G, Di Lorenzo G, et al. A randomized double-blind, cross-over trial of very low-calorie diet in overweight migraine patients: a possible role for ketones? *Nutrients.* (2019) 11:1742. doi: 10.3390/nu11081742

Gross E, Putananickal N, Orsini AL, Schmidt S, Vogt DR, Cichon S, et al. Efficacy and safety of exogenous ketone bodies for preventive treatment of migraine: a study protocol for a single-centred, randomised, placebo-controlled, double-blind crossover trial. *Trials.* (2019) 20:61. doi: 10.1186/s13063-018-3120-7

Moavero R, Elia D, Dionisi Vici C, Papetti L, Ferilli MAN, Ursitti F, et al. *Ketogenic Diet in Pediatric Patients with Chronic Migraine. Abstract SISC.* (2020). Available online at: https://www.sisc.it/upload/atti-congressuali-21- 1.pdf (accessed October 6, 2020).

Ng M, Fleming T, Robinson M, Thomson B, Graetz N, Margono C, et al. Global, regional, and national prevalence of overweight and obesity in children and adults during 1980–2013: a systematic analysis for the Global Burden of Disease Study 2013. *Lancet.* (2014) 384:766–81. doi: 10.1016/S0140-6736(14)60460-8

Ravid S, Shahar E, Schiff A, Gordon S. Obesity in children with headaches: association with headache type, frequency, and disability. *Headache.* (2013) 53:954–61. doi: 10.1111/head.12088

Bigal ME, Liberman JN, Lipton RB. Obesity and migraine: a population study. *Neurology.* (2006) 66:545–50. doi: 10.1212/01.wnl.0000197218. 05284.82

Bigal ME, Gironda M, Tepper SJ, Feleppa M, Rapoport AM, Sheftell FD, et al. Headache prevention outcome and body mass index. *Cephalalgia.* (2006) 26:445–50. doi: 10.1111/j.1468-2982.2005.01054.x

Lu SR, Fuh JL, Wang SJ, Juang KD, Chen SP, Liao YC, et al. Incidence and risk factors of chronic daily headache in young adolescents: a school cohort study. *Pediatrics.* (2013) 132:e9–16. doi: 10.1542/peds.2012-1909

Kinik ST, Alehan F, Erol I, Kanra AR. Obesity and paediatric migraine. *Cephalalgia.* (2010) 30:105–9. doi: 10.1111/j.1468-2982.2009.01907.x

Pinhas-Hamiel O, Frumin K, Gabis L, Mazor-Aronovich K, Modan-Moses D, Reichman B, et al. Headaches in overweight children and adolescents referred to a tertiary-care center in Israel. *Obesity.* (2008) 16:659–63. doi: 10.1038/oby.2007.88

Hershey AD, Powers SW, Nelson TD, Kabbouche MA, Winner P, Yonker M, et al. Obesity in the pediatric headache population: a multicenter study. *Headache.* (2009) 49:170–7. doi: 10.1111/j.1526-4610.2008. 01232.x

Verrotti A, Agostinelli S, D'Egidio C, Di Fonzo A, Carotenuto M, Parisi P, et al. Impact of a weight loss program on migraine in obese adolescents. *Eur J Neurol.* (2013) 20:394–7. doi: 10.1111/j.1468-1331.2012. 03771.x

Verrotti A, Di Fonzo A, Penta L, Agostinelli S, Parisi P. Obesity and headache/ migraine: the importance of weight reduction through lifestyle modifications. *Biomed Res Int.* (2014) 2014:420858. doi: 10.1155/2014/420858

Pakalnis A, Kring D. Chronic daily headache, medication overuse, and obesity in children and adolescents. *J Child Neurol.* (2012) 27:577–80. doi: 10.1177/0883073811420869

Eidlitz-Markus T, Haimi-Cohen Y, Zeharia A. Association of pediatric obesity and migraine with comparison to tension headache and samples from other countries. *J Child Neurol.* (2015) 30:445–50. doi: 10.1177/0883073814553975

Eidlitz Markus T, Toldo I. Obesity and migraine in childhood. *Curr Pain Headache Rep.* (2018) 22:42. doi: 10.1007/s11916-018-0696-2

Shaik MM, Gan SH. Vitamin supplementation as possible prophylactic treatment against migraine with aura and menstrual migraine. *Biomed Res Int.* (2015) 2015:469529. doi: 10.1155/2015/469529

D'Onofrio F, Raimo S, Spitaleri D, Casucci G, Bussone G. Usefulness of nutraceuticals in migraine prophylaxis. *Neurol Sci.* (2017) 38(Suppl. 1):S117–20. doi: 10.1007/s10072-017-2901-1

Ferroni P, Barbanti P, Della-Morte D, Palmirotta R, Jirillo E, Guadagni F. Redox mechanisms in migraine: novel therapeutics and dietary interventions. *Antioxid Redox Signal.* (2018) 28:1144–83. doi: 10.1089/ars.2017.7260

Razeghi Jahromi S, Ghorbani Z, Martelletti P, Lampl C, Togha M; School of advanced studies of the European Headache Federation (EHF- SAS). Association of diet and headache. *J Headache Pain.* (2019) 20:106. doi: 10.1186/s10194-019-1057-1

Moschiano F, Messina P, D'Amico D, Grazzi L, Frediani F, Casucci G. Headache, eating and sleeping behaviors and lifestyle factors in preadolescents and adolescents: preliminary results from an Italian population study. *Neurol Sci.* (2012) 33(Suppl. 1): S87–90. doi: 10.1007/s10072-012-1048-3

Moschiano F, D'Amico D, Ramusino MC, Micieli G. The role of diet and lifestyle in adolescents with headache: a review. *Neurol Sci.* (2013) 34(Suppl. 1):S187–90. doi: 10.1007/s10072-013-1414-9

Chiu CT, Chang YH, Chen CC, Ko MC, Li CY. Mobile phone use and health symptoms in children. *J Formos Med Assoc.* (2015) 114:598–604. doi: 10.1016/j.jfma.2014.07.002

Demir YP, Sumer MM. Effects of smartphone overuse on headache, sleep and quality of life in migraine patients. *Neurosciences.* (2019) 24:115–21. doi: 10.17712/nsj.2019.2.20180037

Neut D, Fily A, Cuvellier JC, Vallée L. The prevalence of triggers in paediatric migraine: a questionnaire study in 102 children and adolescents. *J Headache Pain.* (2012) 13:61–5. doi: 10.1007/s10194-011-0397-2

Xavier MK, Pitangui AC, Silva GR, Oliveira VM, Beltrão NB, Araújo RC. Prevalence of headache in adolescents and association with use of computer and videogames. *Cien Saude Colet.* (2015) 20:3477–86. doi: 10.1590/1413-812320152011.192 72014

Waldie KE, Thompson JM, Mia Y, Murphy R, Wall C, Mitchell EA. Risk factors for migraine and tension-type headache in 11 year old children. *J Headache Pain.* (2014) 15:60. doi: 10.1186/1129-2377-15-60

Russo A, Bruno A, Trojsi F, Tessitore A, Tedeschi G. Lifestyle factors and migraine in childhood. *Curr Pain Headache Rep.* (2016) 20:9. doi: 10.1007/s11916-016-0539-y

Dosi C, Riccioni A, Della Corte M, Novelli L, Ferri R, Bruni O. Comorbidities of sleep disorders in childhood and adolescence: focus on migraine. *Nat Sci Sleep.* (2013) 5:77–85. doi: 10.2147/NSS.S34840

Dosi C, Figura M, Ferri R, Bruni O. Sleep and headache. *Semin Pediatr Neurol.* (2015) 22:105–12. doi: 10.1016/j.spen.2015.04.005

Bruni O, Galli F, Guidetti V. Sleep hygiene and migraine in children and adolescents. *Cephalalgia.* (1999) 19(Suppl. 25):57–9. doi: 10.1177/0333102499019S2516

Bellini B, Panunzi S, Bruni O, Guidetti V. Headache and sleep in children. *Curr Pain Headache Rep.* (2013) 17:335. doi: 10.1007/s11916-013-0335-x

Guidetti V, Dosi C, Bruni O. The relationship between sleep and headache in children: implications for treatment. *Cephalalgia.* (2014) 34:767–76. doi: 10.1177/0333102414541817

Paruthi S, Brooks LJ, D'Ambrosio C, Hall WA, Kotagal S, Lloyd RM, et al. Consensus statement of the American Academy of Sleep Medicine on the recommended amount of sleep for healthy children: methodology and discussion. *J Clin Sleep Med.* (2016) 12:1549–61. doi: 10.5664/jcsm.6288

Carskadon MA. Sleep in adolescents: the perfect storm. *Pediatr Clin North Am.* (2011) 58:637–47. doi: 10.1016/j.pcl.2011.03.003

Carskadon MA, Tarokh L. Developmental changes in sleep biology and potential effects on adolescent behavior and caffeine use. *Nutr Rev.* (2014) 72(Suppl. 1):S60–4. doi: 10.1111/nure.12147

Gelfand AA, Irwin SL. Lifestyle advice for pediatric migraine: blaming the patient, or evidence based. *Semin Neurol.* (2020) 40:277–85. doi: 10.1055/s-0040-1708868

Stovner LJ, Hagen K, Jensen R, Katsarava Z, Lipton RB, Scher AI, et al. The global burden of headache: a documentation of headache prevalence and disability worldwide. *Cephalalgia.* (2007) 23:786–9. doi: 10.1111/j.1468-2982.2007.01288.x

Owens JA, Witmans M. Sleep problems. *Curr Probl Pediatr Adolesc Health Care.* (2004) 34:154–79. doi: 10.1016/j.cppeds.2003.10.003

Merikangas KR. Contributions of epidemiology to our understanding of migraine. *Headache.* (2013) 53:230–46. doi: 10.1111/head.12038

Kelman L, Rains JC. Headache and sleep: examination of sleep patterns and complaints in a large clinical sample of migraineurs. *Headache.* (2005) 45:904–10. doi: 10.1111/j.1526-4610.2005.05159.x

Lovati C, D'Amico D, Raimondi E, Mariani C, Bertora P. Sleep and headache: a bidirectional relationship. *Expert Rev Neurother.* (2010) 10:105– 17. doi: 10.1586/ern.09.135

Bruni O, Fabrizi P, Ottaviano S, Cortesi F, Giannotti F, Guidetti V. Prevalence of sleep disorders in childhood and adolescence with headache: a case-control study. *Cephalalgia.* (1997) 17:492–8. doi: 10.1046/j.1468-2982.1997.1704492.x

Miller VA, Palermo TM, Powers SW, Scher MS, Hershey AD. Migraine headaches and sleep disturbances in children. *Headache.* (2003) 43:362–8. doi: 10.1046/j.1526-4610.2003.03071.x

Barbanti P, Aurilia C, Egeo G, Fofi L, Vanacore N. A case-control study on excessive daytime sleepiness in chronic migraine. *Sleep Med.* (2013) 14:278–81. doi: 10.1016/j.sleep.2012.10.022

Roth-Isigkeit A, Thyen U, Stöven H, Schwarzenberger J, Schmucker P. Pain among children and adolescents: restrictions in daily living and triggering factors. *Pediatrics.* (2005) 115:e152–62. doi: 10.1542/peds.2004-0682

Singh NN, Sahota P. Sleep-related headache and its management. *Curr Treat Options Neurol.* (2013) 15:704–22. doi: 10.1007/s11940-013-0258-1

Armoni Domany K, Nahman-Averbuch H, King CD, Dye T, Xu Y, Hossain M, et al. Clinical presentation, diagnosis and polysomnographic findings in children with migraine referred to sleep clinics. *Sleep Med.* (2019) 63:57–63. doi: 10.1016/j.sleep.2019.04.023

Cerminara C, Compagnone E, Coniglio A, Margiotta M, Curatolo P, Villa MP, et al. Hypnic headache in children. *Cephalalgia.* (2011) 31:1673–6. doi: 10.1177/0333102411427601

Dodick DW. Migraine triggers. *Headache.* (2009) 49:958–61. doi: 10.1111/j.1526-4610.2009.01445.x

Taylor FR. Tobacco, nicotine, and headache. *Headache.* (2015) 55:1028–44. doi: 10.1111/head.12620

Benowitz NL. Drug therapy. Pharmacologic aspects of cigarette smoking and nicotine addiction. *N Engl J Med.* (1988) 319:1318–30. doi: 10.1056/NEJM198811173192005

Rozen T. Clomiphene citrate for treatment refractory chronic cluster headache. *Headache.* (2008) 48:286–90. doi: 10.1111/j.1526-4610.2007. 00995.x

Govare A, Leroux E. Licit and illicit drug use in cluster headache. *Curr Pain Headache Rep.* (2014) 18:413. doi: 10.1007/s11916-014-0413-8

Graham JR, Rogado AZ, Rahman M, Gramer IV. Some physical, physiological characteristics of patients with cluster headaches. In: Cochrane AL, editor. *Background to Migraine.* London: William Heineman (1970). p. 38–52.

Rozen TD. Cluster headache clinical phenotypes: tobacco nonexposed (never smoker and no parental secondary smoke exposure as a child) versus tobacco-exposed: results from the United States Cluster Headache Survey. *Headache.* (2018) 58:688–99. doi: 10.1111/head. 13295

Holmen TL, Barrett-Connor E, Holmen J, Bjermer L. Health problems in teenage daily smokers versus nonsmokers, Norway, 1995–1997: the Nord-Trøndelag Health Study. *Am J Epidemiol.* (2000) 151:148–55. doi: 10.1093/oxfordjournals.aje.a010182

Ghandour RM, Overpeck MD, Huang ZJ, Kogan MD, Scheidt PC. Headache, stomachache, backache, and morning fatigue among adolescent girls in the United States: associations with behavioral, sociodemographic, and environmental factors. *Arch Pediatr Adolesc Med.* (2004) 158:797–803. doi: 10.1001/archpedi.158.8.797

Jurišic′ I, Pavic′ Šimetin I, Dikanovic′ M, Cvitkovic′ A. Headaches and knowledge of the patients. *J Headache Pain.* (2006) 7:188–95. in adolescents-frequency, risk factors and other health complaints: a cross-sectional study in Croatia. *Acta Clin Croat.* (2018) 57:613–7. doi: 10.20471/acc.2018.57.04.01

Dueland AN. Headache and alcohol. *Headache.* (2015) 55:1045–9. doi: 10.1111/head.12621

Aamodt AH, Stovner LJ, Hagen K, Bråthen G, Zwart J. Headache prevalence related to smoking and alcohol use. The Head-HUNT Study. *Eur J Neurol.* (2006) 13:1233–8. doi: 10.1111/j.1468-1331.2006.01492.x

Le H, Tfelt-Hansen P, Skytthe A, Kyvik KO, Olesen J. Association between migraine, lifestyle and socioeconomic factors: a population- based cross-sectional study. *J Headache Pain.* (2011) 12:157–72. doi: 10.1007/s10194-011-0321-9

Domingues RB, Domingues SA. Headache is associated with lower alcohol consumption among medical students. *Arq Neuropsiquiatr.* (2011) 69:620–3. doi: 10.1590/S0004-282X2011000500009

Schramm SH, Obermann M, Katsarava Z, Diener HC, Moebus S, Yoon MS. Epidemiological profiles of patients with chronic migraine and chronic tension-type headache. *J Headache Pain.* (2013) 14:40. doi: 10.1186/1129-2377-14-40

Onderwater GLJ, van Oosterhout WPJ, Schoonman GG, Ferrari MD, Terwindt GM. Alcoholic beverages as trigger factor and the effect on alcohol consumption behavior in patients with migraine. *Eur J Neurol.* (2019) 26:588–95. doi: 10.1111/ene.13861

Panconesi A. Alcohol and migraine: trigger factor, consumption, mechanisms. A review. *J Headache Pain.* (2008) 9:19–27. doi: 10.1007/s10194-008-0006-1

Arruda MA, Guidetti V, Galli F, Albuquerque RC, Bigal ME. Prenatal exposure to tobacco and alcohol are associated with chronic daily headaches at childhood: a population-based study. *Arq Neuropsiquiatr.* (2011) 69:27– 33. doi: 10.1590/S0004-282X2011000100007

Beckmann YY, Seçkin M, Manavgat AI, Zorlu N. Headaches related to psychoactive substance use. *Clin Neurol Neurosurg.* (2012) 114:990–9. doi: 10.1016/j.clineuro.2012.02.041

Marinis MD, Janiri L, Agnoli A. Headache in the use and withdrawal of opi- ates and other associated substances of abuse. *Headache: J Head Face Pain.* (1991) 3:159–63. doi: 10.1111/j.1526-4610.1991.hed3103159.x

Lipton RB, Choy-Kwong M, Solomon S. Headaches in hospitalized cocaine users. *Headache.* (1989) 29:225–8. doi: 10.1111/j.1526-4610.1989.hed22904225.x

El-Mallakh RS, Kranzler HR, Kamanitz JR. Headaches and psychoactive substance use. *Headache.* (1991) 31:584–7. doi: 10.1111/j.1526-4610.1991. hed3109584.x

Lambert GA, Zagami AS. The mode of action of migraine triggers: a hypothesis. *Headache.* (2009) 49:253–75. doi: 10.1111/j.1526-4610. 2008.01230.x

Imbe H, Iwai-Liao Y, Senba E. Stress-induced hyperalgesia: animal models and putative mechanisms. *Front Biosci.* (2006) 11:2179–92. doi: 10.2741/1960

Pielsticker A, Haag G, Zaudig M, Lautenbacher S. Impairment of pain inhibition in chronic tension-type headache. *Pain.* (2005) 118:215–23. doi: 10.1016/j.pain.2005.08.019

Maier SF. Bi-directional immune-brain communication: Implications for understanding stress, pain, and cognition. *Brain Behav Immun.* (2003) 17:69–85. doi: 10.1016/S0889-1591(03)00032-1

Chabriat H, Danchot J, Michel P, Joire JE, Henry P. Precipitating factors of headache. A prospective study in a national control-matched survey in migraineurs and nonmigraineurs. *Headache.* (1999) 39:335–8. doi: 10.1046/j.1526-4610.1999.3905335.x

Zivadinov R, Willheim K, Sepic-Grahovac D, Jurjevic A, Bucuk M, Brnabic-Razmilic O, et al. Migraine and tension-type headache in Croatia: a population-based survey of precipitating factors. *Cephalalgia.* (2003) 23:336– 43. doi: 10.1046/j.1468-2982.2003.00544.x

Karli N, Zarifoglu M, Calisir N, Akgoz S. Comparison of pre-headache phases and trigger factors of migraine and episodic tension-type headache: do they share similar clinical pathophysiology? *Cephalalgia.* (2005) 25:444– 51. doi: 10.1111/j.1468-2982.2005.00880.x

Wöber C, Holzhammer J, Zeitlhofer J, Wessely P, Wöber-Bingöl C. Trigger factors of migraine and tension-type headache: experience doi: 10.1007/s10194-006-0305-3

Kelman L. The triggers or precipitants of the acute migraine attack. *Cephalalgia.* (2007) 27:394–402. doi: 10.1111/j.1468-2982.2007.01303.x

Chakravarty A, Mukherjee A, Roy D. Trigger factors in childhood migraine: a clinic-based study from eastern India. *J Headache Pain.* (2009) 10:375–80. doi: 10.1007/s10194-009-0147-x

Waldie KE. Childhood headache, stress in adolescence, and primary headache in young adulthood: a longitudinal cohort study. *Headache.* (2001) 41:1–10. doi: 10.1046/j.1526-4610.2001.111006001.x

De Benedittis G, Lorenzetti A, Pieri A. The role of stressful life events in the onset of chronic primary headache. *Pain.* (1990) 40:65–75. doi: 10.1016/0304-3959(90)91052-K

Scher AI, Stewart WF, Buse D, Krantz DS, Lipton RB. Major life changes before and after the onset of chronic daily headache: a population- based study. *Cephalalgia.* (2008) 28:868–76. doi: 10.1111/j.1468-2982.2008. 01634.x

Santinello M, Vieno A, Battistella PA. La cefalea nei preadolescenti italiani: correlazioni con lo stress e il sostegno sociale a scuola [Primary headache in Italian early adolescents: correlation with stress and school social support]. *Epidemiol Psichiatr Soc.* (2006) 15:52–8. doi: 10.1017/S1121189X00002037

Kröner-Herwig B, Gassmann J. Headache disorders in children and adolescents: their association with psychological, behavioral, and socio-environmental factors. *Headache.* (2012) 52:1387–401. doi: 10.1111/j.1526-4610.2012.02210.x

Marchenko VG, Stepanchenko KA. The role of family and school in the development of primary headaches in adolescents. *Wiad Lek.* (2018) 71:1492–6.

Liakopoulou-Kairis M, Alifieraki T, Protagora D, Korpa T, Kondyli K, Dimosthenous E, et al. Recurrent abdominal pain and headache– psychopathology, life events and family functioning. *Eur Child Adolesc Psychiatry.* (2002) 11:115–22. doi: 10.1007/s00787-002-0276-0

Gassmann J, Vath N, van Gessel H, Kröner-Herwig B. Risk factors for headache in children. *Dtsch Arztebl Int.* (2009) 106:509–16. doi: 10.3238/arztebl.2009.0509

Hammond NG, Orr SL, Colman I. Early life stress in adolescent migraine and the mediational influence of symptoms of depression and anxiety in a Canadian cohort. *Headache.* (2019) 59:1687–99. doi: 10.1111/head.13644

Aromaa M, Sillanpää M, Rautava P, Helenius H. Pain experience of children with headache and their families: A controlled study. *Pediatrics.* (2000) 106(2 Pt 1):270–5. doi: 10.1542/peds.106.2.270

Campbell JK, Penzien DB, Wall EM. *Evidence Based Guidelines for Migraine Headache: Behavioural and Physical Treatments.* US Headache Consortium (2000). Available online at: https://www.hpmaine.com/images/PDFs/aan-guidelines.pdf (accessed September 11, 2020).

Pickering G, Creac'h C, Radat F, Cardot JM, Alibeu JP, Andre G, et al. Autogenic training in patients treated for chronic headache: a randomised clinical trial. *J Pain Manage.* (2012) 5:195–208. Available online at: http://www.novapublishers.org/catalog/product_info.php?products_id= 37774 (accessed October 6, 2020).

Álvarez-Melcón AC, Valero-Alcaide R, Atín-Arratibel MA, Melcón-Álvarez A, Beneit-Montesinos JV. Effects of physical therapy and relaxation techniques on the parameters of pain in university students with tension-type headache: a randomised controlled clinical trial. Efectos de entrenamiento físico específico y técnicas de relajación sobre los parámetros dolorosos de la cefalea tensional en estudiantes universitarios: un ensayo clínico controlado y aleatorizado. *Neurologia.* (2018) 33:233–43. doi: 10.1016/j.nrl.2016. 06.008

Nestoriuc Y, Martin A. Efficacy of biofeedback for migraine: a meta-analysis. *Pain.* (2007) 128:111–27. doi: 10.1016/j.pain.2006. 09.007

Kang EH, Park JE, Chung CS, Yu BH. Effect of biofeedback-assisted autogenic training on headache activity and mood states in Korean female migraine patients. *J Korean Med Sci.* (2009) 24:936–40. doi: 10.3346/jkms.2009.24.5.936

Hermann C, Kim M, Blanchard EB. Behavioral and prophylactic pharmacological intervention studies of pediatric migraine: an exploratory meta-analysis. *Pain.* (1995) 60:239–55. doi: 10.1016/0304-3959(94) 00210-6

Couturier EG, Laman DM, van Duijn MA, van Duijn H. Influence of caffeine and caffeine withdrawal on headache and cerebral blood flow velocities. *Cephalalgia.* (1997) 17:188–90. doi: 10.1046/j.1468-2982.1997.1703188.x

21

Emotion Regulation in Everyday Life: The Role of Goals and Situational Factors

Rafael Wilms[1], Ralf Lanwehr[2] and Andreas Kastenmüller[1]*

[1] Department of Education Studies and Psychology, University of Siegen, Siegen, Germany, [2] Department of International Management, South Westphalia University of Applied Sciences, Meschede, Germany

***Correspondence:**
Rafael Wilms
rafael.wilms@uni-siegen.de

This study addresses three questions: How often and how consistently do predictors for emotion regulation choice occur in daily life? What predicts emotion regulation choice in daily life? How do predictors for emotion regulation choice interact in daily life? We examined emotion regulation goals (i.e., prohedonic and social goals), situational factors (i.e., perceived control, expected reoccurrence, and emotional intensity), and emotion regulation strategies (i.e., active coping, distraction, rumination, cognitive reappraisal, and expressive suppression) in negative emotion events. A total of 110 individuals (65% female) participated in an experience sampling study and received beeps, five times a day over the course of 9 days. We used a random intercept model to estimate our results. Emotion regulation goals and situational factors vary strongly in different events within the same person. Emotion regulation strategies, effective in changing the emotional experience, are crucial for prohedonic goals, whereas expressive suppression is important for social goals. Perceived control was positively associated with putatively adaptive strategies. Emotional intensity and expected reoccurrence were negatively associated with putatively adaptive strategies. Emotional intensity was positively associated with putatively maladaptive strategies. Emotion regulation strategies were not associated with the interaction of emotion regulation goals and situational factors. We conclude that emotion regulation goals and situational factors are extremely context-dependent, suggesting that they should be treated as states. Emotion regulation goals appear to have a functional association with strategies for prohedonic and social goals. The associations between situational factors and strategies in daily life appear to be largely different from the results found in the laboratory, emphasizing the importance of experience sampling studies.

Keywords: situational factors, emotion regulation, emotion regulation goals, experience sampling study, negative emotions

INTRODUCTION

The way we regulate our emotions has important implications for our well-being (Webb et al., 2012) and our social relationships (Cameron and Overall, 2017). Adaptive emotion regulation requires a flexible alternation between strategies in accordance with personal goals and contextual demands (Bonanno and Burton, 2013; Aldao et al., 2015). Emotion regulation goals (e.g., the goal of feeling better) and situational factors (e.g., emotional intensity) influence the choice for or against particular emotion regulation strategies (Sheppes et al., 2011; Haines et al., 2016; Millgram et al., 2019). These phenomena were primarily investigated in the lab (e.g., Millgram et al., 2019). Even though first studies examined them in daily life (e.g., Haines et al., 2016; English et al., 2017), we are far from having a complete picture of emotion regulation in daily life. We want to contribute to this picture by shedding light on three questions: How often and how consistently do predictors for emotion regulation choice occur in daily life? What predicts emotion regulation choice in daily life? How do predictors for emotion regulation choice interact in daily life?

To address these questions, we conducted an experience sampling study (Beal, 2015) and examined emotion regulation goals, situational factors, and emotion regulation strategies five times a day at negative emotion events. In detail, we included a prohedonic goal, four social goals (i.e., *to avoid conflict, to keep up appearances, to make others feel better*, and *to influence others*), and three situational factors (perceived control over the situation, emotional intensity, and expected reoccurrence of a similar situation) as predictors. As criterions, we used emotion regulation strategies from the entire emotion generative process (Gross, 1998): situation selection/modification (i.e., active coping), attentional deployment (i.e., distraction and rumination), cognitive change (i.e., cognitive reappraisal), and response-modulation (i.e., expressive suppression).

To the authors' knowledge, this is the first study that examines emotion regulation goals and situational factors in combination at negative emotion events. We focus on negative events, as individuals regulate negative emotions more often than positive ones (Brans et al., 2013; English et al., 2017), predictors of emotion regulation have only rarely been studied in daily life in general, and the regulation of negative emotions offers a more solid foundation for theoretical reasoning. Moreover, the current study has a higher resolution of daily life and also collects events with lower emotional intensity. Prior studies (e.g., English et al., 2017; Kalokerinos et al., 2017a) examined the most negative event of the day, whereas we focus on the most negative event of the last 3 h. Thus, this study captures a more realistic picture of emotion regulation in daily life.

Emotion Regulation Goals

Individuals often regulate their emotions to pursue their goals (Tamir et al., 2015; Millgram et al., 2019). Goals are a cognitive representation of an end state (Fishbach and Ferguson, 2007). They typically come up when an individual becomes aware of the discrepancy between a current state and a desired end state (Carver and Schreier, 2000). The detected discrepancy usually motivates people to reduce this gap. The current study investigates two different classes of emotion regulation goals: prohedonic goals and social instrumental goals (Tamir, 2016). These are important to examine because they often occur in everyday life (English et al., 2017; Eldesouky and English, 2018). Prohedonic goals aim at changing the *current* pleasure-to-pain ratio in favor of pleasure, and thus aim to change the feeling component (e.g., experienced pleasure or pain) of an emotion. By contrast, instrumental goals encompass superordinate goals that are potentially, but not necessarily achieved by regulating emotions (Tamir, 2016). One particular class of instrumental goals are social goals, which reflect the pursuit of creating and maintaining positive social relationships (Gable and Berkman, 2008; Netzer et al., 2015; Tamir, 2016). For instance, it may be beneficial to signal empathy for a friend whose girlfriend has left him.

Situational Factors

Situations, in which individuals regulate their emotions, may differ dramatically from each other (Bonanno and Burton, 2013; Aldao et al., 2015; Doré et al., 2016). For example, individuals may regulate their emotions in situations of weak or strong emotional intensity. We refer to specific situational differences as situational factors. Previous studies showed that situational factors affect emotion regulation choice. For example, most individuals prefer cognitive reappraisal (distraction) over distraction (cognitive reappraisal) in situations of low (high) emotional intensity (Sheppes et al., 2011). Since situational factors often determine how individuals regulate their emotions, they are crucial for understanding emotion regulation in daily life.

How Often and How Consistently Do Predictors for Emotion Regulation Choice Occur in Daily Life?

In order to understand emotion regulation in daily life, it is important to understand not only what predicts emotion regulation choices, but also how often and consistently these predictors occur. A strong predictor that occurs very seldom may be less important than a weaker predictor that occurs frequently. Likewise, a predictor that occurs consistently for some people, but not for others may reveal group differences in emotion regulation choice.

Prior daily diary studies examined the fluctuation of emotion regulation goals. They demonstrated that prohedonic goals are the primary reason for emotion regulation, but that social goals also play an important role (English et al., 2017; Kalokerinos et al., 2017c; Eldesouky and English, 2018). These studies examined emotion regulation goals only once a day and targeted the strongest negative event of that day (e.g., English et al., 2017; Kalokerinos et al., 2017b). Consequently, we only have a preliminary understanding of how often and consistently emotion regulation goals occur.

What Predicts Emotion Regulation Choice in Daily Life?

The emotion regulation flexibility framework (Bonanno and Burton, 2013; Aldao et al., 2015) challenges that certain strategies are uniformly more adaptive or efficacious than others and argues instead that a strategy's effectiveness depends on the context. Consistently, individuals show considerable variability in strategy use in everyday life (Blanke et al., 2019). In the following, we develop hypotheses about contexts (i.e., emotion regulation goals and situational factors) that affect the choice for or against a particular emotion regulation strategy.

Hedonic Goals and Emotion Regulation

Individuals expect strategies, effective in changing the emotional experience (Webb et al., 2012), to be more potent for achieving prohedonic goals (Sheppes et al., 2014; Millgram et al., 2019). For example, distraction, instead of rumination, is primarily used when individuals are asked to reduce their negative emotional experience (Millgram et al., 2019).

Based on that, we propose that prohedonic goals are positively associated with active coping, distraction, and cognitive reappraisal, as those are effective in changing the current emotional experience (Webb et al., 2012, 2018). By contrast, prohedonic goals are negatively associated with rumination, since it is effective in increasing or maintaining the negative emotional experience (Webb et al., 2012; Millgram et al., 2019). However, people often believe that this strategy will help them to feel better (Nolen-Hoeksema et al., 2008). So, mixed evidence exists for the relationship between prohedonic goals and rumination. Finally, expressive suppression should not be associated with prohedonic goals (English et al., 2017) because it is not effective in changing the emotional experience (Webb et al., 2012).

> H1: Prohedonic goals are positively associated with active coping.
> H2: Prohedonic goals are positively associated with distraction.
> H3: Prohedonic goals are positively associated with cognitive reappraisal.

Social Goals and Emotion Regulation

We focus on four social goals: *to avoid conflict*, *to keep up appearances*, *to make others feel better*, and *to influence others*.

To keep up appearances requires hiding an emotion from at least one other person. Accordingly, we assume that the goal is positively associated with expressive suppression, as it decreases the degree of facial expression of an emotion (Webb et al., 2012), and positively associated with distraction, as it decreases the emotional experience (Webb et al., 2012), which in turn (potentially) decreases its expression (Gross et al., 2000).

> H4: *To keep up appearances* is positively associated with expressive suppression.
> H5: *To keep up appearances* is positively associated with distraction.

To avoid conflict with others requires a down-regulation of an emotion experience or its expression. For example, experiencing or expressing anger may increase the likelihood of conflict (e.g., Kassinove et al., 2002). As distraction and expressive suppression effectively decrease the experience and the expression of emotions, respectively (Webb et al., 2012), we assume that *to avoid conflict with others* is positively associated with these strategies.

> H6: *To avoid conflict with others* is positively associated with expression suppression.
> H7: *To avoid conflict with others* is positively associated with distraction.

To make others feel better primarily targets emotions of others, and we included only expressive suppression as an interpersonal emotion regulation strategy. However, expressive suppression was not associated with *to make others feel better* in another study (English et al., 2017); we therefore do not expect the goal *to make others feel better* to predict any included strategy.

To influence others requires the passing of information to others, as the transmitter can only influence others if information is passed to the receiver. Expressive suppression reduces the emotional information passed (Greenaway and Kalokerinos, 2017; Kalokerinos et al., 2017a), as it diminishes the emotional expression of the transmitter (Webb et al., 2012). Accordingly, we assume that *to influence others* is negatively associated with expressive suppression.

> H8: *To influence others* is negatively associated with expressive suppression.

Situational Factors and Emotion Regulation

We focus on three characteristics of situations: Individuals may perceive different levels of control over the situation (referred to as perceived control; Haines et al., 2016), experience different degrees of emotional intensities (referred to as emotional intensity; Dixon-Gordon et al., 2015), or perceive different likelihoods of the event repeating itself (referred to as expected reoccurrence; Sheppes et al., 2014). Those situational factors influence emotion regulation choice.

Perceived control may increase the likelihood of using active coping, as trying to change a situation requires at least some control over the situation. By contrast, it may decrease the likelihood of using cognitive reappraisal (Troy et al., 2013; Haines et al., 2016), as reappraising may be more useful, when a situation cannot be changed. For example, if a woman is in a toxic relationship, it may be more detrimental to reappraise the behavior of her boyfriend, compared to actively taking actions (e.g., leaving him). Accordingly, we assume that perceived control is positively associated with active coping and negatively associated with cognitive reappraisal.

> H9: Perceived control is positively associated with active coping.
> H10: Perceived control is negatively associated with cognitive reappraisal.

Emotional intensity influences whether individuals choose to engage in distraction or cognitive reappraisal (Sheppes et al., 2014). In situations with low (high) emotional intensity, most individuals prefer to choose cognitive reappraisal (distraction) over distraction (cognitive reappraisal) (Sheppes et al., 2014; Milyavsky et al., 2019). Further, emotional intensity is positively associated with the use of rumination and active coping (Dixon-Gordon et al., 2015; Van Bockstaele et al., 2019). Accordingly, we expect emotional intensity to be positively associated with active coping, distraction, and rumination, but negatively associated with cognitive reappraisal.

H11: Emotional intensity is positively associated with active coping.
H12: Emotional intensity is positively associated with distraction.
H13: Emotional intensity is positively associated with rumination.
H14: Emotional intensity is negatively associated with cognitive reappraisal.

Expected reoccurrence influences whether individuals choose distraction or cognitive reappraisal. In situations with low (high) expected reoccurrence, individuals choose distraction (cognitive reappraisal) over cognitive reappraisal (distraction). Cognitive reappraisal changes the emotional experience of a stimulus in the long-term, whereas distraction only changes it in the short-term (Sheppes et al., 2014). Similarly, active coping changes (potentially) the long-term emotional reaction to a stimulus by altering it (Gross, 1998; Van Bockstaele et al., 2019). If a person expects to be confronted with the same stimuli again, cognitive reappraisal and active coping are more beneficial than distraction, as they reduce the negative impact of the stimulus. Accordingly, we assume expected reoccurrence to be positively associated with active coping and cognitive reappraisal, but negatively associated with distraction.

H15: Expected reoccurrence is positively associated with active coping.
H16: Expected reoccurrence is positively associated with cognitive reappraisal.
H17: Expected reoccurrence is negatively associated with distraction.

How Do These Predictors Interact in Daily Life?

We propose that the interaction of emotion regulation goals and situational factors predicts the preference for emotion regulation strategies. Our predictions focus on prohedonic goals, as they provide a more solid foundation for our theoretical reasoning (e.g., Sheppes et al., 2014; Millgram et al., 2019; Tamir et al., 2019).

The effect of prohedonic goals on distraction and cognitive reappraisal (Sheppes et al., 2014) is moderated by emotional intensity. That is, we expect that the effect of prohedonic goals on distraction and cognitive reappraisal to be stronger (weaker) with a high (low) emotional intensity.

H18: The positive relationship between prohedonic goals and distraction is moderated by emotional intensity, so that the effect is stronger with a higher emotional intensity and weaker with a lower emotional intensity.
H19: The positive relationship between prohedonic goals and cognitive reappraisal is moderated by emotional intensity, so that the effect is stronger with a higher emotional intensity and weaker with a lower emotional intensity.

The effect of prohedonic goals on active coping, cognitive reappraisal, and distraction is moderated by expected reoccurrence. As cognitive reappraisal and active coping change the reaction to a negative stimulus in the long term, we assume that individuals prefer them, when they want to feel better and the expected reoccurrence is high instead of low. As distraction changes the reaction to a negative stimulus in the short term, we assume that individuals avoid it, when they want to feel better and the expected reoccurrence is low instead of high.

H20: The positive relationship between prohedonic goals and active coping is moderated by expected reoccurrence, so that the effect is stronger with a higher expected reoccurrence and weaker with a lower expected reoccurrence.
H21: The positive relationship between prohedonic goals and distraction is moderated by expected reoccurrence, so that the effect is weaker with a higher expected reoccurrence and stronger with a lower expected reoccurrence.
H22: The positive relationship between prohedonic goals and cognitive reappraisal is moderated by expected reoccurrence, so that the effect is stronger with a higher expected reoccurrence and weaker with a lower expected reoccurrence.

MATERIALS AND METHODS

Participants and Procedure

The participants were 143 students in business-related study programs from three universities in Germany (65% female and 35% male; age M = 21.81 and SD = 2.52) and were recruited by advertising the study at the start of different courses.

The experience sampling study had two parts: The introduction session and the experience sampling phase. First, participants signed the informed consent form and completed different questionnaires unrelated to this study. Second, the authors explained the procedure of the experience sampling study to the participants and outlined how to install the app, RealLifeExp Version 2.5.2, on the participants' own smartphones. Third, the participants were trained on the experience sampling study's protocol.

The participants received beeps at 10 a.m., 1, 4, 7, and 10 p.m. over a period of 9 consecutive days. The participants had to answer the beep within 1.5 h; otherwise, the beep was counted as not-responded. Aiming to reduce the burden of participants (Bolger et al., 2003), we chose these time periods based on information by students from the same universities. Those did not participate in this study. The median response time was 06:22 s (M = 14:58 s; SD = 19:58 s). To incentivize participants, they received a €10 Amazon voucher if they responded to at least 26 beeps.

We excluded participants who did not respond to at least 20 beeps to ensure that participants had sufficient motivation for the experience sampling study (Podsakoff et al., 2012). On average, participants completed 37.92 beeps. One hundred ten participants remained.

Measures

At each beep, items were asked in the following order. First, participants were thanked for their participation, asked about their mood, what they have done since the last beep (or at the first beep, since they have been awake), and if they experienced a negative emotion within the last 3 h. Only if they responded with *yes* to the last question were they instructed to report on the event that elicited the most intense negative emotions, asked which emotion they experienced (unrelated to this study), and answered questions about situational factors, emotion regulation strategies, emotion regulation goals, and emotion regulation direction (unrelated to this study). In 718 of 4171 situations (17.21%), participants reported they experienced at least one negative emotion during the last 3 h.

Situational Factors

Participants were asked to indicate three situational factors. We measured the emotional intensity of the focal event ("How intense was your most negative emotion?"), their perceived control ("To what extent was the event in which you felt the negative emotion(s) under your control?"), and the expected reoccurrence ("How likely is it that this situation will repeat itself or that a very similar one will occur?"). Each of these questions appeared on a separate page. All situational factors were measured on a scale from not at all (1) to very (7).

Emotion Regulation Strategies

Participants were asked to recall the situation that elicited the negative emotion(s) and indicate how intensively they used the following five emotion regulation strategies (e.g., Kalokerinos et al., 2017b): active coping ("I have taken active steps to improve the situation"; Knoll et al., 2005), distraction ("I distracted myself from the situation or my feelings"), rumination ("I dwelled on the situation or my feelings"), cognitive reappraisal ("I tried to change my perspective on the situation or to change how I think about it"), and expressive suppression ("I suppressed my outward expression of my emotions"). All emotion regulation strategies were presented in one block and measured on a scale from not at all (1) to very (7).

Emotion Regulation Goals

Participants were asked to recall the situation that elicited the negative emotion(s) again and indicate the emotion regulation goals, they pursued in this situation. The questions were introduced with "*I tried to influence my emotions ...*," and were largely oriented on the study by English et al. (2017): a prohedonic goal ("to make me feel better"), four social goals ("to avoid conflict," "to keep up appearances," "to make others feel better," and "to influence others") and one performance goal ("to get work done or to learn"; used as a control variable). Further, participants could choose to indicate "other" and "I did not want to influence my emotions." All emotion regulation goals were presented in one block and were dichotomous (0 = not chosen; 1 = chosen) to reduce the participants' burden (Bolger et al., 2003). Participants were free to choose how many goals they endorsed.

DATA ANALYSIS AND RESULTS

We structure the data analysis and the results in three questions: How often and how consistently do predictors for emotion regulation choice occur in daily life? What predicts emotion regulation choice in daily life? How do predictors for emotion regulation choice interact in daily life? All analysis were performed with R Cran (R Core Team, 2015). The data is available in the **Supplementary Material**.

How Often and How Consistently Do Predictors for Emotion Regulation Choice Occur in Daily Life?

Data Analysis

We calculated percentages based on regular averages and on averages of the person-means. The average of the person-means[1] weighs the response of each person equally and is more robust against different numbers of events per person.

We calculated the ICCs based on a three-level model (events within days within persons) and as the ratio of between-variance to total variance (i.e., the sum of between-variance, day-variance, and event-variance; Baguley, 2012). They can be interpreted as follows: A low ICC indicates that the variance observed in a variable is determined by the event and the day; the pattern of the variable varies a lot within individuals. A high ICC indicates that the variance is determined by the individual; in other words, the pattern of the variable is very similar among different events and days within one individual, but very different among individuals.

Results

Table 1 shows the number of events with the goals endorsed, the percentages of events with this goal, based on regular averages and based on averages of the person-means, and the ICCs for emotion regulation goals. The goals *to feel better*, *to keep up appearances*, and *to avoid conflict* were most frequent, whereas *to make others feel better* and *to influence others* were

[1] The group-mean first creates the mean for each person (person-mean) separately and afterward calculates the mean of the person-means.

TABLE 1 | Descriptive statistics on emotion regulation goals.

Goals	*n* events with this goal	% events with this goal	% events with this goal based on person-means	ICC
To feel better	266	0.37	0.34	0.21
To avoid conflict with others	175	0.24	0.24	0.11
To keep up appearances	213	0.30	0.24	0.14
To make others feel better	65	0.09	0.08	0.09
To influence others	17	0.02	0.02	0.02

The abbreviations n and ICC refer to the sample size and intraclass coefficient, respectively.

TABLE 2 | Descriptive statistics on situational factors.

Situational factors	*M*	*SD*	*M* of person-means	*SD* of group mean	ICC
Perceived control	3.54	2.00	3.55	1.42	0.28
Emotional intensity	4.48	1.54	4.42	1.01	0.17
Expected reoccurrence	5.25	1.65	5.04	1.16	0.22

The abbreviations M, SD, and ICC refer to mean, standard deviation, and intraclass coefficient, respectively.

the least frequent. The patterns of the regular averages and the averages of the person-means seem to be very similar, showing consistency between individuals with higher vs. lower response rates.

The ICCs show that emotion regulation goals vary strongly from situation to situation within one person. The most stable goal is *to feel better* with 21% between-person variance. The goals *to keep up appearances* and *to avoid conflict* have a similar level of between-person variance. The goals *to make others feel better* and *to influence others* vary more dramatically from situation to situation.

Table 2 shows the means, standard deviations, and ICCs for situational factors. In descending order, expected reoccurrence, emotional intensity, and perceived control show the highest level of intensity. The patterns of the regular averages and averages of the person-means seem to be very similar, showing consistency between individuals with higher vs. lower response rates.

The ICCs show that situation factors vary substantially more among the events and days than among individuals. Perceived control varies the least and emotional intensity the most among events and days.

What Predicts Emotion Regulation Choice in Daily Life?

Data Analysis

Accounting for the nested structure of our experience sampling data, we conducted multilevel analyses using *lme4* (Bates et al., 2015). We are primarily interested in the within-person effects, and therefore included the person-means (between-person effects) of each independent variable. Those person-means absorb all interindividual differences that may affect within-person effects (Mundlak, 1978).

The within-person effect can be interpreted as a situation specific effect. For example, if a person wants to feel better, the goal may affect choosing cognitive reappraisal in the focal situation but does not provide information about the relationship between habitual prohedonic goals and the habitual use of cognitive reappraisal.

To estimate our results, we included the emotion regulation goals *to feel better, to avoid conflict, to keep up appearances, to make others feel better, to influence others,* and *to get work done or learn* as well as the situational factors *expected reoccurrence, emotional intensity,* and *perceived control* simultaneously as predictors. We used active coping, distraction, rumination, cognitive reappraisal, and expressive suppression as criterions in separate models.

Following the recommendation by Luke (2017) we estimated our linear mixed effects model with the robust maximum likelihood estimator and estimated the degrees of freedom with the Kenward-Roger approximation (Kenward and Roger, 1997) using the package *pbkrtest* (Halekoh and Højsgaard, 2014). We modeled three-level random intercept models (events within days within persons), unless indicated otherwise and used standardized variables to obtain standardized effects.

In case a model suffers from heteroskedasticity, we fitted it again with the package *robustlmm* (Koller, 2016). The package allows a more robust estimation of standard errors than the normal *lme4* package. The function *rlmer* reduces the influence of outliers that may cause heteroskedasticity. Since there is no package available that provides degrees of freedom for this robust estimation, we followed the t-as-z approach. To make our heuristic approach less susceptible to alpha errors, we decided to increase the critical *p*-value to 0.01 (*t*-value of |2.236|) (for a similar approach, see Kornilov et al., 2019).

Finally, we computed the explained within-variance based on the R_1^2 *(approx.)*, developed by Bryk and Raudenbush (1992), which showed a good estimation performance in previous simulation studies (LaHuis et al., 2014).

Results

Table 3 shows the results of what predicts emotion regulation strategies, whereas **Table 4** provides an overview of the supported or unsupported hypotheses. Active coping was positively associated with *to feel better* [H1; $\beta = 0.09$; $F(1, 615.37) = 5.01$; $p = 0.03$] and perceived control [H9; $\beta = 0.09$; $F(1, 615.52) = 4.20$; $p = 0.04$]. Contrary to our hypotheses, active coping was negatively associated with emotional intensity [H11; $\beta = -0.14$; $F(1, 611.61) = 12.69$; $p < 0.00$] and expected reoccurrence [H15; $\beta = -0.09$; $F(1, 611.59) = 4.81$; $p = 0.03$]. The predictors jointly explained the within-variance of active coping [R_1^2 *(approx.)* = 0.07].

Testing the hypotheses for distraction, the day component of the model yields zero variance. Accordingly, we fitted a two-level model (events within persons) for distraction. Distraction was positively associated with *to feel better* [H2; $\beta = 0.19$; $F(1, 611.75) = 24.11$; $p < 0.00$], *to keep up appearances* [H5; $\beta = 0.11$; $F(1, 611.75) = 8.14$; $p < 0.00$], and *to avoid conflict* [H7; $\beta = 0.12$; $F(1, 611.75) = 10.28$; $p < 0.00$]. Contrary to our hypotheses, distraction was not associated with emotional intensity [H12; $\beta = -0.07$; $F(1, 611.75) = 3.58$; $p = 0.06$] and expected reoccurrence [H17; $\beta = -0.04$; $F(1, 611.75) = 1.23$; $p = 0.27$]. Since this model suffered from heteroskedasticity, we also fitted a model with the package *robustlmm* (Koller, 2016). The results of the robust model remained essentially unchanged, except that the non-robust model showed an unexpected and significant positive relationship for *to influence others*, but the robust model did not. The predictors jointly explained the within-variance of distraction [R_1^2 *(approx.)* = 0.08].

Rumination was positively associated with emotional intensity [H13; $\beta = 0.30$; $F(1, 582.35) = 80.42$; $p < 0.00$] and *to feel better* [$\beta = 0.10$; $F(1, 603.15) = 7.80$; $p < 0.01$]. The

TABLE 3 | Emotion regulation goals and situational factors as joint predictors for emotion regulation strategies in random intercept models.

	Active coping	Distraction	Rumination	Cognitive reappraisal	Expressive suppression
Intercept	−0.01	−0.03	−0.01	0.01	−0.06
Emotion Regulation Goals					
To feel better	0.09*	0.19***	0.10**	0.12***	0.04
To avoid conflict	0.05	0.12**	0.03	0.07	0.21***
To keep up appearances	−0.08	0.11**	0.07	0.04	0.40***
To make someone else feel better	0.03	0.10**	0.03	0.09*	0.03
To influence others	0.08*	−0.07*	0.01	0.02	−0.05
Situational Factors					
Perceived control	0.09*	0.03	0.00	0.13**	0.06
Emotional intensity	−0.14***	−0.07	0.30***	−0.11**	−0.08*
Expected reoccurrence	−0.09*	−0.04	0.01	−0.12**	−0.02
Interaction Effects					
To work or learn	0.03	0.02	−0.01	0.04	0.02
To feel better * emotional intensity		0.00		−0.01	
To feel better * expected reoccurrence	0.00	0.02		−0.05	

**p < 0.05. **p < 0.01. ***p < 0.001. Effects reported as standardized regression estimates based on the random intercept model. Significance is estimated by using Kenward–Rogers approximation (Kenward and Roger, 1997), and given the presence of heteroskedasticity, it is based on robust estimation (Koller, 2016). The model included person-means of the focal variables, but for simplicity, we omitted them in the table.*

TABLE 4 | Overview of the supported or unsupported hypotheses.

	Active coping	Distraction	Rumination	Cognitive reappraisal	Expressive suppression
To feel better	✓ (+/+)	✓ (+/+)	(?/+)	✓ (+/+)	–
To avoid conflict	–	✓ (+/+)	–	–	✓ (+/+)
To keep up appearances	–	✓ (+/+)	–	–	✓ (+/+)
To influence others	–	–	–	–	× (–/0)
Perceived control	✓ (+/+)	–	–	× (–/+)	–
Emotional intensity	× (+/–)	× (+/–)	✓ (+/–)	✓ (–/–)	–
Expected reoccurrence	× (+/–)	× (+/–)	–	× (+/–)	–
To feel better * emotional intensity	–	×	–	×	–
To feel better * expected reoccurrence	×	×	–	×	–

The expected/observed direction of the main effects are provided in parentheses. Dashes indicate no hypothesis.

predictors jointly explained the within-variance of distraction [R_1^2 *(approx.)* = 0.13].

Cognitive reappraisal was positively associated with *to feel better* [H3; β = 0.12; $F(1, 610.47) = 9.08$; $p < 0.00$] and emotional intensity [H14; β = −0.11; $F(1, 609.06) = 7.45$; $p = 0.01$]. Contrary to our hypotheses, cognitive reappraisal was positively associated with perceived control [H10; β = 0.13; $F(1, 610.44) = 8.92$; $p < 0.00$] and negatively associated with expected reoccurrence [H16; β = −0.12; $F(1, 604.38) = 9.05$; $p < 0.00$]. Since this model suffered from heteroskedasticity, we estimated a robust model (Koller, 2016). The results remained essentially unchanged. The predictors jointly explained the within-variance of cognitive reappraisal [R_1^2 *(approx.)* = 0.06].

Expressive suppression was positively associated with *to keep up appearances* [H4; β = 0.40; $F(1, 617.81) = 128.08$; $p < 0.00$] and *to avoid conflict* [H6; β = 0.21; $F(1, 618.04) = 35.56$; $p < 0.00$]. Contrary to our hypotheses, it was not negatively associated with *to influence others* [β = −0.05; $F(1, 616.97) = 2.50$; $p = 0.11$]. The predictors jointly explained the within-variance of expressive suppression [R_1^2 *(approx.)* = 0.22].

Testing the assumptions of linear mixed effects model, we checked the normality assumption of residuals visually, heteroskedasticity, and tested for multicollinearity (see **Table A1** for the within-correlations of the predictors). Those assumptions did not seem to be violated.

How Do Predictors for Emotion Regulation Choice Interact in Daily Life?

Results

Table 3 shows the results of the interaction of emotion regulation goals and situational factors. The interaction between emotional intensity and *to feel better* was not positively associated with distraction [H18; β = 0.00; $F(1, 662.67) = 0.01$; $p = 0.93$]. The interaction between emotional intensity and *to feel better* was not negatively associated with cognitive reappraisal [H19; β = −0.01; $F(1, 653.13) = 0.09$; $p = 0.76$].

The interaction between expected reoccurrence and *to feel better* was not positively associated with active coping [H20; β = 0.00; $F(1, 673.33) = 0.00$; $p = 0.97$]. The interaction between expected reoccurrence and *to feel better* was not positively associated with distraction [H21; β = 0.02; $F(1, 659.84) = 0.44$; $p = 0.51$]. The interaction between expected reoccurrence and *to feel better* was not positively associated with cognitive reappraisal [H22; β = −0.05; $F(1, 667.72) = 3.37$; $p = 0.07$].

DISCUSSION

As the choice of emotion regulation strategies has a profound impact on our well-being (Webb et al., 2012) and our social lives (Cameron and Overall, 2017), it is crucial to understand its antecedents. This study addressed three questions: How often and how consistently do predictors for emotion regulation choice occur in daily life? What predicts emotion regulation choice in daily life? How do predictors for emotion regulation choice interact in daily life? Moreover, it complements earlier research, as it examines emotion regulation goals and situational factors in combination and captures a broader range of emotional intensities, compared to other studies (English et al., 2017; Kalokerinos et al., 2017c).

How Often and How Consistently Do Predictors for Emotion Regulation Choice Occur in Daily Life?

Emotion Regulation Goals

We found that emotion regulation goals differ dramatically in their frequencies. The most prevalent goal is *to feel better* (in about every 2.5 events). Further, to keep up appearances and to avoid conflict (in about every third or fourth events) occur slightly less often than to feel better. To make others feel better and to influence others occur the least often (in about every tenth to fiftieth event). Participants reported to make others feel better and to influence others infrequently. One potential explanation is that to make others feel better may be more important in older samples with caring responsibilities (e.g. young children or care of elderly relatives). Similarly, to influence others may be more important in a professional or occupational context. Alternatively, participants could have been reluctant to acknowledge that they want to influence others, since it may be interpreted as socially undesirable. This may explain why we observe these emotion regulation goals relatively infrequently.

In comparison to prior daily diary studies (English et al., 2017; Kalokerinos et al., 2017c), we found lower frequencies in emotion regulation goals. Kalokerinos et al. (2017c) found social motives about once in 10 events, but they used a very broad item. English et al. (2017) used more specific items and found prohedonic goals about every second event, *to avoid conflict* about every third, *to keep up appearances* about every two and a half events, and *to make others feel better* in about every fifth event. However, these studies asked participants only once a day about one emotional situation. We attribute these differences found in our study to its higher resolution. It makes sense that we found lower frequencies, as the likelihood of having a negative emotion event over the course of a day is higher than over the course of 3 h.

Further, we found substantial differences in the ICCs of emotion regulation goals with 0.21, 0.11, 0.14, 0.09, and 0.02 for *to feel better, to avoid conflict with others, to keep up appearances, to make others feel better*, and *to influence others*, respectively. Participants reported *to make others feel better* and *to influence others* infrequently.

In comparison to previous studies (English et al., 2017; Kalokerinos et al., 2017b; Eldesouky and English, 2018), we found lower ICCs in emotion regulation goals. Eldesouky and English (2018) found ICCs between 0.57 and 0.87. English et al. (2017) reported ICCs between 0.18 and 0.38. Kalokerinos et al. (2017a) found ICCs between 0.15 and 0.29. The difference to our study may be attributable to the higher resolution – the more surveys a day, the higher the within-variance (i.e., the lower the ICC) (Podsakoff et al., 2019). Moreover, lower ICCs may also reflect that the current study captures a larger variety of different situations. Prior studies asked about the most negative event of the day, whereas we asked for the most negative event of the last 3 h. Thus, the chance of capturing a situation with lower emotional intensity is higher in our study, and participants may be less motivated to develop an emotion regulation goal for less emotionally intense events (Milyavsky et al., 2019). Emotion regulation goals may vary more strongly among different events for this reason.

A recent meta-analysis examined the ICCs of a wide range of psychological constructs and found an average ICC of about 0.52 (Podsakoff et al., 2019). Accordingly, emotion regulation goals varied considerably more among different situations in our sample, compared to other constructs.

Situational Factors

We found that situational factors differ in their average degree of expression. In descending order, expected reoccurrence, emotional intensity, and perceived control show the strongest average degree of expression in negative emotion events. Compared to another study (Haines et al., 2016), we observed a slightly lower level of perceived controllability in negative emotion events. We are not aware of any study that examined emotional intensity or expected reoccurrence in the context of emotion regulation in an experience sampling study.

Further, we found substantial differences in the ICCs. In descending order, we found 0.28, 0.22, and 0.17 for perceived control, expected reoccurrence, and emotional intensity, respectively. Haines et al. (2016) reported an ICC of 0.35 for perceived control, which is slightly above the value found in this study, but they conducted a two-level model (events nested in persons) for their estimation. Our value may be lower because we used a three-level model instead.

Comparing the situational factors' ICCs to the average ICC among psychological constructs (see above; Podsakoff et al., 2019), situational factors varied considerably more among different situations in our sample, compared to other constructs.

Conclusion: How Often and How Consistently Do Predictors for Emotion Regulation Choice Occur in Daily Life?

All in all, we conclude that certain emotion regulation goals and situational factors are more prevalent than others in negative emotion events. Further, our results suggest that emotion regulation goals and situational factors should be treated as states, but not as dispositional personality traits, as they vary strongly among different events. Overall, our results are consistent with the emotion regulation flexibility framework: Individuals regulate their emotions in vastly different contexts (Aldao, 2013; Bonanno and Burton, 2013; Aldao et al., 2015).

What Predicts Emotion Regulation Choice in Daily Life?

Emotion Regulation Goals

Emotion regulation goals were associated with different emotion regulation strategies. Prohedonic goals were positively associated with the use of active coping, cognitive reappraisal, and distraction, but not with expressive suppression. Our results are broadly consistent with the notion that individuals use emotion regulation strategies that are functional for their goals (Tamir et al., 2015; Eldesouky and English, 2018; Milyavsky et al., 2019). The inclusion of active coping is particularly notable, as it is an understudied strategy.

We found small effect sizes for active coping and cognitive reappraisal, and a medium effect size for distraction. Our results suggest that participants relied more strongly on strategies, which have less cognitive costs. This is in line with the cognitive energetics theory (Kruglanski et al., 2012), which posits that individuals prefer to use emotion regulation strategies that consume less cognitive energy to achieve their goals (Milyavsky et al., 2019).

However, prohedonic goals were positively associated with rumination. This appears to be inconsistent with the notion of a functional association between emotion regulation goals and emotion regulation strategies, but individuals often use rumination to better understand a critical situation, to gain insight, and to solve problems (Nolen-Hoeksema et al., 2008). We could conclude that participants often falsely believe that it will help them to feel better. Alternatively, some kinds of repetitive thoughts are actually constructive (for a review, see Watkins, 2008), for example, when they are more concrete instead of abstract. Since we did not distinguish between concrete and abstract forms of rumination, our item may have captured both. The association between prohedonic goals with a concrete form of rumination may be interpreted as functional, whereas the association with an abstract form of rumination may be interpreted as dysfunctional. However, other studies used a similarly broad item and found that rumination was associated with longer periods of higher negative emotional intensity (Kalokerinos et al., 2017b; Résibois et al., 2018), and with a more explosive trajectory of negative emotional intensity (Résibois et al., 2018). We are therefore inclined to interpret our results as a dysfunctional link between prohedonic goals and rumination, although more evidence is required for a final conclusion.

To keep up appearances and *to avoid conflict* were positively associated with expressive suppression and distraction. Our results suggest a functional association between social goals and emotion regulation strategies, which is largely consistent with other studies (e.g., English et al., 2017; Eldesouky and English, 2018). Participants used strategies that change the immediate expression or experience of an emotion for social goals more often. Since the interaction with another person probably occupies some cognitive resources, participants may have preferred low-cost distraction over high-cost active coping and cognitive reappraisal (Sheppes et al., 2014). For example, when an individual wants to hide an emotion, while talking to a friend, the conversation consumes some of the cognitive resources. Additionally, she could engage in distraction for highly intense emotions, when they may not be able to, or it may be too costly to suppress she emotional expression.

We found a small effect size for distraction and a medium effect size for expressive suppression: Hiding emotional expressions may be more important for these goals than reducing emotional experiences. Our results suggest that participants may have sometimes wanted to maintain (or not alter) a negative emotion, when they pursue social goals, but simply hide them from others.

To influence others was not negatively associated with expressive suppression. Generally, participants reported *to influence others* extremely seldom. We therefore hesitate to interpret the results for this goal.

Conclusion for emotion regulation goals.

All in all, we conclude that our results largely support the notion of the functional association between prohedonic goals, but also social goals, and emotion regulation strategies. Emotion regulation strategies, effective in changing the emotional experience, appear to be particularly important for prohedonic goals, whereas expressive suppression appears to be particularly important for social goals. By contrast, the positive association between prohedonic goals and rumination seems to be dysfunctional. In this case, our results do not support the notion of the functional association between emotion regulation goals and strategies.

Situational Factors

Situational factors were associated with different emotion regulation strategies. Perceived control was positively associated with active coping, and unexpectedly positively with cognitive reappraisal, each with small effect sizes. In more controllable situations, participants relied on emotion regulation strategies that change either the actual situation or the appraisal of that situation, which partly contradicts our predictions. One potential explanation is that active coping and cognitive reappraisal occurred together sometimes ($r_{\text{within}} = 0.20$; $p < 0.001$). For example, participants may have used cognitive reappraisal first to gain or maintain confidence and then deal with the situation actively, or first actively deal with the situation and then change their appraisal on the situation. Overall, our results suggest that perceived control appears to increase the use of putatively adaptive strategies.

Emotional intensity was positively associated with rumination with a medium effect size, which replicates the results from Dixon-Gordon et al. (2015). This result suggests that high emotional intensity triggers the use of rumination. As outlined above, rumination does not necessarily need to be a dysfunctional strategy to regulate emotions (Watkins, 2008), but other studies found that rumination (measured with a similar item) was positively associated with the accumulation of negative emotional intensity (Kalokerinos et al., 2017b; Résibois et al., 2018). Accordingly, if negative emotional intensity is high, the use of rumination preserves this state, which we interpret as a dysfunctional emotion regulation choice in most cases. Alternatively, the result may indicate a mutual reinforcement of emotional intensity and rumination, since rumination also increases the emotional intensity of an event (Kalokerinos et al., 2017b). All in all, this result suggests a dysfunctional association between emotional intensity and rumination.

Emotional intensity was negatively associated with cognitive reappraisal with a small effect size. Several experiments validated: The higher the emotional intensity, the lower the frequency of cognitive reappraisal (Sheppes et al., 2011, 2014). We complement this research by supporting this finding in everyday life.

Unexpectedly, emotional intensity was negatively associated with active coping with a small effect size. A previous study, in which individuals were asked to recall events from the past, found a positive association between emotional intensity and active coping instead (Dixon-Gordon et al., 2015). Our results contradict their findings. The difference could be explained because people recall memories that are short or long in the past with different accuracy.

Likewise, emotional intensity was not associated with distraction. Several experiments validated: The higher the emotional intensity, the more frequently individuals use distraction (Sheppes et al., 2011, 2014). Our experience sampling study does not support the findings from the laboratory and suggests that participants regulated their emotions differently in everyday life. Since the main effect of emotional intensity on distraction was replicated in a German sample (Scheibe et al., 2015), it also appears unlikely that cultural differences caused the observed difference between the laboratory studies and our experience sample study. Overall, our results suggest that emotional intensity appears to reduce the use of putatively adaptive strategies, but to increase the use of maladaptive strategies.

Expected reoccurrence was negatively associated with active coping and cognitive reappraisal with small effect sizes, and not negatively associated with distraction. This contradicts our predictions and broadly the results found in the laboratory (Sheppes et al., 2014). One potential explanation for our results may be temporal discounting (for a review, see Frederick et al., 2002): Individuals increasingly discount the value of an event the further in the future it takes place. In the laboratory, individuals may discount the reoccurrence of a negative stimulus less than in everyday life because they expect to encounter it again sooner (i.e., during the laboratory session). They thus may be more motivated to engage in strategies with long-term effects in the laboratory, but not in everyday life. Alternatively, participants may have assumed that a similar situation reoccurs in the future, but they were unable to act on it immediately in a reasonable way. For example, a student fails an exam, and the next chance to take the exam is 1 year. The student may struggle to act immediately on this event. Overall, our results suggest that expected reoccurrence appears to reduce the use of putatively adaptive strategies.

Conclusion for situational factors

Most of our hypotheses on situational factors were not supported (6 out of 9). We based five of our hypotheses (H11, H12, H14, H16, and H17) on the results of previous laboratory studies (Sheppes et al., 2011, 2014; Milyavsky et al., 2019; Van Bockstaele et al., 2019) and only replicated the relationship between emotional intensity and cognitive reappraisal. We therefore conclude that participants regulated their negative emotions in largely different ways in the laboratory as compared with everyday life, which underscores the importance of experience sampling studies to better understand emotion regulation. All in all, perceived control was positively associated with putatively adaptive strategies, whereas expected reoccurrence was negatively associated with them. Emotional intensity appears to be positively associated with dysfunctional emotion regulation choice.

Conclusion: What Predicts Emotion Regulation Choice in Daily Life?

Consistent with the emotion regulation flexibility framework (Bonanno and Burton, 2013; Aldao et al., 2015), we firstly found a considerable within-person variability in emotion regulation strategies (i.e., ICCs from 0.19 to 0.35). Secondly, we found that different contexts (i.e., emotion regulation goals and situational factors) were associated with different emotion regulation strategies, which suggests that individuals change their emotion regulation as a function of context. However, the majority of effects were small, suggesting either that there are omitted factors, which influence emotion regulation choice or some inherent variability, which is independent from the context.

Hence, we found that emotion regulation goals and perceived control appear to be related to mostly functional emotion regulation choices. By contrast, emotional intensity and expected reoccurrence appear to be related to dysfunctional emotion regulation choice, which does not support findings from the laboratory. Possibly, laboratory stimuli may be easier to handle than the stimuli in participants' everyday life.

How Do Predictors for Emotion Regulation Choice Interact in Daily Life?

We did not find any significant interaction effect in this study. One interpretation of this finding is that the interaction effects do not exist, and only the main effects influence emotion regulation choice. However, interaction effects may be hard to find: The measurement error accumulates in the interaction effect, which reduces its effect size (for a similar argument for the expectancy-value model, see Nagengast et al., 2011).

Limitations and Direction for Future Research

The study has some limitations. First and foremost, we examined emotion regulation goals and situational factors in response to negative events only and therefore cannot draw any conclusions about them in response to positive events. Future studies may address this gap to extend our results to positive events.

Second, we only examined prohedonic and social goals. Examining performance goals, eudaimonic goals, and epistemic goals (Tamir, 2016) would allow better mapping of the frequencies of emotion regulation goals and their (potential) functional or dysfunctional associations with emotion regulation strategies in daily life.

Third, we relied on undergraduate students. Accordingly, it is unclear to what extent our results generalize to other populations. For example, some evidence exists that older individuals pursue prohedonic goals more often than younger ones (Riediger et al., 2009, 2014). Our results would probably look partly different if evaluated in an older sample. Other studies may examine the frequencies of emotion regulation goals and situational factors and their association with emotion regulation strategies in older, less educated samples or working samples. They could then test whether our results can be generalized or are specific to our sample.

Fourth, we relied on non-random sampling, and thus may have over-sampled or under-sampled specific characteristics of the student population. Potentially, the students included in our study (i.e., mostly business-related studies) do not represent the entire student population. It is unclear to what extent our results generalize to the student population in Germany.

Fifth, we relied on a deterministic sampling throughout the day; participants potentially anticipate the scheduled survey and may adjust their momentary experience before it (Beal and Weiss, 2003). Further, negative events could be more likely directly after participants answered a scheduled survey (e.g., because of specific circadian rhythm), which would increase the time between the event participants' report and the report itself. Hence, since we allowed some delay to answer the prompt, our participants potentially did not answer immediately after a negative event, but instead when they had calmed down. All these factors could introduce bias to their responses (Bolger et al., 2003), although we do not assume this effect to be large. All in all, the deterministic sampling approach, which we chose to reduce the burden of participants, diminishes the ecological validity of our results. Future studies may benefit from random sampling over the day (Brans et al., 2013) to capture the emotional life of participants more naturally.

Finally, the examined relationships between emotion regulation goals and emotion regulation strategies, and between situational factors and emotion regulation strategies were correlational in nature: A causal conclusion should not be drawn from the data. It is likely that some of the examined relationships are bidirectional, but experimental designs are needed to disentangle the directionality and show causal relationships.

CONCLUSION

Overall, the findings from this study suggest that, firstly, emotion regulation goals and situational factors are very context-dependent; they should be treated as states, instead of traits. Secondly, emotion regulation goals and perceived control appear to be related to mostly functional emotion regulation choices. In contrast, emotional intensity and expected reoccurrence appear to be related to dysfunctional emotion regulation choices in daily life. These associations differ largely from the results found in the laboratory, which underlines the importance of experience sampling studies. Finally, the interactions of emotion regulation goals and situational factors need further investigation in future studies.

ETHICS STATEMENT

Ethical approval was not provided for this study on human participants because the used questions are not of ethical concern, the data were stored anonymously, and participants had the chance and possibility to quit the study at any time without further consequences. In addition, people had to give their consent to participate in the study, and only then, we used their data for scientific research. The study was not approved by any other ethics committee, as the design of the study is common practice. Following §7.3.1 of the "Ethical guidelines, The Association of German Professional Psychologists" the approval by an ethical committee is optional. The patients/participants provided their written informed consent to participate in this study.

AUTHOR CONTRIBUTIONS

RW designed the concept of manuscript, supervised the data gathering process, analyzed, and interpreted the data, and drafted the manuscript. RL and AK contributed substantially in the process by providing feedback at all stages of the research and the manuscript. All authors contributed to, reviewed, and commented on drafts of the manuscript. All authors read and approved the final manuscript.

REFERENCES

Aldao, A. (2013). The future of emotion regulation research: capturing context. *Perspect. Psychol. Sci.* 8, 155–172. doi: 10.1177/1745691612459518

Aldao, A., Sheppes, G., and Gross, J. J. (2015). Emotion regulation flexibility. *Cogn. Ther. Res.* 39, 263–278. doi: 10.1007/s10608-014-9662-4

Baguley, T. (2012). *Serious Stats: A Guide To Advanced Statistics For The Behavioral Sciences*. New York, NY: Palgrave Macmillan.

Bates, D., Mächler, M., Bolker, B., and Walker, S. (2015). Fitting linear mixed-effects models using lme4. *J. Stat. Soft.* 67, 1–48. doi: 10.18637/jss.v067.i01

Beal, D. J. (2015). ESM 2.0: state of the art and future potential of experience sampling methods in organizational research. *Annu. Rev. Organ. Psychol. Organ. Behav.* 2, 383–407. doi: 10.1146/annurev-orgpsych-032414-111335

Beal, D. J., and Weiss, H. M. (2003). Methods of ecological momentary assessment in organizational research. *Organ. Res. Methods* 6, 440–464. doi: 10.1177/1094428103257361

Blanke, E. S., Brose, A., Kalokerinos, E. K., Erbas, Y., Riediger, M., and Kuppens, P. (2019). Mix it to fix it: emotion regulation variability in daily life. *Emot. Adv. Online Public.* 20, 473–485. doi: 10.1037/emo0000566

Bolger, N., Davis, A., and Rafaeli, E. (2003). Diary methods: capturing life as it is lived. *Annu. Rev. Psychol.* 54, 579–616. doi: 10.1146/annurev.psych.54.101601.145030

Bonanno, G. A., and Burton, C. L. (2013). Regulatory flexibility: an individual differences perspective on coping and emotion regulation. *Perspect. Psychol. Sci.* 8, 591–612. doi: 10.1177/1745691613504116

Brans, K., Koval, P., Verduyn, P., Lim, Y. L., and Kuppens, P. (2013). The regulation of negative and positive affect in daily life. *Emotion* 13, 926–939. doi: 10.1037/a0032400

Bryk, A. S., and Raudenbush, S. W. (1992). *Hierarchical Linear Models: Applications And Data Analysis Methods.* Thousand Oaks, CA: Sage Publications, Inc.

Cameron, L. D., and Overall, N. C. (2017). Suppression and expression as distinct emotion-regulation processes in daily interactions: longitudinal and meta-analyses. *Emotion* 18, 465–480. doi: 10.1037/emo0000334

Carver, C. S., and Schreier, M. (2000). "On the structure of behavioral self-regulation," in *Handbook of Self-Regulation*, eds M. Boekaerts, P. Pintrich, and M. Zeidner (San Diego, CA: Academic Press), 42–85.

Dixon-Gordon, K. L., Aldao, A., and De Los Reyes, A. (2015). Emotion regulation in context: examining the spontaneous use of strategies across emotional intensity and type of emotion. *Pers. Individ. Differ.* 86, 271–276. doi: 10.1016/j.paid.2015.06.011

Doré, B. P., Silvers, J. A., and Ochsner, K. N. (2016). Toward a personalized science of emotion regulation: personalized emotion regulation. *Soc. Personal. Psychol. Compass* 10, 171–187. doi: 10.1111/spc3.12240

Eldesouky, L., and English, T. (2018). Regulating for a reason: emotion regulation goals are linked to spontaneous strategy use. *J. Pers.* 87, 948–961. doi: 10.1111/jopy.12447

English, T., Lee, I. A., John, O. P., and Gross, J. J. (2017). Emotion regulation strategy selection in daily life: the role of social context and goals. *Motiv. Emot.* 41, 230–242. doi: 10.1007/s11031-016-9597-z

Fishbach, A., and Ferguson, M. J. (2007). "The goal construct in social psychology," in *Social Psychology: Handbook of Basic Principles*, 2nd Edn, eds A. W. Kruglanski and E. T. Higgins ((New York, NY: The Guilford Press), 490–515.

Frederick, S., Loewenstein, G., and O'donoghue, T. (2002). Time discounting and time preference: a critical review. *J. Econ. Lit.* 40, 351–401. doi: 10.1257/jel.40.2.351

Gable, S. L., and Berkman, E. T. (2008). "Making connections and avoiding loneliness: Approach and avoidance social motives and goals," in *Handbook of Approach and Avoidance Motivation*, ed A. J. Elliot (Psychology Press), 203–216.

Greenaway, K. H., and Kalokerinos, E. K. (2017). Suppress for success? exploring the contexts in which expressing positive emotion can have social costs. *Eur. Rev. Soc. Psychol.* 28, 134–174. doi: 10.1080/10463283.2017.1331874

Gross, J. J. (1998). The emerging field of emotion regulation: an integrative review. *Rev. Gen. Psychol.* 2, 271–299. doi: 10.1037/1089-2680.2.3.271

Gross, J. J., John, O. P., and Richards, J. M. (2000). The dissociation of emotion expression from emotion experience: a personality perspective. *Pers. Soc. Psychol. Bull.* 26, 712–726. doi: 10.1177/0146167200268006

Haines, S. J., Gleeson, J., Kuppens, P., Hollenstein, T., Ciarrochi, J., Labuschagne, I., et al. (2016). The wisdom to know the difference: strategy-situation fit in emotion regulation in daily life is associated with well-being. *Psychol. Sci.* 27, 1651–1659. doi: 10.1177/0956797616669086

Halekoh, U., and Højsgaard, S. (2014). A kenward-roger approximation and parametric bootstrap methods for tests in linear mixed models - The R package pbkrtest. *J. Stat. Soft.* 59, 1–32. doi: 10.18637/jss.v059.i09

Kalokerinos, E. K., Greenaway, K. H., and Casey, J. P. (2017a). Context shapes social judgments of positive emotion suppression and expression. *Emotion* 17, 169–186. doi: 10.1037/emo0000222

Kalokerinos, E. K., Résibois, M., Verduyn, P., and Kuppens, P. (2017b). The temporal deployment of emotion regulation strategies during negative emotional episodes. *Emotion* 17, 450–458. doi: 10.1037/emo0000248

Kalokerinos, E. K., Tamir, M., and Kuppens, P. (2017c). Instrumental motives in negative emotion regulation in daily life: frequency, consistency, and predictors. *Emotion* 17, 648–657. doi: 10.1037/emo0000269

Kassinove, H., Roth, D., Owens, S. G., and Fuller, J. R. (2002). Effects of trait anger and anger expression style on competitive attack responses in a wartime prisoner's dilemma game. *Aggr. Behav.* 28, 117–125. doi: 10.1002/ab.90013

Kenward, M. G., and Roger, J. H. (1997). Small sample inference for fixed effects from restricted maximum likelihood. *Biometrics* 53, 983–997. doi: 10.2307/2533558

Knoll, N., Rieckmann, N., and Schwarzer, R. (2005). Coping as a mediator between personality and stress outcomes: a longitudinal study with cataract surgery patients. *Eur. J. Pers.* 19, 229–247. doi: 10.1002/per.546

Koller, M. (2016). robustlmm: an R package for robust estimation of linear mixed-effects models. *J. Stat. Softw.* 75, 1–24. doi: 10.18637/jss.v075.i06

Kornilov, S. A., Zhukova, M. A., Ovchinnikova, I. V., Golovanova, I. V., Naumova, O. Yu, Logvinenko, T. I, et al. (2019). Language outcomes in adults with a history of institutionalization: behavioral and neurophysiological characterization. *Sci. Rep.* 9, 1–13. doi: 10.1038/s41598-019-40007-9

Kruglanski, A. W., Bélanger, J. J., Chen, X., Köpetz, C., Pierro, A., and Mannetti, L. (2012). The energetics of motivated cognition: a force-field analysis. *Psychol. Rev.* 119, 1–20. doi: 10.1037/a0025488

LaHuis, D. M., Hartman, M. J., Hakoyama, S., and Clark, P. C. (2014). Explained variance measures for multilevel models. *Organ. Res. Methods* 17, 433–451. doi: 10.1177/1094428114541701

Luke, S. G. (2017). Evaluating significance in linear mixed-effects models in R. *Behav. Res.* 49, 1494–1502. doi: 10.3758/s13428-016-0809-y

Millgram, Y., Sheppes, G., Kalokerinos, E. K., Kuppens, P., and Tamir, M. (2019). Do the ends dictate the means in emotion regulation? *J. Exp. Psychol. Gen.* 148, 80–96. doi: 10.1037/xge0000477

Milyavsky, M., Webber, D., Fernandez, J. R., Kruglanski, A. W., Goldenberg, A., Suri, G., et al. (2019). To reappraise or not to reappraise? Emotion regulation choice and cognitive energetics. *Emotion* 19, 964–981. doi: 10.1037/emo0000498

Mundlak, Y. (1978). On the pooling of time series and cross section data. *Econometrica* 46, 69–85. doi: 10.2307/1913646

Nagengast, B., Marsh, H. W., Scalas, L. F., Xu, M. K., Hau, K.-T., and Trautwein, U. (2011). Who took the " × " out of expectancy-value theory?: a psychological mystery, a substantive-methodological synergy, and a cross-national generalization. *Psychol. Sci.* 22, 1058–1066. doi: 10.1177/0956797611415540

Netzer, L., Van Kleef, G. A., and Tamir, M. (2015). Interpersonal instrumental emotion regulation. *J. Exp. Soc. Psychol.* 58, 124–135. doi: 10.1016/j.jesp.2015.01.006

Nolen-Hoeksema, S., Wisco, B. E., and Lyubomirsky, S. (2008). Rethinking rumination. *Perspect. Psychol. Sci.* 3, 400–424. doi: 10.1111/j.1745-6924.2008.00088.x

Podsakoff, N. P., Spoelma, T. M., Chawla, N., and Gabriel, A. S. (2019). What predicts within-person variance in applied psychology constructs? An empirical examination. *J. Appl. Psychol.* 104, 727–754. doi: 10.1037/apl0000374

Podsakoff, P. M., MacKenzie, S. B., and Podsakoff, N. P. (2012). Sources of method bias in social science research and recommendations on how to control it. *Annu. Rev. Psychol.* 63, 539–569. doi: 10.1146/annurev-psych-120710-100452

R Core Team (2015). *A Language And Environment For Statistical Computing.* Vienna: R Foundation for Statistical Computing.

Résibois, M., Kalokerinos, E. K., Verleysen, G., Kuppens, P., Van Mechelen, I., Fossati, P., et al. (2018). The relation between rumination and temporal features of emotion intensity. *Cogn. Emot.* 32, 259–274. doi: 10.1080/02699931.2017.1298993

Riediger, M., Schmiedek, F., Wagner, G. G., and Lindenberger, U. (2009). Seeking pleasure and seeking pain: differences in prohedonic and contra-hedonic motivation from adolescence to old age. *Psychol. Sci.* 20, 1529–1535. doi: 10.1111/j.1467-9280.2009.02473.x

Riediger, M., Wrzus, C., and Wagner, G. G. (2014). Happiness is pleasant, or is it? Implicit representations of affect valence are associated with contrahedonic motivation and mixed affect in daily life. *Emotion* 14, 950–961. doi: 10.1037/a0037711

Scheibe, S., Sheppes, G., and Staudinger, U. M. (2015). Distract or reappraise? Age-related differences in emotion-regulation choice. *Emotion* 15, 677–681. doi: 10.1037/a0039246

Sheppes, G., Scheibe, S., Suri, G., and Gross, J. J. (2011). Emotion-regulation choice. *Psychol. Sci.* 22, 1391–1396. doi: 10.1177/0956797611418350

Sheppes, G., Scheibe, S., Suri, G., Radu, P., Blechert, J., and Gross, J. J. (2014). Emotion regulation choice: a conceptual framework and supporting evidence. *J. Exp. Psychol. Gen.* 143, 163–181. doi: 10.1037/a0030831

Tamir, M. (2016). Why do people regulate their emotions? A taxonomy of motives in emotion regulation. *Pers. Soc. Psychol. Rev.* 20, 199–222. doi: 10.1177/1088868315586325

Tamir, M., Bigman, Y. E., Rhodes, E., Salerno, J., and Schreier, J. (2015). An expectancy-value model of emotion regulation: implications for motivation, emotional experience, and decision making. *Emotion* 15, 90–103. doi: 10.1037/emo0000021

Tamir, M., Halperin, E., Porat, R., Bigman, Y. E., and Hasson, Y. (2019). When there's a will, there's a way: disentangling the effects of goals and means in emotion regulation. *J. Pers. Soc. Psychol.* 116, 795–816. doi: 10.1037/pspp0000232

Troy, A. S., Shallcross, A. J., and Mauss, I. B. (2013). A person-by-situation approach to emotion regulation: cognitive reappraisal can either help or hurt, depending on the context. *Psychol. Sci.* 24, 2505–2514. doi: 10.1177/0956797613496434

Van Bockstaele, B., Atticciati, L., Hiekkaranta, A. P., Larsen, H., and Verschuere, B. (2019). Choose change: situation modification, distraction, and reappraisal in mild versus intense negative situations. *Motiv. Emot.* doi: 10.1007/s11031-019-09811-8 [Epub ahead of print].

Watkins, E. R. (2008). Constructive and unconstructive repetitive thought. *Psychol. Bull.* 134, 163–206. doi: 10.1037/0033-2909.134.2.163

Webb, T. L., Lindquist, K. A., Jones, K., Avishai, A., and Sheeran, P. (2018). Situation selection is a particularly effective emotion regulation strategy for people who need help regulating their emotions. *Cogn. Emot.* 32, 231–248. doi: 10.1080/02699931.2017.1295922

Webb, T. L., Miles, E., and Sheeran, P. (2012). Dealing with feeling: a meta-analysis of the effectiveness of strategies derived from the process model of emotion regulation. *Psychol. Bull.* 138, 775–808. doi: 10.1037/a0027600

22

The Mechanism of Human Connectedness in Relationship to Physical Health, Mental Health and Cognitive Function among the Elderly

Shicun Xu [1,2,3*], Yuanyuan Wang [4*] and Hui Yu [4]

[1] Northeast Asian Research Center, Jilin University, Changchun, China, [2] Department of Population, Resources and Environment, Northeast Asian Studies College, Jilin University, Changchun, China, [3] China Center for Aging Studies and Social-Economic Development, Jilin University, Changchun, China, [4] Division of Psychology, Faculty of Health and Life Sciences, De Montfort University, Leicester, United Kingdom

***Correspondence:**
Shicun Xu
xushicun@jlu.edu.cn
Yuanyuan Wang
angelayuanyuanwang@gmail.com

Background: Elderly people face particular challenges in their everyday lives, and these are likely to be caused by physical health, mental health, cognitive function, and lack of maintaining a connection to other people. This study aims to explore a meaningful measure of human connectedness among the elderly in rural China and to examine the extent to which it impacts elderly people's physical and mental health as well as their cognitive function.

Methods: Survey data were collected from 483 participants who were aged 60 and older in northeast rural China. The outcome variables included cognitive function, which was assessed by the Short Portable Mental Status Questionnaire; depressive symptoms, which were measured by the 10-item version of the Center for Epidemiologic Studies Depression Scale; and the participants' physical health, which was assessed by a 15-item checklist. On the other hand, human connectedness was constructed by perceived family support, which was measured by the Multidimensional Scale of Perceived Social Support; the sense of community, which was measured by the Brief Sense of Community Scale; and the satisfaction of connectedness with others (i.e., with family members and friends).

Results: Structural equation modeling analysis confirms that perceived family support, community feelings, and perceived satisfactory connections with family and friends constitute a sufficient representation of human connectedness. Moreover, human connectedness also significantly predicted one's mental and physical well-being as well as cognitive function ($b = 0.11$, $SD = 0.02$, $\beta = 0.50$, $p < 0.001$; model fitting indexes $X^2_{(16)} = 17.27$, $p = 0.368$, CFI = 0.998, and RMSEA = 0.013).

Conclusion: The present study is the first attempt to explore the latent structure of human connectedness and its positive impact on cognitive function as well as physical and mental health among elderly people. The implications and the importance of fostering a stronger social support network, especially for the aging population, are discussed.

Keywords: human connectedness, elderly, cognitive function, physical illness, depression

INTRODUCTION

The aging population is one of the most complicated social issues that many societies have to face in the modern era (1). According to the sixth Chinese national census, there were 118.83 million people aged 65 years and older, which counted for 8.87% of the total population, and 50.32% of them lived in rural areas (2). The rapidly increasing aging population in China has attracted research interests (3). It is estimated that a great amount of resources needs to be allocated to address elderly people's physical and mental health problems as well as to compensate for their declined cognitive functions (4). Therefore, it is essential to distinguish those important factors that can help the elderly to maintain their physical and mental health as well as preserve their cognitive functions.

Connecting to others is one of the essential needs for all humans (5), whereas human connectedness can be considered a very broad concept that reflects this basic human need. In a landmark study, House et al. (6) show that the lack of social connection might be as, if not more, detrimental to health than obesity or smoking. However, it may be particularly challenging for elderly people to maintain the level of connectedness with others that they used to have. In the rural areas of China, it may be particularly so as many young people leave their hometowns to seek work opportunities in the big cities. In rural China, it is still popular to believe that it is the filial piety duty of the adult children to take care of their parents and older generations (7). Those elderly who are left behind, therefore, may be subjected to disappointment in addition to loneliness coming from the conflict between beliefs in Chinese filial piety and the absence of their children in their everyday life (8). Previous studies show that the elderly receive limited social support and lack of care suffered from mental problems, such as depression and loneliness (9, 10). Loneliness is demonstrated to be an important factor that undermines general health in the elderly (11). A meta-analysis shows that loneliness is associated with decreased cognitive function in the elderly (12). Furthermore, a study in the elderly also indicates that loneliness negatively impacts mood, especially for those with cognitive impairment (13). That is, those factors appear to interact with each other, and the decrease of human connectedness appears to have detrimental impacts on cognition, emotional feelings, and the physical health of the elderly (11).

Currently, there is an absence of study focusing on the association between human connectedness, mental and physical health, and cognitive functions in the elderly in rural China. As such, understanding the perspective and need for connection from these elderly people living in the rural area is the first crucial step to help them adapt to a rapidly changing environment. In a collectivism culture, family is always in the center of one's social life (14). For example, research shows that elderly people with social support are more likely to engage in physical activities, especially when they receive support from family members (15). In addition, a sense of community feeling is also of ultimate importance in the concept of human connectedness as well as being associated with an individual's function and well-being (16).

In the current study, we aimed to investigate the benefits of human connectedness and how human connectedness can be operationalized. We hypothesize that (1) perceived family support, the sense of community, and the direct measure of one's satisfaction with family and friend connectedness is a good starting point in capturing human connectedness among the elderly in rural China and (2) human connectedness has a significant impact on one's cognitive function as well as physical and mental health.

MATERIALS AND METHODS

Participants

The sample consists of 483 participants from Dongliao County, Liaoyuan City, Jilin Province in northeast China. The inclusion criteria is (1) age 60 years and older, (2) having lived in the village for at least 180 days in the past 12 months, and (3) having a local household registration (rural Hu Kou status). Ethical approval for the study was granted by the Ethics Committee of the University of Hong Kong. Sixteen villages out of 235 villages in Dongliao County were randomly chosen, and about 30 participants from each village were recruited based on referrals from the village commissions. There were 241 males and 228 females in the sample. The mean age of the participants was 69.40 ($SD = 6.21$). Other socio-demographic characters of the sample are shown in **Table 1**.

Measures

Cognitive Function

The Short Portable Mental Status Questionnaire (17) was used to assess participants' cognitive function. Some of the questions were adapted to the Chinese context; for example, "Who is the current president of P. R. China?" and "What day is the Autumn Festival?" Other items of pure cognitive function were directly translated, such as "Count backward from 20 by threes." Participants' responses were rated as correct (score 1) or incorrect/do not know (score 0). The total score of the cognitive function was calculated ranging from 1 to 10 with a higher score indicating a higher cognitive function. The total score was used in the modeling analysis as a continuous variable. In addition, high or low cognitive function was categorized following the established cutoff scores (18, 19); having fewer than one or two errors (total score $\geq$8) in their answers is considered normal cognitive functioning, three of four errors considered mild cognitive impairment; five to seven errors moderate cognitive impairment, and eight or more errors severe cognitive impairment. The categorization was used in the summary of the variable only (see **Table 1**).

Physical Illness

Participants were asked whether they suffered from a range of 15 commonly observed conditions among the elderly, including high blood pressure, diabetes, liver disease, etc., and participants chose from "0" (no) or "1" (yes). This measure was adapted from the China Health and Retirement Longitudinal Study (CHARLS) (20, 21). A composite score of physical illness was calculated by

TABLE 1 | Socio-demographic characters of the sample.

Measure variable	*n*	(%)	Mean	(*SD*)
Age			69.40	(6.21)
60–69	278	(57.56%)		
>70	192	(39.75%)		
Missing data	13	(2.69%)		
Gender				
Male	241	(49.90%)		
Female	228	(47.20%)		
Missing data	14	(2.90%)		
Marital status				
Never married	3	(0.62%)		
Separation/Divorced	3	(0.62%)		
Widow/Widower	132	(27.33%)		
Married	328	(67.91%)		
Others/missing data	17	(3.52%)		
Education level				
<9 years	367	(75.98%)		
9–12 years	96	(19.88%)		
>12 years	3	(0.62%)		
Missing data	17	(3.52%)		
Cognitive test			8.84	(1.56)
1–2 errors	411	(85.09%)		
3–4 errors	44	(9.11%)		
>4 errors	17	(3.52%)		
Missing data	11	(2.28%)		
Physical illness			1.86	(1.74)
Free from any illness	101	(20.91%)		
Suffering from some illness	361	(74.74%)		
Missing data	21	(4.35%)		
Depressive symptoms			6.95	(6.11)
Total score 0–15	415	(85.92%)		
Total score >16	52	(10.77%)		
Missing data	16	(3.31%)		

SD, standard deviation.

adding the responses from the 15 items, ranging from 0 to 15, with a higher score indicating poorer physical health.

Depressive Symptoms

Depressive symptoms were measured by a 10-item version of the Center for Epidemiologic Studies Depression Scale (CES-D-10) (22). Participants were asked to rate the frequency of symptoms that they experience (such as "I feel upset") during the last week on a 0–3 Likert scale with 0 as "almost never" and 3 as "almost every day." The internal consistency of this measure is high with a Cronbach's alpha of 0.85. The total score was calculated, ranging from 0 to 30, with a higher score indicating a greater level of depressive feeling. The total score was used in the modeling analysis as a continuous variable. Summary information was made according to the suggested cutoff score (23): a total score >16 is considered showing depressive symptoms.

Human Connectedness Variables

Human connectedness is conceptualized as receiving good family support, having a warm community feeling, and feeling satisfied with their connectedness to family members and friends.

Perceived Family Support

Perceived family support was measured by four items, taken and adapted from the Multidimensional Scale of Perceived Social Support (24) including (1) my family really tries to help me, (2) I receive emotional help and support from my family, (3) I can talk about my problems with my family, and (4) my family helps me to make important decisions. Participants were asked to indicate how much they agree with the statements on a Likert scale with 1 as "strongly disagree" to 5 as "strongly agree." The internal consistency of this measure is high with a Cronbach's alpha of 0.88. The total score was calculated, ranging from 4 to 20 with a higher score indicating higher perceived family support.

The Community Feeling

This measure is based on essential elements from the Brief Sense of Community Scale (25), but the items and the language were adapted to a Chinese context. The community feeling was measured by five items, including (1) people of different backgrounds in the community get along very well; (2) people respect each other in the community; (3) people help each other in the community; (4) people do not only mind their own business, but also take care of others in the community; (5) the community is like a family, and I am one of the contributing members. Participants were asked to indicate how much they agree with the statements on a Likert scale with 1 as "strongly disagree" to 5 as "strongly agree." The internal consistency of this measure is high with a Cronbach's alpha of 0.95. The total score was calculated, ranging from 5 to 25 with a higher score indicating higher perceived community support.

Satisfaction of the Connectedness With Others

Satisfaction with the connectedness with others was directly measured with three items, including (1) the number and mode of contact with family members, (2) the number and mode of contact with friends, and (3) the quality of communication with children and grandchildren. Participants were asked to indicate how satisfied they were with the abovementioned statements with 1 as very much dissatisfied to 5 as very much satisfied. The internal consistency of this measure is high with a Cronbach's alpha of 0.79. The total score was calculated, ranging from 3 to 15 with a higher score indicating a higher satisfaction of their connectedness with others.

Data Analysis

All analyses were carried out using R version 4.0.3 for Mac. The structural equation model (SEM) was conducted using the Lavaan package for R (26), examining the relationship between human connectedness and the outcome variables, including physical and mental health as well as cognitive function with participants' age and gender controlled. Model fit indexes, including the chi-square test, the comparative fit index (CFI), and the root mean square error of approximation (RMSEA), were used to assess the goodness of the model fit. It is commonly considered that a non-significant chi-square test, a CFI higher than 0.95, and an RMSEA smaller than 0.05 indicate good model fit. A $p < 0.05$ was considered statistically significant in this study.

RESULTS

Descriptive Statistics

Table 1 summarizes the characteristics of the sample. Means, SDs, and the correlations among the study variables are summarized in **Table 2.** It is worth noticing that this sample has a relatively low level of education with 367 participants (75.98%) spending <9 years in formal schooling. On the other hand, for marital status, never being married or separated/divorced was rare with three participants (0.62%) in each of the abovementioned categories. It is also worth noticing that the participants, on average, did not suffer from a lot of physical illness with $M = 1.86/15$ ($SD = 1.74$). Within the sample, 101 participants (20.91%) reported being free from suffering from any physical illness. In addition, the average cognitive function score ($M = 8.84$, $SD = 1.56$) was in the normal mental functioning range. Among all participants, 411 (85.09%) scored eight or above, indicating normal cognitive function; 44 (9.11%) made three or four errors, indicating mild cognitive impairment; 17 participants (3.52%) made more than four errors, indicating a moderate-to-severe cognitive impairment. Indicated by the CES-D-10 score, 52 participants (10.77%) scored higher than 16/30, indicating that they probably show depressive symptoms. Among the testing variables, except for a non-significant correlation between cognitive function and community feeling, all other pairs were significantly correlated with $p < 0.001$.

Structure Equation Modeling

An SEM analysis was conducted to test the effect of human connectedness on the health and function outcome variables with age and gender being controlled as covariates (**Figure 1**). The path estimates are shown in **Table 3**. The model fitting indexes all indicate an adequate model fit with $X^2_{(16)} = 17.27, p = 0.368$, CFI $= 0.998$, and RMSEA $= 0.013$. The standardized factor loading estimates for human connectedness range from 0.70 to 0.86. In addition, human connectedness is significantly associated with cognitive function as well as physical and mental health ($b = 0.11, SD = 0.02, \beta = 0.50, p < 0.001$). Among the covariates' paths, gender has a significant effect on the outcome variable construct ($b = -0.32$, $SD = 0.07$, $\beta = -0.36$, $p < 0.001$) as females show significantly lower levels of cognitive function and health. In addition, the variance explained by the model for the three dependent variables is as follows: $R^2_{\text{cognitive-function}} = 0.14$; $R^2_{\text{depressive-symptom}} = 0.38$; $R^2_{\text{physical-illness}} = 0.26$; and for the construct of "health and function," $R^2 = 0.42$.

DISCUSSION

The present study is one of the first attempts to explore the latent structure of human connectedness and its positive impact on cognitive function as well as physical and mental health among the elderly in rural China. The results support both of our hypotheses. Perceived family support, community feeling, and the direct measure of one's satisfaction on connectedness are closely correlated constructs, and they form a good measurement model for human connectedness. In addition, human connectedness has a significant impact on the outcome variables, which indicate that human connectedness can be considered a powerful protective factor against the decline of cognitive function and physical as well as mental health among the elderly.

Although human connectedness is not a new concept, there has not been an established measure for this important construct. In the current study, we explored combining family support, community feeling, and a direct measure of one's satisfaction on connectedness to capture the essential elements of human connectedness. These indicators prove forming a good operationalization for human connectedness among the elderly people in rural China. Family support is undoubtedly situated at

TABLE 2 | Means, SDs, and bivariate correlation among the study variables.

		Mean	*SD*	Bivariate correlation 1	2	3	4	5
1	Physical illness	1.86	1.74	–				
2	Depressive symptoms	6.95	6.11	0.37***	–			
3	Cognitive function	8.84	1.56	−0.16***	−0.26***	–		
4	Family support	17.59	2.26	−0.23***	−0.23***	0.20***	–	
5	Community feeling	22.17	2.56	−0.21***	−0.18***	0.09	0.62***	–
6	Satisfaction of connectedness	12.64	1.86	−0.20***	−0.34***	0.20***	0.60***	0.51***

*SD, standard deviation; ***p < 0.001.*

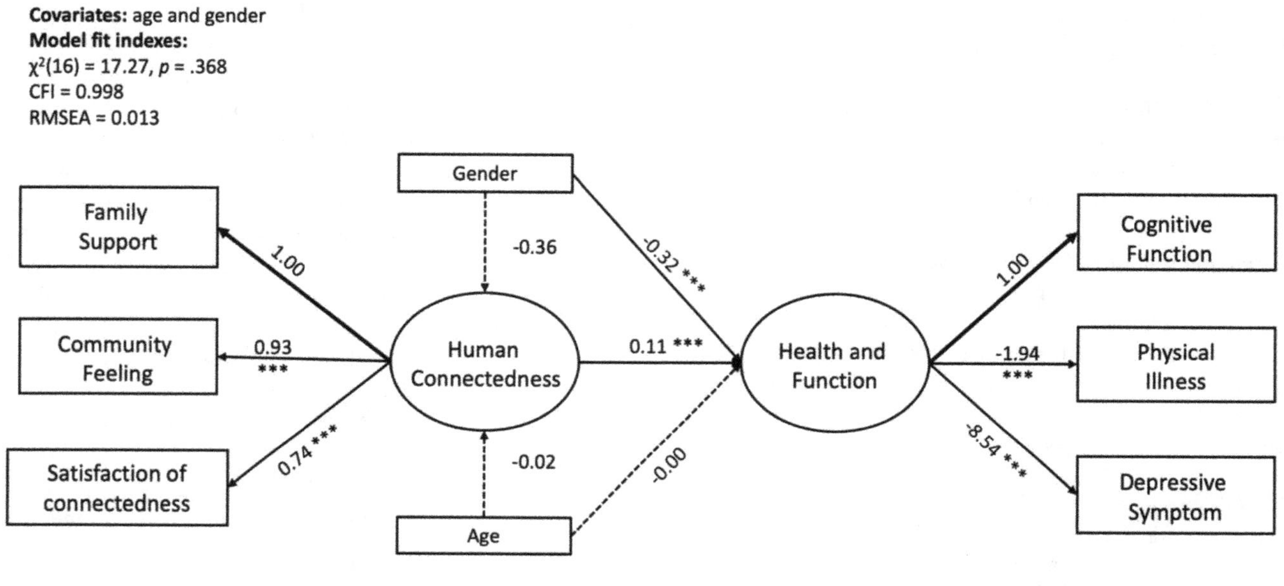

FIGURE 1 | SEM model of human connectedness and health and function with gender and age as covariates. Non-standardized coefficients were reported in the figure; ***$p < 0.001$.

the center of one's connectedness, which is the hub for individuals to turn to in times of both joy and distress. In Chinese tradition, elderly people rely on their children for care and support; in particular, the elderly son, together with his wife and children, is responsible for taking care of his aging parents (27). However, it is reported that family support for the elderly is weakening in rural China due to rapid societal changes (28). For example, many young people are moving to big cities, leaving their children to the care of their grandparents in rural areas. This change not only deprives the elderly of the expected support of their adult children, it also adds additional responsibility to care for the grandchildren (29). As emphasized by a previous study (11), it is important for healthcare professionals to be alert to the loneliness experience of the elderly and pay attention to the adverse health outcomes of a lack of human connectedness.

Conversely, it is worth noticing that the sample in this study reports a relatively high score of community feeling (mean score of 22.17 out of the maximum score of 25), which was more or less expected in the context of the rural area in northeast China, where people traditionally were closely connected. The model in the current study suggests that community feeling incorporates well into the construct of human connectedness. The sense of community feelings are studied in a wide range of contexts, for example, at workplaces (30) and among adolescents (31) as well as in immigrant communities (32). Existing literature suggests that participating actively in their community affairs and a sense of belonging are positively associated with one's overall health (33). Consistent with findings from some previous studies (34), the findings of this study suggest that the latent construct of human connectedness is associated with higher cognitive function, fewer physical illness conditions, and a lower level of depressive feelings among the elderly in rural China.

Among the outcome variables, the current study shows that 74.74% of the elderly participants suffered from one or more physical illness conditions, 12.63% from mild-to-severe levels of cognitive impairment, and 10.77% showed depressive symptoms. It is worth noticing that the measures used were screening tools rather than rigorous diagnostic tests; also, the smallness of the

TABLE 3 | SEM model summary.

Factor/Path	Estimate	*SD*	95% CI	Standardized estimate	*p*
Human connectedness					
Family support	1.00			0.86	
Community feeling	0.93	0.11	[0.71, 1.14]	0.70	**<0.001**
Satisfaction with connectedness	0.74	0.05	[0.64, 0.84]	0.78	**<0.001**
Health and function					
Cognitive function	1.00			0.37	
Physical illness	−1.94	0.40	[−2.72, −1.16]	−0.51	**<0.001**
Depressive symptoms	−8.54	1.62	[−11.72, −5.36]	−0.62	**<0.001**
Predictive path					
Connectedness -> Health and function	0.11	0.02	[0.07, 0.15]	0.50	**<0.001**
Covariates					
Gender -> Health and function	−0.32	0.07	[−0.46, −0.18]	−0.37	**<0.001**
Age -> Health and function	0.00	0.00	[−0.03, 0.01]	−0.03	0.632
Gender -> Human connectedness	−0.36	0.20	[−0.75, 0.03]	−0.09	0.069
Age -> Human connectedness	−0.02	0.02	[−0.06, 0.02]	−0.07	0.190

SD, standard deviation. The bold values indicate that the coefficients are statistically significant.

sample size and the rigor of the sampling method could not support this as a representative sample of the elderly in rural China. Still, our result does signal a strong need for attention to the physical and mental health of elderly people living in rural areas. Previous research also shows that elderly people in rural areas have fewer social resources compared with those in other areas (35). In addition, the current pension system in rural China is extremely insufficient (3), which cannot provide elderly people in rural areas with financial support and security. Combining these results, we see the urgency of providing structural support for elderly people in rural China.

Another interesting finding is that we identified a health disparity in gender comparison with elderly females being at a disadvantage compared with elderly males, which is inconsistent with previous studies in elderly populations in rural China (3, 36). That is, it is important to focus on the elderly population in Chinese rural areas, and specific attention should be given to the more disadvantaged elderly female population. More importantly, females have a longer life expectancy than males, and the disadvantages of elderly females implies that long-term care services should be considered for them (37). Together with the findings in the current study, it is fair to claim that building a stronger social support network focusing on strengthening human connectedness is of ultimate importance for the future of a thriving society.

The current study has some limitations. First, this is a cross-sectional survey; thus, the causality in the measured variables cannot be granted. Future longitudinal study is required to further investigate the mechanism among human connectedness, physical health, mental health, and cognitive function in elderly people. Second, the current sample was recruited from the economically less developed northeast China, which may not represent the other economically developed areas in China. Research indicates that the elderly in urban areas have better living conditions and access to various facilities (38), and it is likely that the elderly in the urban and economically developed regions have better general health. In addition, the sample size was not enough to represent the surveyed economic less developed region. Finally, due to the insufficient resources, we did not offer follow up assessments for participants identified with poor physical, cognitive, and mental health.

CONCLUSIONS

It is with little doubt that, knowing elderly people's needs, fostering and restoring the culture to respect and support the elderly would be of great importance for the entire society to thrive. In conclusion, an improved support system with human connectedness at the center is greatly needed to help the elderly living in rural China cope with the rapidly changing environment in addition to their naturally declining physical and mental health as well as cognitive functioning.

ETHICS STATEMENT

The studies involving human participants were reviewed and approved by Hong Kong University. The patients/participants provided their written informed consent to participate in this study.

AUTHOR CONTRIBUTIONS

SX: study design, data collection, manuscript writing, data analysis, and interpretation. HY: data analysis and interpretation, tables and figures editing, and manuscript writing. YW: literature research, data interpretation, and manuscript writing. All authors reviewed and agreed with the final version of the manuscript.

REFERENCES

Voss P, Kornadt AE, Hess TM, Fung HH, Rothermund K. A world of difference? Domain-specific views on aging in China, the US, and Germany. *Psychol Aging.* (2018) 33:595–606. doi: 10.1037/pag0000237

National Bureau of Statistics of China. *The Sixth National Population Census in 2010.* Beijing (2010).

Liang Y, Niu X, Lu P. The aging population in China: subjective well-being of empty nesters in rural eastern China. *J Health Psychol.* (2020) 25:361– 72. doi: 10.1177/1359105317717599

Brouwer W, Van Baal P, Van Exel J, Versteegh M. When is it too expensive? Cost-effectiveness thresholds and health care decision-making. *Eur J Health Econ.* (2019) 20:175–80. doi: 10.1007/s10198-018-1000-4

Baumeister RF, Leary MR. The need to belong: desire for interpersonal attachments as a fundamental human motivation. *Psychol Bull.* (1995) 117:497–529. doi: 10.1037/0033-2909.117.3.497

House JS, Landis KR, Umberson D. Social relationships and health. *Science.* (1988) 241:540–5. doi: 10.1126/science.3399889

Dai YT, Dimond MF. Filial piety. A cross-cultural comparison and its implications for the well-being of older parents. *J Gerontol Nurs.* (1998) 24:13–8. doi: 10.3928/0098-9134-19980301-05

Leung JC. Family support for the elderly in China: issues and challenges. *J Aging Soc Policy.* (1997) 9:87–101. doi: 10.1300/J031v09n03_05

Liu L-J, Guo Q. Life satisfaction in a sample of empty-nest elderly: a survey in the rural area of a mountainous county in China. *Qual Life Res.* (2008) 17:823–30. doi: 10.1007/s11136-008-9370-1

Cheng P, Jin Y, Sun H, Tang Z, Zhang C, Chen Y, et al. Disparities in prevalence and risk indicators of loneliness between rural empty nest and non-empty nest older adults in Chizhou, China. *Geriatr Gerontol Int.* (2015) 15:356–64. doi: 10.1111/ggi.12277

Liu LJ, Guo Q. Loneliness and health-related quality of life for the empty nest elderly in the rural area of a mountainous county in China. *Qual Life Res.* (2007) 16:1275–80. doi: 10.1007/s11136-007-9250-0

Boss L, Kang D-H, Branson S. Loneliness and cognitive function in the older adult: a systematic review. *Int Psychogeriatr.* (2015) 27:541– 53. doi: 10.1017/S1041610214002749

Holmén K, Ericsson K, Winblad B. Quality of life among the elderly: State of mood and loneliness in two selected groups. *Scand J Caring Sci.* (1999) 13:91–5. doi: 10.1111/j.1471-6712.1999.tb00521.x

Triandis HC, Bontempo R, Villareal MJ, Asai M, Lucca N. Individualism and collectivism: cross-cultural perspectives on self-ingroup relationships. *J Pers Soc Psychol.* (1988) 54:323–38. doi: 10.1037/0022-3514.54.2.323

Smith GL, Banting L, Eime R, O'Sullivan G, Van Uffelen JG. The association between social support and physical activity in older adults: a systematic review. *Int J Behav Nutr Phys Activ.* (2017) 14:56. doi: 10.1186/s12966-017-0509-8

McMillan DW, Chavis DM. Sense of community: a definition and theory. *J Community Psychol.* (1986) 14:6–23.

Pfeiffer E. A short portable mental status questionnaire for the assessment of organic brain deficit in elderly patients. *J Am Geriatr Soc.* (1975) 23:433– 41. doi: 10.1111/j.1532-5415.1975.tb00927.x

Söderqvist A, Strömberg L, Ponzer S, Tidermark J. Documenting the cognitive status of hip fracture patients using the Short Portable Mental Status Questionnaire. *J Clin Nurs.* (2006) 15:308–14. doi: 10.1111/j.1365-2702.2006.01296.x

Liu X, Hou L, Xia X, Liu Y, Zuo Z, Zhang Y. et al. Prevalence of sarcopenia in multi ethnics adults and the association with cognitive impairment: findings from West-China health and aging trend study. *BMC Geriatr.* (2020) 20:1–10. doi: 10.1186/s12877-020-1468-5

Zhao Y, Hu Y, Smith JP, Strauss J, Yang G. Cohort profile: the China health and retirement longitudinal study (CHARLS). *Int J Epidemiol.* (2014) 43:61– 8. doi: 10.1093/ije/dys203

Wen Y, Liu C, Liao J, Yin Y, Wu D. Incidence and risk factors of depressive symptoms in 4 years of follow-up among mid-aged and elderly community-dwelling Chinese adults: findings from the China Health and Retirement Longitudinal Study. *BMJ Open.* (2019) 9:e029529. doi: 10.1136/bmjopen-2019-029529

Andresen EM, Malmgren JA, Carter WB, Patrick DL. Screening for depression in well older adults: evaluation of a short form of the CES-D (Center for Epidemiologic Studies Depression Scale). *Am J Prev Med.* (1994) 10:77– 84. doi: 10.1016/S0749-3797(18)30622-6

Björgvinsson T, Kertz SJ, Bigda-Peyton JS, McCoy KL, Aderka IM. Psychometric properties of the CES-D-10 in a psychiatric sample. *Assessment.* (2013) 20:429–36. doi: 10.1177/1073191113481998

Zimet GD, Dahlem NW, Zimet SG, Farley GK. The multidimensional scale of perceived social support. *J Pers Assess.* (1988) 52:30– 41. doi: 10.1207/s15327752jpa5201_2

Peterson NA, Speer PW, McMillan DW. Validation of a brief sense of community scale: confirmation of the principal theory of sense of community. *J Commun Psychol.* (2008) 36:61–73. doi: 10.1002/jcop.20217

Rosseel Y. Lavaan: an R package for structural equation modeling and more. Version 05–12 (BETA). *J Statist Softw.* (2012) 48:1–36. doi: 10.18637/jss.v048.i02

Wong ST, Yoo GJ, Stewart AL. The changing meaning of family support among older Chinese and Korean immigrants. *J Gerontol Ser B Psychol Sci Soc Sci.* (2006) 61:S4–9. doi: 10.1093/geronb/61.1.s4

Yuan Y. Weakening family support for the elderly in China: a cultural explanation. *Chin Sociol Anthropol.* (2001) 34:26– 34. doi: 10.2753/CSA0009-4625340126

Liu J. Ageing, migration and familial support in rural China. *Geoforum.* (2014) 51:305–12. doi: 10.1016/j.geoforum.2013.04.013

Grant AM, O'Connor SA, Studholme I. Towards a positive psychology of buildings and workplace community: the positive built workplace environment. *Int J Appl Posit Psychol.* (2019) 4:67–89. doi: 10.1007/s41042-019-00019-2

Prati G, Tomasetto C, Cicognani E. Sense of community in early adolescents: validating the scale of sense of community in early adolescents. *J Early Adolesc.* (2021) 41:309–31. doi: 10.1177/0272431620912469

Mannarini T, Talò C, Rochira A. How diverse is this community? Sense of community, ethnic prejudice and perceived ethnic heterogeneity. *J Commun Appl Soc Psychol.* (2017) 27:181–95. doi: 10.1002/casp.2295

Terry R, Townley G, Brusilovskiy E, Salzer MS. The influence of sense of community on the relationship between community participation and mental health for individuals with serious mental illnesses. *J Commun Psychol.* (2019) 47:163–75. doi: 10.1002/jcop.22115

Dinkins CS. Seeing oneself in the face of the other: the value and challenge of human connectedness for older adults. *J Psychosoc Nurs Ment Health Serv.* (2017) 55:13–7. doi: 10.3928/02793695-20170619-03

Norstrand JA, Xu Q. Social capital and health outcomes among older adults in China: the urban–rural dimension. *Gerontologist.* (2012) 52:325– 34. doi: 10.1093/geront/gnr072

Zhou Y, Zhou L, Fu C, Wang Y, Liu Q, Wu H, et al. Socio- economic factors related with the subjective well-being of the rural elderly people living independently in China. *Int J Equity Health.* (2015) 14:5. doi: 10.1186/s12939-015-0136-4

Yi Z, Yuzhi L, George LK. Female disadvantages among the elderly in China. In: Yi Z, Crimmins EM, Carrière Y, Robine JM, editors. *Longer Life and Healthy Aging.* International Studies in Population, vol 2. Dordrecht: Springer (2006). doi: 10.1007/1-4020-4032-6_13

Li M, Zhang Y, Zhang Z, Zhang Y, Zhou L, Chen K. Rural-urban differences in the long-term care of the disabled elderly in China. *PLoS One.* (2013) 8:e79955. doi: 10.1371/journal.pone.0079955

Permissions

All chapters in this book were first published by Frontiers; hereby published with permission under the Creative Commons Attribution License or equivalent. Every chapter published in this book has been scrutinized by our experts. Their significance has been extensively debated. The topics covered herein carry significant findings which will fuel the growth of the discipline. They may even be implemented as practical applications or may be referred to as a beginning point for another development.

The contributors of this book come from diverse backgrounds, making this book a truly international effort. This book will bring forth new frontiers with its revolutionizing research information and detailed analysis of the nascent developments around the world.

We would like to thank all the contributing authors for lending their expertise to make the book truly unique. They have played a crucial role in the development of this book. Without their invaluable contributions this book wouldn't have been possible. They have made vital efforts to compile up to date information on the varied aspects of this subject to make this book a valuable addition to the collection of many professionals and students.

This book was conceptualized with the vision of imparting up-to-date information and advanced data in this field. To ensure the same, a matchless editorial board was set up. Every individual on the board went through rigorous rounds of assessment to prove their worth. After which they invested a large part of their time researching and compiling the most relevant data for our readers.

The editorial board has been involved in producing this book since its inception. They have spent rigorous hours researching and exploring the diverse topics which have resulted in the successful publishing of this book. They have passed on their knowledge of decades through this book. To expedite this challenging task, the publisher supported the team at every step. A small team of assistant editors was also appointed to further simplify the editing procedure and attain best results for the readers.

Apart from the editorial board, the designing team has also invested a significant amount of their time in understanding the subject and creating the most relevant covers. They scrutinized every image to scout for the most suitable representation of the subject and create an appropriate cover for the book.

The publishing team has been an ardent support to the editorial, designing and production team. Their endless efforts to recruit the best for this project, has resulted in the accomplishment of this book. They are a veteran in the field of academics and their pool of knowledge is as vast as their experience in printing. Their expertise and guidance has proved useful at every step. Their uncompromising quality standards have made this book an exceptional effort. Their encouragement from time to time has been an inspiration for everyone.

The publisher and the editorial board hope that this book will prove to be a valuable piece of knowledge for researchers, students, practitioners and scholars across the globe.

List of Contributors

Bin Zhang, Ying Liu, Xiaochun Wang and Xinyan Zheng
Shanghai University of Sport, Shanghai, China

Yuqin Deng
School of Sports Science, Nantong University, Nantong, China

Nicole J. Hegberg
VA Boston Healthcare System, Memory Disorders Research Center, Boston University School of Medicine, Boston, MA, United States

Jasmeet P. Hayes
Department of Psychology, The Ohio State University, Columbus, OH, United States
Chronic Brain Injury Initiative, The Ohio State University, Columbus, OH, United States

Scott M. Hayes
VA Boston Healthcare System, Memory Disorders Research Center, Boston University School of Medicine, Boston, MA, United States
Department of Psychology, The Ohio State University, Columbus, OH, United States
Chronic Brain Injury Initiative, The Ohio State University, Columbus, OH, United States

Shijie Liu, Sitong Chen and Yujun Cai
School of Physical Education and Sport Training, Shanghai University of Sport, Shanghai, China

Qian Yu
Exercise and Mental Health Laboratory, School of Psychology, Shenzhen University, Shenzhen, China

Zaimin Li
School of Wushu, Chengdu Sport University, Chengdu, China

Paolo Marcello Cunha
Metabolism, Nutrition, and Exercise Laboratory, Londrina State University, Londrina, Brazil

Yanjie Zhang
Health and Exercise Science Laboratory, Institute of Sports Science, Seoul National University, Seoul, South Korea

Zhaowei Kong
Faculty of Education, University of Macao, Macao, China

Wang Lin
Department of Physical Education, Wuhan University of Technology, Wuhan, China

Emily Benedetto, Ellie Grossman and Dorosella Kaluma
Department of Primary Care, Cambridge Health Alliance, Cambridge, MA, United States

John Torous
Division of Digital Psychiatry, Department of Psychiatry, Beth Israel Deaconess Medical Center, Boston, MA, United States

Liza Hoffman
Department of Primary Care, Cambridge Health Alliance, Cambridge, MA, United States
Division of Digital Psychiatry, Department of Psychiatry, Beth Israel Deaconess Medical Center, Boston, MA, United States

Hsiang Huang and Ziva Mann
Department of Psychiatry, Cambridge Health Alliance, Cambridge, MA, United States

Patama Gomutbutra
Department of Family Medicine, Faculty of Medicine, Chiang Mai University, Chiang Mai, Thailand
The Northern Neuroscience Center, Faculty of Medicine Chiang Mai University, Chiang Mai, Thailand

Nalinee Yingchankul
Department of Family Medicine, Faculty of Medicine, Chiang Mai University, Chiang Mai, Thailand

Nipon Chattipakorn
Center of Excellence in Cardiac Electrophysiology Research, Faculty of Medicine, Chiang Mai University, Chiang Mai, Thailand

Siriporn Chattipakorn
Center of Excellence in Cardiac Electrophysiology Research, Faculty of Medicine, Chiang Mai University
Department of Oral Biology and Diagnostic Sciences, Faculty of Dentistry, Chiang Mai University, Chiang Mai, Thailand

Manit Srisurapanont
Department of Psychiatry, Faculty of Medicine Chiang Mai University, Chiang Mai, Thailand

Jenifer A. Murphy and Georgina Oliver
Professorial Unit, The Melbourne Clinic, Department of Psychiatry, The University of Melbourne, Melbourne, VIC, Australia

Chee H. Ng
Professorial Unit, The Melbourne Clinic, Department of Psychiatry, The University of Melbourne, Melbourne, VIC, Australia
The Melbourne Clinic, Melbourne, VIC, Australia

Clinton Wain and Jennifer Magennis
The Melbourne Clinic, Melbourne, VIC, Australia

Rachelle S. Opie
Institute for Physical Activity and Nutrition, School of Exercise and Nutrition Sciences, Deakin University, Geelong, VIC, Australia

Amy Bannatyne
Faculty of Health Sciences and Medicine, Bond University, Gold Coast, QLD, Australia

Jerome Sarris
Professorial Unit, The Melbourne Clinic, Department of Psychiatry, The University of Melbourne, Melbourne, VIC, Australia
NICM Health Research Institute, Western Sydney University, Westmead, NSW, Australia

Chengbo Yang, Jingpu Guo and Hu Wang
The Third Department of Physical Education and Training, Chengdu Sport University, Chengdu, China

Ning Luo, Minfeng Liang, Sihong Zhou, Jiabao Zhang, Jiali Yu and Qing Gao
School of Mathematical Sciences, University of Electronic Science and Technology of China, Chengdu, China

Mu Zhang
Information Technology Center, Chengdu Sport University, Chengdu, China

Qian Cui
School of Public Affairs and Administration, University of Electronic Science and Technology of China, Chengdu, China

Huafu Chen
Ministry of Education Key Lab for Neuroinformation, High-Field Magnetic Resonance Brain Imaging Key Laboratory of Sichuan Province, University of Electronic Science and Technology of China, Chengdu, China
The Clinical Hospital of Chengdu Brain Science Institute, School of Life Sciences and Technology, University of Electronic Science and Technology of China, Chengdu, China

Jeroen Deenik and Peter N. van Harten
GGz Centraal, Amersfoort, Netherlands
School for Mental Health and Neuroscience, Maastricht University, Maastricht, Netherlands

Diederik E. Tenback and Harold F. van Driel
GGz Centraal, Amersfoort, Netherlands

Erwin C. P. M. Tak
Tak Advies en Onderzoek, Leiden, Netherlands

Ingrid J. M. Hendriksen
LivIng Active, Santpoort-Zuid, Netherlands

Yuntao Li
Psychological Education and Counselling Centre, Southwest University of Science and Technology, Mianyang, China

Ningxi Yang, Yan Zhang and Li Cai
Department of Applied Psychology, College of Humanities and Social Sciences, Harbin Engineering University, Harbin, China

Wei Xu
Faculty of Psychology, Beijing Normal University, Beijing, China

Yuanyuan Xu, Li Peng, Tong Wu, Tao Wang, Botao Liu, Junpeng Xie, Song Xu and Min Li
School of Psychology, Army Medical University, Chongqing, China

Fang Lu
School of Psychology, Army Medical University, Chongqing, China
School of Nursing, Army Medical University, Chongqing, China

Yongju Yu
Department of Sociology, Sichuan International Studies University, Chongqing, China

Chun Xie and Anmin Li
School of Psychology, Shanghai University of Sport, Shanghai, China

Brandon L. Alderman
Department of Kinesiology and Health, Center of Alcohol and Substance Use Studies, Rutgers, The State University of New Jersey, New Brunswick, NJ, United States

Fanying Meng
Institute of Physical Education, Huzhou University, Huzhou, China

Jingyi Ai
Department of Physical Education, National Taiwan Normal University, Taipei, Taiwan

Yu-Kai Chang
Department of Physical Education, National Taiwan Normal University, Taipei, Taiwan
Institute for Research Excellence in Learning Science, National Taiwan Normal University, Taipei, Taiwan

Sophie Faulkner
School of Health Sciences, University of Manchester, Manchester, United Kingdom
Greater Manchester Mental Health NHS Foundation Trust, Manchester, United Kingdom

Chris Sidey-Gibbons
Patient Reported Outcomes, Value & Experience Center (PROVE), Brigham and Women's Hospital, Boston, MA, United States
Faculty of Surgery, Harvard Medical School, Boston, MA, United States

Tao Xiao
College of Mathematics and Statistics, Shenzhen University, Shenzhen, China

Lin Yang
Cancer Epidemiology and Prevention Research, Alberta Health Services, Calgary, AB, Canada
Departments of Oncology and Community Health Sciences, Cumming School of Medicine, University of Calgary, Calgary, AB, Canada

Lee Smith
Cambridge Centre for Sport and Exercise Sciences, Anglia Ruskin University, Cambridge, United Kingdom

Paul D. Loprinz
Department of Health, Exercise Science and Recreation Management School of Applied Sciences, The University of Mississippi, Oxford, MS, United States

Nicola Veronese
Geriatrics Division, Department of Medicine-DIMED, University of Padova, Padua, Italy

Jie Yao
School of Humanities and Social Sciences, Harbin Institute of Technology (Shenzhen), Shenzhen, China

Zonghao Zhang
College of Physical Education, Soochow University, Suzhou, China

Jane Jie Yu
Department of Sports Science and Physical Education, The Chinese University of Hong Kong, Hong Kong, China

Mirta Fiorio
Department of Neurosciences, Biomedicine and Movement Sciences, University of Verona, Verona, Italy

Angela Marotta
Department of Neurosciences, Biomedicine and Movement Sciences, University of Verona, Verona, Italy
Neurology Unit, Neuroscience Department, Azienda Ospedaliera Universitaria Integrata, Verona, Italy

Eleonora Sarno and Giovanna E. Felis
Department of Biotechnology, University of Verona, Verona, Italy

Antonio Del Casale
Open Innovation Department, Microbion SRL, Verona, Italy

Marco Pane, Luca Mogna and Angela Amoruso
BIOLAB RESEARCH SRL, Novara, Italy

Zhixiong Yan and Xiaohui Hou
Psychology Department, Nanning Normal University, Nanning, China

Xia Zou
Guangxi College for Preschool Education, Nanning, China
Faculty of Industrial Education and Technology, King Mongkut's Institute of Technology Ladkrabang, Bangkok, Thailand

Erin Hoare, Meghan Hockey and Felice N. Jacka
Food & Mood Centre, IMPACT SRC, School of Medicine, Deakin University, Geelong, VIC, Australia

Anu Ruusunen
Food & Mood Centre, IMPACT SRC, School of Medicine, Deakin University, Geelong, VIC, Australia
Department of Psychiatry, Kuopio University Hospital, Kuopio, Finland
Institute of Public Health and Clinical Nutrition, University of Eastern Finland, Kuopio, Finland

Liang Zhou
Department of Reproductive Medicine, Peking University Shenzhen Hospital, Shenzhen, China

Yao Wang
Department of Rehabilitation Medicine, Dapeng New District Nan'ao People's Hospital, Shenzhen, China

Jun Qiao
The Second Rehabilitation Hospital of Shanghai, Shanghai, China

Qing Mei Wang
Stroke Biological Recovery Laboratory, Spaulding Rehabilitation Hospital, The Teaching Affiliate of Harvard Medical School, Boston, MA, United States

Xun Luo
Department of Rehabilitation Medicine, Dapeng New District Nan'ao People's Hospital, Shenzhen, China
Kerry Rehabilitation Medicine Research Institute, Shenzhen, China

Alexandra Berry, Roger T. Webb and Matthew J. Carr
Division of Psychology & Mental Health, School of Health Sciences, Faculty of Biology, Medicine and Health, Manchester Academic Health Sciences Centre (MAHSC), University of Manchester, Manchester, United Kingdom

Richard J. Drake
Greater Manchester Mental Health NHS Foundation Trust, Manchester, United Kingdom
Division of Psychology & Mental Health, School of Health Sciences, Faculty of Biology, Medicine and Health, Manchester Academic Health Sciences Centre (MAHSC), University of Manchester, Manchester, United Kingdom

Darren M. Ashcroft
Division of Pharmacy & Optometry, School of Health Sciences, Faculty of Biology, Medicine and Health, Manchester Academic Health Sciences Centre (MAHSC), University of Manchester, Manchester, United Kingdom

Alison R. Yung
Division of Psychology & Mental Health, School of Health Sciences, Faculty of Biology, Medicine and Health, Manchester Academic Health Sciences Centre (MAHSC), University of Manchester, Manchester, United Kingdom
Greater Manchester Mental Health NHS Foundation Trust, Manchester, United Kingdom
Orygen, The National Centre of Excellence in Youth Mental Health, The University of Melbourne, Parkville, VIC, Australia

Jutta Lindert
Department of Health and Social Work, University of Applied Sciences Emden/Leer, Emden, Germany
Women's Research Center at Brandeis University, Waltham, MA, United States

Kimberley C. Paul and Beate Ritz
Department of Epidemiology, Jonathan and Karin Fielding School of Public Health, University of California, Los Angeles, Los Angeles, CA, United States

Margie E. Lachman
The Heller School for Social Policy and Management, Brandeis University, Waltham, MA, United States

Teresa E. Seeman
The Heller School for Social Policy and Management, Brandeis University, Waltham, MA, United States
Division of Geriatrics, David Geffen School of Medicine at UCLA, Los Angeles, CA, United States

Umberto Raucci, Nicoletta Della Vecchia, Antonino Reale and Alberto Villani
Pediatric Emergency Department, Bambino Gesù Children's Hospital, Institute for Research, Hospitalization and Health Care (IRCCS), Rome, Italy

Alessandra Boni
Department of Pediatrics, Sapienza University, Rome, Italy

Melania Evangelisti, Margherita Velardi, Giovanni Di Nardo and Pasquale Parisi
Department of Pediatrics, Department of Neuroscience, Mental Health & Sense Organs (NESMOS), Faculty of Medicine & Psychology, c/o Sant'Andrea Hospital, Sapienza University, Rome, Italy

Fabiana Ursitti
Division of Neurology, Bambino Gesù Children's Hospital, Institute for Research, Hospitalization and Health Care (IRCCS), Rome, Italy

Gianluca Terrin
Department of Gynecological Obstetric and Urological Sciences, Faculty of Medicine and Dentistry, Sapienza University of Rome, Rome, Italy

Rafael Wilms and Andreas Kastenmüller
Department of Education Studies and Psychology, University of Siegen, Siegen, Germany

Ralf Lanwehr
Department of International Management, South Westphalia University of Applied Sciences, Meschede, Germany

Shicun Xu
Northeast Asian Research Center, Jilin University, Changchun, China
Department of Population, Resources and Environment, Northeast Asian Studies College, Jilin University, Changchun, China
China Center for Aging Studies and Social-Economic Development, Jilin University, Changchun, China

Yuanyuan Wang and Hui Yu
Division of Psychology, Faculty of Health and Life Sciences, De Montfort University, Leicester, United Kingdom

Index